Springer Series in Statistics

Springer
New York
Berlin
Heidelberg
Barcelona
Hong Kong
London
Milan
Paris
Singapore
Tokyo

Springer Series in Statistics

Andersen/Borgan/Gill/Keiding: Statistical Models Based on Counting Processes.
Berger: Statistical Decision Theory and Bayesian Analysis, 2nd edition.
Bolfarine/Zacks: Prediction Theory for Finite Populations.
Borg/Groenen: Modern Multidimensional Scaling: Theory and Applications
Brockwell/Davis: Time Series: Theory and Methods, 2nd edition.
Chen/Shao/Ibrahim: Monte Carlo Methods in Bayesian Computation.
Efromovich: Nonparametric Curve Estimation: Methods, Theory, and Applications.
Fahrmeir/Tutz: Multivariate Statistical Modelling Based on Generalized Linear Models.
Farebrother: Fitting Linear Relationships: A History of the Calculus of Observations 1750-1900.
Federer: Statistical Design and Analysis for Intercropping Experiments, Volume I: Two Crops.
Federer: Statistical Design and Analysis for Intercropping Experiments, Volume II: Three or More Crops.
Fienberg/Hoaglin/Kruskal/Tanur (Eds.): A Statistical Model: Frederick Mosteller's Contributions to Statistics, Science and Public Policy.
Fisher/Sen: The Collected Works of Wassily Hoeffding.
Good: Permutation Tests: A Practical Guide to Resampling Methods for Testing Hypotheses.
Gouriéroux: ARCH Models and Financial Applications.
Grandell: Aspects of Risk Theory.
Haberman: Advanced Statistics, Volume I: Description of Populations.
Hall: The Bootstrap and Edgeworth Expansion.
Härdle: Smoothing Techniques: With Implementation in S.
Hart: Nonparametric Smoothing and Lack-of-Fit Tests.
Hartigan: Bayes Theory.
Hedayat/Sloane/Stufken: Orthogonal Arrays: Theory and Applications.
Heyde: Quasi-Likelihood and its Application: A General Approach to Optimal Parameter Estimation.
Huet/Bouvier/Gruet/Jolivet: Statistical Tools for Nonlinear Regression: A Practical Guide with S-PLUS Examples.
Kolen/Brennan: Test Equating: Methods and Practices.
Kotz/Johnson (Eds.): Breakthroughs in Statistics Volume I.
Kotz/Johnson (Eds.): Breakthroughs in Statistics Volume II.
Kotz/Johnson (Eds.): Breakthroughs in Statistics Volume III.
Küchler/Sørensen: Exponential Families of Stochastic Processes.
Le Cam: Asymptotic Methods in Statistical Decision Theory.
Le Cam/Yang: Asymptotics in Statistics: Some Basic Concepts.
Longford: Models for Uncertainty in Educational Testing.
Miller, Jr.: Simultaneous Statistical Inference, 2nd edition.
Mosteller/Wallace: Applied Bayesian and Classical Inference: The Case of the Federalist Papers.
Parzen/Tanabe/Kitagawa: Selected Papers of Hirotugu Akaike.
Politis/Romano/Wolf: Subsampling.

(continued after index)

Ming-Hui Chen
Qi-Man Shao
Joseph G. Ibrahim

Monte Carlo Methods in Bayesian Computation

With 32 Illustrations

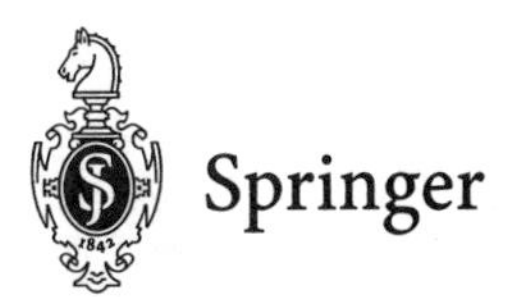

Springer

Ming-Hui Chen
Department of Mathematical Sciences
Worcester Polytechnic Institute
Worcester, MA 01609-2280
USA
mhchen@wpi.edu

Qi-Man Shao
Department of Mathematics
University of Oregon
Eugene, OR 97403-1222
USA
shao@math.uoregon.edu

Joseph G. Ibrahim
Department of Biostatistics
Harvard School of Public Health
and Dana-Farber Cancer Institute
Boston, MA 02115
USA
ibrahim@jimmy.harvard.edu

Library of Congress Cataloging-in-Publication Data
Chen, Ming-Hui, 1961–
Monte Carlo methods in Bayesian computation / Ming-Hui Chen, Qi-Man Shao, Joseph G. Ibrahim
p. cm. — (Springer series in statistics)
Includes bibliographical references and indexes.
ISBN 0-387-98935-8 (hardcover : alk. paper)
1. Bayesian statistical decision theory. 2. Monte Carlo method. I. Shao, Qi-Man. II. Ibrahim, Joseph George. III. Title. IV. Series.
QA279.5.C57 2000
519.5′42—dc21 99-046366

Printed on acid-free paper.

Production managed by A. Orrantia; manufacturing supervised by Jerome Basma.
Photocomposed copy prepared from the authors' LaTeX files.
Printed and bound by Maple-Vail Book Manufacturing Group, York, PA.
Printed in the United States of America.

9 8 7 6 5 4 3 2 1

ISBN 0-387-98935-8 Springer-Verlag New York Berlin Heidelberg SPIN 10745212

To Lan Bai, Jiena Miao, and Mona Ibrahim
Victoria, Paula, and Wenqi

Preface

Sampling from the posterior distribution and computing posterior quantities of interest using Markov chain Monte Carlo (MCMC) samples are two major challenges involved in advanced Bayesian computation. This book examines each of these issues in detail and focuses heavily on computing various posterior quantities of interest from a given MCMC sample. Several topics are addressed, including techniques for MCMC sampling, Monte Carlo (MC) methods for estimation of posterior summaries, improving simulation accuracy, marginal posterior density estimation, estimation of normalizing constants, constrained parameter problems, Highest Posterior Density (HPD) interval calculations, computation of posterior modes, and posterior computations for proportional hazards models and Dirichlet process models. Also extensive discussion is given for computations involving model comparisons, including both nested and nonnested models. Marginal likelihood methods, ratios of normalizing constants, Bayes factors, the Savage–Dickey density ratio, Stochastic Search Variable Selection (SSVS), Bayesian Model Averaging (BMA), the reverse jump algorithm, and model adequacy using predictive and latent residual approaches are also discussed.

The book presents an equal mixture of theory and real applications. Theoretical and applied problems are given in Exercises at the end of each chapter. The book is structured so that the methodology and applications are presented in the main body of each chapter and all rigorous proofs and derivations are placed in Appendices. This should enable a wide audience of readers to use the book without having to go through the technical details. Several types of models are used to demonstrate the various computational methods. We discuss generalized linear models, generalized linear mixed models, order restricted models, models for ordinal response data, semiparametric proportional hazards models, and nonparametric models using the Dirichlet process. Each of these models is demonstrated with real data. The applications are mainly from the health sciences, including food science, agriculture, cancer, AIDS, the environment, and education.

The book is intended as a graduate textbook or a reference book for a one-semester course at the advanced Master's or Ph.D. level. The prerequisites include one course in statistical inference and Bayesian theory at the level of Casella and Berger (1990) and Box and Tiao (1992). Thus, this book would be most suitable for second- or third-year graduate students in statistics or biostatistics. It would also serve as a useful reference book for applied or theoretical researchers as well as practitioners. Moreover, the book presents several open research problems that could serve as useful thesis topics.

We would like to acknowledge the following people, who have helped us in making this book possible. We thank Alan E. Gelfand for sending us the Table of Contents for his book, Jun S. Liu for his help on Multiple-Try Metropolis algorithms, grouped and collapsed Gibbs, grouped move and multigrid MC sampling, and dynamic weighting algorithms for Chapters 2 and 3, Chuanhai Liu for his help on the CA-adjusted MCMC algorithm, Siddhartha Chib for his suggestions on the Metropolis algorithm, Metropolized Carlin–Chib algorithm, marginal likelihood estimation, and other helpful comments, Man-Suk Oh for her extensions to the IWMDE algorithm, and Linghau Peng and her advisor Edward I. George for sending us the copy of her Ph.D. thesis on normalizing constant estimation for discrete distribution simulation, Dipak K. Dey for many helpful discussions and suggestions, Luke Tierney for helpful comments in the early stages of the book, and Xiao-Li Meng for providing us with several useful papers on estimation of normalizing constants.

We also thank Colleen Lewis of the Department of Mathematical Sciences at Worcester Polytechnic Institute for her editorial assistance. Finally, we owe deep thanks to our families for their constant love, patience, understanding, and support. It is to them that we dedicate this book.

July, 1999 Ming-Hui Chen, Qi-Man Shao, and Joseph G. Ibrahim

Contents

1
Introduction

1.1 Aims

There are two major challenges involved in advanced Bayesian computation. These are how to sample from posterior distributions and how to compute posterior quantities of interest using Markov chain Monte Carlo (MCMC) samples. Several books, including Tanner (1996), Gilks, Richardson, and Spiegelhalter (1996), Gamerman (1997), Robert and Casella (1999), and Gelfand and Smith (2000), cover the development of MCMC sampling. Therefore, this book will provide only a quick but sufficient introduction to recently developed MCMC sampling techniques. In particular, the book will discuss several recently developed and useful computational tools in MCMC sampling which may not be presented in other existing MCMC books including those mentioned above.

The main focus of this book will be on the development of advanced Monte Carlo (MC) methods for computing posterior quantities using the samples from the posterior distribution. Typical posterior qualities include the posterior means, posterior modes, posterior standard deviations, Bayesian p-values, marginal posterior densities, marginal likelihoods, Bayes factors, posterior model probabilities, Bayesian credible intervals, and highest probability density (HPD) intervals, and so forth. To compute posterior quantities, the ideal method is exact numerical evaluation. Gelfand and Smith (2000) give an excellent overview of available analytical approximation and numerical integration methods. However, the numerical integration approach may not always be applicable, in particular, when a Bayesian model is complicated, or when the dimension of integration is high. When analytical evaluation is not available, simulation-based approaches can be naturally applied. One of the most widely used MC methods is the importance sampling approach; see Geweke (1989) or Gelfand and Smith (2000) for more details. Similar to the numerical integration approach, importance sampling may also be inefficient for computing posterior quantities. Due to the development of MCMC sampling, many sophisticated but efficient MC methods have been recently developed. As the main objective of this book, we will present the systematic development of efficient MC methods for computing posterior quantities as well as assessing the quality (i.e., simulation precision) of the MC estimates. In particular, the book will discuss the importance weighted marginal density estimation (IWMDE) method, and various efficient MC methods (for example, bridge sampling, path sampling, ratio importance sampling, the Savage–Dicky density ratio, and many others) for estimating normalizing constants or ratios of normalizing constants. The book also emphasizes the applications of MC methods to Bayesian data analysis. To this end, it will cover the development of MC methods for Bayesian inference of constrained parameter problems, Bayesian model comparison and variable selection, Bayesian model adequacy, and Bayesian prediction. In addition, the book will provide the detailed theoretical development of MC methods for challenging computational problems arising from various applications. Several real data examples arising from agriculture, food science, epidemiology, and AIDS will be used throughout the book.

1.2 Outline

Chapter 2 gives an overview of several recently developed MCMC sampling algorithms including the Gibbs sampler, Metropolis–Hastings algorithms, and Hit-and-Run algorithms. It also presents several useful tools for accelerating MCMC sampling algorithms, which include reparameterizations (hierarchical centering and rescaling), grouped and collapsed Gibbs, grouped move and multigrid MCMC sampling, and the covariance-adjusted MCMC algorithm. In addition, the Multiple-Try Metropolis algorithm, the dynamic weighting algorithm, and "black-box" sampling are presented and issues regarding convergence diagnostics are addressed.

Chapter 3 serves as an introduction on how to use MCMC samples to estimate posterior quantities of interest. We discuss various useful posterior summaries for data analysis. Our main focus will be on the general setting of computing posterior summaries instead of specific applications. Basic MC methods will be reviewed. Sophisticated methods for improving the simulation efficiency of MC estimators will be discussed. In order to assess simulation accuracy of an MC estimate, several methods for computing simulation standard errors will also be presented and discussed. In addition, this chapter will address the important issue of how to obtain more efficient MC estimates such as the weighted MC estimates and how to control simulation errors when computing MC estimates.

Posterior marginal density estimation is one of the most important topics in Bayesian computation, and its usefulness and applications have not been fully explored in most of the Bayesian computational literature. Chapter 4 presents some commonly used nonparametric and parametric approaches, such as kernel density estimation and importance weighted marginal density estimation of Chen (1994), and discusses their theoretical properties. A performance study of the marginal posterior density estimate as well as comparisons of different density estimates will also be given. In later chapters, the reader will find that many Bayesian computational problems such as computing marginal likelihoods, Bayes factors, and posterior model probabilities will essentially reduce to the problem of marginal posterior density estimation.

Chapter 5 summarizes all available MC methods for estimating ratios of normalizing constants. This chapter will serve as the foundation of later chapters, and many methods presented in this chapter are very useful and will be revisited later. Another aspect of this chapter is to explore advantages and/or disadvantages of various available methods so that one can have an overall understanding of different MC methods. Discussion will be given to explain when one method may fail and when one method is better than the other.

In Chapter 6, we will focus on Bayesian constrained parameter problems, first considered by Gelfand, Smith, and Lee (1992) and further explored by Chen and Shao (1998). More specifically, this chapter deals with computational problems in which the resulting posterior density contains analytically intractable normalizing constants that depend on hyperparameters. The detailed development of efficient MC methods for such challenging computational problems will be presented, and two examples will be given to motivate and illustrate the methodology.

Chapter 7 is devoted to computation of Bayesian credible intervals and HPD intervals. An overview of various available methods will be given. Detailed treatments of how to estimate Bayesian credible and HPD intervals will be discussed in detail. In particular, we present the MC methods of Chen and Shao (1999b) for computing HPD intervals for parameters of interest as well as functions of the parameters. Various extensions of Chen and Shao's methods and illustrative examples including a simulation study and a real data set from food science are also provided.

Chapters 8 and 9 focus on Bayesian model comparison and model selection. We start with comparing nonnested models in Chapter 8. Several useful methods including marginal likelihood, "super-model" or "sub-model" approaches, and Bayesian criterion based approaches are presented. Examples for selecting links in correlated ordinal response models and for comparing nonnested survival models will also be given. In Chapter 9, we present a comprehensive treatment of Bayesian variable selection. As is well known, Bayesian variable selection is often difficult to carry out because of the challenge in

(i) specifying prior distributions for the regression parameters for all possible models;

(ii) specifying a prior distribution on the model space; and

(iii) computations.

For (i), we discuss classes of informative prior distributions for variable selection that can be elicited in a semiautomatic fashion. Several theoretical and computational properties of the priors will be presented and illustrated with several examples. For (ii), we include methods for specifying an informative prior on the model space, and for (iii) novel methods for computing the marginal distribution and posterior model probabilities will be introduced. In addition, stochastic search variable selection, Bayesian model averaging, and reversible jump MCMC algorithms will be presented.

The last chapter includes other related MC methods commonly used in Bayesian computation. More specifically, we present various Bayesian methods for model adequacy and related computational techniques, including MC estimation of conditional predictive ordinates (CPO) and various Bayesian residuals. This chapter also provides a detailed treatment of the computation of posterior modes, and sampling from posterior distributions for proportional hazards models and mixture of Dirichlet process models.

1.3 Motivating Examples

The following examples will help motivate the various MC methods for statistical inference which are examined later in this book.

Example 1.1. The New Zealand apple data. The New Zealand Apple and Pear Marketing Board (NZAPB) is a statutory body, which amongst other responsibilities, negotiates and arranges all contracts for exporting New Zealand apples throughout the world. In effect, this means that all of the more than 1500 apple growers in New Zealand are joined together as one grower when dealing with the international export market. The NZAPB has recorded total submissions for each grower over the last 30 years, but because the variability is generally too large, ordinary time series modeling does not provide an error bound small enough for practical prediction. It is important to notice that the data recorded consist only of total submissions for each apple variety and for each grower. However, the NZAPB has also recorded the "tree numbers" (i.e., the number of trees at each age) for each grower and for each variety over the last 5 years. For the purposes of NZAPB, ages of trees vary from 2 to 11 where an age "11" tree means eleven or older and is considered to be a mature tree. The year one is not considered because its production is considered nil. Each year these numbers have been scrupulously updated. Thus we have two important pieces of data for each grower and for each variety over the last 5 years; namely the number of trees at each age and the total amount of fruit that grower produced. Using this data set, Chen and Deely (1996) derive a model which will forecast the total crop of apples of any particular variety in the coming year.

For illustrative purposes here we will use only a subset of data arising from one geographical region and for one variety. This is a set of 207 records, each record consisting of the total number of cartons (y) of fruit produced and the number of trees of each year of age. Let x_j = number of trees at age $j+1$ for $j = 1, 2, \ldots, 10$. Table 1.1 gives the first 40 observations. The whole data set is available from the website "http://www.springer-ny.com."

Chen and Deely (1996) use a linear regression model where the quantity of fruit produced is regressed on the tree numbers at each age beginning at physical age 2 for 10 years up to a mature tree, that is,

$$y = \beta_1 x_1 + \beta_2 x_2 + \cdots + \beta_{10} x_{10} + \epsilon, \tag{1.3.1}$$

where $\epsilon \sim N(0, \sigma^2)$, β_j = average number of cartons produced by trees at age $j+1$ for $j = 1, 2, \ldots, 10$, and β_{10} is the average number of cartons produced by all mature trees. Chen and Deely (1996) use an argument based on the Central Limit Theorem to explain that the normal assumption on the error term ϵ is reasonable at least in an asymptotic sense. In order to see this point, let Y_{ijl} be the number of cartons produced by tree l at age $j+1$ from grower i; then the total number of cartons produced by trees from grower i is

$$Y_i = \sum_{j=1}^{10} \sum_{l=1}^{n_{ij}} Y_{ijl},$$

where n_{ij} is the total number trees at age $j+1$ from grower i. Since the n_{ij} are large in our data set, the Central Limit Theorem implies that Y_i is approximately normally distributed.

Furthermore, we note that β_j represents the average over **all** trees of age $j+1$. Since growers do not usually allow poor trees to persist on average, it is realistic to constrain the model by

$$0 \leq \beta_1 \leq \beta_2 \leq \cdots \leq \beta_{10} \tag{1.3.2}$$

which are called monotone constraints. Typically, this assumption is accepted by growers a priori and hence should be included in the analysis of the data used in the forecasting model. Chen and Deely (1996) check such constraints using the available information from the data and they

TABLE 1.1. A Subset of New Zealand Apple Data.

y	x_1	x_2	x_3	x_4	x_5	x_6	x_7	x_8	x_9	x_{10}
181	0	354	480	0	0	0	0	0	344	0
165	0	0	0	224	224	0	0	0	0	0
49	0	16	384	0	544	0	0	0	0	0
60	190	400	105	0	0	0	0	0	0	0
139	0	0	470	0	0	0	0	0	0	0
299	0	880	0	0	182	0	0	0	15	0
8	0	180	0	0	0	0	0	0	0	0
18	98	0	76	0	0	0	0	0	0	0
97	0	500	0	0	0	0	0	0	0	0
36	10	80	0	70	0	0	0	20	0	0
99	0	0	360	0	0	0	0	0	0	0
187	265	0	0	0	195	0	0	0	0	0
134	0	0	0	134	41	35	0	0	0	0
64	0	0	0	0	0	0	0	0	0	154
124	0	0	0	56	0	108	0	0	0	0
24	0	240	0	0	102	0	0	0	0	0
78	0	0	85	0	0	85	0	0	0	0
177	0	0	0	0	0	0	50	66	0	50
119	0	0	260	0	0	0	0	0	0	0
24	72	0	0	24	30	0	0	0	0	0
268	0	0	1324	0	0	0	0	0	0	0
292	365	830	0	0	0	0	0	0	0	0
81	0	0	0	350	0	0	0	0	0	0
48	0	0	0	280	0	0	0	0	0	0
132	0	0	221	216	0	0	0	0	0	0
192	0	0	0	0	168	168	0	0	0	0
50	0	0	0	123	0	0	0	30	0	0
46	387	0	0	0	0	0	0	0	0	0
168	2104	150	0	0	0	0	50	0	0	0
241	0	0	0	450	0	0	0	0	0	0
23	0	0	0	0	57	0	0	0	0	0
24	0	0	560	0	0	0	0	0	0	0
38	0	0	0	200	0	0	0	0	0	0
49	0	0	0	515	0	0	0	0	0	0
37	0	0	0	1200	0	0	0	0	0	0
24	0	0	0	40	0	0	0	0	0	0
642	1000	0	0	453	0	0	192	0	0	0
49	0	800	0	0	0	0	0	0	0	0
379	100	0	0	660	0	0	0	0	0	0
513	0	0	400	0	440	0	0	0	0	0

Source: Chen and Deely (1996).

show that the monotone constraints hold. Using a constrained linear multiple regression model to incorporate the monotonic constraints given by (1.3.2), they utilize the Gibbs sampler to obtain solutions to integration problems associated with Bayesian analysis. Further, the empirical comparison among Bayesian, ordinary and inequality-constrained least squares estimation indicates that the Bayesian model provides the best fit to the data.

Using a slightly different subset of the New Zealand apple data, Robert and Hwang (1996) obtain the maximum likelihood estimation of the regression coefficients under order restriction by the prior feedback method. In this book, we will use this example to illustrate the implementation of MCMC sampling algorithms, such as the Gibbs sampler and the Hit-and-Run algorithm, as well as the computation of marginal posterior density estimation and Bayesian residuals under order restrictions.

Example 1.2. The Meal, Ready-to-Eat (MRE) data. The MRE has twelve meals (menus), each consisting of four to six food items. The system contains 39 distinct foods. Some of these items occur in more than one meal and are regarded as different items in different meals, so the total number of items studied is 52. These items can be classified into five principal types: entrees, pastries, vegetables, fruits, and miscellaneous. Meals were purchased through the military supply procedures of the armed-forces procurement system. On arrival at Natick Laboratories (NLABS) they were inspected for completeness and stored at four different temperatures, 4 °C, 21 °C, 30 °C, 38 °C, then withdrawn and tested at 6, 12, 18, 24, 30, 36, 48, 60 months. Only 23 of the 36 time–temperature combinations were tested. At 4 °C the food was not tested at 6, 18, and 24 months, and at 21 °C the food was not tested at 6 months. Also, upon purchase the foods were immediately tested at room temperature (21 °C), and thus data are only available for time 0 at room temperature.

The meals were opened by test monitors, and each item served to a panel of 36 untrained subjects who judged its acceptability on a nine-point hedonic rating scale where 1 = dislike extremely, 9 = like extremely, and intermediate integer scores have graduated meanings.

Ross, Klicka, Kalick, and Branagan (1987) and Chen, Nandram, and Ross (1996) study results for ten entrees: ham–chicken loaf, barbecued beef, meatballs, chicken, beef patties, turkey, pork sausage, beef in gravy, beef stew, and ham slices. For each of the 23 combinations of time and temperature, there were sensory ratings for each of the 36 panel members, and so the data for each item consisted of 828 scores. The rating scores for ham–chicken loaf are given in Table 1.2. Also we note that each pastry tends to get similar scores as the entree in each meal. Ross et al. (1987) and Chen, Nandram, and Ross (1996) investigate the food shelf-life at each storage temperature of the MRE by using a link with a well-known food

TABLE 1.2. The MRE Sensory Data for Ham–Chicken Loaf.

Temperature	Time (in months)	Rating Scores
4 °C	12	674677567774776476545849257668262669
	30	722648595524643677867377434163374168
	36	417577585521677456878454754477373667
	48	467557627563267461656763537639368737
	60	597764667352474645322645465766692457
21 °C	0	778586477678564845647353165773776776
	12	856757468565462776492366722446847488
	18	877377866744264945834156776437664616
	24	456584471616668968676775744727776388
	30	485682577148775334768337682287637637
	36	837464943577377748472676786577867476
	48	866646177357488778265577374443877855
	60	376755778583237433756485564655456447
30 °C	6	566756367988757482366676666867767777
	12	827746435287914878566663666326357736
	18	573777467738255546734276788746356573
	24	722536537336278672125662731657774577
	30	783755574557574447643667265774683736
	36	726634652246265358235648522448741361
38 °C	6	757873345256787471666746858234656575
	12	674567446666835757554466254147673561
	18	487657774346541254776681471324775636
	24	444473776736523773644453568786428446

Source: Ross et al. (1987) and Chen, Nandram, and Ross (1996).

deterioration equation through nonlinear least squares fitting. However, Ross et al. (1987) use a non-Bayesian nonlinear least squares method while Chen, Nandram, and Ross (1996) fit a hierarchical Bayesian model on the multinomial counts. They show that Bayesian order restricted inference provides improved precision over other methods that are commonly used in food science.

In this book, we will discuss how to analyze the MRE data using latent variable approaches when the resulting posterior contains analytically intractable normalizing constants depending on the hyperparameters. More specifically, we will consider how to compute Bayesian posterior quantities such as posterior moments and HPD intervals.

Example 1.3. Pollen count data. Pollen allergy is a common disease causing hay fever and respiratory discomfort in approximately 10% of the United States population. Although not a life-threatening illness, allergy

TABLE 1.3. Summaries of Variables for Pollen Count Data–Part I.

Year	Variable	Value	Count	Percent
1991	x_1	0	10	10.9
	x_1	1	82	89.1
	x_7	0	27	29.3
	x_7	1	65	70.7
1992	x_1	0	8	9.9
	x_1	1	73	90.1
	x_7	0	30	37.0
	x_7	1	51	63.0
1993	x_1	0	11	12.6
	x_1	1	76	87.3
	x_7	0	29	33.3
	x_7	1	58	66.7
1994	x_1	0	6	8.0
	x_1	1	69	92.0
	x_7	0	25	33.3
	x_7	1	50	66.7

Source: Ibrahim, Chen, and Ryan (1999).

symptoms seem to be increasingly more troublesome, as well as costing society a great deal of money and resources. Therefore, it is becoming increasingly important to identify the important covariates that help predict pollen levels.

Ibrahim, Chen, and Ryan (1999) consider a pollen count data set in which ragweed pollen was collected daily in Kalamazoo, Michigan from 1991 to 1994. Frequentist analyses of these data using standard Poisson regression methods have been conducted by Stark, Ryan, McDonald, and Burge (1997). In this pollen count data set, the response variable y is the pollen count for a particular day in the season for a given year. Ibrahim, Chen, and Ryan (1999) use the 1991, 1992, and 1993 data as the historical data and the 1994 data as the current data to perform Bayesian variable subset selection. The data for each year were collected roughly over a 3 month interval between the months of July and October. However, for each year, the first and last observations were collected on different days. For example, in 1991, the first observation was collected on July 28 and the last was collected on October 27. In 1992, the first observation was collected on August 6 and the last observation on October 26.

The data include seven covariates, which are extensively discussed and motivated by Stark et al. (1997). These are x_1 = rain (which is a binary variable taking the value 0 if there were at least 3 hours of steady rain, and 1 otherwise), x_2 = day in the pollen season , x_3 = log(day). In addition, two covariates, which are functions of temperature, are x_4, the lowess smoothed

TABLE 1.4. Summaries of Variables for Pollen Data–Part II.

Year	Variable	Range	Mean	Std. Dev.
1991	x_2	1.0–92.0	46.5	27.7
	x_3	0.0–4.5	3.6	0.9
	x_4	53.0–73.8	64.6	8.2
	x_5	−13.4–16.1	0.2	6.9
	x_6	0.0–18.0	11.1	3.9
	y	0.0–377	43.1	73.4
1992	x_2	1.0–82.0	41.7	23.9
	x_3	0.0–4.4	3.4	0.9
	x_4	46.2–70.4	61.2	7.7
	x_5	−11.4–13.7	0.5	6.1
	x_6	4.0–24.0	12.8	3.9
	y	0.0–440	53.9	86.3
1993	x_2	1.0–87.0	44.0	25.3
	x_3	0.0–4.5	3.5	0.9
	x_4	49.9–75.2	62.5	9.1
	x_5	−12.6–15.5	0.2	6.2
	x_6	0.0–15.0	8.6	3.5
	y	0–362	47.0	78.8
1994	x_2	1.0–79.0	40.8	23.2
	x_3	0.0–4.4	3.4	0.94
	x_4	50.5–69.3	62.9	6.3
	x_5	−10.0–12.8	0.3	6.0
	x_6	0.0–18.0	10.5	2.8
	y	0–205	32.3	49.1

Source: Ibrahim, Chen, and Ryan (1999).

function of temperature constructed from a nonparametric estimate of the regression of pollen count on average temperature, and x_5 which denotes the deviation from the daily averages temperature to the lowess line. The final two covariates are x_6 = windspeed and x_7 = cold (which is a binary variable taking the value 0 if the overnight temperature dropped below 50 °F, and 1 otherwise).

Tables 1.3 and 1.4 summarize the response variable and covariate data for the 4 years while Table 1.5 contains a subset of the 1994 pollen count data. The entire 1991–1994 pollen count data can be obtained at the website "http://www.springer-ny.com."

Let y_t be a time series of counts for $t = 1, \dots, n$, where each y_t has corresponding 8×1 covariate vector $\boldsymbol{x}_t$. Conditional on $\boldsymbol{\beta} = (\beta_0, \beta_1, \dots, \beta_7)'$ and a stationary unobserved process ϵ_t, the y_t's are assumed to be independent Poisson random variables with mean $\lambda_t = \exp(\epsilon_t + \boldsymbol{x}_t'\boldsymbol{\beta})$, leading to the

TABLE 1.5. A Subset of 1994 Pollen Data.

y	x_1	x_2	x_3	x_4	x_5	x_6	x_7
3	1	1	0	68.432	−6.654	5	1
8	0	2	0.693	68.451	−5.784	8	1
1	1	3	1.099	68.469	−1.656	8	1
8	0	4	1.386	68.486	3.808	8	1
24	1	5	1.609	68.502	−2.969	10	1
18	1	6	1.792	68.519	−2.108	10	1
20	1	7	1.946	68.537	−0.360	10	1
51	1	8	2.079	68.556	3.333	10	1
90	1	9	2.197	68.577	4.757	10	1
34	0	10	2.303	68.601	6.282	11	1
18	1	11	2.398	68.628	2.019	8	1
75	1	12	2.485	68.659	−0.953	8	1
29	1	13	2.565	68.694	2.583	8	1
105	1	14	2.639	68.734	4.155	4	1
205	1	15	2.708	68.779	6.721	6	1
201	1	16	2.773	68.829	10.053	10	1
120	1	17	2.833	68.884	7.763	8	1
147	1	20	2.996	69.068	−2.068	13	1
96	1	21	3.045	69.130	−6.630	18	1
85	1	22	3.091	69.187	−4.298	14	1
57	1	23	3.135	69.236	−9.958	13	0
24	1	24	3.178	69.267	−8.878	12	0
29	1	25	3.219	69.271	−7.438	12	1
133	1	26	3.258	69.234	−9.767	8	0
133	1	27	3.296	69.151	−4.429	9	1
47	1	28	3.332	69.026	−1.581	8	1
56	1	29	3.367	68.862	−1.862	7	1
86	1	30	3.401	68.665	1.335	8	1
77	1	31	3.434	68.438	5.374	7	1
13	1	34	3.526	67.647	5.647	7	1
54	1	35	3.555	67.365	8.690	7	1
133	1	36	3.584	67.083	10.917	8	1
62	1	37	3.611	66.803	12.769	10	1
75	1	38	3.638	66.525	10.357	10	1
25	1	39	3.664	66.249	2.862	10	1
9	1	40	3.689	65.969	0.697	10	1

Source: Stark et al. (1997) and Ibrahim et al. (1999).

conditional density

$$
\begin{aligned}
f(\boldsymbol{y}|\boldsymbol{\beta},\boldsymbol{\epsilon}) &= \prod_{t=1}^{n} f(y_t|\boldsymbol{\beta},\epsilon_t) \\
&= \prod_{t=1}^{n} \exp\{y_t(\epsilon_t + \boldsymbol{x}_t'\boldsymbol{\beta}) - \exp(\epsilon_t + \boldsymbol{x}_t'\boldsymbol{\beta}) - \log(y_t!)\} \\
&= \exp\{\boldsymbol{y}'(\boldsymbol{\epsilon} + X\boldsymbol{\beta}) - J_n'Q(\boldsymbol{\beta},\boldsymbol{\epsilon}) - J_n'C(\boldsymbol{y})\}, \qquad (1.3.3)
\end{aligned}
$$

where $\boldsymbol{y} = (y_1, \ldots, y_n)'$, $\boldsymbol{\epsilon} = (\epsilon_1, \ldots, \epsilon_n)'$, X is the $n \times 8$ matrix of covariates with the tth row equal to $\boldsymbol{x}_t'$, J_n is an $n \times 1$ vector of ones, and $Q(\boldsymbol{\beta}, \boldsymbol{\epsilon})$ is an $n \times 1$ vector with the tth element equal to $q_t = \exp\{\epsilon_t + \boldsymbol{x}_t'\boldsymbol{\beta}\}$, and $C(\boldsymbol{y})$ is an $n \times 1$ vector with the jth element $\log(y_j!)$. Finally, $D = (n, \boldsymbol{y}, X)$ denotes the data.

In (1.3.3), the latent process ϵ_t is assumed to have normal distribution with mean 0. We assume an AR(1) structure for the covariance matrix of $\boldsymbol{\epsilon}$. This structure is well motivated in the statistical literature and is one of the most widely used in the time series setting (see Zeger 1988). Thus, we assume that $\boldsymbol{\epsilon}$ has a multivariate normal distribution with mean 0 and covariance matrix $\sigma^2\Sigma$, where the $(i,j)^{\text{th}}$ element of Σ has the form $\sigma_{ij} = \rho^{|i-j|}$, where $\rho^{|i-j|}$ is the correlation between (ϵ_i, ϵ_j), and $-1 < \rho < 1$. The unobserved process ϵ_t is analogous to a "random effect" in a random effects model, with the exception that the latent process is correlated. We note that the mean and variance of ϵ_t do not depend on t. Zeger (1988) constructs a similar model through the mean and covariance of the latent process, which then defines the estimating equations. Using the above model, Ibrahim, Chen, and Ryan (1999) develop an efficient MCMC sampling algorithm based on the idea of hierarchical centering (Gelfand, Sahu, and Carlin 1996) to compute posterior quantities such as the marginal posterior densities for β. They also derive several key results that lead to efficient calculation of posterior model probabilities. This data set will serve as one of the key examples to illustrate sampling from a Poisson random effects model in Chapter 2, and computing posterior model probabilities in Chapter 9.

Example 1.4. AIDS ACTG019 and ACTG036 data. To motivate the MC methods in Chapter 9, we consider the two landmark AIDS clinical trials, ACTG019 and ACTG036.

The ACTG019 study was a double blind placebo-controlled clinical trial comparing zidovudine (AZT) to placebo in persons with CD4 counts less than 500. The results of this study were published in Volberding et al. (1990). The sample size for this study, excluding cases with missing data,

The ACTG019 study was a double blind placebo-controlled clinical trial comparing zidovudine (AZT) to placebo in persons with CD4 counts less

TABLE 1.6. Summary of AIDS ACTG019 and ACTG036 Data.

ACTG019 Study			ACTG036 Study		
	Mean	Std. Dev.		Mean	Std. Dev.
x_{01}	334.7	109.3	x_1	297.7	130.5
x_{02}	34.64	7.679	x_2	30.43	11.16
x_{03}	AZT	Placebo	x_3	AZT	Placebo
	418	405		89	94
x_{04}	White	Other	x_4	White	Other
	752	71		166	17
			x_5	VIII	Other
				163	20
			x_6	Yes	No
				78	105
y_0	1	0	y	1	0
	55	768		11	172

Source: Chen, Ibrahim, and Yiannoutsos (1999).

than 500. The results of this study were published in Volberding et al. (1990). The sample size for this study, excluding cases with missing data, was $n_0 = 823$. The response variable (y_0) for these data is binary with a 1 indicating death, development of AIDS, or AIDS related complex (ARC), and a 0 indicates otherwise. Several covariates were also measured. The ones we use here are CD4 count (x_{01}) (cell count per mm^3 of serum), age (x_{02}), treatment (x_{03}), and race (x_{04}). The covariates CD4 count and age are continuous, whereas the other covariates are binary.

The ACTG036 study was also a placebo-controlled clinical trial comparing AZT to placebo in patients with hereditary coagulation disorders. The results of this study have been published by Merigan et al. (1991). The sample size in this study, excluding cases with missing data, was $n = 183$. The response variable (y) for these data is binary with a 1 indicating death, development of AIDS, or AIDS related complex (ARC), and a 0 indicates otherwise. Several covariates were measured for these data. The ones we use here are CD4 count (x_1), age (x_2), treatment (x_3), race (x_4), hemophilia factor type (x_5), and monoclonal factor concentrate use (x_6). The covariates CD4 count and age are continuous, whereas the other covariates are binary. The covariate x_5 was coded as 1 if the hemophilia factor type was Factor VIII, 0 otherwise, and the covariate x_6 was coded as 1 if the patient used a monoclonal factor concentrate, 0 otherwise. Table 1.6 summarizes the covariates and response variables for both studies. The data for the ACTG019 and ACTG036 studies can be obtained at the website "http://www.springer-ny.com." Chen, Ibrahim, and Yiannoutsos (1999) use the data from ACTG019 to construct a prior distribution for the parameters in the ACTG036 trial. They also carry out a Bayesian variable selection procedure for identifying important covariates in logistic regression. In this book, we will use these data sets to illustrate how to compute prior and posterior model probabilities in Chapter 9.

1.4 The Bayesian Paradigm

The Bayesian paradigm is based on specifying a probability model for the observed data D, given a vector of unknown parameters $\boldsymbol{\theta}$, leading to the likelihood function $L(\boldsymbol{\theta}|D)$. Then we assume that $\boldsymbol{\theta}$ is random and has a *prior* distribution denoted by $\pi(\boldsymbol{\theta})$. Inference concerning $\boldsymbol{\theta}$ is then based on the *posterior* distribution, which is obtained by Bayes' theorem. The posterior distribution of $\boldsymbol{\theta}$ is given by

$$\pi(\boldsymbol{\theta}|D) = \frac{L(\boldsymbol{\theta}|D)\pi(\boldsymbol{\theta})}{\int_{\Omega} L(\boldsymbol{\theta}|D)\pi(\boldsymbol{\theta})\, d\boldsymbol{\theta}}, \tag{1.4.1}$$

where Ω denotes the parameter space of $\boldsymbol{\theta}$. From (1.4.1) it is clear that $\pi(\boldsymbol{\theta}|D)$ is *proportional* to the likelihood multiplied by the prior,

$$\pi(\boldsymbol{\theta}|D) \propto L(\boldsymbol{\theta}|D)\pi(\boldsymbol{\theta}),$$

and thus it involves a contribution from the observed data through $L(\boldsymbol{\theta}|D)$, and a contribution from prior information quantified through $\pi(\boldsymbol{\theta})$. The quantity $m(D) = \int_{\Omega} L(\boldsymbol{\theta}|D)\pi(\boldsymbol{\theta})\, d\boldsymbol{\theta}$ is the *normalizing constant* of $\pi(\boldsymbol{\theta}|D)$, and is often called the *marginal* distribution of the data or the prior predictive distribution.

In most models and applications, $m(D)$ does not have an analytic closed form, and therefore $\pi(\boldsymbol{\theta}|D)$ does not have a closed form. This dilemma leads us to the following question: How do we sample from the multivariate distribution $\pi(\boldsymbol{\theta}|D)$ when no closed form is available for it? This question had led to an enormous literature for computational methods for sampling from $\pi(\boldsymbol{\theta}|D)$ as well as methods for estimating $m(D)$. Perhaps one of the most popular computational methods for sampling from $\pi(\boldsymbol{\theta}|D)$ is called *the Gibbs Sampler*. The Gibbs sampler is a very powerful simulation algorithm that allows us to sample from $\pi(\boldsymbol{\theta}|D)$ *without* knowing the normalizing constant $m(D)$. We discuss this method along with other MCMC sampling algorithms in detail in Chapter 2.

The quantity $m(D)$ arises in model comparison problems, specifically in the computation of Bayes factors and posterior model probabilities. Thus, in addition to being able to simulate from $\pi(\boldsymbol{\theta}|D)$, one must also estimate the ratio $m_1(D)/m_2(D)$ for comparing two models, say 1 and 2. To this end, there exists extensive literature for efficient estimation of ratios of normalizing constants using samples from the posterior distribution of $\boldsymbol{\theta}$, and therefore this is another major topic discussed in Chapter 5 of this book. For many of the applications discussed in this book, the prior $\pi(\boldsymbol{\theta})$ itself does not have a closed analytic form. This makes sampling from the posterior especially challenging, and novel computational methods are required to carry out the posterior computations. We discuss such methods in Chapters 2, 8, and 9.

A major aspect of the Bayesian paradigm is prediction. Prediction is often an important goal in regression problems, and usually plays an important role in model selection problems. The *posterior predictive* distribution of a future observation vector z given the data D is defined as

$$\pi(z|D) = \int_{\Omega} f(z|\boldsymbol{\theta})\pi(\boldsymbol{\theta}|D)\, d\boldsymbol{\theta}, \tag{1.4.2}$$

where $f(z|\boldsymbol{\theta})$ denotes the sampling density of z, and $\pi(\boldsymbol{\theta}|D)$ is the posterior distribution of $\boldsymbol{\theta}$. We see that (1.4.2) is just the posterior expectation of $f(z|\boldsymbol{\theta})$, and thus sampling from (1.4.2) is easily accomplished via the Gibbs sampler from $\pi(\boldsymbol{\theta}|D)$. This is a nice feature of the Bayesian paradigm since (1.4.2) shows that predictions and predictive distributions are easily computed once samples from $\pi(\boldsymbol{\theta}|D)$ are available. In Chapters 8, 9, and 10, we discuss procedures for sampling from, and summarizing the posterior predictive distribution, and use this distribution to derive several model selection criteria and Bayesian methods for model adequacy.

Exercises

1.1 Classical Order Restricted Inference (Liew 1976; Robertson, Wright, and Dykstra 1988)
Use the following algorithm of Liew (1976) to compute the inequality constrained least squares (ICLS) estimates for the New Zeland Apple data.
Let $\boldsymbol{y} = (y_1, y_2, \ldots, y_n)'$ be an $n \times 1$ vector of a total number of cartons of fruit and let X be the $n \times 10$ matrix of explanatory variables. Also let A be a 10×10 matrix given by

$$A = \begin{pmatrix} 1 & 0 & 0 & \cdots & 0 & 0 \\ -1 & 1 & 0 & \cdots & 0 & 0 \\ 0 & -1 & 1 & \cdots & 0 & 0 \\ \vdots & \vdots & \vdots & \ddots & \vdots & \vdots \\ 0 & 0 & 0 & \cdots & -1 & 1 \end{pmatrix}.$$

Note that the construction of the matrix A is based on the monotone constraints given in (1.3.2). From Liew (1976), the ICLS estimate $\boldsymbol{b}^*$ of $\boldsymbol{\beta}$ is given by

$$\boldsymbol{b}^* = (X'X)^{-1}X'\boldsymbol{y} + (X'X)^{-1}A'\boldsymbol{\lambda}^*,$$

where $\boldsymbol{\lambda}^*$ is the solution of the following dual problem:

$$\boldsymbol{\nu} = W\boldsymbol{\lambda} + \mathbf{q} \begin{bmatrix} \boldsymbol{\nu} \\ \boldsymbol{\lambda} \end{bmatrix} = \mathbf{q},$$

subject to $\boldsymbol{\nu}'\boldsymbol{\lambda} = 0$, $\boldsymbol{\nu} \geq 0$ and $\boldsymbol{\lambda} \geq 0$, where $W = A(X'X)^{-1}A'$ and $\mathbf{q} = A(X'X)^{-1}X'\boldsymbol{y}$.

1.2 Fit an appropriate probit or logistic regression model with storage temperature, time, and their interaction as covariates for the MRE sensory data given in Table 1.2.

1.3 PREDICTING SHELF-LIFE (Chen, Nandram, and Ross 1996; Ross et al. 1987)
From Chen, Nandram, and Ross (1996) and Ross et al (1987), a mathematical model for the behavior of y, the score, as a function of time in months, t, and temperature in °C, H, is

$$y = u + (\nu_3 - u)\exp\{-K(H)t\},$$

where $5 \leq \nu_3 \leq 9$ denotes the unknown food quality at time $t = 0$, and $K(H)$ obeys the Arrhenius relationship

$$K(H) = \exp[-\nu_1 + G(H)\nu_2]$$

with $G(H) = 10(H-27)/(H+273)$, ν_2 is a dimensionless parameter specifying intensity of the temperature effect on $K(H)$, and ν_1 is another dimensionless parameter. The shelf-life, $S(H)$, defined as the time in months at which the score reaches a critical value, y_c (usually $y_c = 5$), is calculated as follows:

$$S(H) = \ln[(\nu_3 - u)/(y_c - u)]/K(H),$$

where u is the limiting value of food quality and $u = 1$ on the nine-point hedonic scale.
Using the MRE sensory data for THE ham–chicken loaf in Table 1.2:

(a) Compute the parameters ν_1, ν_2, and ν_3 so as to minimize the quantity SSQ, which is the sum of squares of differences between model predictions and average data scores at all combinations of time and temperature. Note that the NLIN procedure in SAS can be used here.
(b) Obtain an estimate of $S(H)$ at each of the testing temperatures.

1.4 Compute the marginal mean $E(y_t|\boldsymbol{\beta}, \sigma^2, \rho)$ and the marginal variance, $\text{Var}(y_t|\boldsymbol{\beta}, \sigma^2, \rho)$, for the Poisson random effects model defined by (1.3.3).

1.5 Use the generalized estimating equation approach (GEE) introduced by Liang and Zeger (1986) and Zeger and Liang (1986) to obtain estimates of $\boldsymbol{\beta}$, σ^2, and ρ for the 1994 pollen count data. Note that the

GEE approach has been implemented in the SAS procedure GENMOD. Also, briefly discuss whether there is a potential problem with convergence of the GEE method.

1.6 Suppose that y_1 and y_2 are independent samples from an exponential distribution with density

$$f(y_i|\theta) = \theta \exp(-\theta y_i),$$

where $\theta > 0$ is an unknown parameter. Consider a gamma prior $\pi(\theta)$ with known shape parameter 2 and scale parameter 1 for θ, i.e.,

$$\pi(\theta) \propto \theta \exp(-\theta), \quad \theta > 0.$$

Given the observed data $D = (y_1, y_2) = (1, 3)$:

(a) derive a closed-form expression for the posterior distribution $\pi(\theta|D)$;
(b) compute the posterior mean and variance of θ; and
(c) obtain a closed-form expression for the posterior predictive density $\pi(z|D)$ given in (1.4.2).

1.7 Suppose that y_1 and y_2 are independent samples from a normal distribution with unknown mean θ and known variance 1. Consider an improper uniform prior for θ, i.e., $\pi(\theta) \propto 1$, and suppose we have the observed data $D = (y_1, y_2) = (-2, 1)$.

(a) Write out the posterior density of θ up to a normalizing constant $m(D)$.
(b) Using the grid approximation, compute the normalized constant $m(D)$.
(c) Compute the posterior mean and variance of θ.
(d) Plot the posterior density $\pi(\theta|D)$ and the posterior predictive density $\pi(z|D)$.

1.8 Suppose the probability that a coin yields "heads" is θ. The coin is independently tossed five times, and "heads" appears more than four times. Consider a uniform $U(0, 1)$ prior for θ.

(a) What is the likelihood function of θ?
(b) Is there any evidence against the hypothesis that this is a fair coin?

1.9 Suppose that the posterior density of $\boldsymbol{\theta} = (\theta_1, \theta_2)'$ is a mixture of products of gamma density functions, defined as

$$\pi(\boldsymbol{\theta}|D) = 0.8\theta_1\theta_2 \exp(-\theta_1-\theta_2)+0.2\frac{2^6}{5!}\theta_1^5 \exp(-2\theta_1)\times\frac{3^6}{5!}\theta_2^5 \exp(-3\theta_2)$$

for $\theta_1 > 0$, $\theta_2 > 0$.

(a) Generate a random sample $\{\boldsymbol{\theta}_i,\ i = 1, 2, \ldots, n\}$ with $n = 10,000$ from $\pi(\boldsymbol{\theta}|D)$.

(b) Draw the univariate histogram to obtain an approximation of the marginal distribution for θ_j, $j = 1, 2$. How do these approximate marginal densities compare to the true marginal densities, which can be obtained by integrating out one component of $\boldsymbol{\theta}$ from $\pi(\boldsymbol{\theta}|D)$?

1.10 Suppose that $\{y_1, y_2, \ldots, y_5\}$ is a random sample from an unknown symmetric distribution F with unknown location parameter θ. We take an improper uniform prior for θ, i.e., $\pi(\theta) \propto 1$, and suppose the observed data are $D = (y_1, y_2, \ldots, y_5) = (-4, -2, 0, 1.5, 4.5)$. Consider the following two models for F:

$$F_1: \ y_i|\theta \sim N(\theta, 1)$$

with density

$$f_1(y_i|\theta) = \frac{1}{\sqrt{2\pi}} \exp\{-(y_i - \theta)^2/2\},$$

and

$$F_2: \ y_i|\theta \sim \text{Cauchy}(\theta, 1)$$

with density

$$f_2(y_i|\theta) = \frac{1}{\pi[1 + (y_i - \theta)^2]},$$

where θ is an unknown location parameter, and the scale parameter is equal to 1. Compute the Bayes factor for F_1 against F_2.

(*Hint*: Use the grid approximation to compute the normalizing constants $m_1(D)$ and $m_2(D)$, and then calculate the ratio $m_1(D)/m_2(D)$ to obtain the Bayes factor.)

2

Markov Chain Monte Carlo Sampling

Recently, Monte Carlo (MC) based sampling methods for evaluating high-dimensional posterior integrals have been rapidly developing. Those sampling methods include MC importance sampling (Hammersley and Handscomb 1964; Ripley 1987; Geweke 1989; Wolpert 1991), Gibbs sampling (Geman and Geman 1984; Gelfand and Smith 1990), Hit-and-Run sampling (Smith 1984; Bélisle, Romeijn, and Smith 1993; Chen 1993; Chen and Schmeiser 1993 and 1996), Metropolis–Hastings sampling (Metropolis et al. 1953; Hastings 1970; Green 1995), and hybrid methods (e.g., Müller 1991; Tierney 1994; Berger and Chen 1993). A general discussion of the Gibbs sampler and other Markov chain Monte Carlo (MCMC) methods is given in the *Journal of the Royal Statistical Society, Series B* (1993), and an excellent roundtable discussion on the practical use of MCMC can be found in Kass et al. (1998). Other discussions or instances of the use of MCMC sampling can be found in Tanner and Wong (1987), Tanner (1996), Geyer (1992), Gelman and Rubin (1992), Gelfand, Smith, and Lee (1992), Gilks and Wild (1992), and many others. Further development of state-of-the-arts MCMC sampling techniques include the accelerated MCMC sampling of Liu and Sabatti (1998, 1999), Liu (1998), and Liu and Wu (1997), and the exact MCMC sampling of Green and Murdoch (1999). Comprehensive accounts of MCMC methods and their applications may also be found in Meyn and Tweedie (1993), Tanner (1996), Gilks, Richardson, and Spiegelhalter (1996), Robert and Casella (1999), and Gelfand and Smith (2000). The purpose of this chapter is to give a brief overview of several commonly used MCMC sampling algorithms as well as to present selectively several newly developed computational tools for MCMC sampling.

2.1 Gibbs Sampler

The Gibbs sampler may be one of the best known MCMC sampling algorithms in the Bayesian computational literature. As discussed in Besag and Green (1993), the Gibbs sampler is founded on the ideas of Grenander (1983), while the formal term is introduced by Geman and Geman (1984). The primary bibliographical landmark for Gibbs sampling in problems of Bayesian inference is Gelfand and Smith (1990). A similar idea termed as *data augmentation* is introduced by Tanner and Wong (1987). Casella and George (1992) provide an excellent tutorial on the Gibbs sampler.

Let $\boldsymbol{\theta} = (\theta_1, \theta_2, \ldots, \theta_p)'$ be a p-dimensional vector of parameters and let $\pi(\boldsymbol{\theta}|D)$ be its posterior distribution given the data D. Then, the basic scheme of the Gibbs sampler is given as follows:

Gibbs Sampling Algorithm

Step 0. Choose an arbitrary starting point $\boldsymbol{\theta}_0 = (\theta_{1,0}, \theta_{2,0}, \ldots, \theta_{p,0})'$, and set $i = 0$.

Step 1. Generate $\boldsymbol{\theta}_{i+1} = (\theta_{1,i+1}, \theta_{2,i+1}, \ldots, \theta_{p,i+1})'$ as follows:

- Generate $\theta_{1,i+1} \sim \pi(\theta_1|\theta_{2,i}, \ldots, \theta_{p,i}, D)$;
- Generate $\theta_{2,i+1} \sim \pi(\theta_2|\theta_{1,i+1}, \theta_{3,i}, \ldots, \theta_{p,i}, D)$;

  ... ...
- Generate $\theta_{p,i+1} \sim \pi(\theta_p|\theta_{1,i+1}, \theta_{2,i+1}, \ldots, \theta_{p-1,i+1}, D)$.

Step 2. Set $i = i + 1$, and go to Step 1.

Thus each component of $\boldsymbol{\theta}$ is visited in the natural order and a cycle in this scheme requires generation of p random variates. Gelfand and Smith (1990) show that under certain regularity conditions, the vector sequence $\{\boldsymbol{\theta}_i,\ i = 1, 2, \ldots\}$ has a stationary distribution $\pi(\boldsymbol{\theta}|D)$. Schervish and Carlin (1992) provide a sufficient condition that guarantees geometric convergence. Other properties regarding geometric convergence are discussed in Roberts and Polson (1994). To illustrate the Gibbs sampler, we consider the following two simple examples:

Example 2.1. Bivariate normal model. The purpose of this example is to examine the exact correlation structure of the Markov chain induced by the Gibbs sampler. Assume that the posterior distribution $\pi(\boldsymbol{\theta}|D)$ is a bivariate normal distribution $N_2(\boldsymbol{\mu}, \Sigma)$ with

$$\boldsymbol{\mu} = \begin{pmatrix} \mu_1 \\ \mu_2 \end{pmatrix} \text{ and } \Sigma = \begin{pmatrix} \sigma_1^2 & \rho\sigma_1\sigma_2 \\ \rho\sigma_1\sigma_2 & \sigma_2^2 \end{pmatrix},$$

where μ_j, σ_j, $j = 1, 2$, and ρ are known. Then the Gibbs sampler requires sampling from

$$\theta_1 \sim N\left(\mu_1 + \rho\frac{\sigma_1}{\sigma_2}(\theta_2 - \mu_2), \sigma_1^2(1-\rho^2)\right)$$

and

$$\theta_2 \sim N\left(\mu_2 + \rho\frac{\sigma_2}{\sigma_1}(\theta_1 - \mu_1), \sigma_2^2(1-\rho^2)\right).$$

Let $\{\boldsymbol{\theta}_i = (\theta_{1,i}, \theta_{2,i})', \ i \geq 0\}$ denote the Markov chain induced by the Gibbs sampler for the above bivariate normal distribution. If we start from the stationary distribution, i.e., $\boldsymbol{\theta}_0 \sim N(\mu, \Sigma)$, then each of $\{\theta_{1,i}, \ i \geq 0\}$ and $\{\theta_{2,i}, \ i \geq 0\}$ is an AR(1) process.

To see this, let $\{z_{1,i}, z_{2,i}, \ i \geq 0\}$ be an i.i.d. $N(0,1)$ random variable sequence. Then the structure of the Gibbs sampler implies

$$\begin{aligned}\theta_{1,0} &= \mu_1 + \sigma_1 z_{1,0},\\ \theta_{2,0} &= \mu_2 + \rho\frac{\sigma_2}{\sigma_1}(\theta_{1,0} - \mu_1) + \sigma_2\sqrt{1-\rho^2}z_{2,0},\end{aligned}$$

and

$$\begin{aligned}\theta_{1,i+1} &= \mu_1 + \rho\frac{\sigma_1}{\sigma_2}(\theta_{2,i} - \mu_2) + \sigma_1\sqrt{1-\rho^2}z_{1,i+1},\\ \theta_{2,i+1} &= \mu_2 + \rho\frac{\sigma_2}{\sigma_1}(\theta_{1,i+1} - \mu_1) + \sigma_2\sqrt{1-\rho^2}z_{2,i+1},\end{aligned} \tag{2.1.1}$$

for $i \geq 0$, Now, we consider the first component $\theta_{1,i+1}$. From (2.1.1), for $i \geq 0$,

$$\begin{aligned}\theta_{1,i+1} =& \mu_1 + \rho\frac{\sigma_1}{\sigma_2}\left[\rho\frac{\sigma_2}{\sigma_1}(\theta_{1,i} - \mu_1) + \sigma_2\sqrt{1-\rho^2}z_{2,i}\right]\\ &+ \sigma_1\sqrt{1-\rho^2}z_{1,i+1}\\ =& \mu_1 + \rho^2(\theta_{1,i} - \mu_1) + \rho\sigma_1\sqrt{1-\rho^2}z_{2,i}\\ &+ \sigma_1\sqrt{1-\rho^2}z_{1,i+1}.\end{aligned} \tag{2.1.2}$$

Let $\psi = \rho^2$ and $\sigma_1^{*2} = \sigma_1^2(1-\rho^4)$. Let $\{z_i^*, \ i \geq 0\}$ denote an i.i.d. $N(0,1)$ random variable sequence. Since $z_{1,i}$ and $z_{2,i+1}$ are independently and identically distributed as $N(0,1)$, then we can rewrite (2.1.2) as

$$\theta_{1,0} = \mu_1 + \sigma_1 z_0^*, \tag{2.1.3}$$

$$\theta_{1,i+1} = \mu_1 + \psi(\theta_{1,i} - \mu_1) + \sigma_1^* z_{i+1}^* \quad \text{for } i \geq 0. \tag{2.1.4}$$

Thus, $\{\theta_{1,i}, \ i \geq 0\}$ is an AR(1) process with lag-one autocorrelation $\psi = \rho^2$. Similarly, $\{\theta_{2,i}, \ i \geq 0\}$ is also an AR(1) process with lag-one autocorrelation $\psi = \rho^2$. The only difference is that we use $\sigma_2^* = \sigma_2\sqrt{1-\rho^4}$ instead of σ_1^* in (2.1.4), and use μ_2 and σ_2 instead of μ_1 and σ_1 in (2.1.3).

Roberts and Sahu (1997) obtain a similar result for a general multivariate normal target distribution $\pi(\theta|D)$, that is, the Markov chain induced by the Gibbs sampler is a multivariate AR(1) process.

Example 2.2. Constrained multiple linear regression model. We consider a constrained multiple linear regression model given by (1.3.1) to model the New Zealand apple data described in Example 1.1. Let

$$\Omega = \{\boldsymbol{\beta} = (\beta_1, \beta_2, \ldots, \beta_{10})' : 0 \le \beta_1 \le \beta_2 \le \ldots \le \beta_{10}, \boldsymbol{\beta} \in R^{10}\} \quad (2.1.5)$$

denote the constraints given in (1.3.2). We take a joint prior for $(\boldsymbol{\beta}, \sigma^2)$ of the form

$$\pi(\boldsymbol{\beta}, \sigma^2) \propto \frac{1}{\sigma^2}\pi(\beta_{10}|\mu_{10}, \sigma_{10}^2), \quad (2.1.6)$$

for $\sigma^2 > 0$ and $\boldsymbol{\beta} \in \Omega$, where $\pi(\beta_{10}|\mu_{10}, \sigma_{10}^2)$ is a normal density with mean μ_{10} and variance σ_{10}^2. The modification of the usual flat noninformative prior to include the informative distribution on β_{10} is necessary to prevent too much weight being given to the unconstrained and therefore unbounded parameter β_{10}. Chen and Deely (1996) specify $\mu_{10} = 0.998$, and $\sigma_{10}^2 = 0.089$ by using method-of-moments, a well-known type of empirical Bayes estimation, from the data on growers with mature trees only. Using (2.1.6), the posterior distribution for $(\boldsymbol{\beta}, \sigma^2)$ based on the New Zealand apple data D is given by

$$\pi(\boldsymbol{\beta}, \sigma^2|D) = \frac{\exp\{-(\beta_{10} - \mu_{10})^2/2\sigma_{10}^2\}}{c(D)(\sigma^2)^{(n+1)/2}} \times \exp\left\{-\frac{1}{2\sigma^2}\sum_{i=1}^{n}\left(y_i - \sum_{j=1}^{10} x_{ij}\beta_j\right)^2\right\}, \quad (2.1.7)$$

for $\sigma^2 > 0$ and $\boldsymbol{\beta} \in \Omega$, where y_i is the total number of cartons of fruit produced and x_{ij} = number of trees at age $j+1$ for $j = 1, 2, \ldots, 10$ for the ith grower, $c(D)$ is the normalizing constant, and $n = 207$ denotes the sample size. Due to the constraints, the analytical evaluation of posterior quantities such as the posterior mean and posterior standard deviation of β_j does not appear possible. However, the implementation of the Gibbs sampler for sampling from the posterior (2.1.7) is straightforward. More specifically, we run the Gibbs sampler by taking

$$\beta_j|\beta_1, \ldots, \beta_{j-1}, \beta_{j+1}, \ldots, \beta_{10}, \sigma^2, D \sim N(\theta_j, \delta_j^2) \quad (2.1.8)$$

subject to $\beta_{j-1} \le \beta_j \le \beta_{j+1}$ ($\beta_0 = 0$) for $j = 1, 2, \ldots, 9$,

$$\beta_{10}|\beta_1, \ldots, \beta_9, \sigma^2, D \sim N(\psi\theta_{10} + (1-\psi)\mu_{10}, (1-\psi)\sigma_{10}^2) \quad (2.1.9)$$

subject to $\beta_{10} \geq \beta_9$ and

$$\sigma^2|\boldsymbol{\beta}, D \sim \mathcal{IG}\left(\frac{n}{2}, \frac{\sum_{i=1}^n (y_i - \sum_{j=1}^{10} x_{ij}\beta_j)^2}{2}\right), \tag{2.1.10}$$

where in (2.1.8) and (2.1.9), $\psi = \sigma_{10}^2/(\sigma_{10}^2 + \delta_{10}^2)$,

$$\theta_j = \left(\sum_{i=1}^n x_{ij}^2\right)^{-1} \left[\sum_{i=1}^n \left(y_i - \sum_{l \neq j} x_{il}\beta_l\right) x_{ij}\right], \tag{2.1.11}$$

and

$$\delta_j^2 = \left(\sum_{i=1}^n x_{ij}^2\right)^{-1} \sigma^2 \tag{2.1.12}$$

for $j = 1, \ldots, 10$, and $\mathcal{IG}(\xi, \eta)$ denotes the inverse gamma distribution with parameters (ξ, η), whose density is given by

$$\pi(\sigma^2|\xi, \eta) \propto (\sigma^2)^{-(\xi+1)} e^{-\eta/\sigma^2}.$$

2.2 Metropolis–Hastings Algorithm

The Metropolis–Hastings algorithm is developed by Metropolis et al. (1953) and subsequently generalized by Hastings (1970). Tierney (1994) gives a comprehensive theoretical exposition of this algorithm, and Chib and Greenberg (1995) provide an excellent tutorial on this topic.

Let $q(\boldsymbol{\theta}, \boldsymbol{\vartheta})$ be a proposal density, which is also termed as a *candidate-generating density* by Chib and Greenberg (1995), such that

$$\int q(\boldsymbol{\theta}, \boldsymbol{\vartheta})\, d\boldsymbol{\vartheta} = 1.$$

Also let $U(0, 1)$ denote the uniform distribution over $(0, 1)$. Then, a general version of the Metropolis–Hastings algorithm for sampling from the posterior distribution $\pi(\boldsymbol{\theta}|D)$ can be described as follows:

Metropolis–Hastings Algorithm

Step 0. Choose an arbitrary starting point $\boldsymbol{\theta}_0$ and set $i = 0$.

Step 1. Generate a candidate point $\boldsymbol{\theta}^*$ from $q(\boldsymbol{\theta}_i, \cdot)$ and u from $U(0, 1)$.

Step 2. Set $\boldsymbol{\theta}_{i+1} = \boldsymbol{\theta}^*$ if $u \leq a(\boldsymbol{\theta}_i, \boldsymbol{\theta}^*)$ and $\boldsymbol{\theta}_{i+1} = \boldsymbol{\theta}_i$ otherwise, where the acceptance probability is given by

$$a(\boldsymbol{\theta}, \boldsymbol{\vartheta}) = \min\left\{\frac{\pi(\boldsymbol{\vartheta}|D)q(\boldsymbol{\vartheta}, \boldsymbol{\theta})}{\pi(\boldsymbol{\theta}|D)q(\boldsymbol{\theta}, \boldsymbol{\vartheta})}, 1\right\}. \tag{2.2.1}$$

Step 3. Set $i = i + 1$, and go to Step 1.

The above algorithm is very general. When $q(\boldsymbol{\theta}, \boldsymbol{\vartheta}) = q(\boldsymbol{\vartheta})$, the Metropolis–Hastings algorithm reduces to the *independence chain* Metropolis algorithm (see Tierney 1994). More interestingly, the Gibbs sampler is obtained as a special case of the Metropolis–Hastings algorithm by choosing an appropriate $q(\boldsymbol{\theta}, \boldsymbol{\vartheta})$. This relationship is first pointed out by Gelman (1992) and further elaborated on by Chib and Greenberg (1995).

Another family of proposal densities is given by the form $q(\boldsymbol{\theta}, \boldsymbol{\vartheta}) = q_1(\boldsymbol{\vartheta} - \boldsymbol{\theta})$, where $q_1(\cdot)$ is a multivariate density (see Müller 1991). The candidate $\boldsymbol{\theta}^*$ is thus drawn according to the process $\boldsymbol{\theta}^* = \boldsymbol{\theta} + \boldsymbol{\omega}$, where $\boldsymbol{\omega}$ is called the increment random variable and follows the distribution q_1. Because the candidate is equal to the current value plus noise, Chib and Greenberg (1995) call this case a *random walk chain.* Many other algorithms such as the Hit-and-Run algorithm and dynamic weighting algorithm, which will be presented later in this chapter, are also special cases of this general algorithm.

The performance of a Metropolis–Hastings algorithm depends on the choice of a proposal density q. As discussed in Chib and Greenberg (1995), the spread of the proposal density q affects the behavior of the chain in at least two dimensions: one is the "acceptance rate" (the percentage of times a move to a new point is made), and the other is the region of the sample space that is covered by the chain. If the spread is extremely large, some of the generated candidates will have a low probability of being accepted. On the other hand, if the spread is chosen too small, the chain will take longer to traverse the support of the density. Both of these situations are likely to be reflected in high autocorrelations across sample values. In the context of q_1 (the random walk proposal density), Roberts, Gelman, and Gilks (1997) show that if the target and proposal densities are normal, then the scale of the latter should be tuned so that the acceptance rate is approximately 0.45 in one-dimensional problems and approximately 0.23 as the number of dimensions approaches infinity, with the optimal acceptance rate being around 0.25 in six dimensions. For the *independence chain*, in which we take $q(\boldsymbol{\theta}, \boldsymbol{\vartheta}) = q(\boldsymbol{\vartheta})$, it is important to ensure that the tails of the proposal density $q(\boldsymbol{\vartheta})$ dominate those of the target density $\pi(\boldsymbol{\theta}|D)$, which is similar to a requirement on the importance sampling function in Monte Carlo integration with importance sampling (Geweke 1989).

To illustrate the Metropolis–Hastings algorithm, we consider a problem of sampling a correlation coefficient ρ from its posterior distribution.

Example 2.3. An algorithm for sampling a correlation ρ. Assume that $D = \{\boldsymbol{y}_i = (y_{1i}, y_{2i})',\ i = 1, 2, \ldots, n\}$ is a random sample from a bivariate normal distribution $N_2(0, \Sigma)$, where

$$\Sigma = \begin{pmatrix} 1 & \rho \\ \rho & 1 \end{pmatrix}.$$

Assuming a uniform prior $U(-1, 1)$ for ρ, the posterior density for ρ is given by

$$\pi(\rho|D) \propto (1-\rho^2)^{-n/2} \exp\left\{-\frac{1}{2(1-\rho^2)}(S_{11} - 2\rho S_{12} + S_{22})\right\}, \quad (2.2.2)$$

where $-1 < \rho < 1$, and $S_{rs} = \sum_{i=1}^{n} y_{ri} y_{si}$ for $r, s = 1, 2$. Generating ρ from (2.2.2) is not trivial since $\pi(\rho|D)$ is not log-concave. Therefore, we consider the following Metropolis–Hastings algorithm with a "de-constraint" transformation to sample ρ. Since $-1 < \rho < 1$, we let

$$\rho = \frac{-1 + e^{\xi}}{1 + e^{\xi}}, \quad -\infty < \xi < \infty. \quad (2.2.3)$$

Then

$$\pi(\xi|D) = \pi(\rho|D) \frac{2e^{\xi}}{(1 + e^{\xi})^2}.$$

Instead of directly sampling ρ, we generate ξ by choosing a normal proposal $N(\hat{\xi}, \hat{\sigma}_{\hat{\xi}}^2)$, where $\hat{\xi}$ is a maximizer of the logarithm of $\pi(\xi|D)$, which can be obtained by, for example, the standard Newton–Raphson algorithm or the Nelder–Mead algorithm implemented by O'Neill (1971), and $\hat{\sigma}_{\hat{\xi}}^2$ is minus the inverse of the second derivative of $\log \pi(\xi|D)$ evaluated at $\xi = \hat{\xi}$, that is,

$$\hat{\sigma}_{\hat{\xi}}^{-2} = -\left.\frac{d^2 \log \pi(\xi|D)}{d\xi^2}\right|_{\xi=\hat{\xi}}.$$

The algorithm to generate ξ operates as follows:

Step 1. Let ξ be the current value.

Step 2. Generate a proposal value ξ^* from $N(\hat{\xi}, \hat{\sigma}_{\hat{\xi}}^2)$.

Step 3. A move from ξ to ξ^* is made with probability

$$\min\left\{\frac{\pi(\xi^*|D)\phi\left(\dfrac{\xi - \hat{\xi}}{\hat{\sigma}_{\hat{\xi}}}\right)}{\pi(\xi|D)\phi\left(\dfrac{\xi^* - \hat{\xi}}{\hat{\sigma}_{\hat{\xi}}}\right)}, 1\right\}, \quad (2.2.4)$$

where ϕ is the standard normal probability density function.

After we obtain ξ, we compute ρ by using (2.2.3).

Since the above algorithm does not use a random walk proposal density, the optimal acceptance rate, 0.23, of Roberts, Gelman, and Gilks (1997) cannot be applied here. A detailed study of how this algorithm performs is thus left as an exercise. The above algorithm can also be extended to the cases where $\pi(\rho|D)$ is a conditional posterior distribution that depends on other parameters. For example, the conditional posterior distribution for ρ may be written as $\pi(\rho|\boldsymbol{\theta}, D)$. Then, the Metropolis–Hastings algorithm to sample from $\pi(\rho|\boldsymbol{\theta}, D)$ proceeds in a similar way. The idea of a normal proposal that is matched to the conditional posterior appears for the first time in Chib and Greenberg (1994). A nice feature of this extension is that the normal proposal density for this more general case becomes adaptive since it depends on the values of the other parameters from the current and previous iterations. This semiautomatic updating feature makes the proposal density closer to the true conditional posterior, which may lead to a more efficient Metropolis–Hastings algorithm.

2.3 Hit-and-Run Algorithm

The Hit-and-Run (H&R) algorithm is a special case of the Metropolis–Hastings algorithm. Its original form is proposed independently by Boneh and Golan (1979) and Smith (1980) for generating points uniformly distributed over bounded regions in mathematical programming problems. Smith (1984) calls the H&R a "Mixing Algorithm" and he then proves the convergence of the algorithm. This algorithm has not been studied for about 10 years until Bélisle, Romeijn, and Smith (1993) propose a more general form of the H&R algorithm that generates a sample of points from an arbitrary continuous target distribution. However, Bélisle, Romeijn, and Smith (1993) prove the convergence assuming that the target density is bounded and has bounded support. Chen and Schmeiser (1996) further generalize the H&R algorithm to a general target density for evaluating multidimensional integrals and Chen and Schmeiser (1993) also consider the performance of H&R compared to the Gibbs sampler. In the context of Bayesian computation, Berger and Chen (1993) use the H&R for sampling from a multinomial distribution with a constrained parameter space; Yang and Berger (1994) apply the H&R algorithm for estimation of a covariance matrix using the reference prior; and Yang and Chen (1995) employ the H&R algorithm with parameter transformations for Bayesian analysis of random coefficient regression models using noninformative priors. A slightly different but related algorithm termed *adaptive direction sampling* can be found in Gilks, Roberts, and George (1994) and Roberts and Gilks (1994).

Assume that the posterior distribution $\pi(\boldsymbol{\theta}|D)$ has support Ω. Then, the general H&R algorithm, requiring a distribution for the direction, a density g_i for the signed distance, and an acceptance probability a_i, can be stated as follows:

Hit-and-Run Algorithm

Step 0. Choose an arbitrary starting point $\boldsymbol{\theta}_0$ and set $i = 0$.

Step 1. Generate a direction $\boldsymbol{d}_i$ from a distribution on the surface of the unit sphere.

Step 2. Find the set $\Omega_i = \Omega_i(\boldsymbol{d}_i, \boldsymbol{\theta}_i) = \{\lambda \in R | \boldsymbol{\theta}_i + \lambda \boldsymbol{d}_i \in \Omega\}$.

Step 3. Generate a signed distance λ_i from density $g_i(\lambda | \boldsymbol{d}_i, \boldsymbol{\theta}_i)$, where $\lambda_i \in \Omega_i$.

Step 4. Set $\boldsymbol{\theta}^* = \boldsymbol{\theta}_i + \lambda_i \boldsymbol{d}_i$. Then set

$$\boldsymbol{\theta}_{i+1} = \begin{cases} \boldsymbol{\theta}^*, & \text{with the probability } a_i(\boldsymbol{\theta}^* | \boldsymbol{\theta}_i) \\ \boldsymbol{\theta}_i, & \text{otherwise.} \end{cases} \tag{2.3.1}$$

Step 5. Set $i = i + 1$, and go to Step 1.

Chen and Schmeiser (1996) discuss various choices for the distributions of $\boldsymbol{d}_i$, the densities g_i, and the probabilities a_i. Let the distribution of the direction $\boldsymbol{d}_i$, as used in Step 2 of H&R, have density $r(\boldsymbol{d}_i)$, with the surface of the unit sphere as its support. Then, assume that:

(i) for any density $g_i(\lambda | \boldsymbol{d}_i, \boldsymbol{\theta}_i)$ in Step 3, $g_i(\lambda | \boldsymbol{d}_i, \boldsymbol{\theta}_i) > 0$ and

$$g_i(-\lambda | -\boldsymbol{d}_i, \boldsymbol{\theta}_i) = g_i(\lambda | \boldsymbol{d}_i, \boldsymbol{\theta}_i);$$

(ii) for the distribution of the direction, $r(\boldsymbol{d}_i) > 0$;

(iii) for any a_i in Step 4, $0 < a_i(\boldsymbol{\theta}^* | \boldsymbol{\theta}_i) \leq 1$; and

(iv) for any $\boldsymbol{\theta}, \boldsymbol{\theta}^* \in \Omega$

$$\begin{aligned} &g_i\left(\| \boldsymbol{\theta} - \boldsymbol{\theta}^* \| \left| \frac{\boldsymbol{\theta}^* - \boldsymbol{\theta}}{\| \boldsymbol{\theta}^* - \boldsymbol{\theta} \|}, \theta \right.\right) \cdot a_i(\boldsymbol{\theta}^* | \boldsymbol{\theta}) \pi(\boldsymbol{\theta} | D) \\ &\qquad = g_i\left(\| \boldsymbol{\theta}^* - \boldsymbol{\theta} \| \left| \frac{\boldsymbol{\theta} - \boldsymbol{\theta}^*}{\| \boldsymbol{\theta} - \boldsymbol{\theta}^* \|}, \boldsymbol{\theta}^* \right.\right) \cdot a_i(\boldsymbol{\theta} | \boldsymbol{\theta}^*) \pi(\boldsymbol{\theta}^* | D). \end{aligned}$$

Under the assumptions above, the Markov chain $\{\boldsymbol{\theta}_i,\ i = 0, 1, 2, \dots\}$ converges to its stationary distribution $\pi(\boldsymbol{\theta} | D)$.

The most common choice of $r(\boldsymbol{d}_i)$ is a uniform distribution on the surface of the unit sphere. Common choices of g_i and a_i are given as follows:

Choice I:

$$g_i^{\mathrm{I}}(\lambda | \boldsymbol{d}_i, \boldsymbol{\theta}_i) = \frac{\pi(\boldsymbol{\theta}_i + \lambda \boldsymbol{d}_i | D)}{\int_{\Omega_i(\boldsymbol{d}_i, \boldsymbol{\theta}_i)} \pi(\boldsymbol{\theta}_i + u \boldsymbol{d}_i | D)\, du} \quad \text{for } \lambda \in \Omega_i(\boldsymbol{d}_i, \boldsymbol{\theta}_i),$$

and

$$a_i^{\mathrm{I}}(\boldsymbol{\theta}^*|\boldsymbol{\theta}_i) = a_i^{\mathrm{I}}(\boldsymbol{\theta}_i|\boldsymbol{\theta}^*), \quad 0 < a^{\mathrm{I}}(\boldsymbol{\theta}^*|\boldsymbol{\theta}_i) \leq 1 \text{ for all } \boldsymbol{\theta}_i, \boldsymbol{\theta}^* \in \Omega.$$

Typically $a_i^{\mathrm{I}}(\boldsymbol{\theta}^*|\boldsymbol{\theta}_i) = 1$.

Choice II:

Choose $g_i(\lambda|\boldsymbol{d}_i, \boldsymbol{\theta}_i)$ to be one of the following:

(a) If Ω is bounded, then

$$g_i^{\mathrm{II}}(\lambda|\boldsymbol{d}_i, \boldsymbol{\theta}_i) = \frac{1}{m(\Omega_i(\boldsymbol{d}_i, \boldsymbol{\theta}_i))} \quad \text{for } \lambda \in \Omega_i(\boldsymbol{d}_i, \boldsymbol{\theta}_i),$$

where m denotes Lebesgue measure.

(b) If Ω is unbounded, then choose $g_i^{\mathrm{II}}(\lambda|\boldsymbol{d}_i, \boldsymbol{\theta}_i)$ to be a symmetric-about-zero, continuous distribution with unbounded support $\Omega_i(\boldsymbol{d}_i, \boldsymbol{\theta}_i)$ and shape depending only on $\Omega_i(\boldsymbol{d}_i, \boldsymbol{\theta}_i)$. For example, g_i^{II} can be a normal distribution, Cauchy distribution, or double-exponential distribution with location parameter zero and scale parameter depending only on $\Omega_i(\boldsymbol{d}_i, \boldsymbol{\theta}_i)$.

Independent of the choice (a) or (b), choose $a_i(\boldsymbol{\theta}^*|\boldsymbol{\theta}_i)$ to be either:

(c) Barker's method (Barker 1965)

$$a_i^{\mathrm{II}}(\boldsymbol{\theta}^*|\boldsymbol{\theta}_i) = \frac{\pi(\boldsymbol{\theta}^*|D)}{\pi(\boldsymbol{\theta}_i|D) + \pi(\boldsymbol{\theta}^*|D)}.$$

or

(d) Metropolis's method

$$a_i^{\mathrm{II}}(\boldsymbol{\theta}^*|\boldsymbol{\theta}_i) = \min\left(1, \frac{\pi(\boldsymbol{\theta}^*|D)}{\pi(\boldsymbol{\theta}_i|D)}\right).$$

Choice III:

Choose $g_i^{\mathrm{III}}(\lambda|\boldsymbol{d}_i, \boldsymbol{\theta}_i) = g_i(\boldsymbol{\theta}_i + \lambda \boldsymbol{d}_i)$, where g_i depends only on $\Omega_i(\boldsymbol{d}_i, \boldsymbol{\theta}_i)$, and

$$a_i^{\mathrm{III}}(\boldsymbol{\theta}^*|\boldsymbol{\theta}_i) = \min\{\omega(\boldsymbol{\theta}_i + \lambda \boldsymbol{d}_i)/\omega(\boldsymbol{\theta}_i), 1\},$$

where $\omega(\boldsymbol{\theta}_i) = \pi(\boldsymbol{\theta}_i|D)/g_i(\boldsymbol{\theta}_i)$.

These choices are motivated by Hastings (1970). For a given g_i in Choice III, the results of Peskun (1973) imply that when Ω is a finite set, the choice of a_i^{III} is optimal in the sense of minimizing the asymptotic variance of the sample average $(1/n)\sum_{i=1}^{n} h(\boldsymbol{\theta}_i)$, where $h(\cdot)$ is a real function of $\boldsymbol{\theta}$

satisfying

$$\int_{R^p} |h(\boldsymbol{\theta})|\pi(\boldsymbol{\theta}|D)\, d\boldsymbol{\theta} < \infty.$$

With Choice I, Kaufman and Smith (1998) develop an optimal direction choice algorithm for H&R and prove that there exists a unique optimal direction choice distribution for $r(\cdot)$. The other theoretical properties of H&R can be found in Bélisle, Romeijn, and Smith (1993), and Chen and Schmeiser (1993, 1996). Regarding applications of H&R to Bayesian computation, Berger (1993) comments that

> *"This method is particularly useful when $\boldsymbol{\theta}$ has a sharply constrained parameter space."*

To illustrate the H&R algorithm, we revisit the constrained multiple linear regression model discussed in Section 2.1.

Example 2.4. Constrained multiple linear regression model (Example 2.2 continued). Instead of using the Gibbs sampler to sample $(\boldsymbol{\beta}, \sigma^2)$ from $\pi(\boldsymbol{\beta}, \sigma^2|D)$ given in (2.1.7), we use the H&R algorithm. All eleven dimensions are sampled within a Gibbs sampling framework, with the ten $\boldsymbol{\beta}$ dimensions sampled with H&R and σ^2 sampled from its known conditional gamma density in the Gibbs step. For illustrative purposes, we state the H&R logic for sampling $\boldsymbol{\beta} = (\beta_1, \beta_2, \ldots, \beta_{10})'$ from its conditional posterior distribution for a given value of σ^2 and D:

Step 0. Choose a starting point $\boldsymbol{\beta}_0 \in \Omega$ and set $i = 0$.

Step 1. Generate a uniformly distributed unit-length direction $\boldsymbol{d}_i = (d_{1,i}, d_{2,i}, \ldots, d_{10,i})'$.

Step 2. Find the set $\Omega_i = (R_1^i, R_2^i)$, where

$$R_1^i = \inf_{\lambda}\{\lambda : \boldsymbol{\beta}_i + \lambda \boldsymbol{d}_i \in \Omega\} \text{ and } R_2^i = \sup_{\lambda}\{\lambda : \boldsymbol{\beta}_i + \lambda \boldsymbol{d}_i \in \Omega\}.$$

Step 3. Generate a signed distance λ_i from the density

$$\pi_i(\lambda) = \frac{\pi(\boldsymbol{\beta}_i + \lambda \boldsymbol{d}_i, \sigma^2|D)}{\int_{R_1^i}^{R_2^i} \pi(\boldsymbol{\beta}_i + u\boldsymbol{d}_i, \sigma^2|D)\, du}, \quad \lambda \in (R_1^i, R_2^i). \tag{2.3.2}$$

Step 4. Set $\boldsymbol{\beta}_{i+1} = \boldsymbol{\beta}_i + \lambda_i \boldsymbol{d}_i$.

Step 5. Set $i = i + 1$ and go to Step 1.

Here we use the probability $a_i = 1$. Sampling in each step is straightforward. A random unit-length direction $\boldsymbol{d}_i$ can be generated in Step 2 by independently generating $z_l \sim N(0,1)$ and setting

$$d_{l,i} = z_l \left(\sum_{j=1}^{10} z_j^2 \right)^{-1/2}$$

for $l = 1, 2, ..., 10$; see, for example, Devroye (1986). The density given in (2.3.2) is a truncated normal probability density function, where the mean and variance are easy-to-compute functions of σ^2, $\boldsymbol{\beta}_i$, $\boldsymbol{d}_i$, and D. Computationally, the H&R algorithm is slightly more efficient than the usual (one-coordinate-at-a-time) Gibbs sampler. Implementation difficulty of the two sampling algorithms is similar.

2.4 Multiple-Try Metropolis Algorithm

Liu, Liang, and Wong (1998a) propose a novel algorithm, called the Multiple-Try Metropolis (MTM) algorithm. The algorithm proceeds as follows. Let $T(\boldsymbol{\theta}, \boldsymbol{\vartheta})$ be a proposal transition density function, which may or may not be symmetric. A requirement for $T(\boldsymbol{\theta}, \boldsymbol{\vartheta})$ is that $T(\boldsymbol{\theta}, \boldsymbol{\vartheta}) > 0$ if and only if $T(\boldsymbol{\vartheta}, \boldsymbol{\theta}) > 0$. Furthermore, define

$$w(\boldsymbol{\theta}, \boldsymbol{\vartheta}) = \pi(\boldsymbol{\theta}|D) T(\boldsymbol{\theta}, \boldsymbol{\vartheta}) \lambda(\boldsymbol{\theta}, \boldsymbol{\vartheta}), \tag{2.4.1}$$

where $\lambda(\boldsymbol{\theta}, \boldsymbol{\vartheta})$ is a nonnegative symmetric function in $\boldsymbol{\theta}$ and $\boldsymbol{\vartheta}$ so that $\lambda(\boldsymbol{\theta}, \boldsymbol{\vartheta}) > 0$ whenever $T(\boldsymbol{\theta}, \boldsymbol{\vartheta}) > 0$. Suppose the current state is $\boldsymbol{\theta}_i$. In an MTM transition, the next state is generated as follows:

Multiple-Try Metropolis

Step 1. Generate k trials $\boldsymbol{\vartheta}_1, \boldsymbol{\vartheta}_2, \ldots, \boldsymbol{\vartheta}_k$ from the proposal distribution $T(\boldsymbol{\theta}_i, \boldsymbol{\vartheta})$. Compute $w(\boldsymbol{\vartheta}_j, \boldsymbol{\theta}_i)$ for $j = 1, 2, \ldots, k$.

Step 2. Select $\boldsymbol{\vartheta}_l$ among the $\boldsymbol{\vartheta}_j$'s with probability proportional to $w(\boldsymbol{\vartheta}_j, \boldsymbol{\theta}_i)$, $j = 1, 2, \ldots, k$. Then draw $\boldsymbol{\vartheta}_1^*, \boldsymbol{\vartheta}_1^*, \ldots, \boldsymbol{\vartheta}_{k-1}^*$ from the distribution $T(\boldsymbol{\vartheta}_l, \boldsymbol{\vartheta}^*)$, and let $\boldsymbol{\vartheta}_k^* = \boldsymbol{\theta}_i$.

Step 3. Generate u from $U(0,1)$. Set $\boldsymbol{\theta}_{i+1} = \boldsymbol{\vartheta}_l$ if $u \le a$ and $\boldsymbol{\theta}_{i+1} = \boldsymbol{\theta}_i$ otherwise, where the acceptance probability is given by

$$a = \min \left\{ 1, \frac{w(\boldsymbol{\vartheta}_1, \boldsymbol{\theta}_i) + w(\boldsymbol{\vartheta}_2, \boldsymbol{\theta}_i) + \cdots + w(\boldsymbol{\vartheta}_k, \boldsymbol{\theta}_i)}{w(\boldsymbol{\vartheta}_1^*, \boldsymbol{\vartheta}_l) + w(\boldsymbol{\vartheta}_2^*, \boldsymbol{\vartheta}_l) + \cdots + w(\boldsymbol{\vartheta}_k^*, \boldsymbol{\vartheta}_l)} \right\}.$$

Liu, Liang, and Wong (1998a) show that the MTM transition rule satisfies the detailed balance, and hence, induces a reversible MC with $\pi(\boldsymbol{\theta}|D)$ as its equilibrium distribution. They also present several choices of $\lambda(\boldsymbol{\theta}, \boldsymbol{\vartheta})$ in (2.4.1). When $T(\boldsymbol{\theta}, \boldsymbol{\vartheta})$ is symmetric and $\lambda(\boldsymbol{\theta}, \boldsymbol{\vartheta}) = [T(\boldsymbol{\theta}, \boldsymbol{\vartheta})]^{-1}$, the MTM algorithm reduces to the method of "orientation biased-Monte Carlo" described in Frenkel and Smit (1996), where they provide a specialized proof in the context of simulating molecular structures of materials. As discussed in Liu, Liang, and Wong (1998a), the MTM algorithm is more advantageous, since it allows one to explore more thoroughly the "neighboring region" defined by $T(\boldsymbol{\theta}, \boldsymbol{\vartheta})$, and it is particularly useful when one identifies certain directions of interest but has difficulty implementing a Gibbs sampling type move due to unfavorable conditional distributions. Liu, Liang, and Wong (1998a) also propose several variations of the MTM algorithm. These include a conjugate-gradient MC algorithm, a random-ray algorithm, and a Griddy–Gibbs MTM, which are closely related to the adaptive direction sampling algorithm of Gilks, Roberts, and George (1994) and Roberts and Gilks (1994), the H&R algorithm of Chen and Schmeiser (1993, 1996), and the Griddy–Gibbs algorithm of Ritter and Tanner (1992). For illustrative purposes, we briefly describe the random-ray algorithm as follows. Suppose the current state is $\boldsymbol{\theta}_i$. The random-ray algorithm executes the following update:

- Randomly generate a unit-length direction $\boldsymbol{d}$.
- Draw $\boldsymbol{\vartheta}_1, \boldsymbol{\vartheta}_2, \ldots, \boldsymbol{\vartheta}_k$ from the proposal transition $T_{\boldsymbol{d}}(\boldsymbol{\theta}_i, \boldsymbol{\vartheta})$ along the direction $\boldsymbol{d}$. One possible way to do this is to generate a random sample $\{r_1, r_2, \ldots, r_k\}$ from $N(0, \sigma^2)$, where σ^2 can be chosen large, and set $\boldsymbol{\vartheta}_k = \boldsymbol{\theta}_i + r_j \boldsymbol{d}$. Another approach is to generate $r_j \sim U[-\sigma, \sigma]$.
- Conduct the other MTM steps as described in the Multiple-Try Metropolis algorithm.

The implementational details for the other variations can be found in Liu, Liang, and Wong (1998a), and are omitted here for brevity.

2.5 Grouping, Collapsing, and Reparameterizations

In this section, we discuss several useful tools to improve convergence of MCMC sampling. In particular, we focus on the grouped and collapsed Gibbs techniques of Liu (1994) and Liu, Wong, and Kong (1994), and the hierarchical centering method of Gelfand, Sahu, and Carlin (1995, 1996).

2.5.1 Grouped and Collapsed Gibbs

Liu (1994) proposes a method of "grouping" and "collapsing" when using the Gibbs sampler in which he shows that both grouping and collapsing are beneficial based on operator theory. To illustrate his idea, we consider a three-dimensional posterior distribution $\pi(\boldsymbol{\theta}|D)$, where $\boldsymbol{\theta} = (\theta_1, \theta_2, \theta_3)'$.

Liu (1994) considers the following three variations of the Gibbs sampler to sample from $\pi(\boldsymbol{\theta}|D)$:

Algorithm 1: *Standard (Original) Gibbs Sampler*

The standard Gibbs sampler requires drawing:

(i) $\theta_1 \sim \pi(\theta_1|\theta_2, \theta_3, D)$;

(ii) $\theta_2 \sim \pi(\theta_2|\theta_1, \theta_3, D)$;

(iii) $\theta_3 \sim \pi(\theta_3|\theta_1, \theta_2, D)$.

Algorithm 2: *Grouped Gibbs Sampler*

The grouped Gibbs sampler requires drawing:

(i) $(\theta_1, \theta_2) \sim \pi(\theta_1, \theta_2|\theta_3, D)$;

(ii) $\theta_3 \sim \pi(\theta_3|\theta_1, \theta_2, D)$.

In Algorithm 2, we first group (θ_1, θ_2) together and then simultaneously draw (θ_1, θ_2) from their joint conditional posterior distribution $\pi(\theta_1, \theta_2|\theta_3, D)$.

Algorithm 3: *Collapsed Gibbs Sampler*

The collapsed Gibbs sampler requires drawing:

(i) $(\theta_1, \theta_2) \sim \pi(\theta_1, \theta_2|D)$;

(ii) $\theta_3 \sim \pi(\theta_3|\theta_1, \theta_2, D)$.

The main difference between Algorithms 2 and 3 is the implementation of step (i). In particular, the collapsed Gibbs draws (θ_1, θ_2) from their marginal posterior distribution instead of the conditional posterior distribution as in Algorithm 2. Liu (1994) also mentions that if one uses a "mini-Gibbs" to draw (θ_1, θ_2) in step (i), that is, to sample $\theta_1 \sim \pi(\theta_1|\theta_2, D)$ and then $\theta_2 \sim \pi(\theta_2|\theta_1, D)$, the collapsed Gibbs requires that the chain from the mini-Gibbs sampler converges before step (ii). In practice, it may be difficult or expensive to directly draw (θ_1, θ_2) jointly from $\pi(\theta_1, \theta_2|D)$. In this case, we consider the following modified version of the collapsed Gibbs sampler:

Algorithm 3(a): *Modified Collapsed Gibbs Sampler*

The modified collapsed Gibbs sampler is similar to the original version by changing step (i) to:

(ia) $\theta_1 \sim \pi(\theta_1|\theta_2, D)$;

(ib) $\theta_2 \sim \pi(\theta_2|\theta_1, D)$.

We can show that the modified Gibbs sampler still leaves the target posterior distribution invariant. To see this, let $\boldsymbol{\theta}_i = (\theta_{1,i}, \theta_{2,i}, \theta_{3,i})'$ and $\boldsymbol{\theta}_{i+1} = (\theta_{1,i+1}, \theta_{2,i+1}, \theta_{3,i+1})'$ be two consecutive states. Then the construction of Algorithm 3(a) yields the following transition probability kernel:

$$T(\boldsymbol{\theta}_i, \boldsymbol{\theta}_{i+1}) = \pi(\theta_{1,i+1}|\theta_{2,i}, D)\pi(\theta_{2,i+1}|\theta_{1,i+1}, D) \times \pi(\theta_{3,i+1}|\theta_{1,i+1}, \theta_{2,i+1}, D). \tag{2.5.1}$$

It follows that

$$\int_{R^3} T(\boldsymbol{\theta}_i, \boldsymbol{\theta}_{i+1})\pi(\boldsymbol{\theta}_i|D)\, d\boldsymbol{\theta}_i = \pi(\boldsymbol{\theta}_{i+1}|D). \tag{2.5.2}$$

(The proof of (2.5.2) is left as an exercise.) Thus, $\pi(\boldsymbol{\theta}|D)$ is invariant with respect to the transition probability kernel $T(\boldsymbol{\theta}_i, \boldsymbol{\theta}_{i+1})$. The modified version of the collapsed Gibbs sampler is useful and practically advantageous since drawing from the conditional posterior distributions is usually easier than sampling from the joint unconditional one. This is particularly true when dealing with higher-dimensional problems.

Using norms of the forward and backward operators of the induced Markov chain, Liu (1994) shows that the collapsed Gibbs works better than the grouped Gibbs, while the latter is better than the original Gibbs. It is expected that the collapsed Gibbs may work better than the modified collapsed Gibbs, while the modified version of collapsed Gibbs may be more beneficial than the original Gibbs. However, between the modified collapsed Gibbs and the grouped Gibbs, it is not straightforward to see which one works better. The performance of these two algorithms may depend on the correlations between θ_i and θ_j. If θ_1 and θ_2 are highly correlated, the grouped Gibbs is expected to work better. Otherwise, the modified collapsed Gibbs may have better performance.

The above three-component Gibbs sampler is also studied by Liu, Wong, and Kong (1994) and further discussed by Roberts and Sahu (1997), when the target distribution $\pi(\boldsymbol{\theta}|D)$ is normal. Regarding the grouping or blocking strategy for the Gibbs sampler, Roberts and Sahu (1997) provide a comprehensive study by comparing rates of convergence of various blocking combinations, and thus we refer the reader to their paper for further discussion. In general, grouping or blocking is beneficial, but often more computationally demanding. In particular, Roberts and Sahu (1997) show that if all partial correlations of a normal (Gaussian) target distribution are nonnegative, i.e., all of the off-diagonal elements of the inverse covariance matrix are nonpositive, then the grouped (blocked) Gibbs sampler has a faster rate of convergence than the standard (original) Gibbs sampler. That is, grouping positively correlated parameters in Gibbs sampling is always beneficial. However, Roberts and Sahu (1997) also find some examples showing that blocking can also make an algorithm converge more slowly.

2.5.2 Reparameterizations: Hierarchical Centering and Rescaling

As pointed out by Roberts and Sahu (1997), high correlations among the coordinates of θ diminish the speed of convergence of the Gibbs sampler (see also Hills and Smith 1992). The correlations among the coordinates are determined by the particular parameterization of the problem. Gelfand, Sahu, and Carlin (1995, 1996) argue that a hierarchically centered parameterization leads to faster mixing and convergence because it generally leads to smaller intercomponent correlations among the coordinates in Bayesian linear models. Roberts and Sahu (1997) further examine the hierarchically centered parameterization and they demonstrate that hierarchical centering yields faster mixing Gibbs samplers.

Here we illustrate this idea with a one-way analysis of variance model with random effects.

Example 2.5. One-way analysis of variance with random effects. Gelfand, Sahu, and Carlin (1996) and Roberts and Sahu (1997) consider the following one-way analysis of variance model. Assume that the error variance σ_e^2 is known and suppose that we have a single observation y_i for each population, i.e.,

$$y_i = \mu + \alpha_i + \epsilon_i, \quad i = 1, 2, \ldots, m, \tag{2.5.3}$$

where $\epsilon_i \sim N(0, \sigma_e^2)$, $\alpha_i \sim N(0, \sigma_\alpha^2)$, $\mu \sim N(\mu_0, \sigma_\mu^2)$, and σ_α^2 is also known. We denote the data by $D = \boldsymbol{y} = (y_1, y_2, \ldots, y_m)'$. Gelfand, Sahu, and Carlin (1996) rewrite (2.5.3) in a hierarchical form. Defining $\eta_i = \mu + \alpha_i$, we have

$$y_i|\eta_i \sim N(\eta_i, \sigma_e^2), \quad \eta_i|\mu \sim N(\mu, \sigma_\alpha^2), \quad \text{and} \quad \mu \sim N(\mu_0, \sigma_\mu^2).$$

This transformation from $(\alpha_1, \alpha_2, \ldots, \alpha_m)'$ to $(\eta_1, \eta_2, \ldots, \eta_m)'$ is thus referred to as hierarchical centering. Working in μ–η space, Gelfand, Sahu, and Carlin (1996) obtain

$$\operatorname{corr}(\eta_i, \mu|D) = \left(1 + \frac{b\sigma_\alpha^2}{\sigma_e^2\sigma_\mu^2}\right)^{-1/2} \tag{2.5.4}$$

and

$$\operatorname{corr}(\eta_i, \eta_j|D) = \left(1 + \frac{b\sigma_\alpha^2}{\sigma_e^2\sigma_\mu^2}\right)^{-1}, \tag{2.5.5}$$

where $b = \sigma_e^2 + \sigma_\alpha^2 + m\sigma_\mu^2$. The correlations given in (2.5.4) and (2.5.5) tend to 0 for fixed σ_e^2 and σ_μ^2 if $\sigma_\alpha^2 \to \infty$. On the other hand, if $\sigma_e^2 \to \infty$, the correlations do not approach 0, and in fact will tend to 1 if $\sigma_\mu^2 \to \infty$.

In μ–α space, we can obtain

$$\mathrm{corr}(\alpha_i, \mu | D) = \left(1 + \frac{b\sigma_e^2}{\sigma_\alpha^2 \sigma_\mu^2}\right)^{-1/2} \tag{2.5.6}$$

and

$$\mathrm{corr}(\alpha_i, \alpha_j | D) = \left(1 + \frac{b\sigma_e^2}{\sigma_\alpha^2 \sigma_\mu^2}\right)^{-1}. \tag{2.5.7}$$

The correlations given in (2.5.6) and (2.5.7) tend to 0 as $\sigma_e^2 \to \infty$, but do not approach 0 as $\sigma_\alpha^2 \to \infty$, and in fact will tend to 1 if $\sigma_\mu^2 \to \infty$ as well. In practice, when the random effects are needed, the error variance is much reduced. Thus σ_e^2 will rarely dominate the variability, so that the centered parameterization will likely be preferred. Roberts and Sahu (1997) obtain similar results by studying the rate of convergence of the Gibbs sampler.

Hierarchical centering is also useful for Bayesian nonlinear models. We will address this issue in Section 2.5.4 below. In the same spirit as hierarchical centering, hierarchical rescaling is another useful tool to reduce the correlations between the location coordinates and the scalar coordinates. We will illustrate hierarchical rescaling in the next subsection using ordinal response models.

2.5.3 Collapsing and Reparameterization for Ordinal Response Models

Consider a probit model for ordinal response data. Let $\boldsymbol{y} = (y_1, y_2, \ldots, y_n)'$ denote an $n \times 1$ vector of n independent ordinal random variables. Assume that y_i takes a value of l ($1 \le l \le L$, $L > 2$) with probability

$$p_{il} = \Phi(\gamma_l + \boldsymbol{x}_i'\boldsymbol{\beta}) - \Phi(\gamma_{l-1} + \boldsymbol{x}_i'\boldsymbol{\beta}), \tag{2.5.8}$$

for $i = 1, ..., n$ and $l = 1, \ldots, L$, where $-\infty = \gamma_0 < \gamma_1 \le \gamma_2 < \ldots < \gamma_{L-1} < \gamma_L = \infty$, $\Phi(\cdot)$ denotes the $N(0,1)$ cumulative distribution function (cdf), which defines the link, $\boldsymbol{x}_i$ is a $p \times 1$ column vector of covariates, and $\boldsymbol{\beta} = (\beta_1, \ldots, \beta_p)'$ is a $p \times 1$ column vector of regression coefficients. To ensure identifiability, we take $\gamma_1 = 0$. Let $\boldsymbol{\gamma} = (\gamma_2, \ldots, \gamma_{L-1})'$ and $D = (\boldsymbol{y}, X, n)$ denote the data, where X is the $n \times p$ design matrix with $\boldsymbol{x}_i'$ as its ith row. Thus, the likelihood function is

$$L(\boldsymbol{\beta}, \boldsymbol{\gamma} | D) = \prod_{i=1}^{n} \left[\Phi(\gamma_{y_i} + \boldsymbol{x}_i'\boldsymbol{\beta}) - \Phi(\gamma_{y_i - 1} + \boldsymbol{x}_i'\boldsymbol{\beta})\right]. \tag{2.5.9}$$

We further assume that $(\boldsymbol{\beta}, \boldsymbol{\gamma})$ has an improper uniform prior, i.e., $\pi(\boldsymbol{\beta}, \boldsymbol{\gamma}) \propto 1$. The posterior distribution for $(\boldsymbol{\beta}, \boldsymbol{\gamma})$ takes the form

$$\begin{aligned}\pi(\boldsymbol{\beta}, \boldsymbol{\gamma}|D) &\propto L(\boldsymbol{\beta}, \boldsymbol{\gamma}|D)\pi(\boldsymbol{\beta}, \boldsymbol{\gamma}) \\ &= \prod_{i=1}^{n} \left[\Phi(\gamma_{y_i} + \boldsymbol{x}_i'\boldsymbol{\beta}) - \Phi(\gamma_{y_i-1} + \boldsymbol{x}_i'\boldsymbol{\beta})\right]. \end{aligned} \tag{2.5.10}$$

Chen and Shao (1999a) obtain necessary and sufficient conditions for the propriety of the posterior defined by (2.5.10). To facilitate the Gibbs sampler, Albert and Chib (1993) introduce latent variables z_i such that

$$y_i = l \text{ iff } \gamma_{l-1} \leq z_i < \gamma_l,$$

for $l = 1, 2, \ldots, L$. Let $\boldsymbol{z} = (z_1, z_2, \ldots, z_n)'$. The complete-data likelihood is given by

$$L(\boldsymbol{\beta}, \gamma_2, \boldsymbol{z}|D) \propto \prod_{i=1}^{n} [\exp\{-\tfrac{1}{2}(z_i - \boldsymbol{x}_i'\boldsymbol{\beta})^2\} 1\{\gamma_{y_i-1} \leq z_i < \gamma_{y_i}\}], \tag{2.5.11}$$

where $1\{\gamma_{y_i-1} \leq z_i < \gamma_{y_i}\}$ is the indicator function, and the joint posterior density for $(\boldsymbol{\beta}, \boldsymbol{\gamma}, \boldsymbol{z})$ is given by

$$\pi(\boldsymbol{\beta}, \boldsymbol{\gamma}, \boldsymbol{z}|D) \propto \left\{\prod_{i=1}^{n} [\exp\{-\tfrac{1}{2}(z_i - \boldsymbol{x}_i'\boldsymbol{\beta})^2\} 1\{\gamma_{y_i-1} \leq z_i < \gamma_{y_i}\}]\right\}. \tag{2.5.12}$$

Then, Albert and Chib (1993) incorporate the unknown latent variables $\boldsymbol{z}$ as additional parameters to run the Gibbs sampler. The original Gibbs sampler for the ordinal probit model proposed by Albert and Chib (1993), which is referred to as the Albert–Chib algorithm thereafter, may be implemented as follows:

Albert–Chib Algorithm

Step 1. Draw $\boldsymbol{\beta}$ from

$$\boldsymbol{\beta}|\boldsymbol{z}, \boldsymbol{\gamma} \sim N((X'X)^{-1}X'\boldsymbol{z}, (X'X)^{-1}).$$

Step 2. Draw z_i from

$$z_i \sim N(\boldsymbol{x}_i'\boldsymbol{\beta}, 1), \quad \gamma_{y_i-1} \leq z_i \leq \gamma_{y_i}.$$

Step 3. Draw $\boldsymbol{\gamma}$ from

$$\gamma_l|\boldsymbol{\gamma}^{(-l)}, \boldsymbol{\beta}, \boldsymbol{z} \sim U[a_l, b_l], \tag{2.5.13}$$

where $a_l = \max\left\{\gamma_{l-1}, \max_{y_i=l} z_i\right\}$, $b_l = \min\left\{\gamma_{l+1}, \min_{y_i=l+1} z_i\right\}$, and $\boldsymbol{\gamma}^{(-l)}$ is $\boldsymbol{\gamma}$ with γ_l deleted.

Since, in Step 1 all p components of the regression coefficient vector are drawn simultaneously, the Albert–Chib algorithm is indeed a grouped Gibbs sampler. The implementation of the Albert–Chib algorithm is straightforward since the conditional posterior distributions are normal, truncated normal, or uniform. When the sample size n is not too big, the Albert–Chib algorithm works reasonably well. However, when n is large, say $n \geq 50$, slow convergence of the Albert–Chib algorithm may occur. Cowles (1996) points out this slow convergence problem. Because the interval (a_l, b_l) within which each γ_l must be generated from its full conditional can be very narrow, the cutpoint values may change very little between successive iterations, making the iterates highly correlated. Of course, slower convergence of the γ_l is also associated with the fact that the variance of the latent variables is fixed at one. The empirical study of Cowles (1996) further shows that the slow convergence of the cutpoints may also seriously affect the convergence of $\boldsymbol{\beta}$. To improve convergence of the original Gibbs sampler, she proposes a Metropolis–Hastings algorithm to generate the cutpoints from their conditional distributions; henceforth, this algorithm is called the Cowles algorithm. Instead of directly generating γ_l from (2.5.13), the Cowles algorithm generates $(\boldsymbol{\gamma}, \boldsymbol{z})$ jointly, which is essentially the same idea as the (modified) collapsed Gibbs sampler described in Section 2.5.1. The joint conditional distribution $\pi(\boldsymbol{\gamma}, \boldsymbol{z}|\boldsymbol{\beta}, D)$ can be expressed as the product of the marginal conditional distributions $\pi(\boldsymbol{\gamma}|\boldsymbol{\beta}, D)$ and $\pi(\boldsymbol{z}|\boldsymbol{\gamma}, \boldsymbol{\beta}, D)$. The Cowles algorithm can be described as follows:

Cowles Algorithm

Step 1. Draw $\boldsymbol{\beta}$ from

$$\boldsymbol{\beta}|\boldsymbol{z}, \boldsymbol{\gamma} \sim N((X'X)^{-1}X'\boldsymbol{z}, (X'X)^{-1}).$$

Step 2. Draw z_i from

$$z_i \sim N(\boldsymbol{x}_i'\boldsymbol{\beta}, 1), \quad \gamma_{y_i-1} \leq z_i \leq \gamma_{y_i}.$$

Step 3. Draw $\boldsymbol{\gamma}$ from the conditional distribution

$$\pi(\boldsymbol{\gamma}|\boldsymbol{\beta}, D) \propto \prod_{i=1}^{n} \left[\Phi(\gamma_{y_i} - \boldsymbol{x}_i'\boldsymbol{\beta}) - \Phi(\gamma_{y_i-1} - \boldsymbol{x}_i'\boldsymbol{\beta})\right]. \tag{2.5.14}$$

In the Cowles algorithm, a Metropolis–Hastings scheme is used to draw $\boldsymbol{\gamma}$. That is, given the value $\boldsymbol{\gamma}_{j-1}$ from the previous iteration, a vector of proposal cutpoint values, γ_l^*, $l = 2, 3, \ldots, L-1$, is generated from a truncated normal distribution

$$\gamma_l^*|\gamma_{l-1}^*, \gamma_{l+1,j-1} \sim N(\gamma_{l,j-1}, \sigma_\gamma^2), \tag{2.5.15}$$

where $\gamma_{l-1}^* \le \gamma_l^* \le \gamma_{l+1,j-1}$. The acceptance probability for the vector $\boldsymbol{\gamma}^*$ of new cutpoints is $a = \min\{1, R\}$, where

$$R = \prod_{l=2}^{L-1} \frac{\{\Phi\{(\gamma_{l+1,j-1} - \gamma_{l,j-1})/\sigma_\gamma\} - \Phi\{(\gamma_{l-1}^* - \gamma_{l,j-1})/\sigma_\gamma\}}{\Phi\{(\gamma_{l+1}^* - \gamma_l^*)/\sigma_\gamma\} - \Phi\{(\gamma_{l-1,j-1} - \gamma_l^*)/\sigma_\gamma\}}$$
$$\times \prod_{i=1}^{n} \frac{\Phi(\gamma_{y_i}^* - \boldsymbol{x}_i'\boldsymbol{\beta}) - \Phi(\gamma_{y_i-1}^* - \boldsymbol{x}_i'\boldsymbol{\beta})}{\Phi(\gamma_{y_i,j-1} - \boldsymbol{x}_i'\boldsymbol{\beta}) - \Phi(\gamma_{y_i-1,j-1} - \boldsymbol{x}_i'\boldsymbol{\beta})}. \tag{2.5.16}$$

However, our experience suggests that in the Cowles algorithm, the truncated normal-distribution in (2.5.15) might not serve as a good proposal density for the conditional posterior density in (2.5.14), since it is not spread out enough (see Tierney (1994), and Section 2.2). Further, Cowles (1996) points out that a good σ_γ^2 in (2.5.15) is difficult to obtain even when using a conventional updating scheme.

To overcome the difficulties arising in the Cowles algorithm, Nandram and Chen (1996) develop an improved algorithm using a Dirichlet proposal distribution based on a rescaling transformation. Similar to hierarchical centering, the hierarchically rescaled transformations proposed by Nandram and Chen (1996) are

$$\delta = 1/\gamma_{L-1}, \quad \boldsymbol{\gamma}^* = \delta\boldsymbol{\gamma}, \quad \boldsymbol{\beta}^* = \delta\boldsymbol{\beta}, \quad \text{and} \quad \boldsymbol{z}^* = \delta\boldsymbol{z}. \tag{2.5.17}$$

Note that in (2.5.17), $\gamma_0^* = -\infty < \gamma_1^* = 0 \le \gamma_2^* \le \cdots \le \gamma_{L-2}^* \le \gamma_{L-1}^* = 1 < \gamma_L^* = \infty$, and that effectively there are only $L-3$ unknown cutpoints in the reparameterized model. Let $\boldsymbol{\gamma}^* = (\gamma_2^*, \gamma_3^*, \ldots, \gamma_{L-2}^*)'$. Thus, when $L = 3$, there are no unknown cutpoints in $\boldsymbol{\gamma}^*$, which is advantageous when one deals with a 3-level ordinal response model. For $L = 3$, the Nandram–Chen algorithm can be implemented as follows:

Nandram–Chen Algorithm

Step 1. Draw $\boldsymbol{\beta}^*$ from

$$\boldsymbol{\beta}^* | \boldsymbol{z}^*, \boldsymbol{\gamma}^* \sim N((X'X)^{-1}X'\boldsymbol{z}, \delta^2(X'X)^{-1}).$$

Step 2. Draw z_i^* from

$$z_i^* | \boldsymbol{\beta}^*, \delta \sim N(\boldsymbol{x}_i'\boldsymbol{\beta}^*, \delta^2), \quad \gamma_{y_i-1}^* \le z_i^* < \gamma_{y_i}^*.$$

Step 3. Draw δ^2 from

$$\delta^2 | \boldsymbol{\beta}^*, \boldsymbol{z}^* \sim \mathcal{IG}\left\{\frac{n+p+L-2}{2}, \tfrac{1}{2}[(\boldsymbol{z}^* - X\boldsymbol{\beta}^*)'(\boldsymbol{z}^* - X\boldsymbol{\beta}^*)]\right\}.$$

For $L > 3$, the Nandram–Chen algorithm requires an additional step to draw $\boldsymbol{\gamma}^*$. That is,

Step 4. Draw $\boldsymbol{\gamma}^*$ from the conditional posterior distribution

$$\pi(\boldsymbol{\gamma}^*|\boldsymbol{\beta}^*,\delta^2,D) \propto \prod_{i=1}^{n}\left\{\Phi\left(\frac{\gamma^*_{y_i}-\boldsymbol{x}_i'\boldsymbol{\beta}^*}{\delta}\right)-\Phi\left(\frac{\gamma^*_{y_i-1}-\boldsymbol{x}_i'\boldsymbol{\beta}^*}{\delta}\right)\right\}. \tag{2.5.18}$$

Instead of using a truncated normal proposal density as in the Cowles algorithm, Nandram and Chen (1996) construct a Dirichlet proposal density for $\pi(\boldsymbol{\gamma}^*|\boldsymbol{\beta}^*,\delta^2,D)$. The motivation for the Dirichlet proposal density is given as follows. Let $q_{l-1}=\gamma^*_l-\gamma^*_{l-1}$, $l=2,\ldots,L-1$, and let $\boldsymbol{q}=(q_1,q_2,\ldots,q_{L-2})'$, $q_l\geq 0$, $l=1,2,\ldots,L-2$ and $\sum_{l=1}^{L-2}q_l=1$. By the fundamental mean value theorem,

$$\Phi\left(\frac{\gamma^*_{y_i}-\boldsymbol{x}_i'\boldsymbol{\beta}^*}{\delta}\right)-\Phi\left(\frac{\gamma^*_{y_i-1}-\boldsymbol{x}_i'\boldsymbol{\beta}^*}{\delta}\right)=\frac{1}{\delta}\phi\left(\frac{\xi_{y_i}-\boldsymbol{x}_i'\boldsymbol{\beta}^*}{\delta}\right)q_{y_i-1}, \tag{2.5.19}$$

where ξ_{y_i} is a real number between $\gamma^*_{y_i}$ and $\gamma^*_{y_i-1}$, $i=1,2,3,\ldots,n$, and $\phi(\cdot)$ is the standard normal density function. Then by (2.5.19),

$$\pi(\boldsymbol{\gamma}^*|\boldsymbol{\beta}^*,\delta^2,D)\propto g_1(\xi)g_2(\boldsymbol{q}), \tag{2.5.20}$$

where

$$g_1(\xi)=\prod_{i=1}^{n}\phi\left(\frac{\xi_{y_i}-\boldsymbol{x}_i'\boldsymbol{\beta}^*}{\delta}\right),\quad g_2(\boldsymbol{q})=\prod_{l=1}^{L-2}q_l^{n_{l+1}},\quad \text{and}\quad n_l=\sum_{i=1}^{n}1\{y_i=l\}.$$

for $l=1,2,\ldots,L$. While in the Cowles algorithm the proposal density is based on $g_1(\xi)$, Nandram and Chen (1996) use $g_2(\boldsymbol{q})$ to construct a proposal density. This is quite natural because if there are no covariates, we can associate $\boldsymbol{q}$ with the bin "probabilities." Assigning an improper prior to the bins and treating the bin counts as data, the joint posterior distribution of these bin "probabilities" is a Dirichlet distribution with the bin counts as the posterior parameters.

An approximation of $\pi(\boldsymbol{\gamma}^*|\boldsymbol{\beta}^*,\delta^2,D)$ motivated by (2.5.20) is

$$\pi(\boldsymbol{q}|\boldsymbol{\beta}^*,\delta^2,D)\ \propto\ \prod_{l=1}^{L-2}q_l^{\alpha_l n_{l+1}-1}, \tag{2.5.21}$$

where $0\leq\alpha_l\leq 1$, $l=1,\ldots,L-2$, are the tuning parameters. (That is, $\boldsymbol{q}$ has a Dirichlet distribution.) The proposal density (2.5.21) is attractive because we can draw the entire vector $\boldsymbol{q}$ at once, and it does not depend on $\boldsymbol{\beta}^*$ and δ^2. In addition, the Dirichlet proposal density will be more useful when more complex link functions (e.g., logistic and complementary log-log) are used. Moreover, one can choose the α_l in (2.5.21) by taking the α_l so as to make the dispersion of the posterior distribution of $\boldsymbol{q}$ comparable to or at least as large as that of the distribution of $\boldsymbol{\gamma}^*$. The rest of the implementation for drawing $\boldsymbol{\gamma}^*$ simultaneously from its conditional posterior distribution is the same as the one given in the Cowles algorithm, and thus the details are omitted.

Nandram and Chen (1996) conduct several simulation studies, and their empirical results show that the Nandram–Chen algorithm substantially improves convergence of the Gibbs sampler compared to the Albert–Chib and Cowles algorithms. A partial explanation for this is that:

(a) hierarchical rescaling reduces the correlations between the cutpoints and the latent variables; and

(b) the meaningful choice (from a theoretical or statistical viewpoint) of the proposal density has better properties than the truncated normal proposal density used in the Cowles algorithm.

The Nandram–Chen algorithm works well if the cell counts n_l are relatively balanced. When the cell counts are unbalanced, in particular, if some of those counts are close to zero, $\pi(\boldsymbol{q}|\boldsymbol{\beta}^*, \delta^2, D)$ in (2.5.21) may not serve as a good proposal density. For these cases, Chen and Dey (1996) propose a Metropolis–Hastings algorithm using a "de-constraint" transformation to draw $\boldsymbol{\gamma}^*$. A similar transformation of the cutpoints is also considered in Albert and Chib (1998). Let

$$\gamma_l^* = \frac{\gamma_{l-1}^* + e^{\zeta_l}}{1 + e^{\zeta_l}}, \quad l = 2, \ldots, L-2, \tag{2.5.22}$$

and $\boldsymbol{\zeta} = (\zeta_2, \ldots, \zeta_{L-2})'$. Then the conditional posterior distribution for ζ is

$$\pi(\boldsymbol{\zeta}|\boldsymbol{\beta}^*, \delta^2, D) \propto \pi(\boldsymbol{\gamma}^*|\boldsymbol{\beta}^*, \delta^2, D) \prod_{l=2}^{L-2} \frac{(1-\gamma_{l-1})e^{\zeta_l}}{(1+e^{\zeta_l})^2}, \tag{2.5.23}$$

where $\boldsymbol{\gamma}^*$ is evaluated at $\gamma_l^* = (\gamma_{l-1}^* + e^{\zeta_l})/(1+e^{\zeta_l})$ for $l = 2, 3, \ldots, L-2$. The remaining steps of the Metropolis–Hastings algorithm are the same as the algorithm for sampling ρ as described in Example 2.3. This modified Nandram–Chen algorithm is thus called the *Chen–Dey algorithm.*

2.5.4 Hierarchical Centering for Poisson Random Effects Models

A Poisson regression model with AR(1) random effects is used for modeling the pollen count data in Example 1.3. Using (1.3.3), the complete-data likelihood is given by

$$\begin{aligned} L(\boldsymbol{\beta}, \sigma^2, \rho, \boldsymbol{\epsilon}|D) = & \exp\{\boldsymbol{y}'(X\boldsymbol{\beta} + \boldsymbol{\epsilon}) - J_n' Q(\boldsymbol{\beta}, \boldsymbol{\epsilon}) - J_n' C(\boldsymbol{y})\} \\ & \times (2\pi\sigma^2)^{-n/2}(1-\rho^2)^{-(n-1)/2} \\ & \times \exp\left\{-\frac{1}{2\sigma^2}\boldsymbol{\epsilon}'\Sigma^{-1}\boldsymbol{\epsilon}\right\}, \end{aligned} \tag{2.5.24}$$

where $\boldsymbol{y} = (y_1, \ldots, y_n)'$, $\boldsymbol{\epsilon} = (\epsilon_1, \ldots, \epsilon_n)'$, X is the $n \times 8$ matrix of covariates with the tth row equal to $\boldsymbol{x}_t'$, J_n is an $n \times 1$ vector of ones, and $Q(\boldsymbol{\beta}, \boldsymbol{\epsilon})$ is an $n \times 1$ vector with the tth element equal to $q_t = \exp\{\epsilon_t + \boldsymbol{x}_t'\boldsymbol{\beta}\}$, $C(\boldsymbol{y})$ is an $n \times 1$ vector with the jth element $\log(y_j!)$, and $D = (n, \boldsymbol{y}, X)$. In (2.5.24), $\Sigma = (\sigma_{ij})$ with $\sigma_{ij} = \rho^{|i-j|}$, where $\rho^{|i-j|}$ is the correlation between (ϵ_i, ϵ_j), and $-1 \le \rho \le 1$. Assume that a noninformative prior for $(\boldsymbol{\beta}, \sigma^2, \rho)$ has the form

$$\pi(\boldsymbol{\beta}, \sigma^2, \rho) \propto (\sigma^2)^{-(\delta_0+1)} \exp(-\sigma^{-2}\gamma_0), \tag{2.5.25}$$

where the hyperparameters $\delta_0 > 0$ and $\gamma_0 > 0$ are prespecified. Then, the joint posterior distribution for $(\boldsymbol{\beta}, \sigma^2, \rho, \boldsymbol{\epsilon})$ is given by

$$\pi(\boldsymbol{\beta}, \sigma^2, \rho, \boldsymbol{\epsilon}|D) \propto L(\boldsymbol{\beta}, \sigma^2, \rho, \boldsymbol{\epsilon}|D)(\sigma^2)^{-(\delta_0+1)} \exp(-\sigma^{-2}\gamma_0), \tag{2.5.26}$$

where the likelihood $L(\boldsymbol{\beta}, \sigma^2, \rho, \boldsymbol{\epsilon}|D)$ is defined by (2.5.24). It can be shown that if X^* is of full rank, where X^* is a matrix induced by X and $\boldsymbol{y}$ with its tth row equal to $1\{y_t > 0\}\boldsymbol{x}_t'$, then the posterior distribution $\pi(\boldsymbol{\beta}, \sigma^2, \rho, \boldsymbol{\epsilon}|D)$ is proper.

Unlike the one-way analysis of variance model with random effects in Example 2.5, the Poisson regression model with AR(1) random effects is not a linear model. The exact correlations among the parameters $\boldsymbol{\epsilon}$, $\boldsymbol{\beta}$, σ^2, and ρ are not clear. However, it is expected that the correlation patterns in the Poisson regression model are similar to that of the one-way analysis of variance model. Ibrahim, Chen, and Ryan (1999) observe that the original Gibbs sampler without hierarchical centering results in very slow convergence and poor mixing. In particular, the correlation ρ appears to converge the slowest. They further find that the hierarchical centering technique is perfectly suited for this problem, and appears quite crucial for convergence of the Gibbs sampler.

Similar to the one-way analysis of variance model, a hierarchically centered reparameterization is given by

$$\boldsymbol{\eta} = X\boldsymbol{\beta} + \boldsymbol{\epsilon}. \tag{2.5.27}$$

Using (2.5.25), the reparameterized posterior for $(\boldsymbol{\beta}, \sigma^2, \rho, \boldsymbol{\eta})$ is written as

$$\begin{aligned}\pi(\boldsymbol{\beta}, \sigma^2, \rho, \boldsymbol{\eta}|D) \propto & \exp\{\boldsymbol{y}'\boldsymbol{\eta} - J_n'Q(\boldsymbol{\eta}) - J_n'C(\boldsymbol{y})\} \\ & \times (2\pi\sigma^2)^{-n/2}(1-\rho^2)^{-(n-1)/2} \\ & \times \exp\left\{-\frac{1}{2\sigma^2}(\boldsymbol{\eta} - X\boldsymbol{\beta})'\Sigma^{-1}(\boldsymbol{\eta} - X\boldsymbol{\beta})\right\},\end{aligned} \tag{2.5.28}$$

where $\boldsymbol{\eta} = (\eta_1, \eta_2, \ldots, \eta_n)'$, and $Q(\boldsymbol{\eta})$ is an $n \times 1$ vector with the tth element equal to $q_t = \exp(\eta_t)$.

The Gibbs sampler for sampling from the reparameterized posterior $\pi(\boldsymbol{\beta}, \sigma^2, \rho, \boldsymbol{\eta}|D)$ requires the following steps:

Step 1. Draw $\boldsymbol{\eta}$ from its conditional posterior distribution

$$\pi(\boldsymbol{\eta}|\boldsymbol{\beta}, \sigma^2, \rho, D) \propto \exp\left\{\boldsymbol{y}'\boldsymbol{\eta} - J_n'Q(\boldsymbol{\eta}) - \frac{(\boldsymbol{\eta} - X\boldsymbol{\beta})'\Sigma^{-1}(\boldsymbol{\eta} - X\boldsymbol{\beta})}{2\sigma^2}\right\}. \tag{2.5.29}$$

Step 2. Draw $\boldsymbol{\beta}$ from

$$\boldsymbol{\beta}|\boldsymbol{\eta}, \sigma^2, \rho, D \sim N_8((X'\Sigma^{-1}X)^{-1}X'\Sigma^{-1}\boldsymbol{\eta}, \sigma^2(X'\Sigma^{-1}X)^{-1}).$$

Step 3. Draw σ^2 from its conditional posterior

$$\sigma^2|\boldsymbol{\beta}, \rho, \boldsymbol{\eta}, D \sim \mathcal{IG}(\delta^*, \gamma^*),$$

where $\delta^* = \delta_0 + n/2$, $\gamma^* = \gamma_0 + \frac{1}{2}(\boldsymbol{\eta} - X\boldsymbol{\beta})'\Sigma^{-1}(\boldsymbol{\eta} - X\boldsymbol{\beta})$, and $\mathcal{IG}(\delta^*, \gamma^*)$ is an inverse gamma distribution.

Step 4. Draw ρ from its conditional posterior

$$\pi(\rho|\sigma^2, \boldsymbol{\beta}, \boldsymbol{\eta}, D)$$
$$\propto (1-\rho^2)^{-(n-1)/2} \exp\left\{-\frac{1}{2\sigma^2}(\boldsymbol{\eta} - X\boldsymbol{\beta})'\Sigma^{-1}(\boldsymbol{\eta} - X\boldsymbol{\beta})\right\}.$$

In Step 1, it can be shown that $\pi(\boldsymbol{\eta}|\boldsymbol{\beta}, \sigma^2, \rho, D)$ is log-concave in each component of $\boldsymbol{\eta}$ (see Exercise 2.7). Thus $\boldsymbol{\eta}$ can be drawn using the adaptive rejection sampling algorithm of Gilks and Wild (1992). The implementation of Steps 2 and 3 is straightforward, which may be a bonus of hierarchical centering, since sampling $\boldsymbol{\beta}$ is much more expensive before the reparameterization. In Chapter 9, we will also show that the hierarchical centering reparameterization can greatly ease the computational burden in Bayesian variable selection. In Step 4, we can use the algorithm in Example 2.3 for sampling ρ.

2.6 Acceleration Algorithms for MCMC Sampling

The major problems for many MCMC algorithms are slow convergence and poor mixing. For example, the Gibbs sampler converges slowly even for a simple ordinal response model as discussed in Section 2.5.3. In the earlier sections of this chapter, we discuss several tools for speeding up an MCMC algorithm, which include grouping (blocking) and collapsing (Liu 1994; Liu, Wong, and Kong 1994; Roberts and Sahu 1997), reparameterizations (Gelfand, Sahu, and Carlin 1995 and 1996; Roberts and Sahu 1997). The other useful techniques are adaptive direction sampling (Gilks, Roberts, and George 1994; Roberts and Gilks 1994), Multiple-Try Metropolis (Liu, Liang, and Wong 1998a), auxiliary variable methods (Besag and Green 1993; Damien, Wakefield, and Walker 1999), simulated tempering (Marinari and Parisi 1992; Geyer and Thompson 1995), and working parameter methods (Meng and van Dyk 1999). In this section, we present two special acceleration MCMC algorithms, i.e., grouped move and Multigrid MC sampling (Liu and Wu 1997; Liu and Sabatti 1998 and 1999) and covariance-adjusted MCMC sampling (Liu 1998), which provide us with a general framework of how to further improve mixing and convergence of an MCMC algorithm.

2.6.1 Grouped Move and Multigrid Monte Carlo Sampling

Goodman and Sokal (1989) present a comparative review of the multigrid Monte Carlo (MGMC) method, which is a stochastic generalization of the multigrid (MG) method for solving finite-difference equations. Liu and Wu (1997) and Liu and Sabatti (1998 and 1999) generalize Goodman and Sokal's MGMC via groups of transformations with applications to MCMC sampling. They propose a Grouped Move Multigrid Monte Carlo (GM-MGMC) algorithm and a generalized version of the MGMC algorithm for sampling from a target posterior distribution.

Assume that the target posterior distribution $\pi(\boldsymbol{\theta}|D)$ is defined on Ω and that an MCMC algorithm such as the Gibbs sampler or Metropolis–Hastings algorithm is used to generate a Markov chain $\{\boldsymbol{\theta}_i,\ i = 0, 1, 2, \dots\}$ from the target distribution $\pi(\boldsymbol{\theta}|D)$. We call the MCMC algorithm used to generate the $\boldsymbol{\theta}_i$ the *parent* MCMC algorithm. Let Γ be a locally compact transformation group (Rao 1987) on Ω. Then the GM-MGMC algorithm of Liu and Wu (1997) and Liu and Sabatti (1998) proceeds as follows:

GM-MGMC Algorithm

MCMC Step. Generate an iteration $\boldsymbol{\theta}_i$ from the parent MCMC.

GM Step. Draw the group element g from

$$g \sim \pi(g|\boldsymbol{\theta}_i)H(g) \propto \pi(g(\boldsymbol{\theta}_i)|D)J_g(\boldsymbol{\theta}_i)H(dg), \tag{2.6.1}$$

and *adjust*

$$\boldsymbol{\theta}_i \leftarrow g(\boldsymbol{\theta}_i).$$

In (2.6.1) $H(dg)$ is the right-invariant Haar measure on Ω and $J_g(\boldsymbol{\theta}_i)$ is the Jacobian of g evaluated at $\boldsymbol{\theta}_i$. Liu and Wu (1997) show that if Γ is a locally compact group of transformations for $\boldsymbol{\theta} \in \Omega$ with a unimodular right-invariant Haar measure $H(dg)$, then $g(\boldsymbol{\theta}_i) \sim \pi(\boldsymbol{\theta}|D)$, provided $\boldsymbol{\theta}_i \sim \pi(\boldsymbol{\theta}|D)$ and $g \sim \pi(g|\boldsymbol{\theta}_i)$. This result ensures that the target posterior distribution $\pi(\boldsymbol{\theta}|D)$ is the stationary distribution of the Markov chain induced by the GM-MGMC algorithm. As discussed in Liu and Sabatti (1998), the GM step is flexible: by selecting appropriate groups of transformations one can achieve either the effect of reparameterization or that of "blocking" or "grouping." Liu and Sabatti use several examples to illustrate these points.

In many cases, directly sampling g in the GM step may be difficult or expensive to achieve. For these cases, Liu and Sabatti (1998, 1999) propose a Markov transition. Assume that $T_{\boldsymbol{\theta}}(g', g)H(dg)$ is a Markov transition function, which leaves (2.6.1) invariant and satisfies the *transformation-invariance*, i.e.,

$$T_{\boldsymbol{\theta}}(g', g) = T_{g_0^{-1}\boldsymbol{\theta}}(g'g_0, gg_0) \tag{2.6.2}$$

for all g, g', and g_0 in Γ. Then, the GM-MGMC algorithm can be extended to the following Generalized MGMC algorithm:

Generalized MGMC Algorithm

MCMC Step. Generate an iteration $\boldsymbol{\theta}_i$ from the parent MCMC.

GM Step. Draw the group element g from

$$g \sim T_{\boldsymbol{\theta}_i}(I, g), \tag{2.6.3}$$

and *adjust*

$$\boldsymbol{\theta}_i \leftarrow g(\boldsymbol{\theta}_i).$$

In (2.6.3), I denotes the identity of the group. Similar to the GM-MGMC algorithm, it can be shown that $g(\boldsymbol{\theta}) \sim \pi(\boldsymbol{\theta}|D)$ provided $\boldsymbol{\theta} \sim \pi(\boldsymbol{\theta}|D)$.

In the GM-MGMC algorithm or the generalized MGMC algorithm, one GM step is used. In some situations, multiple GM steps can also be applied. For example, a three-step GM algorithm can be described by the following cycle. Starting with $\boldsymbol{\theta}_i \in \Omega$, which is drawn from a parent MCMC algorithm:

(i) draw g from a proper $T_{\boldsymbol{\theta}_i}(I, g)$, which leaves (2.6.1) invariant and satisfies (2.6.2), and update $\boldsymbol{\theta}^* = g(\boldsymbol{\theta})$;

(ii) draw g^* from a proper $T_{\boldsymbol{\theta}^*}(I, g^*)$ and update $\boldsymbol{\theta}^{**} = g^*(\boldsymbol{\theta}^*)$; and

(iii) draw g^{**} from $T_{\boldsymbol{\theta}^{**}}(I, g^{**})$ and update $\boldsymbol{\theta}_{i+1} = g^{**}(\boldsymbol{\theta}^{**})$.

Then, if $\boldsymbol{\theta}_i \sim \pi(\boldsymbol{\theta}|D)$, then $\boldsymbol{\theta}_{i+1} \sim \pi(\boldsymbol{\theta}|D)$.

The GM-MCMC algorithm is a flexible generalization of the Gibbs sampler or the Metropolis–Hastings algorithm, which enables us to design more efficient MCMC algorithms. The purpose of the GM step is to improve the convergence or mixing rates of the parent MCMC algorithm. The nature of the multiple GM steps allows us to achieve such an improvement in an iterative fashion. That is, if the performance of a parent MCMC algorithm is unsatisfactory, one can design a GM step, and then make an additional draw in each iteration of the parent algorithm. From an implementational standpoint, the GM step requires only adding a subroutine to the existing code and does not require a change in the basic structure of the code. After a one-step adjustment, the new MCMC algorithm induced by the GM step can be viewed as a new parent algorithm. Then, a similar adjustment can be applied to this new parent algorithm. One can repeat this procedure many times until a satisfactory convergence rate is achieved. Therefore, accelerating an MCMC algorithm can be viewed as a continuous improvement process.

Although the GM-MCMC algorithm provides a general framework for speeding up an MCMC algorithm, finding a computationally feasible group of transformations along with a unimodular right-invariant Haar measure $H(dg)$ is a difficult task. Two simple groups are the multiplicative group, i.e., $g(\boldsymbol{\theta}) = g\boldsymbol{\theta}$, and the additive group, i.e., $g(\boldsymbol{\theta}) = \boldsymbol{\theta} + \boldsymbol{g}$. For these two special cases, the associated unimodular right-invariant Haar measures are $H(dg) = 1/g$ for the multiplicative group and $H(d\boldsymbol{g}) = 1$ for the additive group. Although both the multiplicative group and additive group result in unimodular Haar measures, the linear combination of these two group transformations, i.e., $g(\boldsymbol{\theta}) = g_1\boldsymbol{\theta} + \boldsymbol{g}_2$, does not yield a unimodular Haar measure (see Nachbin 1965). In addition, GM-MGMC may not always improve convergence over the parent MCMC algorithm. In fact, Liu and Sabatti (1998) provide an example showing that GM-MGMC can result in a slower convergence rate than the parent MCMC algorithm. However, in many cases, GM-MGMC can achieve a substantial improvement in the convergence and mixing rate over a parent MCMC algorithm; see Liu and Sabatti (1998) and Chen and Liu (1999) for several illustrative examples. In practice, GM-MGMC can be viewed as an advanced experimental technique for improving convergence of an MCMC algorithm, and it can be helpful in getting a better understanding of the problem. As a practical guideline, we suggest using a GM step as long as it is simple and easy to implement.

2.6.2 Covariance-Adjusted MCMC Algorithm

Liu (1998) provides an alternative method for speeding up an MCMC algorithm using the idea of covariance adjustment. Let $\{\boldsymbol{\theta}_i,\ i = 0, 1, 2, \ldots\}$ be generated by the parent MCMC algorithm, having the stationary distribution $\pi(\boldsymbol{\theta}|D)$. Also let $(\boldsymbol{\xi}, \boldsymbol{\delta}) = \mathcal{M}(\boldsymbol{\theta})$ be a one-to-one mapping from Ω on which the target distribution is defined onto the space $\Xi \times \Delta$. Then, the covariance-adjusted MCMC (CA-MCMC) algorithm at the ith iteration consists of the following two steps:

CA-MCMC Algorithm

MCMC Step. Generate an iteration $\boldsymbol{\theta}_i$ from the parent MCMC and compute $(\boldsymbol{\xi}_i, \boldsymbol{\delta}_i) = \mathcal{M}(\boldsymbol{\theta}_i)$.

CA Step. Draw $\boldsymbol{\delta}_i^*$ from the conditional posterior distribution $\pi(\boldsymbol{\delta}|\boldsymbol{\xi}_i, D)$ and *adjust* $\boldsymbol{\theta}_i$ by

$$\boldsymbol{\theta}_i \leftarrow \boldsymbol{\theta}_i^* = \mathcal{M}^{-1}(\boldsymbol{\xi}_i, \boldsymbol{\delta}_i^*), \tag{2.6.4}$$

where $\mathcal{M}^{-1}(\boldsymbol{\xi}, \boldsymbol{\delta})$ is the inverse mapping of $(\boldsymbol{\xi}, \boldsymbol{\delta}) = \mathcal{M}(\boldsymbol{\theta})$.

Liu (1998) shows that the CA-MCMC algorithm converges to the target distribution $\pi(\boldsymbol{\theta}|D)$. That is, if the Markov chain induced by an MCMC algorithm is irreducible, aperiodic, and stationary with the equilibrium distribution $\pi(\boldsymbol{\theta}|D)$, so is the covariance-adjusted Markov chain. We refer the reader to Liu's paper for a formal proof. This result ensures that the CA step guarantees the correctness of the CA-MCMC algorithm. In addition, Liu (1998) also proves that the CA-MCMC algorithm converges at least as fast as its parent MCMC algorithm in the sense that the CA-MCMC algorithm results in a smaller reversed Kullback–Leibler information distance (e.g., Liu, Wong, and Kong 1995). This implies that the Markov sequence induced by the CA-MCMC algorithm has less dependence than that induced by the parent MCMC algorithm. This result essentially distinguishes the CA-MCMC algorithm from the GM-MGMC algorithm since the latter does not always guarantee faster convergence than its parent MCMC algorithm.

The key issue in using the CA-MCMC algorithm is how to construct the $\boldsymbol{\delta}$-variable so that the resulting algorithm is efficient and simple to implement. A general strategy proposed by Liu (1998) is to construct the $\boldsymbol{\delta}$-variable based on parameters and their sufficient statistics. We use an example given in Liu (1998) to illustrate this idea.

Example 2.6. One-way analysis of variance with random effects (Example 2.5 continued). Consider the one-way analysis of the variance model given in Example 2.5. Assume that the error variance σ_e^2 is known and that a single observation y_i for each population, i.e.,

$$y_i = \mu + \alpha_i + \epsilon_i, \quad i = 1, 2, \ldots, m, \tag{2.6.5}$$

where $\epsilon_i \sim N(0, \sigma_e^2)$, $\alpha_i \sim N(0, \sigma_\alpha^2)$, and σ_α^2 is also known. We assume that $\pi(\mu) \propto 1$ and let $\bar{y} = (1/m)\sum_{i=1}^m y_i$ and $D = (y_1, y_2, \ldots, y_m)$.

For this one-way analysis of the variance model, the vector of model parameters is $\boldsymbol{\theta} = (\mu, \alpha_1, \alpha_2, \ldots, \alpha_m)'$. We use the Gibbs sampler as the parent MCMC algorithm. To apply the CA-MCMC algorithm, we need to construct $\boldsymbol{\xi}$ and $\boldsymbol{\delta}$. In this example, μ and $\boldsymbol{\alpha} = (\alpha_1, \alpha_2, \ldots, \alpha_m)'$ may be highly correlated (see (2.5.6) and (2.5.7)), which may cause slow convergence of the original Gibbs sampler. To break down this correlation pattern, we consider the parameter μ. From (2.6.5), it is easy to see that, a posteriori, the sufficient statistic for μ is

$$\bar{\alpha} = \frac{1}{m} \sum_{i=1}^{m} \alpha_i.$$

Let $\xi_i = \alpha_i - \bar{\alpha}$. Define

$$\boldsymbol{\xi} = (\xi_1, \xi_2, \ldots, \xi_m)' \text{ and } \boldsymbol{\delta} = (\mu, \bar{\alpha})', \tag{2.6.6}$$

and let $\Xi = \{\xi : \sum_{i=1}^{m} \xi_i = 0,\ \xi_i \in R \text{ for } i = 1, 2, \ldots, m\}$. Then, (2.6.6) clearly defines a one-to-one mapping from R^{m+1} to $\Xi \times R^2$. The Jacobian of this transformation is $J_{(\mu,\alpha)\to(\mu,\bar{\alpha},\xi_1,\ldots,\xi_{m-1})} = 1$. The CA step requires drawing a $(\mu, \bar{\alpha})$ conditional on ξ_i for $i = 1, 2, \ldots, m$. The complete CA-MCMC algorithm can be stated as follows:

CA-MCMC for One-Way Analysis of Variance with Random Effects

Gibbs Step. Draw $(\mu|\boldsymbol{\alpha}, D) \sim N(\bar{y} - \bar{\alpha}, \sigma_e^2/m)$ and

$$(\alpha_i|\mu, D) \sim N\left(\frac{\sigma_\alpha^2}{\sigma_e^2 + \sigma_\alpha^2}(y_i - \mu), \frac{\sigma_e^2\sigma_\alpha^2}{\sigma_e^2 + \sigma_\alpha^2}\right).$$

CA Step. Draw $(\bar{\alpha}^*|\boldsymbol{\xi}, D) \sim N(0, \sigma_\alpha^2/m)$ and

$$(\mu^*|\bar{\alpha}^*, \boldsymbol{\xi}, D) \sim N\left(\bar{y} - \bar{\alpha}^*, \frac{\sigma_e^2}{m}\right),$$

then *adjust*

$$\mu \leftarrow \mu^* \text{ and } \alpha_i \leftarrow \xi_i + \bar{\alpha}^* \text{ for } i = 1, 2, \ldots, m.$$

From the structure of the above CA-MCMC algorithm, it can be seen that the draws of $(\mu^*, \bar{\alpha}^*, \xi_1 + \bar{\alpha}^*, \xi_2 + \bar{\alpha}^*, \ldots, \xi_m + \bar{\alpha}^*)$ are independent. Thus, the rate of convergence of this CA-MCMC algorithm is 0. Roberts and Sahu (1997) show that the rate of convergence of the Markov chain using the Gibbs step only is $\sigma_\alpha^2/(\sigma_\alpha^2 + \sigma_e^2)$ and that the rate of convergence of the Gibbs sampler based on the hierarchically centered transformation given in Example 2.5 (namely, $\mu = \mu$ and $\eta_i = \mu + \alpha_i$ for $i = 1, 2, \ldots, m$) is $\sigma_e^2/(\sigma_\alpha^2 + \sigma_e^2)$. Thus, CA-MCMC sampling outperforms original Gibbs sampling as well as hierarchical centering. This simple example also illustrates another important feature of the CA-MCMC algorithm, specifically, the concept of sufficient statistics, which can be nicely integrated into MCMC sampling and dramatically improves convergence of the MCMC algorithm.

2.6.3 An Illustration

To illustrate how an MCMC algorithm can be adjusted to achieve faster convergence and better mixing, we consider the following ordinal response data problem. The data are given in Table 2.1.

TABLE 2.1. The Rating Data.

Gender	F	M	F	M	F	M	F	M
Rating	good	fair	good	poor	good	poor	good	good

We code female as $X = 1$ and male as $X = 0$ and we also denote the response (Y) to be 1 for "poor," 2 for "fair," and 3 for "good." We let $\boldsymbol{y} = (y_1, y_2, \ldots, y_8)'$ denote a 8×1 vector of n independent ordinal responses. Assume that y_i takes a value of l ($1 \le l \le 3$) with probability

$$p_{il} = \Phi(\gamma_l + \boldsymbol{x}_i'\boldsymbol{\beta}) - \Phi(\gamma_{l-1} + \boldsymbol{x}_i'\boldsymbol{\beta}),$$

for $i = 1, ..., 8$ and $l = 1, 2, 3$, where $-\infty = \gamma_0 < \gamma_1 \le \gamma_2 < \gamma_3 = \infty$, x_i is a 2×1 column vector of covariates denoting the intercept and gender, and $\boldsymbol{\beta} = (\beta_0, \beta_1)'$ is a 2×1 column vector of regression coefficients. To ensure identifiability, we fix $\gamma_1 = 0$. Let $D = (\boldsymbol{y}, X)$, where X is the 8×2 design matrix with $\boldsymbol{x}_i'$ as its ith row.

Using (2.5.12), the complete-data likelihood is

$$L(\boldsymbol{\beta}, \gamma_2, \boldsymbol{z}|D) \propto \prod_{i=1}^{8} [\exp\{-\tfrac{1}{2}(z_i - \boldsymbol{x}_i'\boldsymbol{\beta})^2\} 1\{\gamma_{y_i-1} \le z_i < \gamma_{y_i}\}], \tag{2.6.7}$$

where $\boldsymbol{z} = (z_1, z_2, \ldots, z_8)'$ is the vector of latent variables such that $y_i = l$ if $\gamma_{l-1} \le z_i < \gamma_l$ for $l = 1, 2, 3$ and $i = 1, 2, \ldots, 8$. Consider a prior distribution for $(\boldsymbol{\beta}, \gamma_2)$ taking the form

$$\pi(\boldsymbol{\beta}, \gamma_2) \propto \exp\Big\{ -\frac{\tau}{2} \boldsymbol{\beta}'\boldsymbol{\beta} \Big\}, \tag{2.6.8}$$

where $\tau > 0$ is a known precision parameter. Here we take $\tau = 0.001$. Using (2.6.7) and (2.6.8), the posterior for $(\boldsymbol{\beta}, \gamma_2, \boldsymbol{z})$ is given by

$$\pi(\boldsymbol{\beta}, \gamma_2, \boldsymbol{z}|D) \propto L(\boldsymbol{\beta}, \gamma_2, \boldsymbol{z}|D)\pi(\boldsymbol{\beta}, \gamma_2). \tag{2.6.9}$$

Using the necessary and sufficient conditions of Chen and Shao (1999a), it can be shown that when $\pi(\boldsymbol{\beta}, \gamma_2) \propto 1$, the posterior given in (2.6.9) is improper. With the choice of $\tau = 0.001$, it is expected that the resulting posterior is essentially flat.

We first implement the original Gibbs sampler, which requires the following steps:

Step 1. Sample $\boldsymbol{\beta}$ from

$$\boldsymbol{\beta}|\boldsymbol{z}, \gamma_2 \sim N_2(\hat{\boldsymbol{\beta}}, B^{-1}),$$

where $B = \tau I_2 + X'X$ and $\hat{\boldsymbol{\beta}} = B^{-1}X'\boldsymbol{z}$.

Step 2. Sample z_i from

$$z_i \sim N(\boldsymbol{x}_i'\boldsymbol{\beta}, 1), \quad \gamma_{y_i-1} \le z_i \le \gamma_{y_i}.$$

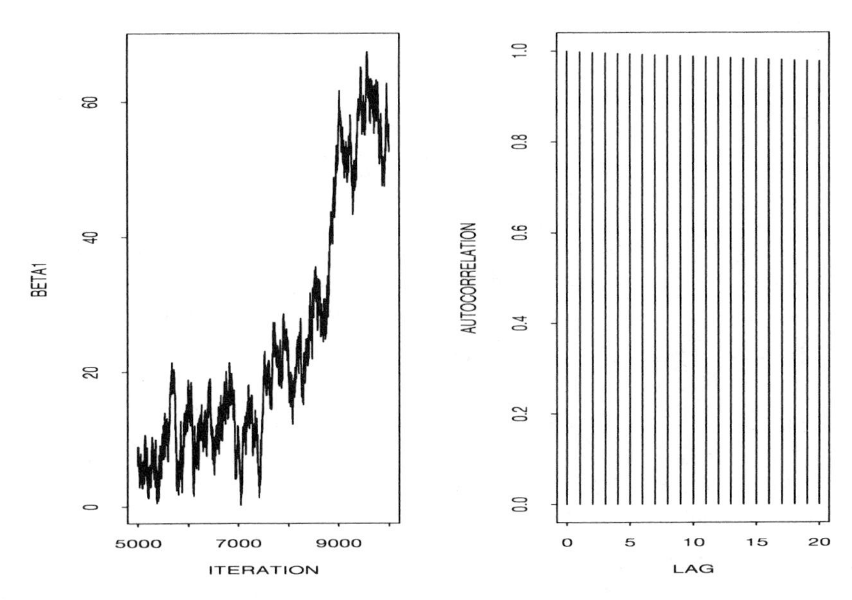

FIGURE 2.1. The original Gibbs sampler sequence of β_1 and its autocorrelation plot.

Step 3. Sample γ_2 from

$$\gamma_2|\boldsymbol{\beta}, \boldsymbol{z} \sim U[a_2, b_2],$$

where $a_2 = \max\left\{0, \max_{y_i=2} z_i\right\}$ and $b_2 = \min_{y_i=3} z_i$.

The trajectory and autocorrelation plots are displayed in Figure 2.1. These plots suggest that the original Gibbs sampler performs very poorly.

To improve the original Gibbs sampling algorithm, we consider the GM-MGMC algorithm. The group transformations proposed by Liu and Sabatti (1998) are

$$g(\boldsymbol{\beta}, \gamma_2, \boldsymbol{z}) = (g\boldsymbol{\beta}, g\gamma_2, g\boldsymbol{z})$$

with $g > 0$. Since the Jacobian $J_g = g^{8+2+1}$ and the Haar measure $H(dg) = dg/g$, the distribution of g is

$$\pi(g|\boldsymbol{\beta}, \gamma_2, \boldsymbol{z})H(dg) \propto g^{10} \exp\{-\tfrac{1}{2}g^2[\tau\boldsymbol{\beta}'\boldsymbol{\beta} + (\boldsymbol{z} - X\boldsymbol{\beta})'(\boldsymbol{z} - X\boldsymbol{\beta})]\}.$$

In addition to the original Gibbs steps, the GM-MGMC algorithm requires the following GM step:

GM Step. Draw the group element g from $\pi(g|\boldsymbol{\beta}, \gamma_2, \boldsymbol{z})H(dg)$ by taking $g = \sqrt{g^2}$, where

$$g^2|\boldsymbol{z}, \boldsymbol{\beta} \sim \mathcal{G}(\tfrac{11}{2}, \tfrac{1}{2}[(\boldsymbol{z} - X\boldsymbol{\beta})'(\boldsymbol{z} - X\boldsymbol{\beta}) + \tau\boldsymbol{\beta}'\boldsymbol{\beta}]),$$

where $\mathcal{G}(\xi, \eta)$ denotes the gamma distribution, whose density is given by

$$\pi(g^2|\xi, \eta) \propto (g^2)^{\xi-1} \exp(-\eta g^2),$$

and *adjust* $\boldsymbol{\beta}$, γ_2, and $\boldsymbol{z}$ by

$$\boldsymbol{\beta} \leftarrow g\boldsymbol{\beta}, \quad \gamma_2 \leftarrow g\gamma_2, \quad \text{and} \quad \boldsymbol{z} \leftarrow g\boldsymbol{z}.$$

The GM-MGMC algorithm has a statistical interpretation in terms of the CA-MCMC of Liu (1998). Given fixed cutpoints, the model reduces to the probit model with the corresponding variance parameter of latent variables fixed at one. The basic idea is to expand this hidden variance by redrawing the following sufficient statistic:

$$S^2 = \sum_{i=1}^{8} (z_i - \boldsymbol{x}_i'\boldsymbol{\beta})^2.$$

To make use of the CA-MCMC algorithm, we consider the following one-to-one mapping:

$$s = S = \sqrt{S^2}, \quad e_i = (z_i - \boldsymbol{x}_i'\boldsymbol{\beta})/S, \quad \eta = \gamma_2/S, \quad \text{and} \quad \boldsymbol{\xi} = \boldsymbol{\beta}/S,$$

with the constraint $\sum_{i=1}^{8} e_i^2 = 1$. Since the Jacobian of this transformation (with fixed $\gamma_1 = 0$) is

$$J_{(z_1,\ldots,z_7,\boldsymbol{\beta},\gamma_2,z_8)\to(e_1,\ldots,e_7,\boldsymbol{\xi},\eta,s)} = s^{10}/\sqrt{e_8^2},$$

given $(e_1, \ldots, e_8, \eta, \boldsymbol{\xi})$ the conditional distribution of s^2 is a gamma distribution:

$$\mathcal{G}(\tfrac{11}{2}, [1 + \tau\boldsymbol{\xi}'\boldsymbol{\xi}]/2).$$

Thus, in addition to the original Gibbs steps, the CA-MCMC algorithm requires the following CA step:

CA Step. Draw s^2 from $\mathcal{G}\left(\frac{11}{2}, [1 + \tau\boldsymbol{\xi}'\boldsymbol{\xi}]/2\right)$ and *adjust* $(\boldsymbol{z}, \boldsymbol{\beta}, \gamma_2)$ by

$$(\boldsymbol{z}, \boldsymbol{\beta}, \gamma_2) \leftarrow (s/S)(\boldsymbol{z}, \boldsymbol{\beta}, \gamma_2),$$

where $S^2 = \sum_{i=1}^{8} (z_i - \boldsymbol{x}_i'\boldsymbol{\beta})^2$.

This version of CA-MCMC leads to the same result as that of the GM-MGMC algorithm.

The trajectory and autocorrelation plots of the GM-MGMC algorithm are displayed in Figure 2.2. From these plots, it is clear that the GM-MGMC algorithm substantially improves the original Gibbs sampler. However, the autocorrelations are still large. For example, the autocorrelation of β_1 at lag 10 is 0.404. This may be mainly due to the lack of information to estimate β_1, the regression coefficient for gender, which results in slow convergence of $\mu = \beta_0 + \beta_1$. To speed up the GM-MGMC algorithm further, we add another CA step that draws the parameter $\mu = \beta_0 + \beta_1$ jointly with its

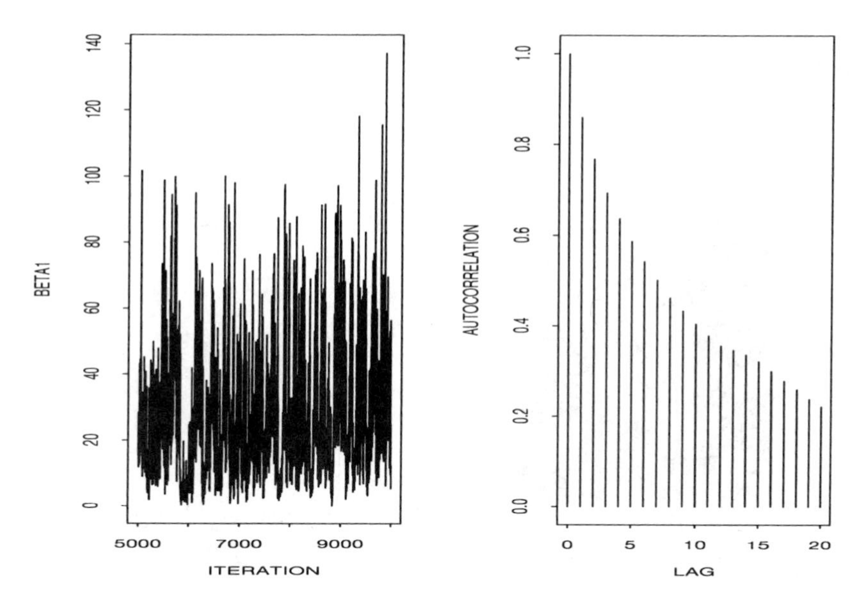

FIGURE 2.2. The GM-MGMC sequence of β_1 and its autocorrelation plot.

sufficient statistic $T = \frac{1}{4}\sum_{x_i=1} z_i$, conditioning on the current draws of $\{z_i : x_i = 0\}$, γ_2, β_0, and $\{z_i^* = z_i - T : x_i = 1\}$. Since the conditional distribution of μ given β_0 from the prior distribution of β is $N(\beta_0, 1/\tau)$, the conditional posterior distribution of (μ, T) given $\{z_i : x_i = 0\}$, γ_2, β_0, and $\{z_i^* = z_i - T : x_i = 1\}$ is

$$N_2\left(\begin{bmatrix}\beta_0\\ \beta_0\end{bmatrix}, \begin{bmatrix}1/\tau & 1/\tau\\ 1/\tau & 1/\tau + \frac{1}{4}\end{bmatrix}\right),$$

where $\max_{x_i=1}(\gamma_2 - z_i^*) \le T < \infty$. Thus, the corresponding CA step in this CA GM-MGMC algorithm can be accomplished by: (i) drawing T from

$$N(\beta_0, 1/\tau + \tfrac{1}{4}),$$

where $\max_{x_i=1}(\gamma_2 - z_i^*) \le T < \infty$, then drawing μ from

$$N\left(\beta_0 + \frac{(1/\tau)}{1/\tau + \frac{1}{4}}(T - \beta_0), \frac{1}{\tau} - \frac{(1/\tau^2)}{1/\tau + \frac{1}{4}}\right),$$

and (ii) adjusting β_1 and $\{z_i : x_i = 1\}$ by

$$\beta_1 \leftarrow \mu - \beta_0 \text{ and } \{z_i : x_i = 1\} \leftarrow \{z_i^* + T : x_i = 1\}.$$

Figure 2.3 indicates that the autocorrelations of β_1 from the CA GM-MGMC algorithm disappear even at lag 1. This simple example illustrates three important points:

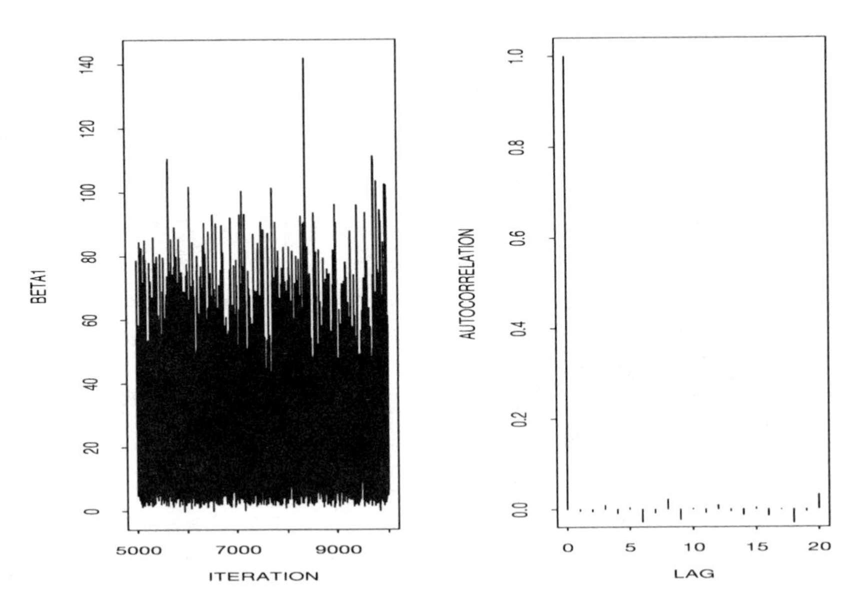

FIGURE 2.3. The CA GM-MGMC sequence of β_1 and its autocorrelation plot.

(i) the adjustment steps can dramatically improve convergence of an MCMC algorithm;

(ii) accelerating an MCMC algorithm is a continuous process; and

(iii) conditioning on sufficient statistics may play a key role in accelerating an MCMC algorithm.

2.7 Dynamic Weighting Algorithm

The *dynamic weighting method* is first introduced by Wong and Liang (1997) and further examined by Liu, Liang, and Wong (1998b). As pointed out by Liu, Liang, and Wong (1998b), the method extends the basic Markov chain equilibrium concept of Metropolis et al. (1953) to a more general weighted equilibrium of a Markov chain. The basic idea of dynamic weighting is to augment the original sample space by a positive scalar w, called a weight function, which can automatically adjust its own value to help the sampler move more freely.

Introducing the importance weights into the dynamic MC process helps make large transitions which are not allowed by the standard Metropolis transition rules. When the distribution has regions of "high" density separated by barriers of very "low" density, for example, when the target distribution is multimodal, the waiting time for a Metropolis process to cross over the barriers will be essentially infinite. In the dynamically weighted Monte Carlo, the process can often move against very steep probability barriers, which apparently violates the Metropolis rule. The weight variable is updated in a way that allows for an adjustment of the bias induced by such non-Metropolis moves.

Similar to the Metropolis algorithm, dynamic weighting starts with an arbitrary Markov transition kernel $T(\boldsymbol{\theta}, \boldsymbol{\vartheta})$ from which the next candidate move is suggested. Suppose the current state is $(\boldsymbol{\theta}, w)$. Liu, Liang, and Wong (1998b) propose two dynamic weighting moves, called the Q-type move and the R-type move. Assume that the target distribution is $\pi(\boldsymbol{\theta}|D)$. Then, these two dynamic weighting schemes are given as follows:

Q-Type Move

Step 1. (Candidate state.) Draw $\boldsymbol{\vartheta} \sim T(\boldsymbol{\theta}, \boldsymbol{\vartheta})$, and compute the Metropolis ratio

$$r(\boldsymbol{\theta}, \boldsymbol{\vartheta}) = \frac{\pi(\boldsymbol{\vartheta}|D)T(\boldsymbol{\vartheta}, \boldsymbol{\theta})}{\pi(\boldsymbol{\theta}|D)T(\boldsymbol{\theta}, \boldsymbol{\vartheta})}.$$

Step 2. (Move?) Choose $\alpha = \alpha(w, \boldsymbol{\theta}) > 0$ and draw $u \sim U(0,1)$. Update $(\boldsymbol{\theta}, w)$ to $(\boldsymbol{\theta}^*, w^*)$ as

$$(\boldsymbol{\theta}^*, w^*) = \begin{cases} (\boldsymbol{\vartheta}, \max\{\boldsymbol{\alpha}, wr(\boldsymbol{\theta}, \boldsymbol{\vartheta})\}) & \text{if } u \le \min\{1, wr(\boldsymbol{\theta}, \boldsymbol{\vartheta})/\alpha\}, \\ (\boldsymbol{\theta}, aw) & \text{otherwise,} \end{cases} \tag{2.7.1}$$

where $a > 1$ can be either a constant or an independent random variable.

R-Type Move

Step 1. (Candidate state.) The same as the Q-type move.

Step 2. (Move?) Choose $\alpha = \alpha(w, \boldsymbol{\theta}) > 0$ and draw $u \sim U(0,1)$. Update $(\boldsymbol{\theta}, w)$ to $(\boldsymbol{\theta}^*, w^*)$ as

$$(\boldsymbol{\theta}^*, w^*) = \begin{cases} (\boldsymbol{\vartheta}, wr(\boldsymbol{\theta}, \boldsymbol{\vartheta}) + \alpha) & \text{if } u \le \dfrac{wr(\boldsymbol{\theta}, \boldsymbol{\vartheta})}{wr(\boldsymbol{\theta}, \boldsymbol{\vartheta}) + \alpha}, \\ (\boldsymbol{\theta}, w(wr(\boldsymbol{\theta}, \boldsymbol{\vartheta}) + \alpha)/\alpha)) & \text{otherwise.} \end{cases} \tag{2.7.2}$$

For practical use of the two dynamic weighting moves, Liu, Liang, and Wong (1998b) suggest that they be applied in a compact space. This can be achieved by preventing the sampler from visiting exceedingly low-probability space. Furthermore, to guard against a possible boundary effect caused by exceedingly small $r(\boldsymbol{\theta}, \boldsymbol{\vartheta})$ (i.e., practically 0), one can modify the weight updating as follows: if $r(\boldsymbol{\theta}, \boldsymbol{\vartheta}) < \epsilon$ for a proposal $\boldsymbol{\vartheta}$, rejection does not induce any change of the weights.

The behavior of both dynamic weighting moves is controlled by the parameter α and the transition kernel $T(\boldsymbol{\theta}, \boldsymbol{\vartheta})$. For example, when $\alpha \to 0$, the Q-type move is identical to the R-type move, and every candidate move will be accepted. Two special cases are of great interest. First, when $T(\boldsymbol{\theta}, \boldsymbol{\vartheta})$ is reversible and stationary with equilibrium distribution $\pi(\boldsymbol{\theta}|D)$, both moves reduce to the standard Metropolis algorithm. Thus, the dynamic weighting method can be viewed as an extension of the standard Metropolis algorithm. Second, when $T(\boldsymbol{\theta}, \boldsymbol{\vartheta})$ is reversible and stationary with equilibrium distribution $g(\boldsymbol{\theta})$,

$$r(\boldsymbol{\theta}, \boldsymbol{\vartheta}) = \frac{\pi(\boldsymbol{\vartheta}|D)g(\boldsymbol{\theta})}{g(\boldsymbol{\vartheta})\pi(\boldsymbol{\theta}|D)} \quad \text{and} \quad w^* = w\frac{\omega(\boldsymbol{\vartheta})}{\omega(\boldsymbol{\theta})},$$

where $w(\boldsymbol{\theta}) = \pi(\boldsymbol{\theta}|D)/g(\boldsymbol{\theta})$. Hence, if we start with $\boldsymbol{\theta}_0$ and $w_0 = c_0\omega(\boldsymbol{\theta}_0)$, then for any $i > 0$, $w_i = c_0\omega(\boldsymbol{\theta}_i)$. These weights are identical to those from the standard importance sampling method with an importance sampling distribution $g(\boldsymbol{\theta})$. Liu, Liang, and Wong (1998b) also study the behavior of the Q-type and R-type moves for several other choices of α and T.

In general, for either the Q-type move or the R-type move, the equilibrium distribution of $\boldsymbol{\theta}$ (if it exists) is not $\pi(\boldsymbol{\theta}|D)$. In this regard, Wong and Liang (1997) propose to use *invariance with respect to importance-weighting* (IWIW) as a principle for validating the above scheme and for designing new transition rules. The formal definition of IWIW is given as follows:

The joint distribution $\pi(\boldsymbol{\theta}, w)$ of $(\boldsymbol{\theta}, w)$ is said to be correctly weighted with respect to $\pi(\boldsymbol{\theta}|D)$ if

$$\int w\pi(\boldsymbol{\theta}, w)\, dw \propto \pi(\boldsymbol{\theta}|D). \tag{2.7.3}$$

A transition rule is said to satisfy IWIW if it maintains the correctly weighted property for the joint distribution of $(\boldsymbol{\theta}, w)$ whenever the initial joint distribution is correctly weighted.

Suppose the starting joint distribution $\pi_1(\boldsymbol{\theta}, w)$ for $(\boldsymbol{\theta}, w)$ is correctly weighted with respect to $\pi(\boldsymbol{\theta}|D)$, i.e., $\int w\pi_1(\boldsymbol{\theta}, w)\, dw \propto \pi(\boldsymbol{\theta}|D)$. It can be shown that after a one-step transition of the R-type move with $\alpha = \alpha(\boldsymbol{\theta}, w) > 0$ for all $(\boldsymbol{\theta}, w)$, the new joint state $(\boldsymbol{\theta}^*, w^*)$ has a joint distribution $\pi_2(\boldsymbol{\theta}^*, w^*)$ that is also correctly weighted with respect to $\pi(\boldsymbol{\theta}|D)$, i.e.,

$$\int w^*\pi_2(\boldsymbol{\theta}^*, w^*)\, dw^* \propto \pi(\boldsymbol{\theta}^*|D). \tag{2.7.4}$$

If $\alpha \to 0$, then the IWIW property holds for both the Q- and R-type moves. However, when $\alpha > 0$, the Q-type move only approximately satisfies the

IWIW property. A more detailed discussion of the properties of the Q-type move can be found in Liu, Liang, and Wong (1998b).

The dynamic reweighting method has been successfully applied to simulation and global optimization problems arising from multimodal sampling, neural network training, high-dimensional integration, the Ising models (Wong and Liang 1997; Liu, Liang, and Wong 1998b), and Bayesian model selection problems (Liu and Sabatti 1999). The applications of IWIW to the computation of posterior quantities of interest will be discussed further in Chapter 3.

2.8 Toward "Black-Box" Sampling

Chen and Schmeiser (1998) propose a random-direction interior-point (RDIP) Markov chain approach to black-box sampling. The purpose of such a black-box sampler is to free the analyst from computational details without paying a large computational penalty, in contrast to specialized samplers such as the Gibbs sampler or the Metropolis–Hastings algorithm.

Assume that the target posterior distribution is of the form

$$\pi(\boldsymbol{\theta}|D) = \frac{L(\boldsymbol{\theta}|D)\pi(\boldsymbol{\theta})}{c(D)}, \tag{2.8.1}$$

where $L(\boldsymbol{\theta}|D)$ is the likelihood function, $\pi(\boldsymbol{\theta})$ is a prior distribution, and $c(D)$ is the normalizing constant. We further assume that $L(\boldsymbol{\theta}|D)$ and $\pi(\boldsymbol{\theta})$ can be computed at any point $\boldsymbol{\theta}$. The key idea of RDIP is to introduce an auxiliary random variable δ so that the joint posterior distribution of $(\boldsymbol{\theta}, \delta)$ has the form

$$\pi(\boldsymbol{\theta}, \delta|D) = \begin{cases} 1/c(D), & \text{if } 0 \le \delta \le \pi(\boldsymbol{\theta}|D), \\ 0, & \text{otherwise.} \end{cases} \tag{2.8.2}$$

Integrating out δ from $\pi(\boldsymbol{\theta}, \delta|D)$ yields the marginal distribution of $\boldsymbol{\theta}$ as $\pi(\boldsymbol{\theta}|D)$. This result implies that if a Markov chain $\{(\boldsymbol{\theta}_i, \delta_i), i = 1, 2, ...\}$ has the unique uniform stationary distribution $\pi(\boldsymbol{\theta}, \delta|D)$, then the "marginal" Markov chain $\{\boldsymbol{\theta}_i, i = 1, 2, ...\}$ has a stationary distribution which is the target posterior $\pi(\boldsymbol{\theta}|D)$.

Let Ω be the interior of the $(p+1)$-dimensional region lying beneath $\pi(\boldsymbol{\theta}|D)$ and over the support of $\pi(\boldsymbol{\theta}|D)$. Then the RDIP sampler has three fundamental characteristics:

(i) Sampling generates points $(\boldsymbol{\theta}, \delta)$ from the interior of Ω.

(ii) The stationary distribution of $(\boldsymbol{\theta}, \delta)$ is uniform over Ω. Therefore, the stationary distribution of $\boldsymbol{\theta}$ is $\pi(\boldsymbol{\theta}|D)$.

(iii) The Markov chain evolution from point to point is based on random directions.

Computationally, whether $\pi(\boldsymbol{\theta}|D)$ integrates to one or not is unimportant. Suppose that $\pi(\boldsymbol{\theta}|D) = L(\boldsymbol{\theta}|D)\pi(\boldsymbol{\theta})$. The advantage of this is that the normalizing constant $c(D)$ need not be computed. Based on this convention, the general version of the RDIP sampler, which essentially defines a class of samplers, can be stated as follows:

The RDIP Sampler

Step 1. (Random direction.) Generate a unit-length $(p+1)$-dimensional direction $\boldsymbol{d} \sim g_1(\boldsymbol{d}|\boldsymbol{\theta}, \delta)$.

Step 2. (Random distance.) Generate $\lambda \sim g_2(\lambda|\boldsymbol{\theta}, \delta, \boldsymbol{d})$.

Step 3. (Candidate point.) Set $(\boldsymbol{\theta}^*, \delta^*) = (\boldsymbol{\theta}, \delta) + \lambda \boldsymbol{d}$.

Step 4. (Candidate posterior density.) Compute $\pi^* = \pi(\boldsymbol{\theta}^*|D)$.

Step 5. (Inside Ω?) If $0 < \delta^* < \pi^*$ is false, go to Step 7.

Step 6. (Move?) Set $(\boldsymbol{\theta}, \delta) = (\boldsymbol{\theta}^*, \delta^*)$ with probability $a(\boldsymbol{\theta}^*, \delta^*|\boldsymbol{\theta}, \delta)$.

Step 7. (Done.) Return $(\boldsymbol{\theta}, \delta)$.

The densities g_1 and g_2 in Steps 1 and 2 and the jump probability a in Step 6 must be chosen to provide a valid sampler. In typical versions, g_1, g_2, and a can be chosen so that the transition kernel of the random sequence of points $\{(\boldsymbol{\theta}_i, \delta_i),\ i \geq 0\}$ is doubly stochastic in Ω, guaranteeing uniformity over Ω in the limit. In general, Steps 1 and 2 can be combined to generate a $(\boldsymbol{d}, \lambda)$ conditional on $(\boldsymbol{\theta}, \delta)$. From the above description, it can be seen that the RDIP sampler is a special case of the H&R sampler.

Chen and Schmeiser (1998) discuss three variations of the general version of the RDIP sampler. One of these variations is called the state-dependent direction-and-radius sampler, which uses the location information of the current state as well as the relative height of the current location without requiring much extra computation. The detailed steps involved in this special case are given as follows:

The State-Dependent Direction-and-Radius Sampler

Step 1. (Random direction.)

- Generate a uniform unit-length p-dimensional direction $(d_1, d_2, \ldots, d_p)$;
- generate $\alpha \sim g_1^*(\alpha|r)$; and
- the $(p+1)$-dimensional random direction is $\boldsymbol{d} = (d_1 \cos\alpha, d_2 \cos\alpha, \ldots, d_p \cos\alpha, \sin\alpha)$.

Step 2. (Random distance.) Generate $\lambda \sim g_2^*(\lambda|\boldsymbol{\theta}, \delta, \boldsymbol{d})$.

Step 3. (Candidate point.) Set $(\boldsymbol{\theta}^*, \delta^*) = (\boldsymbol{\theta}, \delta) + \lambda \boldsymbol{d}$.

Step 4. (Candidate posterior density.) Compute $\pi^* = \pi(\boldsymbol{\theta}^*|D)$ and $r^* = \delta^*/\pi(\boldsymbol{\theta}^*|D)$.

Step 5. (Inside Ω?) If $0 < \delta^* < \pi^*$ is false, go to Step 7.

Step 6. (Move?) Let $\pi(\boldsymbol{\theta}^*, \delta^*|\boldsymbol{\theta}, \delta)$ be the conditional probability density function of the next candidate point $(\boldsymbol{\theta}^*, \delta^*)$ given the current point $(\boldsymbol{\theta}, \delta)$, and let $\pi(\boldsymbol{\theta}, \delta|\boldsymbol{\theta}^*, \delta^*)$ be the conditional probability density function by switching the positions of $(\boldsymbol{\theta}^*, \delta^*)$ and $(\boldsymbol{\theta}, \delta)$. Then set $(\boldsymbol{\theta}, \delta) = (\boldsymbol{\theta}^*, \delta^*)$ with probability $\min\left\{\pi(\boldsymbol{\theta}, \delta|\boldsymbol{\theta}^*, \delta^*)/\pi(\boldsymbol{\theta}^*, \delta^*|\boldsymbol{\theta}, \delta), 1\right\}$.

Step 7. (Done.) Return $(\boldsymbol{\theta}, \delta)$.

Next, we discuss some possible choices of the angle density $g_1^*(\alpha|r)$, the distance density $g_2^*(\lambda|\boldsymbol{\theta}, \delta, \boldsymbol{d})$, the conditional density $\pi(\boldsymbol{\theta}^*, \delta^*|\boldsymbol{\theta}, \delta)$, and the jump probability.

The angle α is with respect to the horizontal plane $\Delta = \delta$. The domain of α is $(-\pi/2, \pi/2)$, with $\alpha = -\pi/2$ corresponding to a move straight down and $\alpha = \pi/2$ corresponding to a move straight up in $p + 1$ dimensions. A reasonable choice of $g_1^*(\alpha|r)$ might be a mixture of beta densities

$$\begin{aligned} g_1^*(\alpha|r) =& P(\text{neg})p(\alpha|\text{neg}) + P(\text{pos})p(\alpha|\text{pos}) \\ =& r\,\frac{(-\alpha)^{a_r-1}((\pi/2)+\alpha)^{b_r-1}}{B(a_r, b_r)(\pi/2)^{a_r+b_r-1}} 1\{-\pi/2 < \alpha < 0\} \\ &+ (1-r)\,\frac{(\alpha)^{a_r-1}((\pi/2)-\alpha)^{b_r-1}}{B(a_r, b_r)(\pi/2)^{a_r+b_r-1}} 1\{0 < \alpha < \pi/2\}, \end{aligned} \tag{2.8.3}$$

where $a_r > 0$, $b_r > 0$, a_r and b_r might depend on r, and $B(a_r, b_r)$ is the beta function. Note that $E(\alpha|r) = [a_r/(a_r + b_r)](\pi/2)(1 - 2r)$. Here we choose the probability of moving down to be $P(\text{neg}) = r$ and the probability of moving up to be $P(\text{pos}) = 1 - r$. The reason for this choice is that if the point $(\boldsymbol{\theta}, \delta)$ is close to the surface $\delta = \pi(\boldsymbol{\theta}|D)$ (i.e., r is close to 1), more probability should be assigned to negative values of α (i.e., the next move should be down), and vice versa. In addition, when r is close to 1, more probability should be assigned to the large absolute value of α, and, therefore, a_r should be large while b_r should be small. Similarly, when r is close to zero, a_r should be small and b_r should be large. Chen and Schmeiser (1998) empirically show that despite choosing a_r and b_r to be constants, the sampler still performs reasonably well.

It is desirable to choose the distance density g_2^* so that it depends upon the current location and the angle α, without incurring expensive computation. One source of almost-free information is to compute the intersection of the line through the point $(\boldsymbol{\theta}, \delta)$ with the direction $\boldsymbol{d}$ and the horizontal plane $\delta = 0$. This intersection is

$$Pt(\boldsymbol{\theta}, \boldsymbol{d}, 0) = (\boldsymbol{\theta} - (\delta \text{cos}\alpha/\text{sin}\alpha)(d_1, d_2, \ldots, d_p), 0)\,.$$

Similarly, the intersection of the line through the point $(\boldsymbol{\theta}, \delta)$ with the direction $\boldsymbol{d}$ and the horizontal plane $\delta = \pi(\boldsymbol{\theta}|D)$ is

$$Pt(\boldsymbol{\theta}, \boldsymbol{d}, \pi(\boldsymbol{\theta}|D)) = (\boldsymbol{\theta} - ((\delta - \pi(\boldsymbol{\theta}|D))\text{cos}\alpha/\text{sin}\alpha)(d_1, d_2, \dots, d_p), \pi(\boldsymbol{\theta}|D)).$$

Then it is easy to compute the distances from the point $(\boldsymbol{\theta}, \delta)$ to $Pt(\boldsymbol{\theta}, \boldsymbol{d}, 0)$ and $Pt(\boldsymbol{\theta}, \boldsymbol{d}, \pi(\boldsymbol{\theta}|D))$, say, λ_1 and λ_2, respectively:

$$\lambda_1 = ||(\boldsymbol{\theta}, \delta) - Pt(\boldsymbol{\theta}, \boldsymbol{d}, 0)|| = \frac{\delta}{|\text{sin}\alpha|}, \tag{2.8.4}$$

$$\lambda_2 = ||(\boldsymbol{\theta}, \delta) - Pt(\boldsymbol{\theta}, \boldsymbol{d}, \pi(\boldsymbol{\theta}|D))|| = \frac{\pi(\boldsymbol{\theta}|D) - \delta}{|\text{sin}\alpha|}. \tag{2.8.5}$$

The distance distribution is chosen based on this information. For example, a gamma distribution might be appropriate when α is positive and a uniform distribution over $(0, \lambda_1)$ might be appropriate when α is negative. More specifically, we can choose

$$g_2^*(\lambda|\theta, \delta, \boldsymbol{d}) = g_{2a}^*(\lambda|\boldsymbol{\theta}, \delta)1\{\alpha < 0\} + g_{2b}^*(\lambda|\boldsymbol{\theta}, \delta)1\{\alpha > 0\}, \tag{2.8.6}$$

where

$$g_{2a}^*(\lambda|\boldsymbol{\theta}, \delta) = \begin{cases} |\text{sin}\alpha|/\delta & \text{for } 0 \le \lambda \le \delta/|\text{sin}\alpha|, \\ 0 & \text{otherwise,} \end{cases}$$

and

$$g_{2b}^*(\lambda|\boldsymbol{\theta}, \delta) = \begin{cases} \dfrac{\lambda^2 \exp\{-6|\text{sin}\alpha|\lambda/(\pi(\boldsymbol{\theta}|D) - \delta)\}}{\Gamma(3)\left((\pi(\boldsymbol{\theta}|D) - \delta)/6|\text{sin}\alpha|\right)^3} & \text{for } \lambda > 0, \\ 0 & \text{otherwise.} \end{cases}$$

That is, $g_2^*(\lambda|\boldsymbol{\theta}, \delta, \boldsymbol{d})$ in (2.8.6) is either the uniform distribution $U(0, \delta/|\text{sin}\alpha|)$ or the gamma distribution with a shape parameter 3 and a scale parameter $(\pi(\boldsymbol{\theta}|D) - \delta)/(6|\text{sin}\alpha|)$.

With the above choices of $g_1^*(\alpha|r)$ and $g_2^*(\lambda|\boldsymbol{\theta}, \delta, \boldsymbol{d})$, the density of the next candidate point $(\boldsymbol{\theta}^*, \delta^*)$ conditional on the current point $(\boldsymbol{\theta}, \delta)$ is

$$\pi(\boldsymbol{\theta}^*, \delta^*|\boldsymbol{\theta}, \delta) \propto \frac{g_1^*(\alpha|r) g_2^*(\lambda|\boldsymbol{\theta}, \delta, \boldsymbol{d})}{|\lambda|^p |\text{cos}\alpha|^{p-1}}, \tag{2.8.7}$$

where $\lambda = ||(\boldsymbol{\theta}^* - \boldsymbol{\theta}, \delta^* - \delta)||$, $\boldsymbol{d} = (\boldsymbol{\theta}^* - \boldsymbol{\theta}, \delta^* - \delta)/\lambda$, $\alpha = \sin^{-1}((\delta^* - \delta)/\lambda)$, and $r = \delta/\pi(\boldsymbol{\theta}|D)$. Let α^*, $\boldsymbol{d}^*$, and λ^* denote the angle, the direction, and the distance from the point $(\boldsymbol{\theta}^*, \delta^*)$ back to the point $(\boldsymbol{\theta}, \delta)$. Then $\lambda^* = ||(\boldsymbol{\theta} - \boldsymbol{\theta}^*, \delta - \delta^*)|| = \lambda$, $\boldsymbol{d}^* = (\boldsymbol{\theta} - \boldsymbol{\theta}^*, \delta - \delta^*)/\lambda = -\boldsymbol{d}$, $\alpha^* = \sin^{-1}((\delta - \delta^*)/\lambda) = -\alpha$, and $r^* = \delta^*/\pi(\boldsymbol{\theta}^*|D)$. Therefore, the jump ratio is

$$\frac{\pi(\boldsymbol{\theta}, \delta|\boldsymbol{\theta}^*, \delta^*)}{\pi(\boldsymbol{\theta}^*, \delta^*|\boldsymbol{\theta}, \delta)} = \left[\frac{g_1^*(-\alpha|r^*)}{g_1^*(\alpha|r)}\right] \cdot \left[\frac{g_2^*(\lambda|\boldsymbol{\theta}^*, \delta^*, -\boldsymbol{d})}{g_2^*(\lambda|\boldsymbol{\theta}, \delta, \boldsymbol{d})}\right]. \tag{2.8.8}$$

With $g_2^*(\lambda|\boldsymbol{\theta}, \delta, \boldsymbol{d})$ given by (2.8.6), (2.8.8) can be further simplified as

$$\frac{\pi(\boldsymbol{\theta}, \delta|\boldsymbol{\theta}^*, \delta^*)}{\pi(\boldsymbol{\theta}^*, \delta^*|\boldsymbol{\theta}, \delta)} = \begin{cases} \dfrac{\pi(\boldsymbol{\theta}|D)}{3\pi(\boldsymbol{\theta}^*|D)} \cdot \left(\dfrac{\pi(\boldsymbol{\theta}|D) - \delta}{6|\text{sin}\alpha|\lambda}\right)^2 \cdot \exp\left\{\dfrac{6|\text{sin}\alpha|\lambda}{\pi(\boldsymbol{\theta}|D) - \delta}\right\} & \text{for } \alpha > 0, \\ \dfrac{3\pi(\boldsymbol{\theta}|D)}{\pi(\boldsymbol{\theta}^*|D)} \cdot \left(\dfrac{6|\text{sin}\alpha|\lambda}{\pi(\boldsymbol{\theta}^*|D) - \delta^*}\right)^2 \cdot \exp\left\{-\dfrac{6|\text{sin}\alpha|\lambda}{\pi(\boldsymbol{\theta}^*|D) - \delta^*}\right\} & \text{for } \alpha < 0. \end{cases} \tag{2.8.9}$$

In Step 1, the uniform distribution for a unit-length p- dimensional direction $(d_1, d_2, \ldots, d_p)$ can be extended to any continuous distribution over the surface of the p-dimensional unit sphere. Additional discussion can be found in Chen and Schmeiser (1996). Chen and Schmeiser (1998) show that with the above choices of $g_1^*(\alpha|r)$ and $g_2^*(\lambda|\boldsymbol{\theta}, \delta, \boldsymbol{d})$, the Markov chain $\{(\boldsymbol{\theta}_i, \delta_i), i = 1, 2, \ldots\}$ induced by the state-dependent direction-and-radius RDIP sampler is irreducible and doubly stochastic, and, therefore, has a unique stationary distribution $\pi(\boldsymbol{\theta}, \delta|D)$. They further empirically study the performance of the RDIP sampler and find that the RDIP sampler works reasonably well for a bimodal distribution as well as for the ordinal response model in Section 2.5.3. The RDIP sampler is the first step toward black-box sampling. Further research in this direction needs to be done in the future.

2.9 Convergence Diagnostics

Convergence diagnostics are one of the most important components in MCMC sampling. For most practical problems, the MCMC sample generated from a user's selected MCMC sampling algorithm will ultimately be used for computing posterior quantities of interest. Thus, if a Markov chain induced by the MCMC algorithm fails to converge, the resulting posterior estimates will be biased and unreliable. As a consequence, an incorrect Bayesian data analysis will be performed and false conclusions may be drawn. Fortunately, many useful diagnostic tools along with their sound theoretical foundations have been developed during the last decade. Although no single diagnostic procedure can guarantee to diagnose convergence successfully, combining several diagnostic tools together may enable us to detect how fast or how slow a Markov chain converges and how well or how poorly a chain is mixing.

By now, the literature on convergence diagnostics is very rich. Excellent and comprehensive reviews are given by Cowles and Carlin (1996), Brooks and Roberts (1998), Mengersen, Robert, and Guihenneuc–Jouyaux (1998), and many other references therein. More recently, Robert (1998, Chap. 2) presents several useful methods on convergence control of MCMC algorithms. In this section, we present several commonly used convergence diagnostic techniques, and we refer the reader to the above review articles for details of other available convergence diagnostic methods.

A simple but effective diagnostic tool is the trace plot. Two kinds of trace plots are useful, which are the trace plot of a single long-run sequence and the trace plots of several short-run sequences with overdispersed starting (initial) points. As discussed in Mengersen, Robert, and Guihenneuc–Jouyaux (1998), there is widespread debate about single run and multiple runs. A single sequence which has difficulty leaving the neighborhood of an attractive mode will exhibit acceptable behavior even though it has failed to explore the whole support of the target distribution $\pi(\boldsymbol{\theta}|D)$. Multiple sequences may have better exploratory power, but depend highly on the choice of starting points. On the other hand, a long-run single sequence may be advantageous in exploring potential coding bugs and the mixing behavior of the Markov chain, while multiple sequences suffer from a large increase in the number of wasted burn-in simulations for estimating posterior quantities. As a practical guideline, we suggest the use of both types of trace plots in exploring convergence and mixing behavior of the chain, and then generate a single long-run sequence with a large number of iterations (say 50,000) for estimation purposes.

For many practical problems, the dimension of the parameter space is high. Thus it may not be feasible to examine the trace plots for all parameters. In this case, we may construct trace plots for several selected parameters, which should include parameters, that are known to converge slowly, functions of parameters of interest, and some nuisance parameters. For example, for the ordinal response models in Section 2.5.3, we may need to monitor the trace plots for the regression coefficients $\boldsymbol{\beta}$, the cutpoints γ, and some of the latent variables z_i's (nuisance parameters). If one is interested in estimating $\xi = h(\boldsymbol{\theta})$, it may be sufficient to monitor the trace plot for ξ only. However, we note that slow convergence of the nuisance parameters may seriously affect the convergence of parameters of interest as discussed in Section 2.5.3. Another related issue is that a simple time series plot for the sequence of ξ may not be effective if ξ is a discrete variable. In this regard, we propose the use of the cumulative sum (CUSUM) plot of Yu and Mykland (1998). The CUSUM plot can be constructed as follows. Given the output $\{\xi_1, \xi_2, \dots, \xi_n\}$, we begin by discarding the initial n_0 iterations, which we believe to correspond to the burn-in period. Then, the following algorithm describes how to produce a CUSUM plot:

The CUSUM Plot

Step 1. Calculate $\bar{\xi} = (n - n_0)^{-1} \sum_{i=n_0+1}^{n} \xi_i$.

Step 2. Calculate the CUSUM

$$S_t = \sum_{i=n_0+1}^{t} (\xi_i - \bar{\xi}) \quad \text{for } t = n_0 + 1, \ldots, n.$$

Step 3. Plot s_t against t for $t = n_0+1, \ldots, n$, connecting successive points by line segments.

Yu and Mykland (1998) argue that the speed with which the chain is mixing is indicated by the smoothness of the resulting CUSUM plot, so that a smooth plot indicates slow mixing, while a "hairy" plot indicates a fast mixing rate for ξ.

The autocorrelation plots are the easiest tool for quantitatively assessing the mixing behavior of a Markov chain. It is important to check not only the within-sequence autocorrelations but also the intraclass (between-sequence) autocorrelations. However, care must be taken in computing autocorrelations. Without discarding iterations corresponding to the burn-in period, the autocorrelations may be under- or over-estimated, which may reflect a false mixing behavior of the Markov chain. For purposes of autocorrelation checking, a long-run single sequence may be more beneficial compared to multiple short-run sequences, since the long-run sequence will lead to more accurate estimates of autocorrelations. The slow decay in the autocorrelation plots indicates a slow mixing. On the other hand, the autocorrelations are also useful in estimating "effective sample size" for studying the convergence rates of the estimates of posterior quantities.

One of the most popular quantitative convergence diagnostics is the variance ratio method of Gelman and Rubin (1992). Gelman and Rubin's method consists of analyzing m independent sequences to form a distributional estimate for what is known about some random variable, given the observations simulated so far. Assume that we independently simulate $m \geq 2$ sequences of length $2n$, each beginning at different starting points from an overdispersed distribution with respect to the target distribution $\pi(\boldsymbol{\theta}|D)$. We discard the first n iterations and retain only the last n. Then, for any scalar function $\xi = h(\boldsymbol{\theta})$ of interest, we calculate the variance between the m sequence means defined by

$$\frac{B}{n} = \frac{1}{m-1} \sum_{i=1}^{m} (\bar{\xi}_{i.} - \bar{\xi}_{..})^2,$$

where

$$\bar{\xi}_{i.} = \frac{1}{n} \sum_{t=n+1}^{2n} \xi_{it}, \quad \bar{\xi}_{..} = \frac{1}{m} \sum_{i=1}^{m} \bar{\xi}_{i.},$$

and $\xi_{it} = h(\boldsymbol{\theta}_{it})$ is the tth observation of ξ from sequence i. Then we calculate the mean of the m within-sequence variances, s_i^2, each of which has $n-1$ degrees of freedom, given by

$$W = \frac{1}{m}\sum_{i=1}^{m} s_i^2,$$

where $s_i^2 = (n-1)^{-1}\sum_{t=n+1}^{2n}(\xi_{it} - \bar{\xi}_{i.})^2$. An estimator of the posterior variance of ξ is

$$\hat{V} = \frac{n-1}{n}W + \left(1 + \frac{1}{m}\right)\frac{B}{n},$$

which is asymptotically equivalent to W. Gelman and Rubin (1992) suggest the use of a t test, deduced from the approximation $B/W \sim \mathcal{F}(m-1, df)$, where $\mathcal{F}(m-1, df)$ denotes the F-distribution with degrees of freedom $(m-1, df)$, $df = 2V^2/\widehat{\text{Var}}(V)$, and

$$\begin{aligned}\widehat{\text{Var}}(V) \quad &= \quad \left(\frac{n-1}{n}\right)^2 \frac{1}{m}\widehat{\text{Var}}(s_i^2) + \left(\frac{m+1}{mn}\right)^2 \frac{2}{m-1}B^2 \\ &\quad + 2\frac{(m+1)(n-1)}{mn^2}\frac{n}{m}[\widehat{\text{Cov}}(s_i^2, \bar{\xi}_{i.}^2) - 2\bar{\xi}_{..}\widehat{\text{Cov}}(s_i^2, \bar{\xi}_{i.})].\end{aligned}$$

Then, we monitor convergence by a *potential scale reduction* (PSR) factor, which is calculated by

$$\hat{R} = (V/W)df/(df-2).$$

A large value of R suggests that either V can be further decreased by more draws, or that further draws will increase W. A value of R close to 1 indicates that each of the m sets of n simulated observations is close to the target distribution, that is, convergence is achieved. The multivariate version of the PSR can be found in Brooks and Gelman (1998). The other quantitative convergence diagnostic methods include the spectral density diagnostic of Geweke (1992), the L^2 convergence diagnostics of Liu, Liu, and Rubin (1992), and Roberts (1994), geometric convergence bounds of Rosenthal (1995a,b) and Cowles and Rosenthal (1998), the convergence rate estimator of Garren and Smith (1995) and Raftery and Lewis (1992), and many others.

As with all statistical procedures, any convergence diagnostic technique can falsely indicate convergence when in fact it has not occurred. In particular, for slowly mixing Markov chains, convergence diagnostics are likely to be unreliable, since their conclusions will be based on output from only a small region of the state space. Therefore, it is important to emphasize that any convergence diagnostic procedure should not be unilaterally relied upon. As in Cowles and Carlin (1996), we recommend using a variety of diagnostic tools rather than any single plot or statistic, and learning as much as possible about the target posterior distribution before applying an MCMC algorithm. In addition, a careful study of the propriety of the posterior distribution is important, since an improper posterior makes Bayesian inference meaningless. Also, we recommend using the acceleration tools described in Sections 2.5 and 2.6 as much as possible, since they can dramatically speed up an MCMC algorithm.

Exercises

2.1 Using the New Zealand apple data in Example 1.1, compute posterior estimates for β and σ^2 for the constrained multiple linear regression model with the prior specification for the model parameters given in Example 2.2, using the Gibbs sampler. Compare the results to those obtained by the classical-order restricted inference in Exercise 1.2.

2.2 SIMULATION STUDY

Construct a simulation study to examine the performance of the algorithm for sampling the correlation ρ given in Example 2.3. More specifically:

(i) generate a data set $D = \{\boldsymbol{y}_i = (y_{1i}, y_{2i})',\ i = 1, 2, \dots, n\}$ from a bivariate normal distribution $N_2(0, \Sigma)$, where $\Sigma = \begin{pmatrix} 1 & \rho \\ \rho & 1 \end{pmatrix}$ with different values of n and ρ;

(ii) implement a Metropolis–Hastings algorithm to obtain a Markov chain of ρ; and

(iii) study the trace plot and autocorrelation of the chain as well as the acceptance probability of the algorithm.

Some other diagnostic tools discussed in Section 2.9 may also be applied here.

2.3 Repeat Problem 2.1 using the Hit-and-Run algorithm described in Section 2.3. Compare the performance of the Gibbs sampler and the H&R algorithm.

2.4 Prove (2.5.2).

2.5 BAYESIAN ANALYSIS FOR SENSORY DATA

(a) Construct a Bayesian probit model using an improper prior for the model parameters to analyze the MRE sensory data given in Table 1.2 with storage temperature, time, and their interaction as possible covariates.

(b) Derive the posterior distribution.

(c) Implement the Albert–Chib, Cowles, Nandram–Chen, and Chen–Dey algorithms described in Section 2.5.3, and compare their performance.

(d) Compute the posterior estimates of the cutpoints and the regression coefficients.

(e) Are the Bayesian results comparable to those obtained from Exercise 1.3?

2.6 Prove that the posterior $\pi(\boldsymbol{\beta}, \sigma^2, \rho, \boldsymbol{\epsilon}|D)$ given in (2.5.26) is proper if $\delta_0 > 0$, $\gamma_0 > 0$, and X^* is of full rank, where X^* is a matrix induced by X and $\boldsymbol{y}$ with its tth row equal to $1\{y_t > 0\}\boldsymbol{x}_t'$.

2.7 Show that the conditional posterior density $\pi(\boldsymbol{\eta}|\boldsymbol{\beta}, \sigma^2, \rho, D)$ given in (2.5.29) for the reparameterized random effects is log-concave in each component of $\boldsymbol{\eta}$.

2.8 Perform a fully Bayesian analysis for the 1994 pollen count data in Example 1.3.

(i) Implement the Gibbs sampler with hierarchical centering described in Section 2.5.4 for sampling from the reparameterized posterior $\pi(\boldsymbol{\beta}, \sigma^2, \rho, \boldsymbol{\eta}|D)$ given in (2.5.28). You may choose $\delta_0 = 0.01$ and $\gamma_0 = 0.01$.
(ii) Obtain the posterior estimates for $\boldsymbol{\beta}$, σ^2, and ρ.
(iii) Compare the Bayesian estimates with those obtained from Exercise 1.5 using the GEE approach.

2.9 A COUNTEREXAMPLE (Liu and Sabatti 1998)
If the transition function T_θ does not satisfy (2.6.2), the target distribution π may not be preserved. Let θ take values in $\{0, 1, 2, 3, 4\}$ and suppose that the target distribution is uniform, i.e., $\pi(\theta|D) = \frac{1}{5}$. The group operation is the translation: $i * j = i + j \pmod 5$. The transition functions T_θ are, respectively, $T_0(i, j) = \frac{1}{3}$ for $|i - j| \le 1$, $i = 1, 2, 3, 4$, $T_0(0, j) = \frac{1}{3}$ for $j = 0, 1, 4$, and $T_0(4, j) = \frac{1}{3}$ for $j = 3, 4, 0$; and $T_k(i, j) = \frac{1}{5}$ for all i, j and $k > 0$.

(a) Show that π is invariant under all T_θ with θ fixed.
(b) Show that the invariant distribution of $T_i(i, j)$ is proportional to $(3, 3, 2, 2, 3)$ instead of π.

2.10 LINEAR REGRESSION MODELS WITH CENSORED DATA
Consider the experiment of improving the lifetime of fluorescent lights (Hamada and Wu 1995). Carried out by a 2^{5-2} fractional factorial design, the experiment was conducted over a time period of 20 days, with inspection every two days. The design and the lifetime data are tabulated in Table 2.2.
Let $\boldsymbol{x}_i$ be the $p \times 1$ column vector of the factor levels, including the intercepts, A, B, C, D, E, AB, and BD, and y_i be the logarithm of the corresponding lifetime for $i = 1, 2, \ldots, n$, where $p = 8$ and $n = 2 \times 2^{5-2} = 16$. Also let $(Y_i^{(l)}, Y_i^{(r)})$ denote the observed censoring interval for y_i, i.e., $y_i \in (Y_i^{(l)}, Y_i^{(r)})$. Hamada and Wu (1995) consider the following model:

$$y_i \overset{\text{i.i.d.}}{\sim} N(\boldsymbol{x}_i'\boldsymbol{\beta}, \sigma^2), \ \ i = 1, 2, \ldots, n,$$

TABLE 2.2. Design and Lifetime Data for Light Experiment.

Run	Design A	B	C	D	E	Data (no. of days)	
1	+	+	+	+	+	(14, 16)	(20, ∞)
2	+	+	−	−	−	(18, 20)	(20, ∞)
3	+	−	+	+	−	(08, 10)	(10, 12)
4	+	−	−	−	+	(18, 20)	(20, ∞)
5	−	+	+	−	+	(20, ∞)	(20, ∞)
6	−	+	−	+	−	(12, 14)	(20, ∞)
7	−	−	+	−	−	(16, 18)	(20, ∞)
8	−	−	−	−	−	(12, 14)	(14, 16)

Source: Hamada and Wu (1995).

with the prior distribution specified by

$$\sigma^2 \sim \mathcal{IG}(\nu_0, \nu_0 s_0/2) \text{ and } \beta|\sigma^2 \sim N(\beta_0, \sigma^2 I_p/\tau_0)$$

for $(\boldsymbol{\beta}, \sigma^2)$, where $\boldsymbol{\beta} = (\beta_0, \beta_1, \ldots, \beta_7)'$ is the vector of regression coefficients with β_0 corresponding to the intercept, $\mathcal{IG}$ denotes the inverse gamma distribution, i.e., $\pi(\sigma^2) \propto (\sigma^2)^{-(\nu_0/2+1)} \exp\{-\nu_0 s_0/(2\sigma^2)\}$, $\nu_0 = 1$, $s_0 = 0.01$, $\boldsymbol{\beta}_0 = (3, 0, \ldots, 0)$, I_p is the $p \times p$ identity matrix, and $\tau_0 = 0.0001$.

(a) Write the posterior distribution for $(\boldsymbol{\beta}, \sigma^2)$ based on the observed data $D_{\text{obs}} = (\{(Y_i^{(l)}, Y_i^{(r)}), \boldsymbol{x}_i\},\ i = 1, 2, \ldots, n)$.
(b) Derive an expression for the posterior distribution based on the complete-observed data $D = ((y_i, \boldsymbol{x}_i),\ i = 1, 2, \ldots, n)$.
(c) Develop an efficient MCMC algorithm for sampling from the posterior distribution.
(*Hint:* Slow convergence of the original Gibbs sampler may occur; so an improved MCMC algorithm such as the GM-MGMC or CA-MCMC algorithm may be required.)
(d) Perform a fully Bayesian analysis for the lifetime data.

2.11 To sample from the posterior distribution in (2.6.9) for the rating data given in Table 2.1, consider the GM-MGMC algorithm with the following additive group transformations:

$$g(\boldsymbol{\beta}, \gamma_2, \boldsymbol{z}) = (\beta_0, \beta_1 + g, \gamma_2, \{z_i : x_i = 0\}, \{z_i + g : x_i = 1\}).$$

(a) Write the GM step.
(b) Study the performance of this version of the GM-MGMC algorithm.

2.12 Prove (2.7.4).

2.13 (i) Explain why the value of the normalizing constant $c(D)$ is not required in the RDIP sampler.

(ii) Derive (2.8.7), (2.8.8), and (2.8.9) for the conditional density and the jump ratio for the state-dependent and direction-and-radius RDIP sampler.

2.14 In Exercise 2.5, compute Gelman and Rubin's PSR factors for all four algorithms with five ($m = 5$) independent sequences of length $2n$ for $n = 500$ and $n = 1000$, and discuss which algorithm converges faster.

3
Basic Monte Carlo Methods for Estimating Posterior Quantities

The fundamental goal of Bayesian computation is to compute posterior quantities of interest. When the posterior distribution $\pi(\boldsymbol{\theta}|D)$ is high dimensional, one is typically driven to do multidimensional integration to evaluate marginal posterior summaries of the parameters. When a Bayesian model is complicated, analytical or exact numerical evaluation may fail to solve this computational problem. In this regard, the Monte Carlo (MC) method, in particular, the Markov chain Monte Carlo (MCMC) approach, may naturally serve as an alternative solution. Many of the MCMC sampling algorithms discussed in Chapter 2 can be applied here to generate an MCMC sample from the posterior distribution. The main objective of this chapter is to provide a comprehensive treatment of how to use an MCMC sample to obtain MC estimates of posterior quantities. In particular, we will present an overview of several basic MC methods for computing posterior quantities as well as assessing simulation accuracy of MC estimates. In addition, several related issues, including how to obtain more efficient MC estimates, such as the weighted MC estimates, and how to control simulation errors when computing MC estimates, will be addressed.

3.1 Posterior Quantities

In Bayesian data analysis, many posterior quantities are of the form

$$E[h(\boldsymbol{\theta})|D] = \int_{R^p} h(\boldsymbol{\theta})\pi(\boldsymbol{\theta}|D)\, d\boldsymbol{\theta}, \tag{3.1.1}$$

where $h(\cdot)$ is a real-valued function of $\boldsymbol{\theta} = (\theta_1, \theta_2, \ldots, \theta_p)'$. We call (3.1.1) an integral-type posterior quantity, or the posterior expectation of $h(\boldsymbol{\theta})$. In (3.1.1), we assume that

$$E(|h(\boldsymbol{\theta})| \mid D) = \int_{R^p} |h(\boldsymbol{\theta})|\pi(\boldsymbol{\theta}|D)\, d\boldsymbol{\theta} < \infty.$$

Integral-type posterior quantities include posterior means, posterior variances, covariances, higher-order moments, and probabilities of sets by taking appropriate functional forms of h. For example, (3.1.1) reduces to:

(a) the posterior mean of $\boldsymbol{\theta}$ when $h(\boldsymbol{\theta}) = \boldsymbol{\theta}$;

(b) the posterior covariance of θ_j and θ_{j^*} if $h(\boldsymbol{\theta}) = (\theta_j - E(\theta_j|D))(\theta_{j^*} - E(\theta_{j^*}|D))'$, where $E(\theta_j|D) = \int_{R^p} \theta_j \pi(\boldsymbol{\theta}|D)\, d\boldsymbol{\theta}$;

(c) the posterior predictive density when $h(\boldsymbol{\theta}) = f(z|\boldsymbol{\theta})$, where $f(z|\boldsymbol{\theta})$ is the predictive density given the parameter $\boldsymbol{\theta}$; and

(d) the posterior probability of a set A if $h(\boldsymbol{\theta}) = 1\{\boldsymbol{\theta} \in A\}$, where $1\{\boldsymbol{\theta} \in A\}$ denotes the indicator function.

In (d), the posterior probability leads to a Bayesian p-value (see Meng 1994) by taking an appropriate form of A. In addition, the marginal posterior densities are also integral-type posterior quantities. See Section 4.3 for details.

Some other posterior quantities such as normalizing constants, Bayes factors, and posterior model probabilities, may not simply be written in the form of (3.1.1). However, they are actually functions of integral-type posterior quantities. We will discuss these quantities in detail in Chapters 5, 8, and 9. Posterior quantiles, Bayesian credible intervals, and Bayesian Highest Posterior Density (HPD) intervals are often viewed as nonintegral-type posterior quantities. Even for these types of posterior quantities, we can express them as functions of integral-type posterior quantities under certain conditions. For example, let $\xi = h(\boldsymbol{\theta})$, and $\xi_{1-\alpha}$ be the $(1-\alpha)$th posterior quantile of ξ with respect to $\pi(\boldsymbol{\theta}|D)$, where $0 < \alpha < 1$ and $h(\cdot)$ is a real-valued function. Then, $\xi_{1-\alpha}$ is the solution of the following equation:

$$\int_{R^p} 1\{h(\boldsymbol{\theta}) \le t\}\pi(\boldsymbol{\theta}|D)\, d\boldsymbol{\theta} = 1 - \alpha.$$

Therefore, the posterior quantile is a function of the posterior expectation of $1\{h(\boldsymbol{\theta}) \le t\}$. We will elaborate further on these types of posterior quantities in Chapter 7.

3.2 Basic Monte Carlo Methods

In Bayesian inference, MC methods are often used to compute the posterior expectation $E(h(\boldsymbol{\theta})|D)$, since the analytical evaluation of $E(h(\boldsymbol{\theta})|D)$

is typically not available. The use of MC methods for computing high-dimensional integrations has a long history. In the MC literature, one of the excellent early references is Hammersley and Handscomb (1964), and many early MC methods such as *importance sampling* and *conditional Monte Carlo*, which are still useful now, can be found therein. Trotter and Tukey (1956) propose a general MC scheme based on the weighted average. More specifically, instead of sampling $\boldsymbol{\theta}$ alone, they suggest generating a pair $(\boldsymbol{\theta}, w)$, where w is a real-valued weight from some joint distribution $\pi(\boldsymbol{\theta}, w)$ so that for all reasonable real-valued functions $h(\boldsymbol{\theta})$,

$$\int_{R^{p+1}} wh(\boldsymbol{\theta})\pi(\boldsymbol{\theta}, w)\, d\boldsymbol{\theta}\, dw = KE(h(\boldsymbol{\theta})|D), \tag{3.2.1}$$

where $K \neq 0$ is an h-independent constant. In fact, by taking $h(\boldsymbol{\theta}) = 1$ (3.2.1) reduces to

$$K = \int_{R^{p+1}} w\pi(\boldsymbol{\theta}, w)\, d\boldsymbol{\theta}\, dw. \tag{3.2.2}$$

Thus, K is the marginal mean of w. In (3.2.1), $h(\cdot)$ is said to be reasonable if

$$\int_{R^{p+1}} |wh(\boldsymbol{\theta})|\pi(\boldsymbol{\theta}, w)\, d\boldsymbol{\theta}\, dw < \infty \quad \text{and} \quad E(|h(\boldsymbol{\theta})| \mid D) < \infty.$$

Interestingly, the IWIW of Wong and Liang (1997) is essentially equivalent to the weighted MC method of Trotter and Tukey (1956), since the IWIW identity given in (2.7.3) implies (3.2.1), and vice versa. Assuming that $\{(\boldsymbol{\theta}_i, w_i),\ i = 1, 2, \ldots, n\}$ is a (dependent or independent) sample from $\pi(\boldsymbol{\theta}, w)$, the weighted MC estimator of $E(h(\boldsymbol{\theta})|D)$ is given by

$$\hat{E}_w(h) = \frac{\sum_{i=1}^n w_i h(\boldsymbol{\theta}_i)}{\sum_{l=1}^n w_l}. \tag{3.2.3}$$

The weighted MC method is very general, which includes, as a special case, the usual sample mean as well as the importance sampling method. By taking $w_i = 1$, the weighted MC estimator (3.2.3) reduces to the usual sample mean of the $h(\boldsymbol{\theta}_i)$, given by

$$\hat{E}_{\text{avg}}(h) = \frac{1}{n}\sum_{i=1}^n h(\boldsymbol{\theta}_i). \tag{3.2.4}$$

Assume that the posterior density $\pi(\boldsymbol{\theta}|D)$ has the form

$$\pi(\boldsymbol{\theta}|D) = \frac{L(\boldsymbol{\theta}|D)\pi(\boldsymbol{\theta})}{c(D)},$$

where $L(\boldsymbol{\theta}|D)$ is the likelihood function, $\pi(\boldsymbol{\theta})$ is the prior, and $c(D)$ is an unknown normalizing constant. Also let $g(\boldsymbol{\theta})$ be an importance sampling density, which is known up to a normalizing constant. Suppose $\{\boldsymbol{\theta}_i,\ i =$

$1, 2, \ldots, n\}$ is a sample from $g(\boldsymbol{\theta})$. Write the importance sampling weight as

$$w_i = \frac{L(\boldsymbol{\theta}_i|D)\pi(\boldsymbol{\theta}_i)}{g(\boldsymbol{\theta}_i)}. \tag{3.2.5}$$

Then, the weighted MC estimator (3.2.3) with w_i given by (3.2.5) gives an importance sampling estimator:

$$\hat{E}_I(h) = \frac{\sum_{i=1}^n h(\boldsymbol{\theta}_i)L(\boldsymbol{\theta}_i|D)\pi(\boldsymbol{\theta}_i)/g(\boldsymbol{\theta}_i)}{\sum_{l=1}^n L(\boldsymbol{\theta}_l|D)\pi(\boldsymbol{\theta}_l)/g(\boldsymbol{\theta}_l)}. \tag{3.2.6}$$

Although $g(\boldsymbol{\theta})$ is not completely known, $\hat{E}_I(h)$ is still well defined, since the unknown normalizing constant in $g(\boldsymbol{\theta})$ cancels out in (3.2.6).

Asymptotic or small sample properties of the weighted MC estimators depend on the choice of the joint distribution $\pi(\boldsymbol{\theta}, w)$ and the algorithm used to generate the weighted sample. Under certain regularity conditions such as *ergodicity*, the weighted MC estimator $\hat{E}_w(h)$ is consistent. However, $\hat{E}_w(h)$ is unbiased only for a few special cases. When $\boldsymbol{\theta}$ and w are independent, i.e., $\pi(\boldsymbol{\theta}, w) = \pi(\boldsymbol{\theta}|D)\pi(w)$, $\hat{E}_w(h)$ is unbiased. In addition, if (3.2.1) holds for $K = 1$, i.e.,

$$\int_{R^{p+1}} wh(\boldsymbol{\theta})\pi(\boldsymbol{\theta}, w)\, d\boldsymbol{\theta}\, dw = E(h(\boldsymbol{\theta})|D), \tag{3.2.7}$$

then $E(h(\boldsymbol{\theta})|D)$ can be estimated by

$$\hat{E}_w^*(h) = \frac{1}{n}\sum_{i=1}^n w_i h(\boldsymbol{\theta}_i). \tag{3.2.8}$$

In this case, it can be shown that $\hat{E}_w^*(h)$ is an unbiased estimator. Further, Trotter and Tukey (1956) claim that if (3.2.1) holds, $\hat{E}_w^*(h)$ is almost always better than $\hat{E}_w(h)$ given by (3.2.3). However, this property has not been theoretically justified. Also note that when $K = 1$, under certain regularity conditions, $(1/n)\sum_{i=1}^n w_i$ converges to 1 almost surely. Therefore, $\hat{E}_w(h)$ is a consistent estimator of $E(h(\boldsymbol{\theta})|D)$.

Other asymptotic properties of the above MC estimators such as asymptotic normality have been studied by many authors, including Geyer (1992), Besag and Green (1993), Tierney (1994), Roberts and Tweedie (1996), and many others. In particular, Geyer (1992) obtains a central limit theorem for $\hat{E}_{\text{avg}}(h)$, when $\{\boldsymbol{\theta}_i,\ i = 1, 2, \ldots,\}$ is a stationary, irreducible, and reversible Markov chain. Roberts and Tweedie (1996) also derive central limit theorems for multidimensional Metropolis–Hastings algorithms. Further, when $\{(\boldsymbol{\theta}_i, w_i),\ i = 1, 2, ...\}$ is a stationary weakly dependent sequence, then under certain regularity conditions such as α-mixing, ρ-mixing, and ϕ-mixing (see, e.g., Lin and Lu 1996), we have

$$n^{1/2}(\hat{E}_w(h) - E(h(\boldsymbol{\theta})|D)) \xrightarrow{d.} N(0, \sigma^2)$$

as $n \to \infty$, where

$$\sigma^2 = b^{-4}\{(E(bw_1 h(\boldsymbol{\theta}_1) - aw_1)^2 + 2\sum_{i=2}^{\infty} E[(bw_1 h(\boldsymbol{\theta}_1) - aw_1)(bw_i h(\boldsymbol{\theta}_i) - aw_i)]\},$$

$a = E(w_1 h(\boldsymbol{\theta}_1))$, and $b = E(w_1)$.

3.3 Simulation Standard Error Estimation

Suppose $\hat{E}(h)$ is a Monte Carlo estimator of $E(h(\boldsymbol{\theta})|D)$ using the weighted sample $\{(\boldsymbol{\theta}_i, w_i),\ i = 1, 2, \ldots, n\}$. Let $\mathrm{Var}(\hat{E}(h))$ be the variance of $\hat{E}(h)$, and let $\widehat{\mathrm{Var}}(\hat{E}(h))$ be an estimate of $\mathrm{Var}(\hat{E}(h))$. Then, the simulation standard error of $\hat{E}(h)$ is defined as

$$\mathrm{se}(\hat{E}(h)) = [\widehat{\mathrm{Var}}(\hat{E}(h))]^{1/2}, \tag{3.3.1}$$

which is the square root of the estimated variance of the MC estimator $\hat{E}(h)$. Computing the simulation standard error is important, since it provides the magnitude of the simulation accuracy of the estimator $\hat{E}(h)$.

Since the sample generated by an MCMC sampling algorithm is often dependent, a complication that arises from the autocorrelation is that $\mathrm{Var}(\hat{E}(h))$ is difficult to obtain. A variety of methods for obtaining a dependent sample based estimate of $\mathrm{Var}(\hat{E}(h))$ are discussed in system simulation textbooks, as, for example, in Bratley, Fox and Schrage (1987), Ripley (1987), or Law and Kelton (1991), with an emphasis on sample averages such as $\hat{E}_{\mathrm{avg}}(h)$ or $\hat{E}_w^*(h)$ given by (3.2.4) and (3.2.8). General point estimators are considered in Schmeiser, Avramidis, and Hashem (1990), who discuss overlapping batch statistics. In the remainder of this section, we discuss using the time series approach as well as the overlapping or nonoverlapping batch statistics methods to estimate $\mathrm{Var}(\hat{E}(h))$.

3.3.1 Time Series Approach

Geyer (1992) proposes three time-series-based methods to estimate the simulation standard error of the sample mean. One of Geyer's approaches is indeed the nonoverlapping batch mean. In the same spirit, Geweke (1992) suggests using the asymptotic variance of the sample mean from spectral analysis. The spectral analysis method for estimating the variance of the sample mean of a dependent sample can also be found in Hannan (1970, pp. 207–210) and Bratley, Fox, and Schrage (1987, pp. 100–103).

Assume that $\{\boldsymbol{\theta}_i,\ i = 1, 2, \ldots\}$ is a stationary, irreducible, and reversible Markov chain. Suppose that our interest is in estimating the variance of the sample mean

$$\hat{E}(h) = \frac{1}{n}\sum_{i=1}^{n} h(\boldsymbol{\theta}_i).$$

Then, the window estimators and the estimators specialized for the Markov chain of Geyer (1992) can be used for computing the simulation standard error of $\hat{E}(h)$. Let

$$\gamma_t = \gamma_{-t} = \text{Cov}(h(\boldsymbol{\theta}_i), h(\boldsymbol{\theta}_{i+t})) \tag{3.3.2}$$

be the lag t autocovariance of the stationary time series $\{h(\boldsymbol{\theta}_i),\ i = 1, 2, \ldots\}$. The natural estimator of the lagged autocovariance γ_t is the empirical autocovariance

$$\hat{\gamma}_{n,t} = \hat{\gamma}_{n,-t} = \frac{1}{n}\sum_{i=1}^{n-t} [h(\boldsymbol{\theta}_i) - \hat{E}(h)][h(\boldsymbol{\theta}_{i+t}) - \hat{E}(h)]. \tag{3.3.3}$$

An argument for using the biased estimate with divisor n rather than the unbiased estimate with divisor $n - t$ is given by Priestley (1981, pp. 323–324). Using (3.3.3), the window estimator is given by

$$\text{se}_{\text{win}} = \frac{\hat{\sigma}_n}{\sqrt{n}}, \tag{3.3.4}$$

where

$$\hat{\sigma}_n^2 = \sum_{-\infty}^{\infty} w_n(t)\hat{\gamma}_{n,t}, \tag{3.3.5}$$

and w_n is some weight function, called a lag window, satisfying $0 \leq w_n(t) \leq 1$, with the choice of the window depending on n. As pointed out by Geyer (1992), under strong enough regularity conditions, the window estimator $\hat{\sigma}_n^2$ is consistent. However, it is not clear whether window estimators $\hat{\sigma}_n^2$ can be shown to be consistent under the weak conditions for which the central limit theorem holds. A large number of weight functions (lag windows) are proposed in the time series literature. For example, Priestley (1981, pp. 437 and 563) discusses many of them. Interestingly, Geweke (1992) also uses the window estimator with a Daniell window and derives the relative numerical efficiency to monitor convergence of the Gibbs sampler.

Standard methods of "simulation output analysis" are not designed specifically for Markov chains. Thus, it is possible to do better by using specific properties of the autocovariances of a Markov chain. Liu, Wong, and Kong (1995) show that if the Markov chain is reversible, all even-lag autocovariances are nonnegative. However, the odd-lag autocovariances need not be positive. Let $\Gamma_m = \gamma_{2m}+\gamma_{2m+1}$ be the sums of adjacent pairs of autocovariances of a stationary, irreducible, and reversible Markov chain. Then, Geyer (1992) shows that Γ_m is a strictly positive, strictly decreasing, and strictly convex function of m. Using this property of the autocovariances, Geyer (1992) derives the following three estimators.

Let $\hat{\Gamma}_{n,m} = \hat{\gamma}_{n,2m} + \hat{\gamma}_{n,2m+1}$, where $\hat{\gamma}_{n,t}$ is given by (3.3.2), be an estimate of Γ_m. Then, the first estimator, called the *initial positive sequence estimator*, is defined by

$$\hat{\sigma}^2_{\text{pos},n} = \hat{\gamma}_{n,0} + 2\sum_{i=1}^{2m+1} \hat{\gamma}_{n,i} = -\hat{\gamma}_{n,0} + 2\sum_{i=0}^{m} \hat{\Gamma}_{n,i}, \tag{3.3.6}$$

where m is chosen to be the largest integer such that

$$\hat{\Gamma}_{n,i} > 0, \quad i = 1, 2, \ldots, m.$$

This estimator is obtained by summing over the longest initial sequence over which the $\hat{\Gamma}_{n,m}$ stay positive. Geyer (1992) points out that it can happen that the estimated autocovariances stay positive for many lags past the point where the noise level is crossed and are nonmonotone or nonconvex so that the estimated curve has a "bump."

By eliminating such "bumps," Geyer (1992) proposes the *initial monotone sequence estimator* $\hat{\sigma}^2_{\text{mono},n}$, and the *initial convex sequence estimator* $\hat{\sigma}^2_{\text{conv},n}$. The estimator $\hat{\sigma}^2_{\text{mono},n}$ is obtained by further reducing the estimated Γ_i to the minimum of the preceding ones so that the estimated sequence is monotone and positive, while $\hat{\sigma}^2_{\text{conv},n}$ is obtained by reducing the estimated Γ_i still further to the greatest convex minorant of the sequence $\hat{\Gamma}_{n,1}, \hat{\Gamma}_{n,2}, \ldots, \hat{\Gamma}_{n,m}, 0$. In both cases, the estimator is the sum like (3.3.6) of the reduced estimates. Although it is not clear that any of these initial sequence estimators is consistent, Geyer (1992) shows that they at least provide consistent overestimates in the following sense:

For almost all sample paths of the MC sequence,

$$\liminf_{n\to\infty} \hat{\sigma}^2_{\text{seq},n} \geq \sigma^2 = \sum_{t=-\infty}^{\infty} \gamma_t,$$

where $\hat{\sigma}^2_{\text{seq},n}$ denotes any of the three initial sequence estimators.

This property is useful in practice, since $\text{se}(\hat{E}(h))$ is always smaller than $\text{se}^*(\hat{E}(h)) = \hat{\sigma}_{\text{seq},n}/\sqrt{n}$, and a small value of $\text{se}^*(\hat{E}(h))$ guarantees the simulation accuracy of $\hat{E}(h)$.

3.3.2 Overlapping Batch Statistics

As discussed in the previous subsection, the time series approach is used only for estimating the variance of the sample mean. To overcome such limitations, we consider using the overlapping batch statistics (obs) of Schmeiser, Avramidis, and Hashem (1990) to estimate the variances of general point estimators, including, the sample mean, the weighted mean, the sample variance, quantiles, and other posterior quantities.

Suppose that $\{(\boldsymbol{\theta}_i, w_i),\ i = 1, 2, \ldots, n\}$ is a dependent sample, from which a point estimator $\hat{\xi}$ of the posterior quantity of interest is computed. The obs estimate of the variance of $\hat{\xi}$ is

$$\hat{V}(m) = \left[\frac{m}{n-m}\right] \frac{\sum_{j=1}^{n-m+1}(\hat{\xi}_j - \hat{\xi})^2}{(n-m+1)}, \tag{3.3.7}$$

where $\hat{\xi}_j$ is defined analogously to $\hat{\xi}$, but is a function of only $(\boldsymbol{\theta}_j, w_j)$, $(\boldsymbol{\theta}_{j+1}, w_{j+1})$, $\ldots$, $(\boldsymbol{\theta}_{j+m-1}, w_{j+m-1})$. Sufficient conditions for obs estimators to be unbiased and have variance inversely proportional to n are given in Schmeiser, Avramidis, and Hashem (1990). Using (3.3.7), the simulation standard error of $\hat{\xi}$ is $\text{se}(\hat{\xi}) = \sqrt{\hat{V}(m)}$. Below we consider two special cases.

Special Case I: Overlapping Batch Means

Specializing $\hat{\xi}$ to the sample mean $\hat{E}_{\text{avg}}(h)$ given in (3.2.4) yields the overlapping batch mean (obm) estimator, which is given by

$$\hat{\xi}_j = m^{-1} \sum_{i=j}^{j+m-1} h(\boldsymbol{\theta}_i).$$

Song (1988) shows that the obm estimator is a spectral estimator with the spectral window

$$w_m^{(0)}(t) = \begin{cases} n^2(n-m+1)^{-1}(n-m)^{-1}(1-|t|/m) & \text{if } t = 1, \ldots, m, \\ 0 & \text{otherwise,} \end{cases}$$

which is essentially the Bartlett window when $n^2(n-m+1)^{-1}(n-m)^{-1} \simeq 1$. Therefore, ignoring end effects, obm can be viewed as an efficient computational method for the Bartlett window at zero frequency. Computation is $O(n)$, as discussed in Meketon and Schmeiser (1984). Schmeiser and Song (1987) give a Fortran subroutine for computing the obm estimate $\hat{V}_{\text{obm}}(m)$, and Song and Schmeiser (1993) discuss generalizations.

The statistical properties of $\hat{V}_{\text{obm}}(m)$ depend upon the batch size m. The bias decreases and the variance increases with m. Asymptotically, the bias of obm is that of the nonoverlapping batch means (nbm) estimator and has two-thirds of the variance of nbm. Song and Schmeiser (1995) show that the mse-optimal asymptotic batch size is $m^* = 1 + (\frac{9}{8} c_g n)^{1/3}$, where c_g is the center of gravity of the absolute value of the autocorrelation lags.

Special Case II: Overlapping Batch Variances

Specializing $\hat{\xi}$ to the sample variance yields the overlapping batch variance (obv) estimator, which is based on $\hat{\xi}_j = S^2_{j,m}$, the sample variance of

$\{h(\boldsymbol{\theta}_j), \ldots, h(\boldsymbol{\theta}_{j+m-1})\}$. The obv estimator is

$$\hat{V}_{\text{obv}}(m) = \frac{m}{n-m} \left[\frac{1}{n-m+1} \sum_{j=1}^{n-m+1} (S_{j,m}^2 - S^2)^2 \right],$$

where $2 \leq m \leq n-1$ is the batch size. Schmeiser, Avramidis, and Hashem (1990) provide a Fortran subroutine for the obv estimator $\hat{V}_{\text{obv}}(m)$ that requires $O(n)$ time for any given value of m.

The primary difficulty in using the obs estimator is the choice of the batch size m to balance bias and variance, since no optimal batch size formula is known for obs estimators other than obm. Schmeiser (1982) discusses the trade-off in the context of confidence intervals for nonoverlapping batch means. Song and Schmeiser (1988a, b) consider variances and covariances of estimators of the variance of the sample mean. Limiting behavior for sample means is discussed by Goldsman and Meketon (1986) and Song and Schmeiser (1995). For many situations, choosing m so that $10 \leq n/m \leq 20$ is reasonable.

Example 3.1. Bivariate normal model (Example 2.1 continued). We now study the empirical performance of obs estimators for the bivariate normal model discussed in Example 2.1. From (2.1.4), the Gibbs sampler sample path $\theta_{1,i}$ is an AR(1) process with marginal variance ${\sigma^*}_1^2 = \sigma_1^2(1-\rho^4)$ and lag-one autocorrelation $\psi = \rho^2$, where σ_1^2 is the marginal posterior variance of θ_1, and ρ is the posterior correlation between θ_1 and θ_2. Let

$$\hat{\mu}_1 = \frac{1}{n} \sum_{i=1}^{n} \theta_{1,i} \quad \text{and} \quad \hat{\sigma}_1^2 = \frac{1}{n-1} \sum_{i=1}^{n} (\theta_{1,i} - \hat{\mu}_1)^2. \tag{3.3.8}$$

Then, we have

$$n \ \text{Var}(\hat{\mu}_1) = {\sigma^*}_1^2 \left[\frac{1+\psi}{1-\psi} - \frac{2\psi(1-\psi^n)}{n(1-\psi)^2} \right], \tag{3.3.9}$$

and the standard error is

$$\text{se}(\hat{\mu}_1) = \frac{\sigma_1^*}{\sqrt{n}} \sqrt{\frac{1+\psi}{1-\psi} - \frac{2\psi(1-\psi^n)}{n(1-\psi)^2}}. \tag{3.3.10}$$

Further, it can be shown that

$$\begin{aligned} (n-1)^2 \ \text{Var}(\hat{\sigma}_1^2) = 2n{\sigma^*}_1^4 \Bigg[& \frac{1+\psi^2}{1-\psi^2} - \frac{2\psi^2(1-\psi^{2n})}{n(1-\psi^2)^2} \\ & - \frac{(1+\psi)^2 + 4\psi^{n+1}}{n(1-\psi)^2} - \frac{4\psi^2(1-\psi^{2n})}{n^2(1-\psi)^2(1-\psi^2)} \\ & + \frac{4\psi(1+\psi)(1-\psi^n)}{n^2(1-\psi)^3} + \frac{4\psi^2(1-\psi^n)^2}{n^3(1-\psi)^4} \Bigg], \end{aligned} \tag{3.3.11}$$

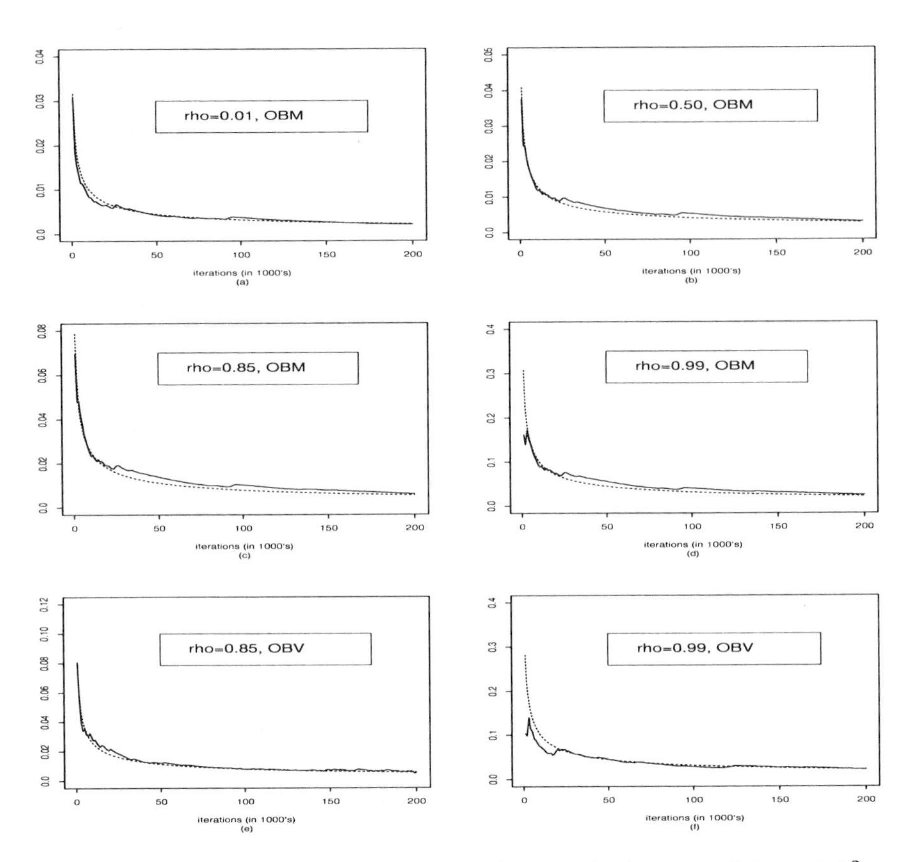

FIGURE 3.1. A single Gibbs trajectory for standard errors of $\hat{\mu}_1$ and $\hat{\sigma}_1^2$.

and the standard error of $\hat{\sigma}_1^2$ is

$$\text{se}(\hat{\sigma}_1^2) = \frac{\sqrt{2}{\sigma^*}_1^2}{\sqrt{n}}\sqrt{\frac{1+\psi^2}{1-\psi^2}} + O\left(\frac{1}{n}\right). \tag{3.3.12}$$

The proofs of (3.3.9) and (3.3.11) are left as an exercise.

Using (3.3.10) and (3.3.12), we are able to check directly whether or not the obm and obv standard error estimates are consistent with the analytical values $\text{se}(\hat{\mu}_1)$ and $\text{se}(\hat{\sigma}_1^2)$. Figure 3.1 shows the obm and obv estimates and the true standard errors for $\hat{\mu}_1$ and $\hat{\sigma}_1^2$ from a single Gibbs run of 200,000 iterations for the bivariate normal distribution with $\mu_1 = \mu_2 = 0$, $\sigma_1^2 = 1$, $\sigma_2^2 = 2$, and $\rho = 0.01, 0.5, 0.85, 0.99$. Graphs (a), (b), (c), and (d) show obm estimates and the true values; graphs (e) and (f) show obv estimates and the true values. In Figure 3.1, the dashed curves are true standard errors; the solid curves are overlapping batch statistics standard error estimates.

Here we choose the batch size $m = \max\{n/20, (1+\rho^2)/(1-\rho^2)\}$. This crude batch size works reasonably well in this case. For the smaller correlations $|\rho| = 0.01, 0.5, 0.85$, the obm and obv estimators are consistent with the analytical values (see graphs (a), (b), (c), and (e)), even for small numbers of iterations n. For a large correlation $|\rho| = 0.99$, the obm and obv estimators are also consistent with the true standard errors (see graphs (d) and (f)) except for small values of n.

3.4 Improving Monte Carlo Estimates

As with any simulation method, variance reduction techniques can often significantly reduce the sample size required for accurate estimates. Tierney (1994) presents a general strategy of how standard variance reduction methods such as importance sampling, conditioning, antithetic variates, control variates, and common variates (e.g., Bratley, Fox, and Schrage 1987, Chap. 2) can be used with Markov chain methods. Suppose that our objective is to compute $E(h(\boldsymbol{\theta})|D)$ given in (3.1.1) using an MCMC sample $\{\boldsymbol{\theta}_i,\ i = 1, 2, \ldots, n\}$ from the posterior distribution $\pi(\boldsymbol{\theta}|D)$. More accurate MC estimates can be obtained by using:

(i) all the simulated random variables involved in MCMC sampling;

(ii) the variance-reduction MCMC sampling technique; and

(iii) the weighted MC estimates in (3.2.3).

For (i), Casella and Robert (1996) propose a Rao–Blackwellization method that integrates over the uniform random variables involved in the acceptance–rejection and Metropolis algorithms. In the same spirit, Casella and Robert (1998) propose an alternative method for constructing estimators from accept-reject samples by incorporating the variables rejected by the algorithm. Robert (1998) and Robert and Casella (1999) also provide a detailed description and illustrative examples for this method. Thus we refer the reader to their article and their books for further discussion. The Rao–Blackwellization method of Casella and Robert (1996) is essentially the conditional MC method of Hammersley and Handscomb (1964). Here, we note that the Rao–Blackwellized estimators may not always reduce variance in MCMC methods when the dependence in the Markov chain is taken into account. See Geyer (1995a) for a detailed discussion and Exercise 3.4 for an example. In the remainder of this section, we will focus on (ii) and (iii).

3.4.1 Variance-Reduction MCMC Sampling

The variance-reduction technique can be generically integrated into MCMC sampling algorithms for estimating $E(h(\boldsymbol{\theta})|D)$. In the context of the Hit-

and-Run (H&R) algorithm described in Section 2.3, Schmeiser and Chen (1991) propose a conditional-expectation sampling algorithm. Suppose $\{\boldsymbol{\theta}_i, \ i = 1, 2, \ldots, n\}$ is an MCMC sample generated by the H&R algorithm. Then a consistent estimator of $E(h(\boldsymbol{\theta})|D)$ is given by

$$\hat{E}_{\text{avg}}(h) = \frac{1}{n} \sum_{i=1}^{n} h(\boldsymbol{\theta}_i). \tag{3.4.1}$$

In (3.4.1), the other available information such as the random direction $\boldsymbol{d}_i$ and the random signed distance λ_i at the ith iteration has not been used in computing $\hat{E}_{\text{avg}}(h)$. In the same spirit as the Rao–Blackwellization method of Casella and Robert (1996), using

$$h_{i+1} = E(h(\boldsymbol{\theta}_{i+1})|\boldsymbol{d}_i, \boldsymbol{\theta}_i),$$

instead of $h(\boldsymbol{\theta}_{i+1})$, may give an improved estimate of $E(h(\boldsymbol{\theta})|D)$. Since $E(h(\boldsymbol{\theta}_{i+1})|\boldsymbol{d}_i, \boldsymbol{\theta}_i)$ is a one-dimensional integral, numerical evaluation of h_{i+1} is reasonable. The expected value of each observation is unchanged since

$$E(h_{i+1}) = E[E(h(\boldsymbol{\theta}_{i+1})|\boldsymbol{d}_i, \boldsymbol{\theta}_i)] = E(h(\boldsymbol{\theta}_{i+1})).$$

From the H&R algorithm in Section 2.3, given $\boldsymbol{\theta}_i$ and $\boldsymbol{d}_i$, $\boldsymbol{\theta}_{i+1} = \boldsymbol{\theta}_i + \lambda \boldsymbol{d}_i$, where the random signed distance λ has density and mass

$$q_i(\lambda|\boldsymbol{d}_i, \boldsymbol{\theta}_i) = \begin{cases} g_i(\lambda|\boldsymbol{d}_i, \boldsymbol{\theta}_i) a(\boldsymbol{\theta}_i + \lambda \boldsymbol{d}_i|\boldsymbol{\theta}_i) & \text{if } \lambda \neq 0, \lambda \in \Omega_i(\boldsymbol{d}_i, \boldsymbol{\theta}_i), \\ 1 - \int_{\Omega_i(\boldsymbol{d}_i, \boldsymbol{\theta}_i)} g_i(u|\boldsymbol{d}_i, \boldsymbol{\theta}_i) a(\boldsymbol{\theta}_i + u\boldsymbol{d}_i|\boldsymbol{\theta}_i) \, du & \text{if } \lambda = 0. \end{cases}$$

Let $Q_i(\lambda|\boldsymbol{d}_i, \boldsymbol{\theta}_i)$ denote the cumulative distribution function of λ. Then, the conditional-expectation H&R algorithm is given as follows:

Conditional-Expectation Hit-and-Run Algorithm

Step 0. Choose a starting point $\boldsymbol{\theta}_0$, and set $i = 0$.

Step 1. Generate a random direction $\boldsymbol{d}_i$ from a distribution on the surface of the unit sphere.

Step 2. Find the set $\Omega_i(\boldsymbol{d}_i, \boldsymbol{\theta}_i) = \{\lambda \in R | \boldsymbol{\theta}_i + \lambda \boldsymbol{d}_i \in \Omega\}$, where Ω is the support of $\pi(\boldsymbol{\theta}|D)$.

Step 3. Compute $h_{i+1} = \int_{\Omega_i(\boldsymbol{d}_i, \boldsymbol{\theta}_i)} h(\boldsymbol{\theta}_i + \lambda \boldsymbol{d}_i) \, dQ_i(\lambda|\boldsymbol{d}_i, \boldsymbol{\theta}_i)$.

Step 4. Generate a signed distance λ_i from the density $g_i(\lambda|\boldsymbol{d}_i, \boldsymbol{\theta}_i)$, where $\lambda_i \in \Omega_i(\boldsymbol{d}_i, \boldsymbol{\theta}_i)$.

Step 5. Set $\boldsymbol{\theta}^* = \boldsymbol{\theta}_i + \lambda_i \boldsymbol{d}_i$. Then set

$$\boldsymbol{\theta}_{i+1} = \begin{cases} \boldsymbol{\theta}^* & \text{with the probability } a(\boldsymbol{\theta}^*|\boldsymbol{\theta}_i), \\ \boldsymbol{\theta}_i & \text{otherwise,} \end{cases}$$

Step 6. Set $i = i + 1$, and go to Step 1.

The candidate sets and the assumptions for $g_i(\lambda|\boldsymbol{d}_i, \boldsymbol{\theta}_i)$, and $a(\boldsymbol{\theta}^*|\boldsymbol{\theta}_i)$ are the same as for the original H&R algorithm given in Section 2.3. Let $h_1, h_2, \ldots, h_n$ be a sample from the conditional-expectation H&R algorithm. Then, we can use

$$\hat{E}_{\text{cond}}(h) = \frac{1}{n}\sum_{i=1}^{n} h_i \tag{3.4.2}$$

as an estimator of $E(h(\boldsymbol{\theta})|D)$. Under ergodicity and nonnegative conditional correlations, Schmeiser and Chen (1991) show that

$$\lim_{n\to\infty} E(\hat{E}_{\text{cond}}(h)) = E(h(\boldsymbol{\theta})|D) \tag{3.4.3}$$

and

$$\text{Var}\left[\sum_{i=1}^{n} E(h(\boldsymbol{\theta}_i|\boldsymbol{d}_{i-1}, \boldsymbol{\theta}_{i-1}))\right] \le \text{Var}\left[\sum_{i=1}^{n} h(\boldsymbol{\theta}_i)\right]. \tag{3.4.4}$$

These results indicate that $\hat{E}_{\text{cond}}(h)$ is an asymptotically unbiased estimator of $E(h(\boldsymbol{\theta})|D)$ and the variance of the estimator is reduced by using the conditional expectation. Tierney (1994) also considers a similar conditional MC method for variance reduction. An example given in Tierney (1994) shows that the conditional MC method substantially improves the simulation accuracy of the MC estimates over the usual sample mean estimates.

Similar to the conditional MC method, the external control-variate technique (e.g., see Bratley, Fox, and Schrage 1987 or Nelson 1990) can also be used in MCMC sampling. Let $\pi_N(\boldsymbol{\theta})$ denote the probability density function (pdf) of a normal distribution $N_p(\boldsymbol{\mu}, \Sigma)$ with mean μ and covariance matrix Σ. Furthermore, assume

$$\xi_N = E_{\pi_N}(h) = \int_{R^p} h(\boldsymbol{\theta})\pi_N(\boldsymbol{\theta})\, d\boldsymbol{\theta}$$

is available, i.e., ξ_N can be analytically evaluated. Let $\{\boldsymbol{\theta}_i,\ i = 1, 2, \ldots, n\}$ and $\{\boldsymbol{z}_i,\ i = 1, 2, \ldots, n\}$ be the two MCMC samples from $\pi(\boldsymbol{\theta}|D)$ and $\pi_N(\boldsymbol{\theta})$, respectively. Then the control-variate estimator of $E(h(\boldsymbol{\theta})|D)$ is

$$\hat{E}_{\text{cv}}(h) = \hat{E}_{\text{avg}}(h) - \hat{\beta}(\hat{\xi}_N - \xi_N), \tag{3.4.5}$$

where

$$\hat{E}_{\text{avg}}(h) = \frac{1}{n}\sum_{i=1}^{n} h(\boldsymbol{\theta}_i), \quad \hat{\xi}_N = \frac{1}{n}\sum_{i=1}^{n} h(\boldsymbol{z}_i), \tag{3.4.6}$$

and $\hat{\beta}$ is a control-variate weight, which is typically some function of $\{\boldsymbol{\theta}_i\}$ and $\{\boldsymbol{z}_i\}$.

Inducing positive correlation between $\hat{E}_{\text{avg}}(h)$ and $\hat{\xi}_N$ is central for obtaining

$$\text{Var}(\hat{E}_{\text{cv}}(h)) < \text{Var}(\hat{E}_{\text{avg}}(h)).$$

We hope to obtain such a positive correlation by obtaining a sample path $\{\boldsymbol{\theta}_i\}$ that is similar to the sample path $\{\boldsymbol{z}_i\}$. Similar sample paths can arise by using the same $U(0,1)$ random numbers to obtain $\{\boldsymbol{\theta}_i\}$ and $\{\boldsymbol{z}_i\}$. For example, in the original H&R algorithm in Section 2.3, we might use one random number stream to generate random directions, another to generate random signed distances from g using the inverse transformation, and a third to accept or reject $\boldsymbol{\theta}^*$ based on $a(\boldsymbol{\theta}^*|\boldsymbol{\theta}_i)$. The sample paths are more similar if $a(\boldsymbol{\theta}^*|\boldsymbol{\theta}_i) = 1$, and in this case, the third stream is unnecessary.

Next, we present an adaptive external control-variate sampling algorithm for which we first obtain the initialized estimates of the optimal control-variate weight $\beta = \text{Cov}(h(\boldsymbol{\theta}_i), h(\boldsymbol{z}_i))/\text{Var}(h(\boldsymbol{z}_i))$, the normal mean $\boldsymbol{\mu}$, and covariance matrix Σ. Assume that an MCMC sampling algorithm such as the Gibbs sampler, the Metropolis–Hastings algorithm, or the H&R algorithm is used for generating $\{\boldsymbol{\theta}_i\}$ and $\{\boldsymbol{z}_i\}$. Then the following three steps are required:

Step 1. Initialization

Choose a starting normal distribution $N(\boldsymbol{\mu}, \Sigma)$. Let n_0 denote the number of iterations of the MCMC sampling algorithm. Let $\{\boldsymbol{\theta}_i^0,\ i = 1, 2, \ldots, n_0\}$ and $\{\boldsymbol{z}_i^0,\ i = 1, 2, \ldots, n_0\}$ be the two MCMC samples from $\pi(\boldsymbol{\theta}|D)$ and $\pi_N(\boldsymbol{\theta})$, respectively. Let $h_i^0 = h(\boldsymbol{\theta}_i^0), C_i^0 = h(\boldsymbol{z}_i^0), i = 1, 2, \ldots, n_0$, $H^0 = (h_1^0, h_2^0, \ldots, h_{n_0}^0)'$, and $C^0 = (C_1^0, C_2^0, \ldots, C_{n_0}^0)'$. Choose

$$\hat{\beta}^* = \frac{S_{C^0 H^0}}{S_{C^0 C^0}},$$

where

$$S_{C^0 C^0} = (n_0 - 1)^{-1} \sum_{i=1}^{n_0} (C_i^0 - \bar{C}^0)^2,$$

$$S_{C^0 H^0} = (n_0 - 1)^{-1} \sum_{i=1}^{n_0} (C_i^0 - \bar{C}^0)(h_i^0 - \bar{h}^0),$$

$$\bar{C}^0 = \frac{1}{n_0} \sum_{i=1}^{n_0} C_i^0, \text{ and } \bar{h}^0 = \frac{1}{n_0} \sum_{i=1}^{n_0} h_i^0.$$

Step 2. Updating

Choose

$$\hat{\boldsymbol{\mu}} = \frac{1}{n_0} \sum_{i=1}^{n_0} \boldsymbol{\theta}_i^0 \text{ and } \hat{\Sigma} = \frac{1}{n_0^2} \sum_{i=1}^{n_0} \sum_{j=1}^{n_0} (\boldsymbol{\theta}_i^0 - \hat{\boldsymbol{\mu}})(\boldsymbol{\theta}_j^0 - \hat{\boldsymbol{\mu}})'.$$

Let $\hat{\pi}_N(\theta)$ be the pdf of $N(\hat{\boldsymbol{\mu}}, \hat{\Sigma})$, and let

$$\xi_N = E_{\hat{\pi}_N}(h) = \int_{R^p} h(\boldsymbol{\theta})\hat{\pi}_N(\boldsymbol{\theta})\, d\boldsymbol{\theta}.$$

We assume ξ_N can be analytically evaluated. Then, we generate $\boldsymbol{z}_0^1 \sim N(\hat{\boldsymbol{\mu}}, \hat{\Sigma})$, and set $\boldsymbol{\theta}_0^1 = \boldsymbol{z}_0^1$. We restart the same MCMC sampling algorithm and use the same $U(0,1)$ random number stream to generate $\{\boldsymbol{\theta}_i^1,\ i = 1, 2, \ldots, n\}$ and $\{\boldsymbol{z}_i^1,\ i = 1, 2, \ldots, n\}$ from $\pi(\boldsymbol{\theta}|D)$ and $\hat{\pi}_N(\boldsymbol{\theta})$.

Step 3. Estimation

Compute $\hat{\xi}_N = (1/n)\sum_{i=1}^n h(\boldsymbol{z}_i^1)$, $\hat{E}_{\text{avg}}(h) = (1/n)\sum_{i=1}^n h(\boldsymbol{\theta}_i^1)$, and

$$\hat{E}_{\text{cv}}(h) = \hat{E}_{\text{avg}}(h) - \hat{\beta}^*(\hat{\xi}_N - \xi_N). \tag{3.4.7}$$

For the control-variate estimator $\hat{E}_{\text{cv}}(h)$, Schmeiser and Chen (1991) show that under the moment and ergodicity conditions,

$$\lim_{n\to\infty} \hat{E}_{\text{cv}}(h) = E(h(\boldsymbol{\theta})|D), \text{ almost surely.}$$

In the above control-variate sampling algorithm, the normal distribution $\pi_N(\boldsymbol{\theta})$ can be replaced by any other importance sampling distribution $g(\boldsymbol{\theta})$ as long as $\xi_g = \int_{R^p} h(\boldsymbol{\theta})g(\boldsymbol{\theta})\, d\boldsymbol{\theta}$ can be analytically computed.

3.4.2 Weighted Monte Carlo Estimates

In Section 3.2, we discussed the general weighted MC method of Trotter and Tukey (1956) and its variations. Ideally, the pair $(\boldsymbol{\theta}, w)$ should be sampled jointly from some distribution $\pi(\boldsymbol{\theta}, w)$. In general, it is difficult to construct $\pi(\boldsymbol{\theta}, w)$. The dynamic weighting algorithm of Wong and Liang (1997), discussed in Section 2.8, is an attempt in this regard. However, many of the weighted transition rules proposed by Liu, Liang, and Wong (1998b) lead to a marginal weight distribution that is long-tailed. This long-tailed weight distribution makes the resulting weighted estimates $\hat{E}_w(h)$ converge very slowly. To improve the weighted estimation, Wong and Liang (1997) suggest a *stratified truncation* method, and Liu, Liang, and Wong (1998b) provide theoretical support for the method. The stratified truncation method can be described as follows:

> *Suppose it is of interest to estimate $E(h(\boldsymbol{\theta})|D)$. First, the sample points $(\boldsymbol{\theta}_i, w_i)$ are stratified according to the value of the function $h(\boldsymbol{\theta})$. Within each stratum, the function h should be as close to constant as possible and the sizes of the strata should be comparable. The highest $k\%$ (usually $k = 1$ or 2) of the weights within each stratum are then trimmed down to the value of the $(100-k)^{\text{th}}$ percentile of the weights within the stratum.*

The examples given in Liu, Liang, and Wong (1998b) empirically show that this method works to a satisfactory degree of accuracy. But it is still not clear whether this method can be better than a usual MC method, that is, constructing an estimate of $E(h(\boldsymbol{\theta})|D)$ using a stationary MCMC sample $\{\boldsymbol{\theta}_i\}$ from $\pi(\boldsymbol{\theta}|D)$. Further research in this direction needs to be done in the future.

Next, we consider a situation in which only the stationary MCMC sample $\{\boldsymbol{\theta}_i\}$ from $\pi(\boldsymbol{\theta}|D)$ is available. Again, it is of interest to estimate the posterior expectation $E(h(\boldsymbol{\theta})|D)$. In practice, one of the most commonly used estimates is the usual sample mean $\hat{E}_{\text{avg}}(h)$ given in (3.2.4). Alternatively, we can also construct a weighted MC estimator

$$\hat{E}_w(h) = \sum_{i=1}^{n} w_i h(\boldsymbol{\theta}_i), \tag{3.4.8}$$

where the w_i's are the fixed weights subject to

$$\sum_{i=1}^{n} w_i = 1. \tag{3.4.9}$$

Then, we are led to the following theorem:

Theorem 3.4.1 *Let Σ denote the covariance matrix of $h(\boldsymbol{\theta}_1)$, $h(\boldsymbol{\theta}_2)$, $\ldots$, $h(\boldsymbol{\theta}_n)$. Then, the value of $\boldsymbol{w} = (w_1, w_2, \ldots, w_n)'$ that minimizes the variance of $\hat{E}_w(h)$ in (3.4.8) is*

$$\boldsymbol{w}_{\text{opt}} = \frac{\Sigma^{-1}\mathbf{1}}{\mathbf{1}'\Sigma^{-1}\mathbf{1}}, \tag{3.4.10}$$

where $\mathbf{1} = (1, 1, \ldots, 1)'$, and the optimal weighted MC estimator is given by

$$\hat{E}_{\text{opt}}(h) = (h(\boldsymbol{\theta}_1), h(\boldsymbol{\theta}_2), \ldots, h(\boldsymbol{\theta}_n))\boldsymbol{w}_{\text{opt}} \tag{3.4.11}$$

with variance

$$\text{Var}(\hat{E}_{\text{opt}}(h)) = \frac{1}{\mathbf{1}'\Sigma^{-1}\mathbf{1}}. \tag{3.4.12}$$

The proof of this theorem simply follows from the Lagrange multiplier method, and thus it is left as an exercise. We note that this result is also derived by Peng (1998).

In Theorem 3.4.1, the covariance matrix can be expressed as

$$\Sigma = \sigma^2(\rho_{jj^*}), \tag{3.4.13}$$

where ρ_{jj^*} denotes the correlation between $h(\boldsymbol{\theta}_j)$ and $h(\boldsymbol{\theta}_{j^*})$, and σ^2 is the variance of $h(\boldsymbol{\theta}_i)$. This is true because $\{\boldsymbol{\theta}_i\}$ is a stationary MCMC sample, and thus all of the $h(\boldsymbol{\theta}_i)$'s have the same marginal variances. In addition, if $\Sigma = \sigma^2 I_n$, i.e., the $\boldsymbol{\theta}_i$'s are i.i.d. observations, then $\boldsymbol{w}_{\text{opt}} = (1/n)\mathbf{1}$, and the optimal weighted MC estimate $\hat{E}_{\rm opt}(h)$ reduces to

$$\hat{E}_{\rm avg}(h) = \frac{1}{n}\sum_{i=1}^{n} h(\boldsymbol{\theta}_i)$$

with variance σ^2/n. Thus, for i.i.d. samples, the usual sample mean of the $h(\boldsymbol{\theta}_i)$ is the best estimate of $E(h(\boldsymbol{\theta})|D)$.

In practice, the covariance matrix Σ is unknown. Note that σ^2 in (3.4.13) need not be known since it cancels in (3.4.11). Therefore, if Σ is a banded matrix, then the correlations ρ_{jj^*}'s in (3.4.13) can be approximated by the sample correlations of the $h(\boldsymbol{\theta}_i)$'s. The resulting approximate optimal weighted MC estimate can still be computed numerically. However, its asymptotic properties need to be investigated further in future research.

It is easy to verify that the optimal weights given in (3.4.10) satisfy the restriction (3.4.9). But each component of $\boldsymbol{w}_{\rm opt}$ is not necessarily nonnegative. This property is indeed advantageous. Allowing negative weights leads to the following illustrative example:

Example 3.2. Independent sample versus dependent sample. In MC estimation, it is usually believed that only negative correlations help improve the MC estimates. In this example, we will illustrate that with the optimal weights, positive correlations can also be helpful.

Let θ_1, θ_2, and θ_3 be i.i.d. observations with a common variance σ^2. Then the usual sample mean is

$$\hat{\theta} = \frac{1}{3}\sum_{i=1}^{3} \theta_i$$

with variance

$$\text{Var}(\hat{\theta}) = \frac{\sigma^2}{3}.$$

Also let ξ_1, ξ_2, and ξ_3 be dependent observations with covariance matrix

$$\Sigma = \sigma^2 \begin{pmatrix} 1 & 0.7 & 0 \\ 0.7 & 1 & 0.7 \\ 0 & 0.7 & 1 \end{pmatrix}.$$

Then ξ_i has the same marginal variance as θ_i. Using (3.4.10), (3.4.11), and (3.4.12), the optimal weighted MC estimator is given by

$$\hat{\xi}_{\rm opt} = 1.5\xi_1 - 2\xi_2 + 1.5\xi_3$$

with variance

$$\text{Var}(\hat{\xi}_{\rm opt}) = \frac{\sigma^2}{10}.$$

Therefore,

$$\frac{\mathrm{Var}(\hat{\theta})}{\mathrm{Var}(\hat{\xi}_{\mathrm{opt}})} = \frac{10}{3}.$$

Thus, the optimal weighted MC estimate with the dependent sample has a variance that is less one-third of the variance of the optimal estimate with the independent sample.

As discussed earlier, the usual sample mean is the best estimate for i.i.d. observations. When $\{\boldsymbol{\theta}_i\}$ is an MCMC sample so that $\Sigma \neq \sigma^2 I_n$, $\hat{E}_{\mathrm{opt}}(h)$ given in (3.4.11) is not equal to the sample mean $\hat{E}_{\mathrm{avg}}(h)$. Therefore, it is interesting to investigate how much improvement can be made by using the optimal estimate over the usual sample mean. In this regard, we consider the sample mean of ξ_1, ξ_2, and ξ_3 given in Example 3.2. Let

$$\hat{\xi}_{\mathrm{avg}} = \tfrac{1}{3}(\xi_1 + \xi_2 + \xi_3).$$

Then the variance of $\hat{\xi}_{\mathrm{avg}}$ is given by

$$\mathrm{Var}(\hat{\xi}_{\mathrm{avg}}) = 5.8\sigma^2/9.$$

and

$$\frac{\mathrm{Var}(\hat{\xi}_{\mathrm{avg}})}{\mathrm{Var}(\hat{\xi}_{\mathrm{opt}})} = \frac{58}{9}.$$

Thus, the optimal weighted MC estimate is much better than the usual sample mean. However, when n is large, this advantage may disappear. We use a dependent sample from an AR(1) process to illustrate the idea.

Example 3.3. A dependent sample from an AR(1) process. Assume that $\{\theta_1, \theta_2, \ldots, \theta_n\}$ is a dependent sample from an AR(1) process with marginal variance σ^2 and lag-one autocorrelation ρ. Consider $h(\theta) = \theta$. Then, using (3.3.9), the variance of the usual sample mean of the $h(\theta_i)$ can be expressed as

$$\mathrm{Var}(\hat{E}_{\mathrm{avg}}(h)) = \frac{\sigma^2}{n}\left[\frac{1+\rho}{1-\rho} - \frac{2\rho(1-\rho^n)}{n(1-\rho)^2}\right].$$

Using (3.4.10) and (3.4.11), it can be shown that the optimal fixed weighted estimator is given by

$$\hat{E}_{\mathrm{opt}}(h) = \frac{\theta_1 + (1-\rho)\sum_{i=2}^{n-1}\theta_i + \theta_n}{n-(n-2)\rho}$$

with variance

$$\mathrm{Var}(\hat{E}_{\mathrm{opt}}(h)) = \frac{\sigma^2(1+\rho)}{n-(n-2)\rho}.$$

Thus,

$$\lim_{n\to\infty}[\mathrm{Var}(\hat{E}_{\mathrm{opt}}(h))/\mathrm{Var}(\hat{E}_{\mathrm{avg}}(h))] = 1,$$

which implies that the usual sample mean is as efficient as the optimal weighted estimator asymptotically.

From Example 3.3 and previous discussions, it is clear that the weighted estimator cannot substantially improve the simulation efficiency over the usual sample mean if the weight w_i is fixed (not random). Thus, in order to obtain a better weighted estimator, the weight w_i must be random or depend on the sample $\boldsymbol{\theta}_i$ in a particular functional form. Chen and Shao (1999c) propose a new weighted estimator by partitioning the support of the posterior distribution, and they show that this new estimator can always be better than the usual sample mean for an i.i.d. sample.

Let $\boldsymbol{\theta}_1$, $\boldsymbol{\theta}_2$, ..., $\boldsymbol{\theta}_n$ denote n i.i.d. random variables from $\pi(\boldsymbol{\theta}|D)$ defined on a p-dimensional Euclidean space R^p, and let h be a real-valued function. Assume that $\mu = E[h(\boldsymbol{\theta})] \neq 0$ and $\sigma^2 = \mathrm{Var}(h(\boldsymbol{\theta})) < \infty$, where the expectation and variance are taken with respect to the posterior distribution $\pi(\boldsymbol{\theta}|D)$. Let $\Omega \subset R^p$ denote the support of $\pi(\boldsymbol{\theta}|D)$, and let $A_1, A_2, \ldots, A_\kappa$ be a partition of Ω such that: (i) $\cup_{l=1}^{\kappa} A_1 = \Omega$; (ii) $A_l \cap A_{l^*} = \emptyset$ for $l \neq l^*$; and (iii) $\int_{A_l} \pi(\boldsymbol{\theta}|D)\, d\boldsymbol{\theta} > 0$ for $l = 1, 2, \ldots, \kappa$. Also, let

$$\mu_l = E\left[h(\boldsymbol{\theta})1\{\boldsymbol{\theta} \in A_l\}\right] \quad \text{and} \quad b_l = E\left[h^2(\boldsymbol{\theta})1\{\boldsymbol{\theta} \in A_l\}\right]. \tag{3.4.14}$$

Then the new weighted MC estimator of $\mu = E[h(\boldsymbol{\theta})]$ proposed by Chen and Shao (1999c) is of the form

$$\hat{E}_a(h) = \frac{1}{n}\sum_{i=1}^{n}\sum_{l=1}^{\kappa} a_l h(\boldsymbol{\theta}_i)1\{\boldsymbol{\theta}_i \in A_l\}, \tag{3.4.15}$$

where $a = (a_1, a_2, \ldots, a_\kappa)'$ is a vector of fixed weights subject to

$$\sum_{l=1}^{\kappa} a_l \mu_l = \mu. \tag{3.4.16}$$

The constraint given in (3.4.16) guarantees the unbiasedness of the weighted estimator $\hat{E}_a(h)$. It follows from straightforward algebra that the variance of $\hat{E}_a(h)$ is given by

$$\mathrm{Var}(\hat{E}_a(h)) = \frac{1}{n}\left(\sum_{l=1}^{\kappa} a_l^2 b_l - \mu^2\right). \tag{3.4.17}$$

Since the $\boldsymbol{\theta}_i$'s are i.i.d. observations, the variance of the usual sample mean estimator is σ^2/n. The following theorem states that the weighted estimator given by (3.4.15) can be always better than the usual sample mean:

Theorem 3.4.2 *The value of $a = (a_1, a_2, \ldots, a_\kappa)'$ that minimizes the variance of $\hat{E}_a(h)$ in (3.4.17) is given by*

$$a_{\text{opt},l} = \frac{\mu_l}{b_l} \frac{\mu}{\sum_{j=1}^{\kappa} \mu_j^2 / b_j} \quad \textit{for } l = 1, 2, \ldots, \kappa. \tag{3.4.18}$$

Let $a_{\text{opt}} = (a_{\text{opt},1}, a_{\text{opt},2}, \ldots, a_{\text{opt},\kappa})'$. Then, the optimal weighted estimator $\hat{E}_{a_{\text{opt}}}(h)$ has variance

$$\text{Var}(\hat{E}_{a_{\text{opt}}}(h)) = \frac{1}{n}\Big(\frac{\mu^2}{\sum_{l=1}^{\kappa} \mu_l^2 / b_l} - \mu^2\Big), \tag{3.4.19}$$

and

$$\text{Var}(\hat{E}_{a_{\text{opt}}}(h)) \leq \text{Var}(\hat{E}_{\text{avg}}(h)) = \frac{\sigma^2}{n}, \tag{3.4.20}$$

where μ_l and b_l are defined by (3.4.14).

The proof of Theorem 3.4.2 is given in the Appendix. We note that equality in (3.4.20) holds if and only if

$$b_l = c_0 |\mu_l| \quad \text{for } l = 1, 2, \ldots, \kappa, \tag{3.4.21}$$

and $|\mu| = \sum_{l=1}^{\kappa} |\mu_l|$, where $c_0 = E(h^2(\theta))/|\mu|$ is a constant. Although a_l is a fixed weight, the estimate $\hat{E}_a(h)$ indeed uses random weights. Let $w_i = \sum_{l=1}^{\kappa} a_l 1\{\theta_i \in A_l\}$. Then, we can rewrite (3.4.15) as

$$\hat{E}_a(h) = \sum_{i=1}^{n} w_i h(\boldsymbol{\theta}_i).$$

Clearly, w_i is random, and in fact, it is a function of $\boldsymbol{\theta}_i$.

From (3.4.19), it can be observed that if $h(\boldsymbol{\theta}_i)$ is nearly constant for $\boldsymbol{\theta}_i \in A_l$, then $\mu_l^2/b_l \approx \pi(A_l|D)$, where $\pi(A_l|D)$ is the posterior probability of A_l. Thus, the resulting optimal variance is approximately 0. This is a useful feature, since it can be used as a guideline for choosing the partition $\{A_l,\ l = 1, 2, \ldots, \kappa\}$ of Ω. In (3.4.18), the optimal weights, $a_{\text{opt},l}$'s, depend on the unknown posterior quantity μ. The optimal weighted estimator $\hat{E}_{a_{\text{opt}}}(h)$ appears to be not directly useful. However, if $\mu_l = p_l \mu$, where p_l is known or it can be estimated, $\hat{E}_{a_{\text{opt}}}(h)$ can be attractive. In fact, this will be the case when our interest is in estimating ratios of normalizing constants. We will discuss this application in detail in Section 5.11.

3.5 Controlling Simulation Errors

If samples are generated by an MCMC sampling algorithm, the factors that influence the quality of point estimators include *sampling error*, *estimation bias*, and *systematic bias.* Sampling error arises from the difference between the observed sample and the underlying population; estimator bias arises from using either a biased estimator or a nonrepresentative sample (caused by the initial transient); systematic bias arises from programming error, numerical error, or the use of pseudo-random numbers.

In our experience, the Gibbs sampler seems more sensitive than Metropolis–Hastings algorithms (such as H&R) to systematic bias. Using the same (uniform) random number and (nonuniform) random variate generators, Chen and Schmeiser (1993) find examples where the empirical Gibbs sampler behavior does not match known asymptotic behavior, while the H&R sampler behaves as expected; changing generators causes both algorithms to behave as expected. The straightforward logic of the Gibbs sampler might explain this sensitivity. The $(i(p-1)+j)^{\text{th}}$ random number $U_{i(p-1)+j}$ is transformed into $\theta_{(i),j}$, so lack of p-dimensional uniformity in the pseudorandom number generator is passed directly to the Gibbs sampler results. Note that, here, p is the dimension of the vector θ. Other MCMC sampling algorithms, such as the H&R, use more complicated transformations, which might ameliorate this effect. Systematic bias can be tested by comparing with known solutions for simple problems or by comparing with the known asymptotic performance. In the following discussion, we assume that the experiment has no systematic error.

Now consider sampling error and estimation bias as a function of autocorrelation. Suppose $\{\boldsymbol{\theta}_i, i \geq 1\}$ is a stationary Markov process. Let $\mu = E(h(\boldsymbol{\theta}_i))$, $\sigma^2 = \text{Var}(h(\boldsymbol{\theta}_i))$, and $\rho_t = \text{Corr}(h(\boldsymbol{\theta}_i), h(\boldsymbol{\theta}_{i+t}))$, where $h(\cdot)$ is a real-valued function. Then, the usual estimates of the mean and variance of $h(\boldsymbol{\theta}_i)$ are the sample mean and sample variance

$$\hat{\mu} = \frac{1}{n}\sum_{i=1}^{n} h(\boldsymbol{\theta}_i) \quad \text{and} \quad \hat{\sigma}^2 = \frac{1}{n-1}\sum_{i=1}^{n}(h(\boldsymbol{\theta}_i) - \hat{\mu})^2.$$

If $\{\boldsymbol{\theta}_i, 1 \leq i \leq n\}$ is a random sample, then the standard error of $\hat{\mu}$ is $\sigma/\sqrt{n}$. But now, because of dependence,

$$n \ \text{Var}(\hat{\mu}) = \sigma^2 \left[1 + 2\sum_{t=1}^{n-1}\left(1 - \frac{t}{n}\right)\rho_t\right]. \tag{3.5.1}$$

Since ρ_t is often positive (Tierney 1994; Liu, Wong, and Kong 1995; Schmeiser and Chen 1991), the standard error for dependent observations is larger than that for i.i.d. observations. Furthermore,

$$\begin{aligned} E(\hat{\sigma}^2) &= \frac{1}{n-1}\left[n\sigma^2 - n \ \text{Var}(\hat{\mu})\right] \\ &= \sigma^2 \left[1 - \frac{2}{n-1}\sum_{t=1}^{n-1}\left(1 - \frac{t}{n}\right)\rho_t\right]. \end{aligned} \tag{3.5.2}$$

So, the autocorrelation obtained by an MCMC sampling algorithm increases the standard error (se) of $\hat{\mu}$ and gives a biased estimator, $\hat{\sigma}^2$, of σ^2. Furthermore, from (3.5.1) and (3.5.2), we have the asymptotic result

$$(\text{se}(\hat{\mu}))^2 \doteq |\text{bias}(\hat{\sigma}^2)|,$$

for large n. We recommend using these results to verify simulation experiments when checking programming, numerical, and initial-transient errors.

Next, we discuss the choice of experimental design (which $\boldsymbol{\theta}$ observations to generate) and the choice of point estimator (primarily, which $\boldsymbol{\theta}$ observations to include when computing the point estimator). We consider estimation bias and the standard error arising in three experimental designs.

First, at one extreme, as described by Tierney (1994), we can independently generate n parallel Markov chains of length m, denoted by $\boldsymbol{\theta}_{i,j}$ for $j = 1, 2, \ldots, m$ and $i = 1, 2, \ldots, n$. Then, we use only the last observation $\boldsymbol{\theta}_{i,m}$ from the ith chain to compute the point estimator. The disadvantage is the difficulty of determining a value of m that balances the initial-transient estimation bias with the wasted data. In addition, a large amount of data is wasted.

Second, at the other extreme, we can generate a single long run of length nm, using all observations $\boldsymbol{\theta}_1, \ldots, \boldsymbol{\theta}_{nm}$ in the point estimator, possibly after discarding the j_0 initial observations $\boldsymbol{\theta}_{-j_0+1}, \ldots, \boldsymbol{\theta}_0$. Although exceptions can occur, a single long run usually provides the best point estimator for a fixed number of observations nm, since a single long run simultaneously reduces the standard error and the bias. Whitt (1991) discusses this issue, focusing on queueing simulations. The disadvantage is that the autocorrelation between observations complicates standard-error estimation. Estimating standard errors of general point estimators from stationary autocorrelated data requires (either implicitly or explicitly) including the autocorrelations in the standard error estimate. Several methods are discussed in Section 3.3.

Third, between these two extremes, we can use each of n i.i.d. chains of length m to obtain n point estimates, each based on $\boldsymbol{\theta}_{i,1}$, $\boldsymbol{\theta}_{i,2}$, $\ldots$, $\boldsymbol{\theta}_{i,m}$. These n independent point estimates are averaged to obtain a single point estimator with an easy-to-compute standard error estimate. The advantage and disadvantage of the third approach is that it combines the best and worst of the first two approaches. Consider, for example, estimating the marginal variance σ^2. Let $\hat{\sigma}^2(i)$ be the estimate of σ^2 from the ith chain of length m. Then the estimate of σ^2 is $(1/n)\sum_{i=1}^{n} \hat{\sigma}^2(i)$, which has the same bias as a single $\hat{\sigma}^2(i)$, since the bias depends only on the run length m.

Appendix

Proof of Theorem 3.4.2. The derivation of the optimal a_{opt}, given in (3.4.18), directly follows from the Lagrange multiplier method. We obtain (3.4.19) by plugging a_{opt} into (3.4.17). Noting that $\sum_{l=1}^{\kappa} b_l = E[h^2(\boldsymbol{\theta})]$, we have, by the Cauchy–Schwarz inequality,

$$\begin{aligned}\frac{\mu^2}{\sum_{l=1}^{\kappa}\mu_l^2/b_l} &= \frac{\mu^2}{(\sum_{l=1}^{\kappa}|\mu_l|)^2}\frac{\left(\sum_{l=1}^{\kappa}b_l^{1/2}|\mu_l|/b_l^{1/2}\right)^2}{\sum_{l=1}^{\kappa}\mu_l^2/b_l}\\ &\le \frac{\mu^2}{(\sum_{l=1}^{\kappa}|\mu_l|)^2}\sum_{l=1}^{\kappa}b_l\\ &\le E[h^2(\boldsymbol{\theta})].\end{aligned}$$

This shows that the variance of $\hat{E}_{a_{\text{opt}}}(h)$ is always less than or equal to σ^2/n. □

Exercises

3.1 For the Poisson random effects model discussed in Section 2.6.4, after hierarchical centering, (2.5.28) gives the joint posterior distribution for the model parameters $\boldsymbol{\theta} = (\boldsymbol{\beta}, \sigma^2, \rho, \boldsymbol{\eta})$. That is,

$$\begin{aligned}\pi(\boldsymbol{\theta}|D) \propto &\exp\{\boldsymbol{y}'\boldsymbol{\eta} - J_n'Q(\boldsymbol{\eta}) - J_n'C(\boldsymbol{y})\}\\ &\times (2\pi\sigma^2)^{-n/2}(1-\rho^2)^{-(n-1)/2}\\ &\times \exp\left\{-\frac{1}{2\sigma^2}(\boldsymbol{\eta} - X\boldsymbol{\beta})'\Sigma^{-1}(\boldsymbol{\eta} - X\boldsymbol{\beta})\right\},\end{aligned}$$

where $\boldsymbol{y} = (y_1, \ldots, y_n)'$, $\Sigma = (\sigma_{ij})$ with $\sigma_{ij} = \rho^{|i-j|}$, X is an $n \times p$ matrix, β is a p-dimensional vector of regression coefficients, $\boldsymbol{\eta} = (\eta_1, \eta_2, \ldots, \eta_n)'$, and $Q(\boldsymbol{\eta})$ is an $n \times 1$ vector with the tth element equal to $q_t = \exp(\eta_t)$.

(a) Let $\pi(\boldsymbol{\beta}^*|D)$ be the marginal posterior density of $\boldsymbol{\beta}$ evaluated at $\boldsymbol{\beta}^*$. Show that $\pi(\boldsymbol{\beta}^*|D)$ is an integral-type posterior quantity, i.e., there exists an $h(\boldsymbol{\beta}^*, \boldsymbol{\theta})$ such that

$$\pi(\boldsymbol{\beta}^*|D) = \int h(\boldsymbol{\beta}^*, \boldsymbol{\theta})\pi(\boldsymbol{\theta}|D)\, d\boldsymbol{\theta}.$$

(b) Is the choice of h in Part (a) unique? If not, list all possible choices of h.

3.2 Prove (3.3.9) and (3.3.11).

3.3 For the weighted MC estimate, $\hat{E}_w(h)$, given by (3.2.3), derive an expression for the simulation standard error $\text{se}(\hat{E}_w(h))$ using the overlapping batch statistics method.

3.4 Let $\{\boldsymbol{\theta}_i, i = 1, 2, ...\}$ be a stationary sequence and also let

$$\hat{E}_{n,\text{avg}}(h) = \frac{1}{n}\sum_{i=1}^{n} h(\boldsymbol{\theta}_i) \tag{3.E.1}$$

denote the sample mean of $h(\boldsymbol{\theta}_i)$. Assume that

$$\sum_{i=1}^{\infty} |\text{Cov}(h(\boldsymbol{\theta}_1), h(\boldsymbol{\theta}_i))| < \infty. \tag{3.E.2}$$

Prove that the variance of $\hat{E}_{n,\text{avg}}(h)$ is approximately equal to σ^2/n, where

$$\sigma^2 = \text{Var}(h(\boldsymbol{\theta}_1)) + 2\sum_{i=2}^{\infty} \text{Cov}(h(\boldsymbol{\theta}_1), h(\boldsymbol{\theta}_i)). \tag{3.E.3}$$

3.5 Asymptotic Approach of Standard Error Estimation (Peligrad and Shao 1994, 1995)
Let

$$\sigma_{n,1}^2 = \frac{1}{\ln(n)}\sum_{i=1}^{n} (\hat{E}_{i,\text{avg}}(h) - \hat{E}_{n,\text{avg}}(h))^2$$

and

$$\sigma_{n,2}^2 = \frac{1}{n^{1/2}}\sum_{i=1}^{n-n^{1/2}} (\hat{E}^*_{i,\text{avg}}(h) - \hat{E}_{n,\text{avg}}(h))^2,$$

where $\hat{E}_{n,\text{avg}}(h)$ is given by (3.E.1), and

$$\hat{E}^*_{i,\text{avg}}(h) = n^{-1/2}\sum_{l=i+1}^{i+n^{1/2}} h(\boldsymbol{\theta}_l).$$

(a) Prove that under the assumption (3.E.2), $\sigma_{n,1}^2$ and $\sigma_{n,2}^2$ are asymptotically unbiased estimators of σ^2, i.e.,

$$\lim_{n\to\infty} E\left(\sigma_{n,j}^2\right) = \sigma^2 \text{ for } j = 1, 2.$$

(b) Use Part (a) and Exercise 3.4 to obtain the simulation standard error of $\hat{E}_{n,\text{avg}}(h)$ based on $\sigma_{n,1}^2$ or $\sigma_{n,2}^2$.

3.6 Let $\{\boldsymbol{\theta}_i, i = 1, 2, ...\}$ be an independent sequence from the same population, and let $\sigma_{n,1}^2$ and $\sigma_{n,2}^2$ be defined as in Exercise 3.5. Prove that $\sigma_{n,1}^2$ and $\sigma_{n,2}^2$ are weak consistent estimators of σ^2 if $E[h^4(\boldsymbol{\theta}_1)] < \infty$, i.e., for $\forall \epsilon > 0$,

$$P\left(\lim_{n\to\infty} |\sigma^2_{n,1} - \sigma^2| \geq \epsilon\right) = 0, \quad j = 1, 2.$$

Under what conditions is the above result still true for a stationary sequence?

3.7 CONDITIONING IN MCMC (Geyer 1995a)
Suppose $\pi(\boldsymbol{\theta}|D) = \pi(\theta_1, \theta_2|D)$ is a bivariate normal distribution with mean 0 and covariance matrix $\begin{pmatrix} 1 & \rho \\ \rho & 1 \end{pmatrix}$. Using the Gibbs sampler described in Section 2.1, (2.1.1) defines the Gibbs sampling path

$$\begin{aligned}\theta_{1,i+1} &= \rho\theta_{2,i} + \sqrt{1-\rho^2}z_{1,i+1},\\ \theta_{2,i+1} &= \rho\theta_{1,i+1} + \sqrt{1-\rho^2}z_{2,i+1},\end{aligned}$$

for $i \geq 0$, where $z_{j,i+1}$, $i \geq 0$ and $j = 1, 2$, are i.i.d. $N(0, 1)$ random variables.

(a) Show that

$$\begin{aligned}\mathrm{Cov}(\theta_{1,i}, \theta_{1,i+t}) &= \rho^{2t},\\ \mathrm{Cov}(\theta_{2,i}, \theta_{2,i+t}) &= \rho^{2t},\\ \mathrm{Cov}(\theta_{1,i}, \theta_{2,i+t}) &= \rho^{2t+1},\\ \mathrm{Cov}(\theta_{2,i}, \theta_{1,i+t}) &= \rho^{|2t-1|}.\end{aligned}$$

(b) Consider integrating a linear function $h(\theta_1, \theta_2) = \theta_1 - b\theta_2$, where b is some constant, and compare this to integrating

$$g(\theta_1, \theta_2) = E(h(\theta_1, \theta_2)|\theta_2, D) = (\rho - b)\theta_2.$$

Show that the autocovariances for these functionals sum to

$$\begin{aligned}\sigma^2(h) &= \gamma_0 + 2\sum_{t=1}^{\infty}\gamma_t\\ &= (1 + b^2) - 2\rho b + 2\frac{\rho}{1-\rho^2}[(1+b^2)\rho - b(1+\rho^2)],\end{aligned}$$

where $\gamma_t = \mathrm{Cov}(h(\boldsymbol{\theta}_i), h(\boldsymbol{\theta}_{i+t}))$, and

$$\sigma^2(g) = (\rho - b)^2\frac{1+\rho^2}{1-\rho^2}.$$

(c) Use a plot of $\sigma^2(g)/\sigma^2(h)$ versus (ρ, b) to show that $\sigma^2(g)$ can be larger than $\sigma^2(h)$, and therefore, conditioning does worse.

3.8 Consider the bivariate normal model discussed in Examples 2.1 and 3.1. Let $\{\boldsymbol{\theta}_i = (\theta_{1,i}, \theta_{2,i}),\ i = 1, 2, \ldots, n\}$ denote a sample generated by the Gibbs sampler. Then, a consistent estimator of $E(\theta_1^2)$ is given by

$$\hat{E}_{\text{avg}}(\theta_1^2) = \frac{1}{n}\sum_{i=1}^{n} \theta_{1,i}^2. \tag{3.E.4}$$

As an alternative to (3.E.4), the Rao–Blackwellized estimator of $E(\theta_1^2)$ is given by

$$\hat{E}_{\text{cond}}(\theta_1^2) = \frac{1}{n}\sum_{i=1}^{n} E(\theta_1^2|\theta_{2,i}), \tag{3.E.5}$$

where the conditional expectation is taken with respect to the conditional distribution $N(\mu_1 + \rho(\sigma_1/\sigma_2)(\theta_{2,i} - \mu_2), \sigma_1^2(1-\rho^2))$.

(a) Obtain a closed-form expression of $\hat{E}_{\text{cond}}(\theta_1^2)$.
(b) Find $\text{Var}(\hat{E}_{\text{avg}}(\theta_1^2))$ and $\text{Var}(\hat{E}_{\text{cond}}(\theta_1^2))$.
(c) Compare $\text{Var}(\hat{E}_{\text{avg}}(\theta_1^2))$ to $\text{Var}(\hat{E}_{\text{cond}}(\theta_1^2))$. Does the Rao–Blackwellized estimator result in a smaller variance?

3.9 Prove that if the conditional covariance of $h(\boldsymbol{\theta}_i)$ and $h(\boldsymbol{\theta}_j)$ given d_{j-1} and $\boldsymbol{\theta}_{j-1}$ is finite and nonnegative for $i > j$, then (3.4.4) holds.

3.10 Prove Theorem 3.4.1.

3.11 Let $\{\boldsymbol{\theta}_i = (\theta_{1,i}, \theta_{2,i}),\ i = 1, 2, \ldots, n\}$ denote a sample generated by the Gibbs sampler from the bivariate normal model discussed in Examples 2.1 and 3.1. Then, a weighted MC estimator of $E(\theta_1^2)$ is given by

$$\hat{E}_w(\theta_1^2) = \frac{1}{n}\sum_{i=1}^{n} w_i \theta_{1,i}^2,$$

where $\sum_{i=1}^{n} w_i = 1$.

(a) Obtain a closed-form expression for w_{opt} given by (3.4.10) for $\hat{E}_w(\theta_1^2)$.
(b) Use (3.4.12) to compute $\text{Var}(\hat{E}_{\text{opt}}(\theta_1^2))$.
(c) How does the optimal weighted MC estimator compare to the Rao–Blackwellized estimator $\hat{E}_{\text{cond}}(\theta_1^2)$ given in Exercise 3.8?

3.12 It is common to use pseudo (uniform) random number generators in the implementation of MCMC sampling or to perform a simulation study. As is well known, the simulation results depend on the choice of *initial* random number seed(s).

Suppose that we want to implement ten multiple runs in MCMC sampling or to run ten simulations in a simulation study. Consider the following two experimental designs:

Experiment I	Experiment II
iseed1	iseed
run 1	run 1
iseed2	run2
run 2	
...	...
iseed10	run10
run 10	

In Experiment I, ten initial pseudo-random number seeds (iseed1 to iseed10) are used, while only one initial random number seed (iseed) is used in Experiment II. Which experiment is preferable and why?

4

Estimating Marginal Posterior Densities

In Bayesian inference, a joint posterior distribution is available through the likelihood function and a prior distribution. One purpose of Bayesian inference is to calculate and display marginal posterior densities because the marginal posterior densities provide complete information about parameters of interest. As shown in Chapter 2, a Markov chain Monte Carlo (MCMC) sampling algorithm, such as the Gibbs sampler or a Metropolis–Hastings algorithm, can be used to draw MCMC samples from the posterior distribution. Chapter 3 also demonstrates how we can easily obtain posterior quantities such as posterior means, posterior standard deviations, and other posterior quantities from MCMC samples. However, when a Bayesian model becomes complicated, it may be difficult to obtain a reliable estimator of a marginal posterior density based on the MCMC sample. A traditional method for estimating marginal posterior densities is kernel density estimation. Since the kernel density estimator is nonparametric, it may not be efficient. On the other hand, the kernel density estimator may not be applicable for some complicated Bayesian models. In the context of Bayesian inference, the joint posterior density is typically known up to a normalizing constant. Using the structure of a posterior density, a number of authors (e.g., Gelfand, Smith, and Lee 1992; Johnson 1992; Chen 1993 and 1994; Chen and Shao 1997c; Chib 1995; Verdinelli and Wasserman 1995) propose parametric marginal posterior density estimators based on the MCMC sample. In this chapter, we present several available Monte Carlo (MC) methods for computing marginal posterior density estimators, and we also discuss how well marginal posterior density estimation works using the Kullback–Leibler (K–L) divergence as a performance measure.

4.1 Marginal Posterior Densities

Let $\boldsymbol{\theta}$ be a p-dimensional column vector of parameters. Assume that the joint posterior density, $\pi(\boldsymbol{\theta}|D)$, is of the form

$$\pi(\boldsymbol{\theta}|D) = \frac{L(\boldsymbol{\theta}|D)\pi(\boldsymbol{\theta})}{c(D)}, \tag{4.1.1}$$

where D denotes *data*, $L(\boldsymbol{\theta}|D)$ is the likelihood function given data D, $\pi(\boldsymbol{\theta})$ is the prior, and $c(D)$ is the unknown normalizing constant. Let Ω denote the support of the joint posterior density $\pi(\boldsymbol{\theta}|D)$. Also let

$$\boldsymbol{\theta}^{(j)} = (\theta_1, \dots, \theta_j)' \quad \text{and} \quad \boldsymbol{\theta}^{(-j)} = (\theta_{j+1}, \dots, \theta_p)'$$

be the first j and last $p - j$ components of $\boldsymbol{\theta}$, respectively. The support of the conditional joint marginal posterior density of $\boldsymbol{\theta}^{(j)}$ given $\boldsymbol{\theta}^{(-j)}$ is denoted by

$$\Omega_j(\boldsymbol{\theta}^{(-j)}) = \{(\theta_1, \dots, \theta_j)' : \ (\theta_1, \dots, \theta_j, \theta_{j+1}, \dots, \theta_p)' \in \Omega\}, \tag{4.1.2}$$

and the subspace of Ω, given the first j components $\boldsymbol{\theta}^{*(j)} = (\theta_1^*, \dots, \theta_j^*)'$, is denoted by

$$\Omega_{-j}(\boldsymbol{\theta}^{*(j)}) = \left\{(\theta_{j+1}, \dots, \theta_p)' : \ (\theta_1^*, \dots, \theta_j^*, \theta_{j+1}, \dots, \theta_p)' \in \Omega\right\}. \tag{4.1.3}$$

Then the marginal posterior density of $\boldsymbol{\theta}^{(j)}$ evaluated at $\boldsymbol{\theta}^{*(j)}$ has the form

$$\pi(\boldsymbol{\theta}^{*(j)}|D) = \int_{\Omega_{-j}(\boldsymbol{\theta}^{*(j)})} \pi(\boldsymbol{\theta}^{*(j)}, \boldsymbol{\theta}^{(-j)}|D) \, d\boldsymbol{\theta}^{(-j)}. \tag{4.1.4}$$

Let $\{\boldsymbol{\theta}_i, \ i = 1, 2, \dots, n\}$ be an MCMC sample from $\pi(\boldsymbol{\theta}|D)$. Our goal is to describe how to use the MCMC sample to estimate the marginal posterior density $\pi(\boldsymbol{\theta}^{*(j)}|D)$.

Example 4.1. Marginal density versus predictive density. Consider the constrained multiple linear regression model given by (1.3.1) to model the New Zealand apple data in Example 1.1. From (2.1.7), the joint posterior density of $(\boldsymbol{\beta}, \sigma^2)$ is given by

$$\begin{aligned}\pi(\boldsymbol{\beta}, \sigma^2|D) =& \frac{\exp\{-(\beta_{10} - \mu_{10})^2/2\sigma_{10}^2\}}{c(D)(\sigma^2)^{(207+1)/2}} \\ & \times \exp\left\{-\frac{1}{2\sigma^2}\sum_{i=1}^{207}\left(y_i - \sum_{l=1}^{10} x_{il}\beta_l\right)^2\right\},\end{aligned}$$

for $\sigma^2 > 0$ and $\boldsymbol{\beta} \in \Omega$, where Ω is defined in (2.1.5). The marginal posterior density of β_j evaluated at β_j^* is

$$\pi(\beta_j^*|D) = \int_0^\infty \int_{\Omega_{-j}(\beta_j^*)} \frac{\exp\{-(\beta_{10} - \mu_{10})^2/2\sigma_{10}^2\}}{c(D)(\sigma^2)^{(207+1)/2}} \times \exp\left\{-\frac{1}{2\sigma^2}\sum_{i=1}^{207}\left(y_i - \sum_{l\neq j} x_{il}\beta_l - x_{ij}\beta_j^*\right)^2\right\} d\boldsymbol{\beta}^{(-j)}\, d\sigma^2, \tag{4.1.5}$$

where $\boldsymbol{\beta}^{(-j)} = (\beta_1, \ldots, \beta_{j-1}, \beta_{j+1}, \ldots, \beta_{10})'$, and

$$\Omega_{-j}(\beta_j^*) = \{\boldsymbol{\beta}^{(-j)} : 0 \leq \beta_1 \leq \cdots \leq \beta_{j-1} \leq \beta_j^* \leq \beta_{j+1} \leq \cdots \leq \beta_{10}, \\ \boldsymbol{\beta} \in R^{10}, \text{for a fixed } \beta_j^*\}.$$

From (4.1.5), the analytical evaluation of $\pi(\beta_j^*|D)$ does not appear possible.

To predict the amount of fruit to be produced by an individual grower for the coming year, we need to derive the predictive distribution. Let z denote the total number of cartons of fruit produced in the coming year by tree number $\boldsymbol{x}_\nu$. Then the conditional probability density function of z given $\boldsymbol{\beta}$, σ^2, and $\boldsymbol{x}_\nu$ has the form

$$f(z|\boldsymbol{\beta}, \sigma^2, \boldsymbol{x}_\nu) = \frac{1}{\sqrt{2\pi}\sigma} \exp\left\{-\frac{(z - \boldsymbol{x}_\nu'\boldsymbol{\beta})^2}{2\sigma^2}\right\}, \tag{4.1.6}$$

and thus the predictive density of z is

$$f_\nu(z|D) = \int_0^\infty \int_\Omega f(z|\boldsymbol{\beta}, \sigma^2, \boldsymbol{x}_\nu)\pi(\boldsymbol{\beta}, \sigma^2|D)\, d\boldsymbol{\beta}\, d\sigma^2. \tag{4.1.7}$$

Although it does not appear possible to evaluate $f_\nu(z|D)$ analytically, it is relatively straightforward to obtain an MC estimator of $f_\nu(z|D)$. Assume that $\{(\boldsymbol{\beta}_i, \sigma_i^2),\ i = 1, 2, \ldots, n\}$ is an MCMC sample from $\pi(\boldsymbol{\beta}, \sigma^2|D)$ using the Gibbs sampler described in Section 2.1. Then an estimator of $f_\nu(z|D)$ is simply given by

$$\hat{f}_\nu(z|D) = \frac{1}{n}\sum_{i=1}^n f(y_\nu|\boldsymbol{\beta}_i, \sigma_i^2, \boldsymbol{x}_\nu), \tag{4.1.8}$$

where $f(z|\boldsymbol{\beta}, \sigma^2, \boldsymbol{x}_\nu)$ is given by (4.1.6). However, a similar approach does not apply for obtaining an estimator of the marginal posterior density $\pi(\beta_j^*|D)$. Thus, computing a marginal posterior density is more difficult than a predictive density in general. In the next two sections, we consider two kinds of density estimation methods for obtaining an MC estimator of $\pi(\boldsymbol{\theta}^{*(j)}|D)$.

4.2 Kernel Methods

A widely used nonparametric density estimator is the kernel density estimator, which has the form

$$\hat{\pi}_{\text{kernel}}(\boldsymbol{\theta}^{*(j)}|D) = \frac{1}{nh_n^j}\sum_{i=1}^{n}\mathcal{K}\left(\frac{\boldsymbol{\theta}^{*(j)} - \boldsymbol{\theta}_i^{(j)}}{h_n}\right), \tag{4.2.1}$$

where $\boldsymbol{\theta}_i = (\boldsymbol{\theta}_i^{(j)}, \boldsymbol{\theta}_i^{(-j)})$, the kernel $\mathcal{K}$ is a bounded density on R^j, and h_n is the bandwidth. Assume that $j = 1$ and $\{\boldsymbol{\theta}_i,\ i = 1, 2, \ldots, n\}$ is a random sample. Then, if $\pi(\boldsymbol{\theta}^{(j)}|D)$ is uniformly continuous on R and as $n \to \infty$, $h_n \to 0$, and $nh_n(\ln n)^{-1} \to \infty$, we have $\lim_{n\to\infty}\hat{\pi}_{\text{kernel}}(\boldsymbol{\theta}^{*(j)}|D) \overset{\text{a.s.}}{=} \pi(\boldsymbol{\theta}^{*(j)}|D)$ (see Silverman (1986, p. 72)). Under slightly stronger regularity conditions, similar consistent results can be obtained for $j > 1$ (see Devroye and Wagner 1980). As discussed in Silverman (1986), the use of a single smoothing parameter h_n in (4.2.1) implies that the version of the kernel placed on each data point is scaled equally in all directions. If the spread of the data points is much greater in one of the coordinate directions than the others, it is probably best to prescale the data to avoid extreme differences of spread in the various coordinate directions. The performance of the kernel density estimator $\hat{\pi}_{\text{kernel}}(\boldsymbol{\theta}^{*(j)}|D)$ highly depends on the choice of the kernel $\mathcal{K}$ and the bandwidth h_n. Silverman (1986) provides a detailed discussion on choosing the smoothing parameter. For example, when $j = 1$, if a Gaussian kernel, i.e., $\mathcal{K}(t) = (1/\sqrt{2\pi})e^{-t^2/2}$, is used, the optimal choice for h_n is $1.06\sigma^* n^{-1/5}$, where σ^* is the sample standard deviation of the $\boldsymbol{\theta}_i^{(j)}$'s, provided that the $\boldsymbol{\theta}_i^{(j)}$'s are independent.

Further, the kernel method, in addition to depending on $\mathcal{K}$ and h_n, becomes dramatically worse as the dimension (here j) increases and so it is sometimes quite useful to use different bandwidths in different directions. Gelfand and Smith (1990) introduce the kernel density estimator for calculating a marginal posterior density and they also provide a conditional version of the kernel marginal posterior density estimator. The conditional kernel density estimator is given by

$$(1/n)\sum_{i=1}^{n} E(\hat{\pi}_{\text{kernel}}(\boldsymbol{\theta}^{*(j)}|D)|\boldsymbol{\theta}_i^{(-j)}).$$

However, the conditional kernel density estimator might not be better than the crude kernel density estimator since the Rao–Blackwell theorem may not hold in this case due to the dependence of $E(\hat{\pi}_{\text{kernel}}(\boldsymbol{\theta}^{*(j)}|D)|\boldsymbol{\theta}_i^{(-j)})$. See Geyer (1995a) or Exercise 3.7 for a detailed discussion. Further, the conditional kernel estimator may not be applicable since $E(\hat{\pi}_{\text{kernel}}(\boldsymbol{\theta}^{*(j)}|D)|$ $\boldsymbol{\theta}_i^{(-j)})$ may not be analytically available or may be computationally expensive. Therefore, we will not discuss the conditional kernel density estimator any further in this chapter.

4.3 IWMDE Methods

There are a number of parametric marginal posterior density estimators available in the literature. Assume that the analytical evaluation of the conditional posterior density, $\pi(\boldsymbol{\theta}^{(j)}|\boldsymbol{\theta}^{(-j)}, D)$, is available. Then (4.1.4) can be rewritten as

$$\pi(\boldsymbol{\theta}^{*(j)}|D) = \int_{\Omega} \pi(\boldsymbol{\theta}^{*(j)}|\boldsymbol{\theta}^{(-j)}, D)\pi(\boldsymbol{\theta})\, d\boldsymbol{\theta}. \tag{4.3.1}$$

Using the above identity, Gelfand, Smith, and Lee (1992) propose the conditional marginal density estimator (CMDE) of $\pi(\boldsymbol{\theta}^{*(j)}|D)$, which has the form

$$\hat{\pi}_{\text{CMDE}}(\boldsymbol{\theta}^{*(j)}|D) = \frac{1}{n}\sum_{i=1}^{n} \pi(\boldsymbol{\theta}^{*(j)}|\boldsymbol{\theta}_i^{(-j)}, D), \tag{4.3.2}$$

where $\{\boldsymbol{\theta}_i = (\boldsymbol{\theta}_i^{(j)}, \boldsymbol{\theta}_i^{(-j)}),\ i = 1, 2, \ldots, n\}$ is an MCMC sample from the joint posterior distribution $\pi(\boldsymbol{\theta}|D)$. It can be shown that under some minor regularity conditions, $\hat{\pi}_{\text{CMDE}}(\boldsymbol{\theta}^{*(j)}|D)$ is an unbiased and consistent estimator of $\pi(\boldsymbol{\theta}^{*(j)}|D)$, i.e.,

$$E(\hat{\pi}_{\text{CMDE}}(\boldsymbol{\theta}^{*(j)}|D)) = \pi(\boldsymbol{\theta}^{*(j)}|D)$$

and

$$\lim_{n\to\infty} \hat{\pi}_{\text{CMDE}}(\boldsymbol{\theta}^{*(j)}|D) \overset{\text{a.s.}}{=} \pi(\boldsymbol{\theta}^{*(j)}|D).$$

Verdinelli and Wasserman (1995) and Chib (1995) also propose marginal posterior density estimators. Verdinelli and Wasserman (1995) use the numerical integration method. Chib's estimator is obtained by using the Gibbs sample, and Chib (1995) shows that an estimate of the posterior density is available if all complete conditional densities used in the Gibbs sampler have closed-form expressions. Their methods are closely related to the CMDE.

The CMDE method is simple; however, it requires knowing the closed form of the conditional posterior density. Unfortunately, for many Bayesian models, especially when the parameter space is constrained, the conditional posterior densities are known up only to a normalizing constant. To overcome this difficulty, Chen (1994) proposes an importance weighted marginal density estimation (IWMDE) method. Instead of using (4.3.1) for the CMDE, we consider the following identity:

$$\pi(\boldsymbol{\theta}^{*(j)}|D) = \int_{\Omega} \frac{w(\boldsymbol{\theta}^{*(j)}|\boldsymbol{\theta}^{(-j)})\pi(\boldsymbol{\theta}^{*(j)}, \boldsymbol{\theta}^{(-j)}|D)}{\pi(\boldsymbol{\theta}|D)} \pi(\boldsymbol{\theta}|D)\, d\boldsymbol{\theta}, \tag{4.3.3}$$

where $w(\boldsymbol{\theta}^{(j)}|\boldsymbol{\theta}^{(-j)})$ is a completely known conditional density whose support is contained in, or equal to, the support, $\Omega_j(\boldsymbol{\theta}^{(-j)})$, of the conditional density $\pi(\boldsymbol{\theta}^{(j)}|\boldsymbol{\theta}^{(-j)}, D)$. Here, "*completely* known" means that

$w(\boldsymbol{\theta}^{(j)}|\boldsymbol{\theta}^{(-j)})$ can be evaluated at any point of $(\boldsymbol{\theta}^{(j)}, \boldsymbol{\theta}^{(-j)})$. In other words, the kernel *and* the normalizing constant of this conditional density are available in closed form. Using the identity (4.3.3), the IWMDE of $\pi(\boldsymbol{\theta}^{*(j)}|D)$ is defined by

$$\hat{\pi}_{\text{IWMDE}}(\boldsymbol{\theta}^{*(j)}|D) = \frac{1}{n}\sum_{i=1}^{n} w(\boldsymbol{\theta}_i^{(j)}|\boldsymbol{\theta}_i^{(-j)})\frac{\pi(\boldsymbol{\theta}^{*(j)}, \boldsymbol{\theta}_i^{(-j)}|D)}{\pi(\boldsymbol{\theta}_i^{(j)}, \boldsymbol{\theta}_i^{(-j)}|D)}. \tag{4.3.4}$$

In (4.3.4), w plays the role of a weight function. Further, $\hat{\pi}_{\text{IWMDE}}(\boldsymbol{\theta}^{*(j)}|D)$ does not depend on the unknown normalizing constant $c(D)$, since $c(D)$ cancels in the ratio $\pi(\boldsymbol{\theta}^{*(j)}, \boldsymbol{\theta}_i^{(-j)}|D)/\pi(\boldsymbol{\theta}_i^{(j)}, \boldsymbol{\theta}_i^{(-j)}|D)$. In fact, using (4.1.1), we can rewrite (4.3.4) as

$$\begin{aligned}
&\hat{\pi}_{\text{IWMDE}}(\boldsymbol{\theta}^{*(j)}|D)\\
&= \frac{1}{n}\sum_{i=1}^{n} w(\boldsymbol{\theta}_i^{(j)}|\boldsymbol{\theta}_i^{(-j)})\frac{L(\boldsymbol{\theta}^{*(j)}, \boldsymbol{\theta}_i^{(-j)}|D)\pi(\boldsymbol{\theta}^{*(j)}, \boldsymbol{\theta}_i^{(-j)})}{L(\boldsymbol{\theta}_i|D)\pi(\boldsymbol{\theta}_i)}.
\end{aligned} \tag{4.3.5}$$

The IWMDE has several nice properties. First, $\hat{\pi}_{\text{IWMDE}}(\boldsymbol{\theta}^{*(j)}|D)$ is an unbiased estimator of $\pi(\boldsymbol{\theta}^{*(j)}|D)$. This can be shown using the fact that

$$E\left(w(\boldsymbol{\theta}_i^{(j)}|\boldsymbol{\theta}_i^{(-j)})\frac{L(\boldsymbol{\theta}^{*(j)}, \boldsymbol{\theta}_i^{(-j)}|D)\pi(\boldsymbol{\theta}^{(j)}, \boldsymbol{\theta}_i^{(-j)})}{L(\boldsymbol{\theta}_i|D)\pi(\boldsymbol{\theta}_i)}\right) = \pi(\boldsymbol{\theta}^{*(j)}|D). \tag{4.3.6}$$

Unbiasedness is a desirable property for an estimator of the marginal posterior density. Unlike the IWMDE, the kernel estimator $\hat{\pi}_{\text{kernel}}(\boldsymbol{\theta}^{*(j)}|D)$ given in (4.2.1) does not have this property. Second, Chen (1994) shows that under the ergodicity condition, $\hat{\pi}_{\text{IWMDE}}(\boldsymbol{\theta}^{*(j)}|D)$ is consistent. This ensures that the IWMDE is asymptotically valid. Third, Verdinelli and Wasserman (1995) point out that under the uniform ergodicity and the finite second posterior moment of

$$w(\boldsymbol{\theta}^{*(j)}|\boldsymbol{\theta}^{(-j)})\frac{L(\boldsymbol{\theta}^{*(j)}, \boldsymbol{\theta}^{(-j)}|D)\pi(\boldsymbol{\theta}^{*(j)}, \boldsymbol{\theta}^{(-j)})}{L(\boldsymbol{\theta}|D)\pi(\boldsymbol{\theta})},$$

the central limit theorem holds for $\hat{\pi}_{\text{IWMDE}}(\boldsymbol{\theta}^{*(j)}|D)$. Fourth, the IWMDE is a generalization of the CMDE in (4.3.2), which can be observed by choosing $w = w(\boldsymbol{\theta}^{(j)}|\boldsymbol{\theta}^{(-j)}) = \pi(\boldsymbol{\theta}^{(j)}|\boldsymbol{\theta}^{(-j)}, D)$ (see Exercise 4.1).

The only requirement for obtaining the asymptotic convergence of the IWMDE is that w is a conditional density on $\Omega_j(\boldsymbol{\theta}^{(-j)})$. Therefore we can have many IWMDEs by choosing different w's. In this regard, Chen (1994) shows that the CMDE is the best among all IWMDEs. Denote

$$\Pi_{i,j}(\boldsymbol{\theta}^{*(j)}|D) = w(\boldsymbol{\theta}_i^{(j)}|\boldsymbol{\theta}_i^{(-j)})\frac{\pi(\boldsymbol{\theta}^{*(j)}, \boldsymbol{\theta}_i^{(-j)}|D)}{\pi(\boldsymbol{\theta}_i|D)},$$

for $i = 1, 2, \dots, n$. Then $\hat{\pi}(\boldsymbol{\theta}^{*(j)}|D)$ is the sample mean of $\{\Pi_{j,i}(\boldsymbol{\theta}^{*(j)}|D), 1 \le i \le n\}$. Let $\hat{V}_w$ denote the sample variance of $\{\Pi_{j,i}(\boldsymbol{\theta}^{*(j)}|D), 1 \le i \le n\}$

and let

$$V_w(\hat{\pi}(\boldsymbol{\theta}^{*(j)}|D)) = \int_\Omega \left[w(\boldsymbol{\theta}^{(j)}|\boldsymbol{\theta}^{(-j)}) \frac{\pi(\boldsymbol{\theta}^{*(j)}, \boldsymbol{\theta}^{(-j)}|D)}{\pi(\boldsymbol{\theta}|D)} \right]^2 \pi(\boldsymbol{\theta}|D)\, d\boldsymbol{\theta} - (\pi(\boldsymbol{\theta}^{*(j)}|D))^2, \tag{4.3.7}$$

which is the variance of $\Pi_{i,j}(\boldsymbol{\theta}^{*(j)}|D)$ when $\boldsymbol{\theta}_i$ has the stationary distribution $\pi(\boldsymbol{\theta}|D)$. Therefore the *Ergodic* theorem implies that if $V_w(\hat{\pi}(\boldsymbol{\theta}^{*(j)}|D)) < \infty$, then

$$\lim_{n\to\infty} \hat{V}_w \overset{\text{a.s.}}{=} V_w(\hat{\pi}(\boldsymbol{\theta}^{*(j)}|D)).$$

The derivation of the closed form for the variance of the sample mean $\hat{\pi}(\boldsymbol{\theta}^{*(j)}|D)$ is difficult. It depends on the correlations between $\Pi_{i,j}(\boldsymbol{\theta}^{*(j)}|D)$ and $\Pi_{i+l,j}(\boldsymbol{\theta}^{*(j)}|D)$ for $l = 1, \ldots, n-i$ and $i = 1, \ldots, n$. Liu, Wong, and Kong (1995) present a detailed study of the correlation structure for the Gibbs sampler. However, here it is even more difficult to examine the correlation structure of the sequence $\{\Pi_{i,j}(\boldsymbol{\theta}^{*(j)}|D), 1 \le i \le n\}$, since the IWMDE involves a general Markov chain sampler and a weight conditional density w. Therefore, we obtain the "best" w only based on the stationary variance $V_w(\hat{\pi}(\boldsymbol{\theta}^{*(j)}|D))$. Of course, for large n, $\hat{V}_w$ is approximately $V_w(\hat{\pi}(\boldsymbol{\theta}^{*(j)}|D))$.

Letting

$$w_C(\boldsymbol{\theta}^{(j)}|\boldsymbol{\theta}^{(-j)}) = \pi(\boldsymbol{\theta}^{(j)}|\boldsymbol{\theta}^{(-j)}, D),$$

the following theorem indicates that w_C is the best conditional density in the sense of minimizing $V_w(\hat{\pi}(\boldsymbol{\theta}^{*(j)}|D))$.

Theorem 4.3.1 *If $V_{w_C}(\hat{\pi}(\boldsymbol{\theta}^{*(j)}|D)) < \infty$ and w is an arbitrary conditional density on $\Omega_j(\boldsymbol{\theta}^{(-j)})$, then*

$$V_{w_C}(\hat{\pi}(\boldsymbol{\theta}^{*(j)}|D)) \le V_w(\hat{\pi}(\boldsymbol{\theta}^{*(j)}|D)). \tag{4.3.8}$$

The proof of this theorem is given in the Appendix. According to Theorem 4.3.1, when the CMDE is available, it is the best IWMDE. However the CMDE is often not available due to the complexity of the conditional marginal posterior density; or sometimes it is very expensive to compute the CMDE due to the overflow/underflow in implementing the conditional density function. For these cases, we can use an IWMDE instead of the CMDE by choosing a simple weight conditional density w.

Based on the expression of the IWMDE given in (4.3.4) or (4.3.5), the weight conditional density w appears to be an importance sampling density. However, $w(\boldsymbol{\theta}^{(j)}|\boldsymbol{\theta}^{(-j)})$ depends on $\boldsymbol{\theta}^{(-j)}$; and by Theorem 4.3.1, a good w should be chosen to have a shape similar to the conditional marginal density of $\boldsymbol{\theta}^{(j)}$ given $\boldsymbol{\theta}^{(-j)}$, which implies that a good w will vary from one iteration to another. Therefore, a good w is generally not chosen in the same way as a good importance sampling density is. On the other hand, empirical results given in Chen (1994) show that if a w is chosen to have a shape roughly similar to the conditional marginal density, the IWMDE will converge to the marginal posterior density rapidly. Therefore, it is not necessary to choose a w that precisely mimics the conditional marginal density. Although the shape of the conditional marginal density is often not known, it can be roughly assessed by the posterior moments. These posterior moments can be approximated using MCMC samples from the joint posterior distribution $\pi(\boldsymbol{\theta}|D)$ or using the Laplace approximation method (see Tierney and Kadane 1986). Chen (1994) proposes an empirical procedure for choosing a good w using a common distribution, which mimics the conditional marginal density.

Guidelines for choosing an importance sampling density can be found in Geweke (1989) and Rubinstein (1981). For example, we can choose a p-dimensional multivariate normal $N_p(\boldsymbol{\mu}, \Sigma)$ as a joint importance sampling density. Then the conditional marginal density of the fitted multivariate normal distribution $N_p(\boldsymbol{\mu}, \Sigma)$ is used as a w. Here, $\boldsymbol{\mu}$ and Σ can be chosen as the posterior mode and the negative Hessian matrix evaluated at $\boldsymbol{\mu}$. Alternatively, we can run the Markov chain to get n_0 observations $\{\boldsymbol{\theta}_i,\ 1 \leq i \leq n_0\}$, and $\boldsymbol{\mu}$ and Σ are taken to be

$$\begin{aligned}
\boldsymbol{\mu} &= \frac{1}{n_0} \sum_{i=1}^{n_0} \boldsymbol{\theta}_i, \\
\Sigma &= \frac{1}{n_0(n_0-1)} \sum_{i=1}^{n_0} \sum_{l=1}^{n_0} (\boldsymbol{\theta}_i - \boldsymbol{\mu})(\boldsymbol{\theta}_l - \boldsymbol{\mu})'.
\end{aligned}$$

A multivariate Student t distribution $t(df, \mu, \Sigma)$, which has a heavier tail than the multivariate normal distribution, can also be used as a joint importance sampling density. Using the Markov chain preprocessing procedure (see Gelman and Rubin 1992), the degrees of freedom, df, the location vector, μ, and the covariance matrix, Σ, can be approximated.

If Ω is a constrained parameter space, the choice of w is quite complicated. For illustrative purposes, we consider choosing a w for estimating a one-dimensional posterior marginal density, say, for θ_1, and for simplicity, we assume the support $\Omega_1(\boldsymbol{\theta}^{(-1)})$ defined in (4.1.2) is a finite or infinite interval.

If the support $\Omega_1(\boldsymbol{\theta}^{(-1)})$ is a finite interval with two endpoints a_1 and b_1, which are functions of $\theta_2, \ldots, \theta_p$, then we use a simple power-function distribution to mimic the conditional posterior marginal distribution by fitting moments. The form for the density of the power-function distribution is

$$w = \frac{\alpha(\theta_1 - a_1)^{\alpha-1}}{(b_1 - a_1)^{\alpha}} \text{ or } w = \frac{\alpha(b_1 - \theta_1)^{\alpha-1}}{(b_1 - a_1)^{\alpha}} \quad \text{for } a_1 < \theta_1 < b_1. \tag{4.3.9}$$

The corresponding means of the above power-function distributions are

$$\mu_w = a_1 + \frac{\alpha}{\alpha+1}(b_1 - a_1) \text{ or } \mu_w = a_1 + \frac{1}{\alpha+1}(b_1 - a_1). \tag{4.3.10}$$

The parameter α and the form of a power-function density can be determined by:

(i) obtaining the estimated posterior means $\hat{a}_1$, $\hat{b}_1$, and $\hat{\theta}_1$ for a_1, b_1, and θ_1 using the first few Markov chain iterations or entire simulated Markov chain if possible; and

(ii) using $w = \alpha(\theta_1 - a_1)^{\alpha-1}/(b_1 - a_1)^{\alpha}$ if $\hat{\theta}_1 \geq (\hat{a}_1 + \hat{b}_1)/2$ and $\alpha = (\hat{\theta}_1 - \hat{a}_1)/(\hat{b}_1 - \hat{\theta}_1)$; otherwise, using the second form for w and $\alpha = (\hat{b}_1 - \hat{\theta}_1)/(\hat{\theta}_1 - \hat{a}_1)$.

If the support $\Omega_1(\boldsymbol{\theta}^{(-1)})$ is a half-open interval, say, with the form (a_1, ∞), then an exponential distribution is used to fit the conditional distribution. Then w is chosen as

$$w = \lambda e^{-\lambda(\theta_1 - a_1)},$$

where $\lambda = 1/(\hat{\theta}_1 - \hat{a}_1)$ and $\hat{\theta}_1$ and $\hat{a}_1$ are obtained by fitting moments.

The power-function and exponential distributions are used as the candidates of w since the least information, i.e., posterior means, is used; and such a w is also very easy and cheap to compute. If more information such as the posterior covariance matrix is available, then the weighting conditional density w can be chosen to be a beta or gamma density. However, more computing time is often required for such a w.

The foregoing procedure can be extended from one dimension to higher dimensions. 0For example, suppose the joint marginal posterior density of $(\theta_1, \theta_2, \ldots, \theta_j)$ is of interest. Since

$$\begin{aligned} w(\theta_1, \theta_2, \ldots, \theta_j | \theta_{j+1}, \ldots, \theta_p) =& w(\theta_j | \theta_{j+1}, \ldots, \theta_p) \cdot w(\theta_{j-1} | \theta_j, \ldots, \theta_p) \times \cdots \\ & \times w(\theta_1 | \theta_2, \cdots, \theta_p), \end{aligned} \tag{4.3.11}$$

then the joint weighting conditional density w could be selected as a product of j one-dimensional weighting conditional densities by applying the empirical procedure for the one-dimensional case. The choice of such a w is not unique since there are $j!$ ways to express the joint conditional density as the product of one-dimensional conditional densities. However, a w is required to be roughly similar to the conditional posterior distribution. Therefore, we can use one of these w's; or we can average the $j!$ w's.

As an alternative to the above extension, Oh (1999) proposes a more efficient approach using a sequence of one-dimensional conditional distributions to construct an estimator of the joint marginal posterior density. Oh's method is essentially similar to the method of Ritter and Tanner (1992) for the Gibbs stopper (see Section 5.8.5 for details). For ease of exposition, consider $\boldsymbol{\theta}^{(2)} = (\theta_1, \theta_2)'$. Then, Oh (1999) derives the following identity:

$$\begin{aligned}
\pi(\boldsymbol{\theta}^{*(2)}|D) &= \int_{\Omega_{-2}(\boldsymbol{\theta}^{*(2)})} \pi(\boldsymbol{\theta}^{*(2)}, \boldsymbol{\theta}^{(-2)}|D)\ d\boldsymbol{\theta}^{(-2)} \\
&= \int_{\Omega_{-2}(\boldsymbol{\theta}^{*(2)})} \pi(\theta_1^*|\theta_2^*, \boldsymbol{\theta}^{(-2)}, D)\pi(\theta_2^*, \boldsymbol{\theta}^{(-2)}|D)\ d\boldsymbol{\theta}^{(-2)} \\
&= \int_{\Omega_{-2}(\boldsymbol{\theta}^{*(2)})} \pi(\theta_1^*|\theta_2^*, \boldsymbol{\theta}^{(-2)}, D) \\
&\quad \times \left[\int_{\Omega_1(\theta_2^*, \boldsymbol{\theta}^{(-2)})} \pi(\theta_1, \theta_2^*, \boldsymbol{\theta}^{(-2)}|D)\ d\theta_1\right]\ d\boldsymbol{\theta}^{(-2)} \\
&= \int_{\Omega_{-2}(\boldsymbol{\theta}^{*(2)})} \pi(\theta_1^*|\theta_2^*, \boldsymbol{\theta}^{(-2)}, D) \\
&\quad \times \left[\int_{\Omega_1(\theta_2^*, \boldsymbol{\theta}^{(-2)})} \pi(\theta_2^*|\theta_1, \boldsymbol{\theta}^{(-2)}, D)\pi(\theta_1, \boldsymbol{\theta}^{(-2)}|D)\ d\theta_1\right]\ d\boldsymbol{\theta}^{(-2)} \\
&= E[\pi(\theta_1^*|\theta_2^*, \boldsymbol{\theta}^{(-2)}, D)\pi(\theta_2^*|\theta_1, \boldsymbol{\theta}^{(-2)}, D)], \qquad (4.3.12)
\end{aligned}$$

where the expectation is taken with respect to $\pi(\boldsymbol{\theta}|D)$.

When closed forms of the conditional densities $\pi(\theta_1^*|\theta_2^*, \boldsymbol{\theta}^{(-2)}, D)$ and $\pi(\theta_2^*|\theta_1, \boldsymbol{\theta}^{(-2)}, D)$ are known, the joint marginal density, $\pi(\boldsymbol{\theta}^{*(2)}|D)$, can be estimated by

$$\hat{\pi}(\boldsymbol{\theta}^{*(2)}|D) = \frac{1}{n}\sum_{i=1}^{n} \pi(\theta_1^*|\theta_2^*, \boldsymbol{\theta}_i^{(-2)}, D)\pi(\theta_2^*|\theta_{1,i}, \boldsymbol{\theta}_i^{(-2)}, D), \quad (4.3.13)$$

where $\{\boldsymbol{\theta}_i = (\theta_{1,i}, \boldsymbol{\theta}_i^{(-1)}),\ i = 1, 2, \ldots, n\}$ is an MCMC sample from $\pi(\boldsymbol{\theta}|D)$.

When some closed-forms of the conditional densities are not known, we can use the IWMDE method for the unknown conditionals. To examine this approach, we assume $\pi(\theta_2^*|\theta_{1,i}, \boldsymbol{\theta}_i^{(-2)}, D)$ is unknown. Then we can rewrite (4.3.12) as

$$\begin{aligned}
\pi(\boldsymbol{\theta}^{*(2)}|D) &= E\Bigg[\pi(\theta_1^*|\theta_2^*, \boldsymbol{\theta}^{(-2)}, D) \\
&\quad \times\ w(\theta_2|\theta_1, \boldsymbol{\theta}^{(-2)})\frac{\pi(\theta_1, \theta_2^*, \boldsymbol{\theta}^{(-2)}|D)}{\pi(\boldsymbol{\theta}|D)}\Bigg], \qquad (4.3.14)
\end{aligned}$$

where $w(\theta_2|\theta_1, \boldsymbol{\theta}^{(-2)})$ is a completely known conditional density whose support is contained in, or equal to, the support of the conditional density $\pi(\theta_2|\theta_1, \boldsymbol{\theta}^{(-2)}, D)$. Since $w(\theta_2|\theta_1, \boldsymbol{\theta}^{(-2)})$ is a one-dimensional conditional density, a good choice of w is easily available. Once w is chosen, an estimator of $\pi(\boldsymbol{\theta}^{*(2)}|D)$ is given by

$$\hat{\pi}(\boldsymbol{\theta}^{*(2)}|D) = \frac{1}{n}\sum_{i=1}^{n}\Bigg[\pi(\theta_1^*|\theta_2^*,\boldsymbol{\theta}_i^{(-2)},D)w(\theta_{2,i}|\theta_{1,i},\boldsymbol{\theta}_i^{(-2)}) \times \frac{\pi(\theta_{1,i},\theta_2^*,\boldsymbol{\theta}_i^{(-2)}|D)}{\pi(\boldsymbol{\theta}_i|D)}\Bigg]. \tag{4.3.15}$$

The above procedure can be easily extended to an arbitrary dimension. This is left as an exercise.

4.4 Illustrative Examples

In this section, we discuss two examples to illustrate the derivation of IWMDEs.

Example 4.2. Bivariate normal model. In this example, we apply the IWMDE method for computing the marginal density of a bivariate normal distribution $N_2(\boldsymbol{\mu},\Sigma)$, where $\boldsymbol{\mu}=(0,0)'$, and

$$\Sigma = \begin{pmatrix} 1 & 0.1\times\sqrt{2} \\ 0.1\times\sqrt{2} & 2 \end{pmatrix}.$$

Let $\boldsymbol{\theta} = (\theta_1,\theta_2)' \sim N_2(\boldsymbol{\mu},\Sigma)$. We use the Gibbs sampler to generate $\{\boldsymbol{\theta}_i, 0 \le i \le n\}$ from the above bivariate normal distribution $N_2(\boldsymbol{\mu},\Sigma)$. Since the distribution of the ith Gibbs iteration converges to the stationary distribution at a geometric rate, the IWMDE of the marginal density converges to the true marginal density almost surely.

In Figure 4.1, the IWMDEs of the marginal density of θ_1 are based on $n=500$ (the dotted curve), $n=100$ (the dashed curve), and $n=50$ (the long dashed curve) Gibbs iterations. Also, in Figure 4.1, the solid curve is the true marginal density ($n=\infty$). The conditional density w is chosen as the density of a uniform distribution $U(-2,2)$. The absolute differences between the estimated and true marginal densities are less than 0.035 for $n=50$, 0.024 for $n=100$, and 0.009 for $n=500$. So, the IWMDE works well even for small sample sizes. Note that the support of the conditional density of θ_1 is R^1 while the support of w is $(-2,2)$. Therefore the support of w may differ from that of the true conditional density.

Example 4.3. Constrained multiple linear regression model (Example 2.2 continued). We revisit the constrained multiple linear regression model given by (1.3.1) to model the New Zealand apple data. The joint posterior density of $(\boldsymbol{\beta},\sigma^2)$ is given by (2.1.7). For illustrative

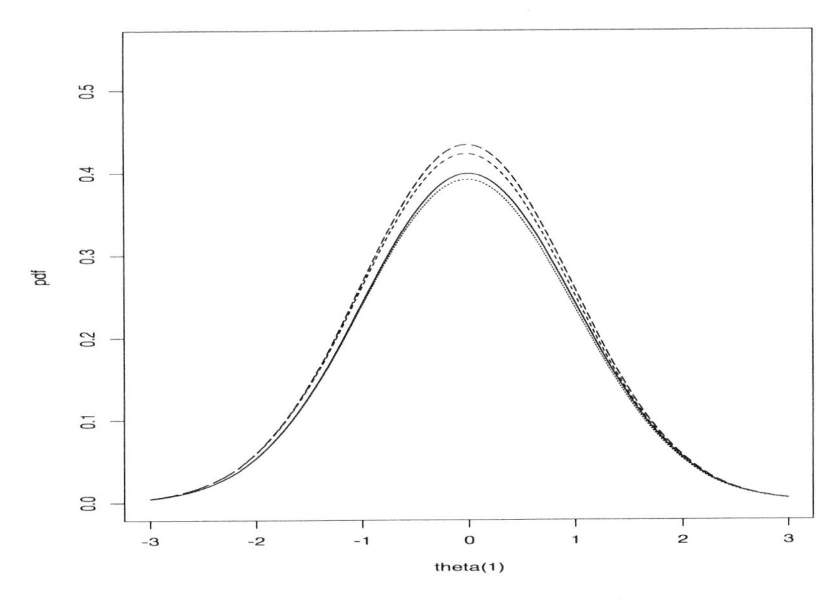

FIGURE 4.1. The IWMDEs for θ_1.

purposes, we consider only estimating the marginal posterior densities of β_1 and β_2 using the IWMDE method.

Using the Gibbs sampler described in Section 2.1, Chen and Deely (1996) derive the posterior means $\hat{\beta}_1 = 0.0131$, $\hat{\beta}_2 = 0.0249$, and $\hat{\beta}_3 = 0.1776$. The support of the conditional posterior density of β_1 given $\beta_2, \ldots, \beta_{10}$, and σ^2 is

$$\Omega_1(\beta_2, \ldots, \beta_{10}, \sigma^2) = \{\beta_1 : 0 \leq \beta_1 \leq \beta_2\}.$$

For this case, $\hat{a}_1 = 0$, $\hat{b}_1 = 0.0249$, and $\hat{\beta}_1 = 0.0131$. Since $\hat{\beta}_1$ is roughly half of $\hat{\beta}_2$, then w can be chosen as the power-function distribution with $\alpha = 1$, which is a uniform distribution $U(0, \beta_2)$. For β_2,

$$\Omega_{\{2\}}(\beta_1, \beta_3, \ldots, \beta_{10}, \sigma^2) = \{\beta_2 : 0 \leq \beta_1 \leq \beta_2 \leq \beta_3\}.$$

Then $\hat{a}_1 = 0.0131$, $\hat{b}_1 = 0.1776$, and $\hat{\beta}_2 = 0.0249$. Since $\hat{\beta}_2 < (\hat{a}_1 + \hat{b}_1)/2$, then $\alpha = (\hat{b}_1 - \hat{\theta}_2)/(\hat{\theta}_2 - \hat{a}_1) = 12.94068 \simeq 13$. Thus

$$w(\beta_2 | \beta_1, \beta_3, \ldots, \beta_{10}, \sigma^2) = \frac{13(\beta_3 - \beta_2)^{12}}{(\beta_3 - \beta_1)^{13}} \quad \text{for } \beta_1 < \beta_2 < \beta_3. \tag{4.4.1}$$

In Figure 4.2, we use 50,000 Gibbs iterations to get the IWMDEs of the marginal posterior densities for β_1 and β_2 with the uniform $U(0, \beta_2)$ density and the power-function density given in (4.4.1) as two weight conditional densities w's. We evaluate the IWMDEs at 101 and 201 grid points for β_1

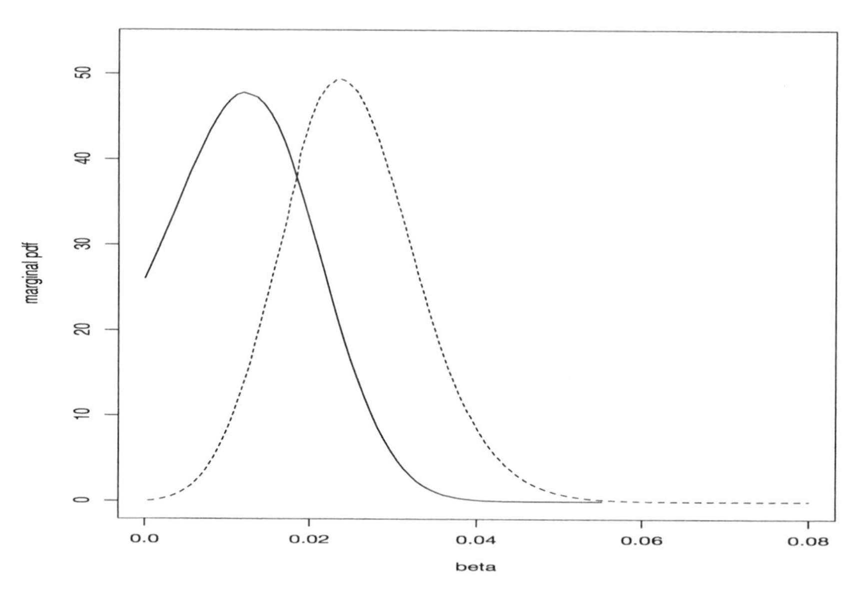

FIGURE 4.2. The IWMDE's for β_1 and β_2.

and β_2, respectively. In Figure 4.2, the solid curve is for β_1 and the dotted curve is for β_2.

Next, we obtain the IWMDE of the joint marginal posterior density of (β_1, β_2). The support of the conditional marginal posterior density of (β_1, β_2), given $(\beta_3, \ldots, \beta_{10}, \sigma^2)$, is

$$\Omega_2(\beta_3, \ldots, \beta_{10}, \sigma^2) = \{(\beta_1, \beta_2) : 0 < \beta_1 \leq \beta_2 \leq \beta_3\}.$$

For this two-dimensional normal case, computation of the normalization constant of the conditional marginal posterior density is expensive, and therefore the CMDE is difficult to obtain.

Using (4.3.11), a joint weighting conditional density w can be chosen as the product of two one-dimensional weighting conditional densities $w(\beta_1|\beta_2, \ldots, \beta_{10}, \sigma^2)$ and $w(\beta_2|\beta_3, \ldots, \beta_{10}, \sigma^2)$. Based on the posterior means of β, we choose $w(\beta_1|\beta_2, \ldots, \beta_{10}, \sigma^2) = 1/\beta_2$. Since $\hat{\beta}_2 = 0.0249$ is less than half of $\hat{\beta}_3 = 0.1776$, we can use the power-function distribution $\alpha(\beta_3 - \beta_2)^{\alpha-1}/\beta_3^{\alpha}$ as $w(\beta_2|\beta_3, \ldots, \beta_{10}, \sigma^2)$. By using the method of moments, $\alpha = (\hat{\beta}_3/\hat{\beta}_2) - 1 = 0.1776/0.0249 - 1 \simeq 6$. Thus, $w(\beta_2|\beta_3, \ldots, \beta_{10}, \sigma^2) = 6(\beta_3 - \beta_2)^5/\beta_3^6$. Therefore

$$w(\beta_1, \beta_2|\beta_3, \ldots, \beta_{10}, \sigma^2) = \frac{6(\beta_3 - \beta_2)^5}{\beta_2 \beta_3^6} \quad \text{for } 0 < \beta_1 \leq \beta_2 \leq \beta_3. \quad (4.4.2)$$

In Figure 4.3, we use 10,000 Gibbs iterations to get the IWMDE of the joint marginal posterior densities for β_1 and β_2 with the weight condi-

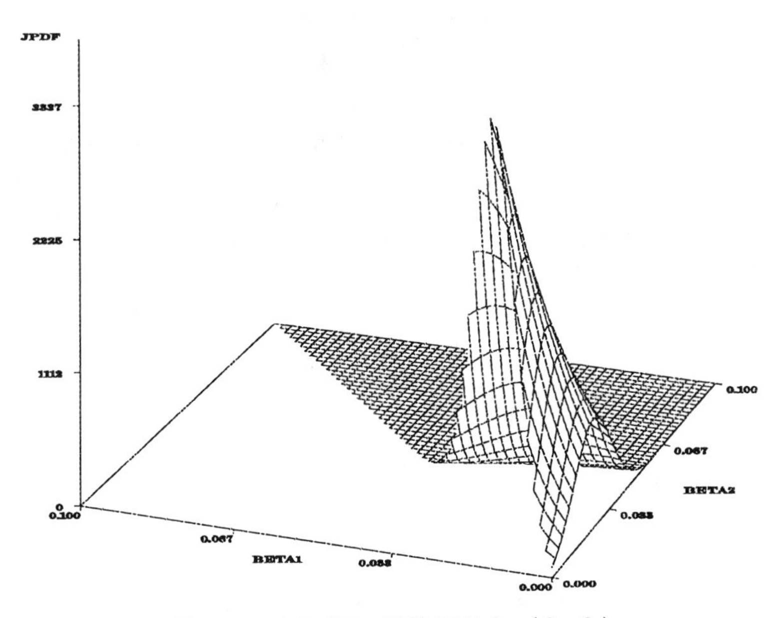

FIGURE 4.3. The IWMDE for (β_1, β_2).

tional density w given in (4.4.2). We evaluate the IWMDE at 2500 grid points for β_1 and β_2. A similar figure is also obtained, but is not shown here, using the w chosen as the product of two one-dimensional densities $w(\beta_2|\beta_1, \beta_3, \ldots, \beta_{10}, \sigma^2)$ and $w(\beta_1|\beta_3, \ldots, \beta_{10}, \sigma^2)$.

4.5 Performance Study Using the Kullback–Leibler Divergence

In Section 4.3, we discuss kernel and IWMDE methods for estimating the marginal posterior density $\pi(\boldsymbol{\theta}^{*(j)}|D)$. The kernel method depends on the choice of the kernel $\mathcal{K}$ and the smoothing parameter h_n, while the IWMDE method depends on the weight conditional density w. Therefore, it is important to study how a kernel estimator or an IWMDE performs when a good h_n or w is chosen, and how many MCMC iterations are needed to obtain a reliable marginal posterior density estimator.

Between the kernel method and the CMDE (the best IWMDE), Gelfand, Smith, and Lee (1992) point out that the CMDE is better than the kernel density estimator under a wide range of loss functions; but they do not provide any theoretical justification or empirical evidence. Chen (1994) proposes two heuristic methods regarding the choice of w for the IWMDE.

The first method is to monitor the area under the estimated density. If it is close to one, then the choice of w may be viewed as a good one. The second method is to estimate the numerical standard deviations at the grid points. The better choice of w will result in a smaller sum of standard deviations over the grid times the mesh of the grid. However, Chen (1994) does not provide any theoretical justification of these two methods.

More recently, Chen and Shao (1997c) introduce the Kullback–Leibler (K–L) divergence as a performance measure for assessing the performance of a marginal density estimator. They show that the K–L divergence can be used to compare two density estimators as well as to assess convergence of a marginal density estimator. In this section, we present the full description and detailed discussion of the K–L divergence method of Chen and Shao (1997c).

Let $\hat{\pi}(\boldsymbol{\theta}^{(j)}|D)$ be an estimator of $\pi(\boldsymbol{\theta}^{(j)}|D)$. The K–L divergence between $\hat{\pi}(\boldsymbol{\theta}^{(j)}|D)$ and $\pi(\boldsymbol{\theta}^{(j)}|D)$ is defined as

$$\Delta(\pi(\boldsymbol{\theta}^{(j)}|D), \hat{\pi}(\boldsymbol{\theta}^{(j)}|D)) = \int_{R^j} \pi(\boldsymbol{\theta}^{(j)}|D) \ln \pi(\boldsymbol{\theta}^{(j)}|D)\, d\boldsymbol{\theta}^{(j)} - \int_{R^j} \pi(\boldsymbol{\theta}^{(j)}|D) \ln \hat{\pi}(\boldsymbol{\theta}^{(j)}|D)\, d\boldsymbol{\theta}^{(j)}. \tag{4.5.1}$$

The K–L divergence is often called the *relative entropy* (see, e.g., Cover and Thomas (1991)). Using Jensen's inequality, it can be shown that if $\hat{\pi}(\boldsymbol{\theta}^{(j)}|D)$ is a density function, i.e., $\int_{R^j} \hat{\pi}(\boldsymbol{\theta}^{(j)}|D)\, d\boldsymbol{\theta}^{(j)} = 1$, then

$$\Delta(\pi(\boldsymbol{\theta}^{(j)}|D), \hat{\pi}(\boldsymbol{\theta}^{(j)}|D)) \geq 0$$

with equality if and only if $\hat{\pi}(\boldsymbol{\theta}^{(j)}|D) = \pi(\boldsymbol{\theta}^{(j)}|D)$.

As noted by Cover and Thomas (1991), the K–L divergence is not a distance because it is not symmetric and does not satisfy the triangle inequality. However, the relative entropy is conventionally used to measure the distance between two densities. There are a number of divergence measures other than the Kullback–Leibler, which include:

(i) the L_1-divergence ($\int_{R^j} |\hat{\pi}(\boldsymbol{\theta}^{(j)}|D) - \pi(\boldsymbol{\theta}^{(j)}|D)|\, d\boldsymbol{\theta}^{(j)}$);

(ii) the L_2-divergence ($\int_{R^j} (\hat{\pi}(\boldsymbol{\theta}^{(j)}|D) - \pi(\boldsymbol{\theta}^{(j)}|D))^2\, d\boldsymbol{\theta}^{(j)}$); and

(iii) the χ^2-divergence ($\int_{R^j} (\hat{\pi}(\boldsymbol{\theta}^{(j)}|D) - \pi(\boldsymbol{\theta}^{(j)}|D))^2 \times [\pi(\boldsymbol{\theta}^{(j)}|D)]^{-1}\, d\boldsymbol{\theta}^{(j)}$).

The primary reasons for choosing the K–L divergence are as follows. First, the K–L divergence measures how much information $\hat{\pi}(\boldsymbol{\theta}^{(j)}|D)$ carries about $\pi(\boldsymbol{\theta}^{(j)}|D)$ and, as discussed in Hall (1987), the K–L divergence is purpose-built for discriminating against $\hat{\pi}(\boldsymbol{\theta}^{(j)}|D)$. In contrast, Hall (1992) points out that it would be most inappropriate to use the mean integrated square error (MISE) as a global criterion for measuring the performance of $\hat{\pi}(\boldsymbol{\theta}^{(j)}|D)$ when $\pi(\boldsymbol{\theta}^{(j)}|D)$ has heavy tails. Second, the second term on the right-hand side of (4.5.1) can be estimated by using MCMC samples. Suppose that $\{\boldsymbol{\theta}_l^*,\ l = 1, 2, \ldots, m\}$ is another MCMC sample from $\pi(\boldsymbol{\theta}|D)$, which is independent of the MCMC sample $\{\boldsymbol{\theta}_i,\ i = 1, 2, \ldots, n\}$. We also write $\boldsymbol{\theta}_l^* = (\boldsymbol{\theta}_l^{*(j)}, \boldsymbol{\theta}_l^{*(-j)})$. Then $\int_{R^j} \pi(\boldsymbol{\theta}^{(j)}|D) \ln \hat{\pi}(\boldsymbol{\theta}^{(j)}|D)\ d\boldsymbol{\theta}^{(j)}$ can be approximated by

$$\frac{1}{m} \sum_{l=1}^{m} \ln \hat{\pi}(\boldsymbol{\theta}_l^{*(j)}|D). \tag{4.5.2}$$

This is a very attractive feature, since we can compare two different marginal posterior density estimators, in which we do not know the first term on the right-hand side of (4.5.1). However, the L_1-divergence and the χ^2-divergence do not have the same properties as the K–L divergence. Although the L_2-divergence shares some nice properties with the K–L divergence, it has some undesirable features when it is used to compare two different marginal posterior density estimators. To see this, we rewrite the L_2-divergence as

$$\begin{aligned} &\int_{R^j} (\hat{\pi}(\boldsymbol{\theta}^{(j)}|D) - \pi(\boldsymbol{\theta}^{(j)}|D))^2\ d\boldsymbol{\theta}^{(j)} \\ &\quad = \int_{R^j} \hat{\pi}^2(\boldsymbol{\theta}^{(j)}|D)\ d\boldsymbol{\theta}^{(j)} - 2\int_{R^j} \hat{\pi}^2(\boldsymbol{\theta}^{(j)}|D)\pi(\boldsymbol{\theta}^{(j)}|D)\ d\boldsymbol{\theta}^{(j)} \\ &\quad\quad + \int_{R^j} \pi^2(\boldsymbol{\theta}^{(j)}|D)\ d\boldsymbol{\theta}^{(j)}. \end{aligned} \tag{4.5.3}$$

The third term on the right-hand side of (4.5.3) can be canceled out and the second term can be estimated in a similar way as the K–L divergence. However, the first term is difficult and expensive to evaluate when $\boldsymbol{\theta}^{(j)}$ is high-dimensional.

If $\hat{\pi}(\boldsymbol{\theta}^{(j)}|D)$ is a kernel estimator, then, $\Delta(\pi(\boldsymbol{\theta}^{(j)}|D), \hat{\pi}(\boldsymbol{\theta}^{(j)}|D))$ is always nonnegative. However, $E[\Delta(\pi(\boldsymbol{\theta}^{(j)}|D), \hat{\pi}(\boldsymbol{\theta}^{(j)}|D))]$ may not exist when $\pi(\boldsymbol{\theta}^{(j)}|D)$ has particularly heavy tails. To remedy this potential problem, Hall (1987) proposes a choice of $\mathcal{K}$ that is proportional to

$$\exp[-\tfrac{1}{2}\{\ln(1 + (\boldsymbol{\theta}^{(j)})'\boldsymbol{\theta}^{(j)})\}^2].$$

On the other hand, if $\hat{\pi}(\boldsymbol{\theta}^{(j)}|D)$ is an IWMDE, then $\Delta(\pi(\boldsymbol{\theta}^{(j)}|D), \hat{\pi}(\boldsymbol{\theta}^{(j)}|D))$ may not be nonnegative. In practice, $\hat{\pi}(\boldsymbol{\theta}^{(j)}|D)$ is often evaluated over a set of grid points. Thus, $\hat{\pi}(\boldsymbol{\theta}^{(j)}|D)$ may be normalized by dividing the sum over the grid of $\hat{\pi}(\boldsymbol{\theta}^{(j)}|D)$ times the mesh of the grid. However, without normalization, the expected value of the K–L divergence for an IWMDE is always nonnegative. Most notably, under certain regularity conditions, the expected value of the K–L divergence for an IWMDE is finite. We present this result as follows:

Theorem 4.5.1 *Assume that*

$$E|\ln \pi(\boldsymbol{\theta}^{(j)}|D)| < \infty \tag{4.5.4}$$

and

$$E\left|\ln\left(\frac{w(\boldsymbol{\theta}^{*(j)}|\boldsymbol{\theta}^{*(-j)})L(\boldsymbol{\theta}^{(j)},\boldsymbol{\theta}^{*(-j)}|D)\pi(\boldsymbol{\theta}^{(j)},\boldsymbol{\theta}^{*(-j)})}{L(\boldsymbol{\theta}^*|D)\pi(\boldsymbol{\theta}^*)}\right)\right| < \infty, \tag{4.5.5}$$

where $\boldsymbol{\theta}^{(j)} \sim \pi(\boldsymbol{\theta}^{(j)}|D)$, $\boldsymbol{\theta}^* \sim \pi(\boldsymbol{\theta}|D)$, *and* $\boldsymbol{\theta}^{(j)}$ *and* $\boldsymbol{\theta}^* = (\boldsymbol{\theta}^{*(j)},\boldsymbol{\theta}^{*(-j)})$ *are independent. Then, for an IWMDE given by* (4.3.4),

$$0 \le E[\Delta(\pi(\boldsymbol{\theta}^{(j)}|D), \hat{\pi}_{\text{IWMDE}}(\boldsymbol{\theta}^{(j)}|D))] < \infty. \tag{4.5.6}$$

In addition, if

$$\int_{R^j} \frac{1}{\pi(\boldsymbol{\theta}^{(j)}|D)} \cdot \left(\int_\Omega w^2(\boldsymbol{\theta}^{*(j)}|\boldsymbol{\theta}^{*(-j)})\frac{\pi^2(\boldsymbol{\theta}^{(j)},\boldsymbol{\theta}^{*(-j)}|D)}{\pi(\boldsymbol{\theta}^*|D)}d\boldsymbol{\theta}^*\right) d\boldsymbol{\theta}^{(j)} < \infty \tag{4.5.7}$$

and $\{\boldsymbol{\theta}_i,\ i = 1, 2, \ldots, n\}$ *is a random sample, then we have*

$$\begin{aligned} E[\Delta(\pi(\boldsymbol{\theta}^{(j)}|D), \hat{\pi}_{\text{IWMDE}}(\boldsymbol{\theta}^{(j)}|D))] &= \frac{1}{n}\left[\int_{R^j} \frac{1}{\pi(\boldsymbol{\theta}^{(j)}|D)}\right. \\ &\times \left.\left(\int_\Omega w^2(\boldsymbol{\theta}^{*(j)}|\boldsymbol{\theta}^{*(-j)})\frac{\pi^2(\boldsymbol{\theta}^{(j)},\boldsymbol{\theta}^{*(-j)}|D)}{\pi(\boldsymbol{\theta}^*|D)}\,d\boldsymbol{\theta}^*\right)\,d\boldsymbol{\theta}^{(j)} - 1\right] \\ &+ o\left(\frac{1}{n}\right). \end{aligned} \tag{4.5.8}$$

The proof is given in the Appendix.

Next we discuss how to use the K–L divergence to compare two marginal density estimators, and to assess convergence of a marginal density estimator. Let $\hat{\pi}_{n,\nu}(\boldsymbol{\theta}^{(j)}|D)$, $\nu = 1, 2$, be two estimators of $\pi(\boldsymbol{\theta}^{(j)}|D)$. To compare these two estimators, we introduce the difference between two K–L divergences, $\Delta(\pi(\boldsymbol{\theta}^{(j)}|D), \hat{\pi}_{n,\nu}(\boldsymbol{\theta}^{(j)}|D))$, $\nu = 1, 2$, defined as

$$\delta(\hat{\pi}_{n,1}, \hat{\pi}_{n,2}) = \int_{R^j} \ln\left(\frac{\hat{\pi}_{n,2}(\boldsymbol{\theta}^{(j)}|D)}{\hat{\pi}_{n,1}(\boldsymbol{\theta}^{(j)}|D)}\right)\pi(\boldsymbol{\theta}^{(j)}|D)\,d\boldsymbol{\theta}^{(j)}. \tag{4.5.9}$$

From (4.5.9), it can be seen that $\delta(\hat{\pi}_{n,1}, \hat{\pi}_{n,2})$ is not a statistic since it depends on the unknown density $\pi(\boldsymbol{\theta}^{(j)}|D)$. Therefore, we need to estimate $\delta(\hat{\pi}_{n,1}, \hat{\pi}_{n,2})$. One possible approach is the smoothed bootstrap (see Scott 1992) which, however, requires a bootstrap sample from $\hat{\pi}_{n,\nu}$. This does not appear to be easy to generate. Another possible approach is to use the available sample $\{\boldsymbol{\theta}_i,\ i = 1, 2, \ldots, n\}$ to estimate $\delta(\hat{\pi}_{n,1}, \hat{\pi}_{n,2})$ by

$$\hat{\delta}(\hat{\pi}_{n,1}, \hat{\pi}_{n,2}) = \frac{1}{n}\sum_{i=1}^n \ln\left(\frac{\hat{\pi}_{n,2}(\boldsymbol{\theta}_i^{(j)}|D)}{\hat{\pi}_{n,1}(\boldsymbol{\theta}_i^{(j)}|D)}\right). \tag{4.5.10}$$

Alternatively, we can replace (4.5.10) by using a jackknife-type estimator with the available sample $\{\boldsymbol{\theta}_i\}$. Since the sample $\{\boldsymbol{\theta}_i\}$ has already been used for estimating the $\hat{\pi}_{n,\nu}$, it can be shown that $\hat{\delta}(\hat{\pi}_{n,1}, \hat{\pi}_{n,2})$ given in (4.5.10), or a similar jackknife estimator, is a degenerate U-statistic. Since the limiting distribution of this degenerate U-statistic is associated with a series of eigenvalues that depend on the forms of $\hat{\pi}_{n,\nu}$, $\nu = 1, 2$, and the unknown marginal posterior distribution of $\boldsymbol{\theta}^{(j)}$ (see Serfling (1980, pp. 193–194)), it is difficult to estimate the standard error of $\hat{\delta}(\hat{\pi}_{n,1}, \hat{\pi}_{n,2})$. One simple remedy is to use an additional sample from $\pi(\boldsymbol{\theta}|D)$ to obtain a Monte Carlo estimate of $\delta(\hat{\pi}_{n,1}, \hat{\pi}_{n,2})$. Let $\{\boldsymbol{\theta}_l^*,\ l = 1, 2, \ldots, m\}$ be another sample from $\pi(\boldsymbol{\theta}|D)$ that is independent of the $\{\boldsymbol{\theta}_i,\ i = 1, 2, \ldots, n\}$. Further, we assume that both $\{\boldsymbol{\theta}_i\}$ and $\{\boldsymbol{\theta}_l^*\}$ are independent. Then $\delta(\hat{\pi}_{n,1}, \hat{\pi}_{n,2})$ can be approximated by

$$\hat{\delta}_m(\hat{\pi}_{n,1}, \hat{\pi}_{n,2}) = \frac{1}{m} \sum_{l=1}^{m} \ln \left(\frac{\hat{\pi}_{n,2}(\boldsymbol{\theta}_l^{*(j)}|D)}{\hat{\pi}_{n,1}(\boldsymbol{\theta}_l^{*(j)}|D)} \right), \tag{4.5.11}$$

and the sign of $\hat{\delta}_m(\hat{\pi}_{n,1}, \hat{\pi}_{n,2})$ determines which of the two density estimators is better.

In order to obtain an estimate of the variance of $\hat{\delta}_m(\hat{\pi}_{n,1}, \hat{\pi}_{n,2})$, we assume that $\hat{\pi}_{n,\nu}$ has the following form:

$$\hat{\pi}_{n,\nu}(\boldsymbol{\theta}^{(j)}|D) = \frac{1}{n} \sum_{i=1}^{n} f_\nu(\boldsymbol{\theta}^{(j)}, \boldsymbol{\theta}_i), \tag{4.5.12}$$

where $f_\nu(\boldsymbol{\theta}^{(j)}, \boldsymbol{\theta}_i)$ is a function of $\boldsymbol{\theta}^{(j)}$ and $\boldsymbol{\theta}_i$, which may depend on n. In (4.5.12), $\hat{\pi}_{n,\nu}(\boldsymbol{\theta}^{(j)}|D)$ reduces to a kernel density estimator or an IWMDE if we take

$$f_\nu(\boldsymbol{\theta}^{(j)}, \boldsymbol{\theta}_i) = \frac{1}{h_n^j} \mathcal{K}\left(\frac{\boldsymbol{\theta}^{(j)} - \boldsymbol{\theta}_i^{(j)}}{h_n} \right)$$

or

$$f_\nu(\boldsymbol{\theta}^{(j)}, \boldsymbol{\theta}_i) = w(\boldsymbol{\theta}_i^{(j)}|\boldsymbol{\theta}_i^{(-j)}) \frac{L(\boldsymbol{\theta}^{(j)}, \boldsymbol{\theta}_i^{(-j)}|D)\pi(\boldsymbol{\theta}^{(j)}, \boldsymbol{\theta}_i^{(-j)})}{L(\boldsymbol{\theta}_i|D)\pi(\boldsymbol{\theta}_i)}.$$

Then, we have the following asymptotic result:

Theorem 4.5.2 *Let* $\hat{\pi}_{n,\nu}$, $\nu = 1, 2$, *be two unbiased estimators of* $\pi(\boldsymbol{\theta}^{(j)}|D)$. *Assume that* (4.5.4),

$$E(|\ln f_\nu(\boldsymbol{\theta}^{*(j)}, \boldsymbol{\theta})|) < \infty, \quad \nu = 1, 2, \tag{4.5.13}$$

and

$$E[E(f_\nu(\boldsymbol{\theta}^{*(j)}, \boldsymbol{\theta})/\pi(\boldsymbol{\theta}^{*(j)}|D) \,|\, \boldsymbol{\theta})]^2 < \infty, \quad \nu = 1, 2 \tag{4.5.14}$$

are satisfied, where $\boldsymbol{\theta}^{*(j)} \sim \pi(\boldsymbol{\theta}^{(j)}|D)$, $\boldsymbol{\theta} \sim \pi(\boldsymbol{\theta}|D)$, *and* $\boldsymbol{\theta}^{*(j)}$ *and* $\boldsymbol{\theta}$ *are independent. If* $m \geq n$ *and* $f_\nu(\boldsymbol{\theta}^{*(j)}, \boldsymbol{\theta}_i)$, $\nu = 1, 2$, *do not depend on* n, *then*

$$n \operatorname{Var}(\hat{\delta}_m(\hat{\pi}_{n,1}, \hat{\pi}_{n,2})) \longrightarrow E\left[E\left(\frac{f_2(\boldsymbol{\theta}^{*(j)}, \boldsymbol{\theta}) - f_1(\boldsymbol{\theta}^{*(j)}, \boldsymbol{\theta})}{\pi(\boldsymbol{\theta}^{*(j)}|D)} \,\middle|\, \boldsymbol{\theta}\right)\right]^2 \quad \text{as } n \to \infty. \tag{4.5.15}$$

The proof is given in the Appendix. Theorem 4.5.2 cannot be directly applied to the kernel estimator since a kernel estimator is not an unbiased estimator of $\pi(\boldsymbol{\theta}^{(j)}|D)$ and $f_l(\boldsymbol{\theta}^{(j)}, \boldsymbol{\theta}_i)$ in the kernel estimator does depend on n. However, when one of the density estimators is kernel and another is an IWMDE, we have the following asymptotic result:

Corollary 4.5.1 *Assume that* $\hat{\pi}_{n,1}$ *is a kernel estimator, i.e.,*

$$f_1(\boldsymbol{\theta}^{(j)}, \boldsymbol{\theta}_i) = \frac{1}{h_n^j}\mathcal{K}\left(\frac{\boldsymbol{\theta}^{(j)} - \boldsymbol{\theta}_i^{(j)}}{h_n}\right)$$

and $\hat{\pi}_{n,2}$ *is an IWMDE. Suppose that* (4.5.4), (4.5.13), *and* (4.5.14) *are satisfied. If* $m \geq n$, *then*

$$n \operatorname{Var}(\hat{\delta}_m(\hat{\pi}_{n,1}, \hat{\pi}_{n,2})) \longrightarrow \operatorname{Var}\left[E\left(\frac{f_2(\boldsymbol{\theta}^{*(j)}, \boldsymbol{\theta})}{\pi(\boldsymbol{\theta}^{*(j)}|D)} \,\middle|\, \boldsymbol{\theta}\right)\right] \quad \text{as } n \to \infty. \tag{4.5.16}$$

The proof is provided in the Appendix.

Now we can obtain an approximate standard error of $\hat{\delta}_m(\hat{\pi}_{n,1}, \hat{\pi}_{n,2})$ by Theorem 4.5.2 or Corollary 4.5.1 using the available Monte Carlo outputs $\{\boldsymbol{\theta}_i,\ i = 1, 2, \ldots, n\}$ and $\{\boldsymbol{\theta}_l^*,\ l = 1, 2, \ldots, m\}$. For example, when the $\hat{\pi}_{n,\nu}$'s are unbiased, the standard error of $\hat{\delta}_m(\hat{\pi}_{n,1}, \hat{\pi}_{n,2})$ can be approximated by

$$\sqrt{1/n}\left[\frac{1}{n}\sum_{i=1}^n\left(\frac{1}{m}\sum_{l=1}^m \frac{f_2(\boldsymbol{\theta}_l^{*(j)}, \boldsymbol{\theta}_i) - f_1(\boldsymbol{\theta}_l^{*(j)}, \boldsymbol{\theta}_i)}{\hat{\pi}_{n+m}(\boldsymbol{\theta}_l^{*(j)}|D)}\right)^2\right]^{1/2}, \tag{4.5.17}$$

where $\hat{\pi}_{n+m}(\boldsymbol{\theta}_l^{*(j)}|D)$ is an estimator of $\pi(\boldsymbol{\theta}_l^{*(j)}|D)$ using the combined Monte Carlo samples $\{\boldsymbol{\theta}_i\}$ and $\{\boldsymbol{\theta}_l^*\}$. In (4.5.17), $\hat{\pi}_{n+m}(\boldsymbol{\theta}_l^{*(j)}|D)$ may be chosen as either $\hat{\pi}_{n+m,1}(\boldsymbol{\theta}_l^{*(j)}|D)$ or $\hat{\pi}_{n+m,2}(\boldsymbol{\theta}_l^{*(j)}|D)$. Since the combined Monte Carlo samples yield a larger sample size, $\hat{\pi}_{n+m}(\boldsymbol{\theta}_l^{*(j)}|D)$ is expected to be a good approximation of $\pi(\boldsymbol{\theta}_l^{*(j)}|D)$ for each $\boldsymbol{\theta}_l^{*(j)}$. When $\hat{\pi}_{n,1}$ is a kernel estimator, the standard error of $\hat{\delta}_m(\hat{\pi}_{n,1}, \hat{\pi}_{n,2})$ can be approximated by

$$\sqrt{1/n}\left[\frac{1}{n}\sum_{i=1}^n\left(\frac{1}{m}\sum_{l=1}^m \frac{f_2(\boldsymbol{\theta}_l^{*(j)}, \boldsymbol{\theta}_i)}{\hat{\pi}_{n+m,2}(\boldsymbol{\theta}_l^{*(j)}|D)} - 1\right)^2\right]^{1/2}. \tag{4.5.18}$$

Finally, we consider assessing convergence of a marginal posterior density estimator. In this case, we need to take n^* additional random observations from $\pi(\boldsymbol{\theta}|D)$. Let $\{\boldsymbol{\theta}_i, i = n+1, \ldots, n+n^*\}$ be these n^* observations and assume that $\{\boldsymbol{\theta}_i, i = n+1, \ldots, n+n^*\}$, $\{\boldsymbol{\theta}_i, i = 1, \ldots, n\}$, and $\{\boldsymbol{\theta}_l^*, l = 1, \ldots, m\}$ are independent. Let $\hat{\pi}_n(\boldsymbol{\theta}^{(j)}|D)$ and $\hat{\pi}_{n+n^*}(\boldsymbol{\theta}^{(j)}|D)$ denote two estimators of $\pi(\boldsymbol{\theta}^{(j)}|D)$ associated with sample sizes n and $n+n^*$. Suppose that

$$\hat{\pi}_n(\boldsymbol{\theta}^{(j)}|D) = \frac{1}{n}\sum_{i=1}^{n} f(\boldsymbol{\theta}^{(j)}, \boldsymbol{\theta}_i)$$

and

$$\hat{\pi}_{n+n^*}(\boldsymbol{\theta}^{(j)}|D) = \frac{1}{n+n^*}\sum_{i=1}^{n+n^*} f(\boldsymbol{\theta}^{(j)}, \boldsymbol{\theta}_i),$$

where $f(\boldsymbol{\theta}^{(j)}, \boldsymbol{\theta})$ is a function of $\boldsymbol{\theta}^{(j)}$ and $\boldsymbol{\theta}$, which is similar to f_ν in (4.5.12). Thus, the difference between the two K–L divergences $\Delta(\pi(\boldsymbol{\theta}^{(j)}|D), \hat{\pi}_n\,(\boldsymbol{\theta}^{(j)}\,|D))$ and $\Delta(\pi(\boldsymbol{\theta}^{(j)}|D), \hat{\pi}_{n+n^*}(\boldsymbol{\theta}^{(j)}|D))$ is of the form

$$\delta(\hat{\pi}_n, \hat{\pi}_{n+n^*}) = \int_{R^j} \ln\left(\frac{\hat{\pi}_{n+n^*}(\boldsymbol{\theta}_i^{(j)}|D)}{\hat{\pi}_n(\boldsymbol{\theta}_i^{(j)}|D)}\right) \pi(\boldsymbol{\theta}^{(j)}|D)\; d\boldsymbol{\theta}^{(j)},$$

which can be approximated by

$$\hat{\delta}_m \overset{\text{def}}{=} \hat{\delta}_m(\hat{\pi}_n, \hat{\pi}_{n+n^*}) = \frac{1}{m}\sum_{l=1}^{m} \ln\left(\frac{\hat{\pi}_{n+n^*}(\boldsymbol{\theta}_l^{*(j)}|D)}{\hat{\pi}_n(\boldsymbol{\theta}_l^{*(j)}|D)}\right). \tag{4.5.19}$$

Therefore, if $\hat{\pi}_n(\boldsymbol{\theta}^{(j)}|D)$ converges with sample size n, $\hat{\delta}_m(\hat{\pi}_n, \hat{\pi}_{n+n^*})$ should be reasonably small. Otherwise, a larger sample size n must be taken. Note that the above procedure may not give a reliable result if n^* is too small. We recommend that n^* is chosen to be at least as large as n so that $\hat{\pi}_{n+n^*}(\boldsymbol{\theta}^{(j)}|D)$ is approximately the true marginal density $\pi(\boldsymbol{\theta}^{(j)}|D)$. Similar to (4.5.15), we have the following asymptotic result:

Theorem 4.5.3 *Assume that for any given* $\boldsymbol{\theta}_{(l)}$,

$$E[f(\boldsymbol{\theta}^{*(j)}, \boldsymbol{\theta})] = \pi(\boldsymbol{\theta}^{*(j)}|D),$$

where the expectation is taken with respect to $\pi(\boldsymbol{\theta}|D)$ *and* $f(\boldsymbol{\theta}^{*(j)}, \boldsymbol{\theta})$ *does not depend on* n *and* n^*. *Assume that* (4.5.4),

$$E(|\ln f(\boldsymbol{\theta}^{*(j)}, \boldsymbol{\theta})|) < \infty$$

and

$$E[E(f(\boldsymbol{\theta}^{*(j)}, \boldsymbol{\theta})/\pi(\boldsymbol{\theta}^{*(j)}|D)\ |\boldsymbol{\theta})]^2 < \infty$$

are satisfied. Then, if $m \geq n + n^*$, we have

$$\frac{n(n+n^*)}{n^*} \operatorname{Var}(\hat{\delta}_m)$$
$$\longrightarrow E\left[E\left(\frac{f(\boldsymbol{\theta}^{*(j)}, \boldsymbol{\theta}) - \pi(\boldsymbol{\theta}^{*(j)}|D)}{\pi(\boldsymbol{\theta}^{*(j)}|D)}\middle|\boldsymbol{\theta}\right)\right]^2 \quad \text{as } n \to \infty, \tag{4.5.20}$$

where $\hat{\delta}_m$ is defined by (4.5.19), $\boldsymbol{\theta}^{*(j)} \sim \pi(\boldsymbol{\theta}^{*(j)}|D)$, $\boldsymbol{\theta} \sim \pi(\boldsymbol{\theta}|D)$, and $\boldsymbol{\theta}^{*(j)}$ and $\boldsymbol{\theta}$ are independent.

The proof is similar to that of Theorem 4.5.2. Using Theorem 4.5.3 and the available Monte Carlo samples, the standard error of $\hat{\delta}_m$ can be approximated by

$$\sqrt{n^*/(n(n+n^*))}\left[\frac{1}{n+n^*}\sum_{i=1}^{n+n^*}\left(\frac{1}{m}\sum_{l=1}^{m}\frac{f(\boldsymbol{\theta}_l^{*(j)}, \boldsymbol{\theta}_i)}{\hat{\pi}_{n+n^*+m}(\boldsymbol{\theta}_l^{*(j)}|D)} - 1\right)^2\right]^{1/2}, \tag{4.5.21}$$

where $\hat{\pi}_{n+n^*+m}(\boldsymbol{\theta}_l^{*(j)}|D)$ is an estimator of $\pi(\boldsymbol{\theta}_l^{*(j)}|D)$ using all the Monte Carlo samples $\{\boldsymbol{\theta}_i\}$ and $\{\boldsymbol{\theta}_l^*\}$. Since $n + n^* + m$ is large, $\hat{\pi}_{n+n^*+m}(\boldsymbol{\theta}_l^{*(j)}|D)$ is expected to be a good approximation of $\pi(\boldsymbol{\theta}_l^{*(j)}|D)$.

Example 4.4. Constrained Multiple Linear Regression Model (Example 4.3 continued). For the constrained multiple linear regression model and the corresponding joint posterior density for $(\boldsymbol{\beta}, \sigma^2)$ given by (1.3.1) and (2.1.7), we study the performance of the marginal posterior density estimators for β_1 and β_2 obtained in Example 4.3.

First, we consider β_1. In Example 4.3, we chose

$$w(\beta_1|\beta_j, j \geq 2, \sigma^2) = \frac{1}{\beta_2}, \quad 0 < \beta_1 < \beta_2,$$

to obtain an IWMDE of the marginal posterior density for β_1. In this case, the CMDE is available, since the conditional posterior distribution of β_1 is a truncated normal distribution over the interval $(0, \beta_2)$ with mean

$$\frac{\sum_{i=1}^{207}(y_i - \sum_{l=2}^{10} x_{il}\beta_l)x_{i1}}{\sum_{i=1}^{207} x_{i1}^2}$$

and variance

$$\frac{\sigma^2}{\sum_{i=1}^{207} x_{i1}^2}.$$

We obtain a kernel density estimator by taking $\mathcal{K}$ in (4.2.1) equal to the $N(0, 1)$ density and $h_n = 1.06s(\hat{\beta}_1)n^{-1/5}$, where n is the size of the Monte Carlo sample and the posterior standard deviation of β_1 is $s(\hat{\beta}_1) = 0.0081$.

TABLE 4.1. Performance Comparisons of the Kernel Estimator, IWMDE and CMDE for β_1.

	$n = 50$	$n = 100$	$n = 500$
$\hat{\delta}$ (IWMDE, CMDE)	0.0151	0.0131	0.008
(Std. Err.)	(0.050)	(0.041)	(0.035)
$\hat{\delta}$ (Kernel, CMDE)	0.0533	0.0411	0.0240
(Std. Err.)	(0.046)	(0.035)	(0.015)

To compare the performance of the kernel estimator, IWMDE and CMDE, using (4.5.11), (4.5.17), and (4.5.18), we obtain the estimated differences between two K–L divergences and their simulation standard errors. We consider three different sample sizes, namely, $n = 50$, 100, and 500, and use $m = 1000$ in our calculations. The results are given in Table 4.1. From Table 4.1, it can be seen that the IWMDEs and CMDEs are virtually the same even for $n = 50$ while the CMDEs are better than the kernel estimates for all three n's as are the IWMDEs. We further investigate convergence of IWMDE and CMDE and obtain the $\hat{\delta}(\hat{\pi}_n, \hat{\pi}_{n+n^*})$'s and their simulation standard errors using (4.5.19) and (4.5.21) for $n = n^* = 50$, 100, and 500. The results are given in Table 4.2. Again, we use $m = 1000$ in our calculations. From Table 4.2, we see that both IWMDE and CMDE converge as early as $n = 50$, since the estimated differences of the two K–L divergences are essentially zero for all three n's.

Second, we consider β_2. For the kernel estimate, IWMDE, and CMDE we obtain similar performance comparison results as for β_1. Therefore, we focus on investigating the performance of the IWMDE for different choices of the weight conditional density w. Note that the posterior mean and the posterior standard deviation of β_2 are $\hat{\beta}_2 = 0.0249$ and $s(\hat{\beta}_2) = 0.0082$ and the posterior mean of β_3 is $\hat{\beta}_3 = 0.1776$. We consider three choices of w as follows. The first w is simply chosen as a uniform distribution over the interval (β_1, β_3). That is,

$$w_1(\beta_2|\beta_j, j \neq 2, \sigma^2) = \frac{1}{\beta_3 - \beta_1}, \quad \beta_1 < \beta_2 < \beta_3.$$

TABLE 4.2. Convergence Study of IWMDE and CMDE for β_1.

	$n = n^* = 50$	$n = n^* = 100$	$n = n^* = 500$
$\hat{\delta}$ (IWMDE)	0.0384	−0.0020	−0.0094
(Std. Err.)	(0.0424)	(0.0298)	(0.0147)
$\hat{\delta}$ (CMDE)	−0.0017	−0.0004	0.0009
(Std. Err.)	(0.0043)	(0.0038)	(0.0019)

TABLE 4.3. Performance Comparison of Three IWMDEs for β_2.

	$n = 100$	$n = 500$
$\hat{\delta}$ (IWMDE$_1$, CMDE) (Std. Err.)	1.714 (0.243)	1.328 (0.144)
$\hat{\delta}$ (IWMDE$_2$, CMDE) (Std. Err.)	0.185 (0.191)	0.091 (0.135)
$\hat{\delta}$ (IWMDE$_3$, CMDE) (Std. Err.)	0.153 (0.110)	0.034 (0.058)

We follow the empirical procedure described in Section 4.3 to obtain the second w_2, which is given in (4.4.1). The third choice (w_3) is a truncated normal density over the interval (β_1, β_3) with a mean of $\hat{\beta}_2$ and a standard deviation of $s(\hat{\beta}_2)$. The IWMDEs corresponding to w_1, w_2, and w_3 are denoted by IWMDE$_1$, IWMDE$_2$, and IWMDE$_3$, respectively. Note that the CMDE is also available and is a truncated normal distribution over the interval (β_1, β_3) with mean

$$\frac{\sum_{i=1}^{207}(y_i - \sum_{l=1, l\neq 2}^{10} x_{il}\beta_l)x_{i2}}{\sum_{i=1}^{207} x_{i2}^2}$$

and variance

$$\frac{\sigma^2}{\sum_{i=1}^{207} x_{i2}^2}.$$

Therefore, IWMDE$_3$ is not CMDE. Since $\hat{\beta}_2$ is much closer to $\hat{\beta}_1$ than $\hat{\beta}_3$, w_1 may be a bad choice, since w_1 does not have a shape similar to that of the conditional posterior density of β_2 given the other parameters. On the other hand, w_3 may be a better choice, since the conditional distribution of β_2 given the other β_j's and σ^2 is normal. Again, using (4.5.11) and (4.5.17) we obtain the estimated differences between the two K–L divergences and their simulation standard errors. We consider three different sample sizes, namely, $n = 100$ and 500, and we use $m = 5000$ in our calculations. The results are given in Table 4.3. From Table 4.3, we can see that IWMDE$_3$ is marginally better than IWMDE$_2$. Also IWMDE$_2$ is much better than IWMDE$_1$, which is expected. From these results, we can also see that the K–L divergence measure proposed in this section can detect whether a "good" w or a "bad" w is chosen.

Chen and Shao (1997c) also study the performance of the IWMDE for estimating the joint distribution of β_1 and β_2. They find that the IWMDE given in (4.4.2) is better than a two-dimensional kernel estimate suggested by Silverman (1986, Chap. 4). All of the above results indicate that the empirical procedure for choosing a w for the IWMDE given in Section 4.3 works well, and this procedure indeed provides a good choice of w.

Appendix

Proof of Theorem 4.3.1. If $V_w(\hat{\pi}(\boldsymbol{\theta}^{*(j)}|D)) = \infty$, the inequality (4.3.8) automatically holds. Now we assume

$$V_w(\hat{\pi}(\boldsymbol{\theta}^{*(j)}|D)) < \infty.$$

Since the CMDE is a special case of the IWMDE, by (4.3.7), it suffices to prove that

$$\begin{aligned}\int_\Omega \left[\frac{w_C(\boldsymbol{\theta}^{(j)}|\boldsymbol{\theta}^{(-j)})\pi(\boldsymbol{\theta}^{*(j)},\boldsymbol{\theta}^{(-j)}|D)}{\pi(\boldsymbol{\theta}|D)}\right]^2 \pi(\boldsymbol{\theta}|D)\ d\boldsymbol{\theta}^{(j)}\ d\boldsymbol{\theta}^{(-j)} \\ \leq \int_\Omega \left[\frac{w(\boldsymbol{\theta}^{(j)}|\boldsymbol{\theta}^{(-j)})\pi(\boldsymbol{\theta}^{*(j)},\boldsymbol{\theta}^{(-j)}|D)}{\pi(\boldsymbol{\theta}|D)}\right]^2 \pi(\boldsymbol{\theta}|D)\ d\boldsymbol{\theta}^{(j)}\ d\boldsymbol{\theta}^{(-j)}.\end{aligned} \tag{4.A.1}$$

Let $\pi(\boldsymbol{\theta}^{(-j)}|D)$ denote the marginal posterior density of $\boldsymbol{\theta}^{(-j)}$. Then

$$w_C(\boldsymbol{\theta}^{(j)}|\boldsymbol{\theta}^{(-j)}) = \frac{\pi(\boldsymbol{\theta}|D)}{\pi(\boldsymbol{\theta}^{(-j)}|D)}.$$

Thus, the left-hand side of inequality (4.A.1) is equal to

$$\begin{aligned}\int_{\Omega_{-j}(\boldsymbol{\theta}^{*(j)})} \frac{\pi^2(\boldsymbol{\theta}^{*(j)},\boldsymbol{\theta}^{(-j)}|D)}{\pi^2(\boldsymbol{\theta}^{(-j)}|D)} \left[\int_{\Omega_j(\boldsymbol{\theta}^{(-j)})} \pi(\boldsymbol{\theta}|D)\ d\boldsymbol{\theta}^{(j)}\right] d\boldsymbol{\theta}^{(-j)} \\ = \int_{\Omega_{-j}(\boldsymbol{\theta}^{*(j)})} \frac{\pi^2(\boldsymbol{\theta}^{*(j)},\boldsymbol{\theta}^{(-j)}|D)}{\pi(\boldsymbol{\theta}^{(-j)}|D)}\ d\boldsymbol{\theta}^{(-j)}.\end{aligned} \tag{4.A.2}$$

By the Cauchy–Schwarz inequality, we have

$$\begin{aligned}1 &= \left[\int_{\Omega_j(\boldsymbol{\theta}^{(-j)})} w(\boldsymbol{\theta}^{(j)}|\boldsymbol{\theta}^{(-j)})\ d\boldsymbol{\theta}^{(j)}\right]^2 \\ &= \left[\int_{\Omega_j(\boldsymbol{\theta}^{(-j)})} \sqrt{\pi(\boldsymbol{\theta}|D)}\frac{w(\boldsymbol{\theta}^{(j)}|\boldsymbol{\theta}^{(-j)})}{\sqrt{\pi(\boldsymbol{\theta}|D)}}\ d\boldsymbol{\theta}^{(j)}\right]^2 \\ &\leq \left[\int_{\Omega_j(\boldsymbol{\theta}^{(-j)})} \pi(\boldsymbol{\theta}|D) d\boldsymbol{\theta}^{(j)}\right]\left[\int_{\Omega_j(\boldsymbol{\theta}^{(-j)})} \frac{w^2(\boldsymbol{\theta}^{(j)}|\boldsymbol{\theta}^{(-j)})}{\pi(\boldsymbol{\theta}|D)}\ d\boldsymbol{\theta}^{(j)}\right] \\ &= \pi(\boldsymbol{\theta}^{(-j)}|D)\left[\int_{\Omega_j(\boldsymbol{\theta}^{(-j)})} \frac{w^2(\boldsymbol{\theta}^{(j)}|\boldsymbol{\theta}^{(-j)})}{\pi(\boldsymbol{\theta}|D)}\ d\boldsymbol{\theta}^{(j)}\right].\end{aligned} \tag{4.A.3}$$

Theorem 4.3.1 now follows from (4.A.2) and (4.A.3). □

Proof of Theorem 4.5.1. It is easy to observe that (4.5.4) implies

$$\int_{R^j} \pi(\boldsymbol{\theta}^{(j)}|D) \ln \pi(\boldsymbol{\theta}^{(j)}|D)\ d\boldsymbol{\theta}^{(j)} < \infty.$$

Below we show that

$$L \stackrel{\text{def}}{=} E\left\{\int_{R^j} \pi(\boldsymbol{\theta}^{(j)}|D) |\ln \hat{\pi}_{\text{IWMDE}}(\boldsymbol{\theta}^{(j)}|D)|\ d\boldsymbol{\theta}^{(j)}\right\} < \infty, \tag{4.A.4}$$

which will immediately imply that

$$\int_{R^j} \pi(\boldsymbol{\theta}^{(j)}|D) |\ln \hat{\pi}_{\text{IWMDE}}(\boldsymbol{\theta}^{(j)}|D)|\ d\boldsymbol{\theta}^{(j)} < \infty \quad \text{a.s.}$$

Note that

$$\begin{aligned} L \leq & E\left\{\int_{R^j} \pi(\boldsymbol{\theta}^{(j)}|D) \ln(1 + \hat{\pi}_{\text{IWMDE}}(\boldsymbol{\theta}^{(j)}|D))\ d\boldsymbol{\theta}^{(j)}\right\} \\ & + E\left\{\int_{R^j} \pi(\boldsymbol{\theta}^{(j)}|D) |\ln \hat{\pi}_{\text{IWMDE}}(\boldsymbol{\theta}^{(j)}|D)|\, 1\{\hat{\pi}_{\text{IWMDE}}(\boldsymbol{\theta}^{(j)}|D) \leq 1\}\ d\boldsymbol{\theta}^{(j)}\right\} \\ \stackrel{\text{def}}{=} & L_1 + L_2, \end{aligned} \tag{4.A.5}$$

where the indicator function $1\{\hat{\pi}_{\text{IWMDE}}(\boldsymbol{\theta}^{(j)}|D) \leq 1\}$ is 1 if $\hat{\pi}_{\text{IWMDE}}(\boldsymbol{\theta}^{(j)}|D) \leq 1$ and 0 otherwise. From Jensen's inequality it follows that

$$\begin{aligned} L_1 \leq & \int_{R^j} \pi(\boldsymbol{\theta}^{(j)}|D) \ln E(1 + \hat{\pi}_{\text{IWMDE}}(\boldsymbol{\theta}^{(j)}|D))\ d\boldsymbol{\theta}^{(j)} \\ = & \int_{R^j} \pi(\boldsymbol{\theta}^{(j)}|D) \ln(1 + \pi(\boldsymbol{\theta}^{(j)}|D))\ d\boldsymbol{\theta}^{(j)} < \infty. \end{aligned}$$

As for L_2, we have

$$\begin{aligned} L_2 \leq & E\Big\{\int_{R^j} \pi(\boldsymbol{\theta}^{(j)}|D) \Big| \ln\Big(w(\boldsymbol{\theta}^{*(j)}|\boldsymbol{\theta}^{*(-j)}) \frac{L(\boldsymbol{\theta}^{(j)}, \boldsymbol{\theta}^{*(-j)}|D)\pi(\boldsymbol{\theta}^{(j)}, \boldsymbol{\theta}^{*(-j)})}{nL(\boldsymbol{\theta}^*|D)\pi(\boldsymbol{\theta}^*)}\Big)\Big| \\ & \times\ 1\{w(\boldsymbol{\theta}^{*(j)}|\boldsymbol{\theta}^{*(-j)}) \frac{L(\boldsymbol{\theta}^{(j)}, \boldsymbol{\theta}^{*(-j)}|D)\pi(\boldsymbol{\theta}^{(j)}, \boldsymbol{\theta}^{*(-j)})}{nL(\boldsymbol{\theta}^*|D)\pi(\boldsymbol{\theta}^*)} \leq 1\}\ d\boldsymbol{\theta}^{(j)}\Big\} \\ \leq & \ln n + E\Big\{\int_{R^j} \pi(\boldsymbol{\theta}^{(j)}|D) \Big| \ln\Big(w(\boldsymbol{\theta}^{*(j)}|\boldsymbol{\theta}^{*(-j)}) \\ & \times\ \frac{L(\boldsymbol{\theta}^{(j)}, \boldsymbol{\theta}^{*(-j)}|D)\pi(\boldsymbol{\theta}^{(j)}, \boldsymbol{\theta}^{*(-j)})}{L(\boldsymbol{\theta}^*|D)\pi(\boldsymbol{\theta}^*)}\Big)\Big|\ d\boldsymbol{\theta}^{(j)}\Big\} \\ = & \ln n + E\Big| \ln\Big(w(\boldsymbol{\theta}^{*(j)}|\boldsymbol{\theta}^{*(-j)}) \frac{L(\boldsymbol{\theta}^{(j)}, \boldsymbol{\theta}^{*(-j)}|D)\pi(\boldsymbol{\theta}^{(j)}, \boldsymbol{\theta}^{*(-j)})}{L(\boldsymbol{\theta}^*|D)\pi(\boldsymbol{\theta}^*)}\Big)\Big| \\ < & \infty. \end{aligned}$$

This proves (4.A.4).

Using Jensen's inequality again, we have

$$
\begin{aligned}
&E[\Delta(\pi(\boldsymbol{\theta}^{(j)}|D), \hat{\pi}_{\mathrm{IWMDE}}(\boldsymbol{\theta}^{(j)}|D))] \\
&\qquad \geq \int_{R^j} \pi(\boldsymbol{\theta}^{(j)}|D) \ln \pi(\boldsymbol{\theta}^{(j)}|D)\, d\boldsymbol{\theta}^{(j)} \\
&\qquad\quad - \int_{R^j} \pi(\boldsymbol{\theta}^{(j)}|D) \ln E[\hat{\pi}_{\mathrm{IWMDE}}(\boldsymbol{\theta}^{(j)}|D)]\, d\boldsymbol{\theta}^{(j)}.
\end{aligned} \tag{4.A.6}
$$

Since $\hat{\pi}_{\mathrm{IWMDE}}(\boldsymbol{\theta}^{(j)}|D)$ is an unbiased estimator of $\pi(\boldsymbol{\theta}^{(j)}|D)$, the right-hand side of (4.A.6) is zero. This proves (4.5.6).

Next we prove (4.5.8). Observe that

$$
\ln \hat{\pi}_{\mathrm{IWMDE}}(\boldsymbol{\theta}^{(j)}|D) = \ln \pi(\boldsymbol{\theta}^{(j)}|D) + \ln\left(1 + \frac{\hat{\pi}_{\mathrm{IWMDE}}(\boldsymbol{\theta}^{(j)}|D) - \pi(\boldsymbol{\theta}^{(j)}|D)}{\pi(\boldsymbol{\theta}^{(j)}|D)}\right).
$$

Using a Taylor series expansion along with condition (4.5.7), we have

$$
\begin{aligned}
&E[\Delta(\pi(\boldsymbol{\theta}^{(j)}|D), \hat{\pi}_{\mathrm{IWMDE}}(\boldsymbol{\theta}^{(j)}|D))] \\
&\quad = \int_{R^j} \pi(\boldsymbol{\theta}^{(j)}|D) \ln \pi(\boldsymbol{\theta}^{(j)}|D)\, d\boldsymbol{\theta}^{(j)} \\
&\qquad - \int_{R^j} \pi(\boldsymbol{\theta}_{(l)}|D) E[\ln \hat{\pi}_{\mathrm{IWMDE}}(\boldsymbol{\theta}^{(j)}|D)]\, d\boldsymbol{\theta}^{(j)} \\
&\quad = - \int_{R^j} \pi(\boldsymbol{\theta}^{(j)}|D) E\left[\ln\left(1 + \frac{\hat{\pi}_{\mathrm{IWMDE}}(\boldsymbol{\theta}^{(j)}|D) - \pi(\boldsymbol{\theta}^{(j)}|D)}{\pi(\boldsymbol{\theta}^{(j)}|D)}\right)\right] d\boldsymbol{\theta}^{(j)} \\
&\quad = \int_{R^j} E\left(\frac{\hat{\pi}_{\mathrm{IWMDE}}(\boldsymbol{\theta}^{(j)}|D) - \pi(\boldsymbol{\theta}^{(j)}|D)}{\pi(\boldsymbol{\theta}^{(j)}|D)}\right)^2 \pi(\boldsymbol{\theta}^{(j)}|D)\, d\boldsymbol{\theta}^{(j)} + o\left(\frac{1}{n}\right) \\
&\quad = \frac{1}{n}\left[\int_{R^j} \frac{1}{\pi(\boldsymbol{\theta}^{(j)}|D)} \left(\int_{\Omega} w^2(\boldsymbol{\theta}^{*(j)}|\boldsymbol{\theta}^{*(-j)}) \right.\right. \\
&\qquad \left.\left. \times \frac{\pi^2(\boldsymbol{\theta}^{(j)}, \boldsymbol{\theta}^{*(-j)}|D)}{\pi(\boldsymbol{\theta}^*|D)}\, d\boldsymbol{\theta}^*\right) d\boldsymbol{\theta}^{(j)} - 1\right] \\
&\qquad + o\left(\frac{1}{n}\right).
\end{aligned}
$$

This proves Theorem 4.5.1. □

Proof of Theorem 4.5.2. Let $\hat{\delta}$ denote $\hat{\delta}_m(\hat{\pi}_{n,1}, \hat{\pi}_{n,2})$. Observe that

$$\begin{aligned}
\operatorname{Var}(\hat{\delta}) &= \operatorname{Var}[E(\hat{\delta}|\boldsymbol{\theta}_i, 1 \le i \le n)] + E[\operatorname{Var}(\hat{\delta}|\boldsymbol{\theta}_i, 1 \le i \le n)] \\
&= \operatorname{Var}\left[E\left\{\ln\left(\frac{\hat{\pi}_{n,2}(\boldsymbol{\theta}^{*(j)}|D)}{\hat{\pi}_{n,1}(\boldsymbol{\theta}^{*(j)}|D)}\right)\middle|\, \boldsymbol{\theta}_i, 1 \le i \le n\right\}\right] \\
&\quad + \frac{1}{m}E\left[\operatorname{Var}\left\{\ln\left(\frac{\hat{\pi}_{n,2}(\boldsymbol{\theta}^{*(j)}|D)}{\hat{\pi}_{n,1}(\boldsymbol{\theta}^{*(j)}|D)}\right)\middle|\, \boldsymbol{\theta}_i, 1 \le i \le n\right\}\right] \\
&\stackrel{\text{def}}{=} J_1 + J_2/m.
\end{aligned} \tag{4.A.7}$$

Using $\ln(1+x) = x + o(x)$ as $x \to 0$, we have

$$\begin{aligned}
J_1 &= \operatorname{Var}\left[E\left(\frac{\hat{\pi}_{n,2}(\boldsymbol{\theta}^{*(j)}|D) - \hat{\pi}_{n,1}(\boldsymbol{\theta}^{*(j)}|D)}{\pi(\boldsymbol{\theta}^{*(j)}|D)}\middle|\, \boldsymbol{\theta}_i, 1 \le i \le n\right)\right] + o\left(\frac{1}{n}\right) \\
&= \frac{1}{n}\operatorname{Var}\left[E\left(\frac{f_2(\boldsymbol{\theta}^{*(j)}, \boldsymbol{\theta}) - f_1(\boldsymbol{\theta}^{*(j)}, \boldsymbol{\theta})}{\pi(\boldsymbol{\theta}^{*(j)}|D)}\middle|\, \boldsymbol{\theta}\right)\right] + o\left(\frac{1}{n}\right)
\end{aligned} \tag{4.A.8}$$

and

$$\begin{aligned}
J_2 &= E\left[\operatorname{Var}\left(\frac{\hat{\pi}_{n,2}(\boldsymbol{\theta}^{*(j)}|D) - \hat{\pi}_{n,1}(\boldsymbol{\theta}^{*(j)}|D)}{\pi(\boldsymbol{\theta}^{*(j)}|D)}\middle|\, \boldsymbol{\theta}_i, 1 \le i \le n\right)\right] + o\left(\frac{1}{n}\right) \\
&= E\left[\int_{R^j}\left(\frac{1}{n}\sum_{i=1}^n \frac{f_2(\boldsymbol{\theta}^{*(j)}, \boldsymbol{\theta}_i) - f_1(\boldsymbol{\theta}^{*(j)}, \boldsymbol{\theta}_i)}{\pi(\boldsymbol{\theta}^{*(j)}|D)}\right)^2 \pi(\boldsymbol{\theta}^{*(j)}|D)\, d\boldsymbol{\theta}^{*(j)}\right] \\
&\quad - E\left(\frac{1}{n}\sum_{i=1}^n \int_{R^j} \frac{f_2(\boldsymbol{\theta}^{*(j)}, \boldsymbol{\theta}_i) - f_1(\boldsymbol{\theta}^{*(j)}, \boldsymbol{\theta}_i)}{\pi(\boldsymbol{\theta}^{*(j)}|D)} \pi(\boldsymbol{\theta}^{*(j)}|D)\, d\boldsymbol{\theta}^{*(j)}\right)^2 \\
&\quad + o\left(\frac{1}{n}\right) \\
&= \frac{1}{n}\int_{R^j} E\left(\frac{f_2(\boldsymbol{\theta}^{*(j)}, \boldsymbol{\theta}) - f_1(\boldsymbol{\theta}^{*(j)}, \boldsymbol{\theta})}{\pi(\boldsymbol{\theta}^{*(j)}|D)}\right)^2 \pi(\boldsymbol{\theta}^{*(j)}|D)\, d\boldsymbol{\theta}^{*(j)} \\
&\quad - \frac{1}{n}E\left(\int_{R^j} \frac{f_2(\boldsymbol{\theta}^{*(j)}, \boldsymbol{\theta}) - f_1(\boldsymbol{\theta}^{*(j)}, \boldsymbol{\theta})}{\pi(\boldsymbol{\theta}^{*(j)}|D)} \pi(\boldsymbol{\theta}^{*(j)}|D)\, d\boldsymbol{\theta}^{*(j)}\right)^2 + o\left(\frac{1}{n}\right) \\
&= \frac{1}{n}E\left[\operatorname{Var}\left(\frac{f_2(\boldsymbol{\theta}^{*(j)}, \boldsymbol{\theta}) - f_1(\boldsymbol{\theta}^{*(j)}, \boldsymbol{\theta})}{\pi(\boldsymbol{\theta}^{*(j)}|D)}\middle|\, \boldsymbol{\theta}\right)\right] + o\left(\frac{1}{n}\right).
\end{aligned} \tag{4.A.9}$$

Since $m \ge n$, Theorem 4.5.2 follows from (4.A.7) to (4.A.9). □

Proof of Corollary 4.5.1. For J_1 in (4.A.7), we have

$$\begin{aligned} J_1 &= \frac{1}{n} \operatorname{Var}\left[E\left(\frac{f_2(\boldsymbol{\theta}^{*(j)}, \boldsymbol{\theta}) - f_{n,1}(\boldsymbol{\theta}^{*(j)}, \boldsymbol{\theta})}{\pi(\boldsymbol{\theta}^{*(j)}|D)} \middle| \boldsymbol{\theta} \right) \right] + o\left(\frac{1}{n}\right) \\ &= \frac{1}{n} \operatorname{Var}\left[E\left(\frac{f_2(\boldsymbol{\theta}^{*(j)}, \boldsymbol{\theta})}{\pi(\boldsymbol{\theta}^{*(j)}|D)} - 1 \middle| \boldsymbol{\theta} \right) \right] + o\left(\frac{1}{n}\right) \\ &= \frac{1}{n} \operatorname{Var}\left[E\left(\frac{f_2(\boldsymbol{\theta}^{*(j)}, \boldsymbol{\theta})}{\pi(\boldsymbol{\theta}^{*(j)}|D)} \middle| \boldsymbol{\theta} \right) \right] + o\left(\frac{1}{n}\right). \end{aligned} \tag{4.A.10}$$

To estimate J_2 in (4.A.7), let

$$f_1^*(\boldsymbol{\theta}^{(j)}) = E(f_1|\boldsymbol{\theta}^{(j)}) = \int_{R^j} \mathcal{K}(\boldsymbol{\theta}^{*(j)}) \pi(\boldsymbol{\theta}^{(j)} + h_n \boldsymbol{\theta}^{*(j)}|D) \, d\boldsymbol{\theta}^{*(j)}.$$

Then $\lim_{n\to\infty} f_1^*(\boldsymbol{\theta}^{(j)}) = \pi(\boldsymbol{\theta}^{(j)}|D)$ and

$$\begin{aligned} J_2 &= \int_{R^j} E\left(\frac{1}{n} \sum_{i=1}^n \frac{f_2(\boldsymbol{\theta}_{(j)}, \boldsymbol{\theta}_i) - f_1(\boldsymbol{\theta}^{(j)}, \boldsymbol{\theta}_i)}{\pi(\boldsymbol{\theta}^{(j)}|D)} \right)^2 \pi(\boldsymbol{\theta}^{(j)}|D) \, d\boldsymbol{\theta}^{(j)} \\ &\quad - E\left(\frac{1}{n} \sum_{i=1}^n \int_{R^j} \frac{f_2(\boldsymbol{\theta}^{(j)}, \boldsymbol{\theta}_i) - f_1(\boldsymbol{\theta}^{(j)}, \boldsymbol{\theta}_i)}{\pi(\boldsymbol{\theta}^{(j)}|D)} \pi(\boldsymbol{\theta}^{(j)}|D) \, d\boldsymbol{\theta}^{(j)} \right)^2 \\ &\quad + o\left(\frac{1}{n}\right) \\ &= \int_{R^j} \frac{(\pi(\boldsymbol{\theta}^{(j)}|D) - f_1^*(\boldsymbol{\theta}^{(j)}))^2}{\pi(\boldsymbol{\theta}^{(j)}|D)} \, d\boldsymbol{\theta}^{(j)} \\ &\quad + \frac{1}{n h_n^j} \int_{R^j} \mathcal{K}^2(\boldsymbol{\theta}^{(j)}) \, d\boldsymbol{\theta}^{(j)} + o\left(\frac{1}{n}\right). \end{aligned} \tag{4.A.11}$$

Note that in (4.A.11), the first term goes to zero as n goes to infinity. Therefore, Corollary 4.5.1 follows from (4.A.10) and (4.A.11). □

Exercises

4.1 Prove the identity (4.3.3) for the IWMDE. Also prove that (4.3.3) reduces to (4.3.1) when $w(\boldsymbol{\theta}^{(j)}|\boldsymbol{\theta}^{(-j)}) = \pi(\boldsymbol{\theta}^{(j)}|\boldsymbol{\theta}^{(-j)}, D)$.

4.2 Prove (4.3.6) and thus show that the IWMDE is unbiased.

4.3 Derive an estimate of the standard error of $\hat{\pi}(\boldsymbol{\theta}^{*(j)}|D)$ for the CMDE and IWMDE based on the asymptotic variance.

4.4 For the constrained multiple linear regression model in (1.3.1), the joint posterior density of $(\boldsymbol{\beta}, \sigma^2)$ is given in (2.1.7). Chen and Deely (1996) obtain the posterior means of β_4, β_5, β_6, β_9, and β_{10} as $\hat{\beta}_4 = 0.3113$, $\hat{\beta}_5 = 0.5542$, $\hat{\beta}_6 = 0.7806$, $\hat{\beta}_9 = 1.0410$, and $\hat{\beta}_{10} = 1.2282$.

(i) Using the guidelines described in Section 4.3, derive the weight conditional densities (i.e., w's) for estimating the univariate marginal posterior densities of β_5 and β_{10}, respectively.

(ii) Using (4.3.11), derive an expression of w for computing the joint marginal posterior density of (β_5, β_{10}).

(iii) Use the w's obtained in (i) and (ii) to obtain the univariate marginal posterior densities as well as the joint marginal posterior density of β_5 and β_{10}.

4.5 Assume that the function $\xi = g(\boldsymbol{\theta}^{(j)})$ has continuous partial derivatives at all points $\boldsymbol{\theta}^{(j)}$, and the determinant $\left|\partial g(\boldsymbol{\theta}^{(j)})/\partial \boldsymbol{\theta}^{(j)}\right| \neq 0$. Further, assume that $\{\boldsymbol{\theta}_i,\ i = 1, 2, \ldots, n\}$ is an MCMC sample from the joint posterior distribution $\pi(\boldsymbol{\theta}|D)$.

(i) Using (4.3.4), derive a generalized version of the IWMDE for estimating the posterior density of ξ.

(ii) Construct two different versions of the kernel estimators of the posterior density for ξ based on the MCMC sample $\{\boldsymbol{\theta}_i,\ i = 1, 2, \ldots, n\}$.

(iii) For the IWMDE and kernel methods, which method is more convenient for estimating the posterior density for a function of the model parameters?

4.6 For the Poisson random effects models discussed in Section 2.5.4, obtain an expression of the CMDE for the joint marginal posterior density of $\boldsymbol{\beta}$ (the vector of regression coefficients) after hierarchical centering, based on an MCMC sample from the joint posterior distribution $\pi(\boldsymbol{\beta}, \sigma^2, \rho, \eta|D)$ given in (2.5.28). Discuss whether the hierarchical centering technique is advantageous for computing marginal posterior densities.

4.7 Show that the optimal IWMDE is still CMDE in the sense of minimizing the asymptotic expectation of the K–L divergence of $\hat{\pi}_{\text{IWMDE}}(\boldsymbol{\theta}^{(j)}|D)$. More specifically, show that if w is a density function such that (4.5.5) and (4.5.7) hold, and

$$\int_{\Omega} \frac{\pi^2(\boldsymbol{\theta}|D)}{\pi(\boldsymbol{\theta}^{(j)}|D)\pi(\boldsymbol{\theta}^{(-j)}|D)}\, d\boldsymbol{\theta} < \infty,$$

then the first term on the right-hand side of (4.5.8) is minimized at

$$w(\boldsymbol{\theta}^{(j)}|\boldsymbol{\theta}^{(-j)}) = \pi(\boldsymbol{\theta}^{(j)}|\boldsymbol{\theta}^{(-j)}, D).$$

That is, the optimal w is the conditional posterior density of $\boldsymbol{\theta}^{(j)}$ given $\boldsymbol{\theta}^{(-j)}$ with respect to the posterior $\pi(\boldsymbol{\theta}|D)$.

4.8 Prove the identity in (4.3.14).

4.9 Obtain similar expressions to (4.3.12), (4.3.13), (4.3.14), and (4.3.15) for $j > 2$.

4.10 For the bivariate normal model discussed in Example 4.2, derive an explicit expression of the CMDE based on the Gibbs sample.

4.11 For the constrained multiple linear regression model in Example 4.3, derive an estimate of the joint marginal posterior density of (β_1, β_2) using Oh's method given in Section 4.3.

4.12 Consider the bivariate normal model in Example 4.2. Let

$$\boldsymbol{\theta} = (\theta_1, \theta_2) \sim N_2(\boldsymbol{\mu}, \Sigma).$$

Assume that $\{\boldsymbol{\theta}_i = (\theta_{i1}, \theta_{i2})', 1 \le i \le n\}$ and $\{\boldsymbol{\theta}_i^* = (\theta_{i1}^*, \theta_{i2}^*)', 1 \le i \le n\}$ are two independent random samples from the above bivariate normal distribution $N_2(\boldsymbol{\mu}, \Sigma)$. Letting

$$f_1(\theta_1, \boldsymbol{\theta}_i) = \tfrac{1}{2} e^{-|\theta_{i1}|} \frac{L(\theta_1, \theta_{i2}|D)\pi(\theta_1, \theta_{i2})}{L(\boldsymbol{\theta}_i|D)\pi(\boldsymbol{\theta}_i)}$$

and

$$f_2(\theta_1, \boldsymbol{\theta}_i) = n^{1/2} \exp(-|\theta_1 - \theta_{i1}|n^{1/2}),$$

define $\hat{\pi}_{n,v}$ in (4.5.12) as the corresponding IWMDE and kernel estimators. Compare the K–L divergences of these two estimators.

5

Estimating Ratios of Normalizing Constants

5.1 Introduction

A computational problem arising frequently in Bayesian inference is the computation of normalizing constants for posterior densities from which we can sample. Typically, we are interested in the ratios of such normalizing constants. For example, a Bayes factor is defined as the ratio of posterior odds versus prior odds, where posterior odds is simply a ratio of the normalizing constants of two posterior densities. Mathematically, this problem can be formulated as follows. Let $\pi_l(\boldsymbol{\theta})$, $l = 1, 2$, be two densities, each of which is known up to a normalizing constant:

$$\pi_l(\boldsymbol{\theta}) = \frac{q_l(\boldsymbol{\theta})}{c_l}, \quad \boldsymbol{\theta} \in \Omega_l,$$

where Ω_l is the support of π_l, and the unnormalized density $q_l(\boldsymbol{\theta})$ can be evaluated at any $\boldsymbol{\theta} \in \Omega_l$ for $l = 1, 2$. Then, the ratio of two normalizing constants is defined as

$$r = \frac{c_1}{c_2}. \tag{5.1.1}$$

In this chapter, we also use the parameter $\boldsymbol{\lambda}$ to index different densities:

$$\pi(\boldsymbol{\theta}|\boldsymbol{\lambda}_l) = \frac{q(\boldsymbol{\theta}|\boldsymbol{\lambda}_l)}{c(\boldsymbol{\lambda}_l)} \quad \text{for } l = 1, 2,$$

where $q(\boldsymbol{\theta}|\boldsymbol{\lambda}_l)$ is known, and the ratio is

$$r = \frac{c(\boldsymbol{\lambda}_1)}{c(\boldsymbol{\lambda}_2)}. \tag{5.1.2}$$

Estimating ratios of normalizing constants is extremely challenging and very important, particularly in Bayesian computations. Such problems often arise in likelihood inference, especially in the presence of missing data (Meng and Wong 1996), in computing intrinsic Bayes factors (Berger and Pericchi 1996), in the Bayesian comparison of econometric models considered by Geweke (1994), and in estimating marginal likelihood (Chib 1995). For example, in likelihood inference, this ratio is viewed as the likelihood ratio and in Bayesian model selection, the ratio is called the Bayes factor.

The $\pi_l(\boldsymbol{\theta})$ or $\pi(\boldsymbol{\theta}|\boldsymbol{\lambda}_l)$ are often very complicated and therefore, the ratio defined by either (5.1.1) or (5.1.2) is analytically intractable (Meng and Wong 1996; Gelman and Meng 1998; Geyer 1994). However, without knowing the normalizing constants, c_l or $c(\boldsymbol{\lambda}_l)$, $l = 1, 2$, the distributions, $\pi_l(\boldsymbol{\theta})$ or $\pi(\boldsymbol{\theta}|\boldsymbol{\lambda}_l)$, $l = 1, 2$, can be sampled by means of MCMC methods, for example, the Metropolis–Hastings algorithm, the Gibbs sampler, and the various hybrid algorithms (Chen and Schmeiser 1993; Müller 1991; Tierney 1994). Therefore, simulation-based methods for estimating the ratio, r, seem to be very attractive because of their general applicability.

Recently, several Monte Carlo (MC) methods for estimating normalizing constants have been developed, which include bridge sampling of Meng and Wong (1996), path sampling of Gelman and Meng (1998), ratio importance sampling of Chen and Shao (1997a), Chib's method for computing marginal likelihood (Chib 1995), and reverse logistic regression of Geyer (1994). We start with importance sampling (IS) in Section 5.2. Sections 5.3–5.5 present bridge sampling (BS), path sampling (PS), and ratio importance sampling (RIS). A theoretical illustration is given in Section 5.6 and extensions to posterior densities with different dimensions are considered in Section 5.8. Section 5.7 presents a comprehensive treatment of how to compute simulation standard errors. The estimation of normalizing constants after transformation as well as some other related MC methods are discussed in Sections 5.9 and 5.10. An application of the weighted MC estimators discussed in Section 3.4.2 to the computation of the ratio of normalizing constants is given in Section 5.11. We conclude this chapter with a brief discussion in Section 5.12.

5.2 Importance Sampling

A standard and simple method for estimating the ratios of normalizing constants is importance sampling (see, e.g., Geweke 1989). We present two versions of the importance sampling methods.

5.2.1 Importance Sampling–Version 1

Choose two importance sampling densities $\pi_l^{\mathrm{I}}(\boldsymbol{\theta})$, $l = 1, 2$, which are completely known, for $\pi_i(\boldsymbol{\theta})$, $l = 1, 2$, respectively. Let $\{\boldsymbol{\theta}_{l,1}, \boldsymbol{\theta}_{l,2}, \ldots, \boldsymbol{\theta}_{l,n_l}\}$, $l = 1, 2$, be two independent samples from $\pi_l^{\mathrm{I}}(\boldsymbol{\theta})$, $l = 1, 2$, respectively. Then an IS estimator of r is defined as

$$\hat{r}_{\mathrm{IS}_1} = \frac{(1/n_1)\sum_{i=1}^{n_1} q_1(\boldsymbol{\theta}_{1,i})/\pi_1^{\mathrm{I}}(\boldsymbol{\theta}_{1,i})}{(1/n_2)\sum_{i=1}^{n_2} q_2(\boldsymbol{\theta}_{2,i})/\pi_2^{\mathrm{I}}(\boldsymbol{\theta}_{2,i})}. \tag{5.2.1}$$

From the law of large numbers, it is easy to see that

$$\hat{r}_{\mathrm{IS}_1} \rightarrow r \ \text{ a.s. } \ \text{as } n_1, n_2 \rightarrow \infty.$$

To examine the performance of the estimator, $\hat{r}$, we introduce the relative mean-square error (RE^2) as a measure of accuracy:

$$\mathrm{RE}^2(\hat{r}_{\mathrm{IS}_1}) = \frac{E(\hat{r}_{\mathrm{IS}_1} - r)^2}{r^2}, \tag{5.2.2}$$

where the expectation is taken over all random samples. The exact calculation of (5.2.2) does not appear possible since it depends on the choice of the $\pi_i^{\mathrm{I}}(\boldsymbol{\theta})$. However, when both n_1 and n_2 are large, we can approximate (5.2.2) by the first-order term of its asymptotic expansion.

Theorem 5.2.1 *Let* $n = n_1 + n_2$, $s_{l,n} = n_l/n$. *Suppose that* $\lim_{n\rightarrow\infty} s_{l,n} > 0$ *for* $l = 1, 2$. *Then we have*

$$\mathrm{RE}^2(\hat{r}_{\mathrm{IS}_1}) = \sum_{l=1}^{2} \frac{1}{n_l} E_l^{\mathrm{I}} \left(\frac{\pi_l(\boldsymbol{\theta}) - \pi_l^{\mathrm{I}}(\boldsymbol{\theta})}{\pi_l^{\mathrm{I}}(\boldsymbol{\theta})} \right)^2 + o\left(\frac{1}{n}\right), \tag{5.2.3}$$

where the expectation E_l^{I} *is taken with respect to* $\pi_l^{\mathrm{I}}(\boldsymbol{\theta})$ *for* $l = 1, 2$.

The proof of Theorem 5.2.1 follows directly from the δ-method. From (5.2.3), it is easy to observe that the performance of the estimator, $\hat{r}_{\mathrm{IS}_1}$, depends heavily on the choice of $\pi_l^{\mathrm{I}}(\boldsymbol{\theta})$. If $\pi_l^{\mathrm{I}}(\boldsymbol{\theta})$ is a good approximation to $\pi_l(\boldsymbol{\theta})$, this IS method works well. However, it is often difficult to find $\pi_l^{\mathrm{I}}(\boldsymbol{\theta})$, $l = 1, 2$, which serve as good IS densities (see Geyer 1994; Green 1992; Gelman and Meng 1998). When the parameter spaces, Ω_l, $l = 1, 2$, are constrained, good completely known IS densities, $\pi_l^{\mathrm{I}}(\boldsymbol{\theta})$, $l = 1, 2$, are not available or are extremely difficult to obtain (see Gelfand, Smith, and Lee 1992 for practical examples).

5.2.2 Importance Sampling–Version 2

Let $\boldsymbol{\theta}$ be a random variable from π_2. When $\Omega_1 \subset \Omega_2$, we have the identity,

$$r = \frac{c_1}{c_2} = E_2\left\{\frac{q_1(\boldsymbol{\theta})}{q_2(\boldsymbol{\theta})}\right\}. \tag{5.2.4}$$

Here, and in the sequel, E_2 denotes the expected value with respect to π_2. Let $\{\boldsymbol{\theta}_{2,1}, \boldsymbol{\theta}_{2,2}, \ldots, \boldsymbol{\theta}_{2,n}\}$ be a random sample from π_2. Then the ratio r can be estimated by

$$\hat{r}_{\text{IS}_2} = \frac{1}{n} \sum_{i=1}^{n} \frac{q_1(\boldsymbol{\theta}_{2,i})}{q_2(\boldsymbol{\theta}_{2,i})}. \tag{5.2.5}$$

Unlike the estimator $\hat{r}_{\text{IS}_1}$ of r given in (5.2.1), it is easy to show that $\hat{r}_{\text{IS}_2}$ is an unbiased and consistent estimator of r and direct calculations yield

$$\text{RE}^2(\hat{r}_{\text{IS}_2}) = \frac{\text{Var}(\hat{r}_{\text{IS}_2})}{r^2} = \frac{1}{n} E_2 \left(\frac{\pi_1(\boldsymbol{\theta}) - \pi_2(\boldsymbol{\theta})}{\pi_2(\boldsymbol{\theta})} \right)^2. \tag{5.2.6}$$

Thus it is easy to see that when the two densities π_1 and π_2 have very little overlap (i.e., $E_2(\pi_1(\boldsymbol{\theta}))$ is very small), this IS-based method will work poorly.

5.3 Bridge Sampling

The generalization of (5.2.4) given by Meng and Wong (1996) is

$$r = \frac{c_1}{c_2} = \frac{E_2\{q_1(\boldsymbol{\theta})\alpha(\boldsymbol{\theta})\}}{E_1\{q_2(\boldsymbol{\theta})\alpha(\boldsymbol{\theta})\}}, \tag{5.3.1}$$

where $\alpha(\boldsymbol{\theta})$ is an arbitrary function defined on $\Omega_1 \cap \Omega_2$ such that

$$0 < \left| \int_{\Omega_1 \cap \Omega_2} \alpha(\boldsymbol{\theta}) q_1(\boldsymbol{\theta}) q_2(\boldsymbol{\theta}) \, d\boldsymbol{\theta} \right| < \infty. \tag{5.3.2}$$

The identity given in (5.3.1) unifies many identities used in the literature for simulating normalizing constants or other similar computations. As discussed in Meng and Wong (1996), the most general one is given by Bennett (1976), who proposes (5.3.1) in the context of simulating free-energy differences with $q_l = \exp(-U_l)$, where U_l is the temperature-scaled potential energy and $l = 1, 2$ indexes two canonical ensembles on the same configuration space. Taking $\alpha(\boldsymbol{\theta}) = q_2^{-1}(\boldsymbol{\theta})$ leads to (5.2.4), assuming $\Omega_1 \subset \Omega_2$. When $\Omega_1 = \Omega_2$ and Ω_1 has a finite Lebesgue measure, taking $\alpha(\boldsymbol{\theta}) = [q_1(\boldsymbol{\theta}) q_2(\boldsymbol{\theta})]^{-1}$ leads to a generalization of the "harmonic rule" given in Newton and Raftery (1994) and Gelfand and Dey (1994):

$$r = \frac{E_2[q_2^{-1}(\boldsymbol{\theta})]}{E_1[q_1^{-1}(\boldsymbol{\theta})]}.$$

Before discussing the optimal choice of $\alpha(\boldsymbol{\theta})$, we first define the BS estimator, denoted by $\hat{r}_{\text{BS}}(\alpha)$, of r. Letting $\{\boldsymbol{\theta}_{l,1}, \boldsymbol{\theta}_{l,2}, \ldots, \boldsymbol{\theta}_{l,n_l}\}$ be a random sample from π_l for $l = 1, 2$, a BS estimator of r is given by

$$\hat{r}_{\text{BS}} = \hat{r}_{\text{BS}}(\alpha) = \frac{(1/n_2)\sum_{i=1}^{n_2} q_1(\boldsymbol{\theta}_{2,i})\alpha(\boldsymbol{\theta}_{2,i})}{(1/n_1)\sum_{i=1}^{n_1} q_2(\boldsymbol{\theta}_{1,i})\alpha(\boldsymbol{\theta}_{1,i})}. \tag{5.3.3}$$

Similar to $\hat{r}_{\text{IS}_1}$ in (5.2.1), the law of large numbers yields that $\hat{r}_{\text{BS}}$ is a consistent estimator of r. Let $n = n_1 + n_2$ and $s_{l,n} = n_l/n$, and assume $s_l = \lim_{n\to\infty} s_{l,n} > 0$, $l = 1, 2$. Analogous to Theorem 5.2.1, the δ-method yields

$$\begin{aligned} \text{RE}^2(\hat{r}_{\text{BS}}) =& \frac{1}{ns_1s_2}\left\{\frac{\int_{\Omega_1\cap\Omega_2} \pi_1(\boldsymbol{\theta})\pi_2(\boldsymbol{\theta})(s_1\pi_1(\boldsymbol{\theta}) + s_2\pi_2(\boldsymbol{\theta}))\alpha^2(\boldsymbol{\theta})\, d\boldsymbol{\theta}}{(\int_{\Omega_1\cap\Omega_2} \pi_1(\boldsymbol{\theta})\pi_2(\boldsymbol{\theta})\alpha(\boldsymbol{\theta})\, d\boldsymbol{\theta})^2} - 1\right\} \\ &+ o\Big(\frac{1}{n}\Big). \end{aligned} \tag{5.3.4}$$

Meng and Wong (1996) provide the so-called (asymptotically) optimal choice of α, which is given by the following theorem:

Theorem 5.3.1 *The first term of the right side of* (5.3.4)*, as a function of* α*, is minimized at*

$$\alpha_{\text{opt}}(\boldsymbol{\theta}) \;\propto\; \frac{1}{s_1\pi_1(\boldsymbol{\theta}) + s_2\pi_2(\boldsymbol{\theta})}, \qquad \boldsymbol{\theta} \in \Omega_1 \cap \Omega_2, \tag{5.3.5}$$

with the minimum value

$$\frac{1}{ns_1s_2}\left[\left\{\int_{\Omega_1\cap\Omega_2} \frac{\pi_1(\boldsymbol{\theta})\pi_2(\boldsymbol{\theta})}{s_1\pi_1(\boldsymbol{\theta}) + s_2\pi_2(\boldsymbol{\theta})}\, d\boldsymbol{\theta}\right\}^{-1} - 1\right]. \tag{5.3.6}$$

The proof of the theorem is given in the Appendix. This asymptotically optimal choice is intuitively appealing. It represents the inverse of the mixture of π_1 and π_2 with mixture proportions determined by the sampling rates of the two distributions. But, it is not of direct use because α_{opt} depends on the unknown ratio $r = c_1/c_2$. Furthermore, it depends on the ratio of the two sample sizes, because $\alpha_{\text{opt}}(\boldsymbol{\theta}) \propto 1/(\pi_1(\boldsymbol{\theta}) + (n_2/n_1)\pi_2(\boldsymbol{\theta}))$. To overcome this problem, Meng and Wong (1996) construct the following iterative estimator:

$$\hat{r}^{(t+1)}_{\text{BS,opt}} = \frac{(1/n_2)\sum_{i=1}^{n_2} q_1(\boldsymbol{\theta}_{2,i})/(s_1q_1(\boldsymbol{\theta}_{2,i}) + s_2\hat{r}^{(t)}_{\text{BS,opt}}q_2(\boldsymbol{\theta}_{2,i}))}{(1/n_1)\sum_{i=1}^{n_1} q_2(\boldsymbol{\theta}_{1,i})/(s_1q_1(\boldsymbol{\theta}_{1,i}) + s_2\hat{r}^{(t)}_{\text{opt}}q_2(\boldsymbol{\theta}_{1,i}))}, \tag{5.3.7}$$

with an initial guess of r, $\hat{r}^{(0)}_{\text{BS,opt}}$. They show that for each $t \geq 0$, $\hat{r}^{(t+1)}_{\text{BS,opt}}$ provides a consistent estimator of r and that the unique limit, $\hat{r}_{\text{BS,opt}}$, achieves the asymptotic minimal relative mean-square error with the first-order term given in (5.3.6). By the construction of $\hat{r}^{(t+1)}_{\text{BS,opt}}$ given in (5.3.7), it can be shown that $\hat{r}_{\text{BS,opt}}$ must be a root of the following "score" function:

$$S(r) = \sum_{i=1}^{n_1} \frac{s_2rq_2(\boldsymbol{\theta}_{1,i})}{s_1q_1(\boldsymbol{\theta}_{1,i}) + s_2rq_2(\boldsymbol{\theta}_{1,i})} - \sum_{i=1}^{n_2} \frac{s_1q_1(\boldsymbol{\theta}_{2,i})}{s_1q_1(\boldsymbol{\theta}_{2,i}) + s_2rq_2(\boldsymbol{\theta}_{2,i})}. \tag{5.3.8}$$

Since $S(0) = -n_2 < 0$, $S(\infty) = n_1 > 0$, and

$$\frac{dS(r)}{dr} = \sum_{i=1}^{n_1} \frac{s_1 s_2 q_1(\boldsymbol{\theta}_{1,i}) q_2(\boldsymbol{\theta}_{1,i})}{[s_1 q_1(\boldsymbol{\theta}_{1,i}) + s_2 r q_2(\boldsymbol{\theta}_{1,i})]^2} + \sum_{i=1}^{n_2} \frac{s_1 s_2 q_1(\boldsymbol{\theta}_{2,i}) q_2(\boldsymbol{\theta}_{2,i})}{[s_1 q_1(\boldsymbol{\theta}_{2,i}) + s_2 r q_2(\boldsymbol{\theta}_{2,i})]^2} > 0$$

for all $r \geq 0$, $S(r)$ has a unique root. This property yields another approach to finding $\hat{r}_{\text{BS,opt}}$ instead of using the iterative procedure of Meng and Wong (1996), which requires an initial guess for an estimator of r. We solve the equation

$$S(r) = 0$$

to get $\hat{r}_{\text{BS,opt}}$ by, for example, a simple bisection method. Now, the only issue for a BS estimator is the choice of the sample sizes n_l. This issue is discussed in detail in Meng and Wong (1996), and it is shown that when $\Omega_1 = \Omega_2$ and $\alpha(\boldsymbol{\theta}) = [q_1(\boldsymbol{\theta}) q_2(\boldsymbol{\theta})]^{-1/2}$ is used, the optimal allocation of sample sizes, given $n_1 + n_2 = n$, is $n_1 = n_2 = n/2$. When sampling from the two densities requires a similar amount of time per sample, equal-sample-size allocation is also recommended by Bennett (1976). To obtain a simulation efficient BS estimator, the optimal choice of α is often more essential than the optimal allocation of sample sizes. However, equal-sample-size allocation may not be a good idea for the cases in which we know that the locations of both densities are roughly the same while one density has heavier tails than the other. Sometimes, it is even better that we just take random samples only from one density if it has extremely heavier tails. See Section 5.6 for an illustrative example.

Similar to the IS estimator $\hat{r}_{\text{IS}_2}$, the BS estimator $\hat{r}_{\text{BS}}$ given in (5.3.3) will become inefficient when π_1 and π_2 have little overlap; see Section 5.4.3 for further explanation. For such cases, the PS method of Gelman and Meng (1998) presented in Section 5.4, as well as the BS method after transformation as given in Section 5.9, will substantially improve the simulation efficiency.

5.4 Path Sampling

In this section, we let $q(\boldsymbol{\theta}|\boldsymbol{\lambda}_l)$ denote the unnormalized density and denote Ω to be the support of $\pi(\boldsymbol{\theta}|\boldsymbol{\lambda}_l)$ for $l = 1, 2$. As discussed in Gelman and Meng (1998), we can often construct a continuous path to link $q(\boldsymbol{\theta}|\boldsymbol{\lambda}_1)$ and $q(\boldsymbol{\theta}|\boldsymbol{\lambda}_2)$. Instead of directly working on r, Gelman and Meng (1998) propose the PS method to estimate the natural logarithm of r, i.e.,

$$\xi = -\ln(r) = -\ln(c(\boldsymbol{\lambda}_1)/c(\boldsymbol{\lambda}_2)).$$

5.4.1 Univariate Path Sampling

We first consider λ to be a scalar quantity, i.e., λ is one dimensional. Without loss of generality, assume that $\lambda_1 < \lambda_2$. Gelman and Meng (1998) develop the following identity:

$$\xi = -\ln\left\{\frac{c(\lambda_1)}{c(\lambda_2)}\right\} = E\left[\frac{U(\boldsymbol{\theta}, \lambda)}{\pi_\lambda(\lambda)}\right], \tag{5.4.1}$$

where $U(\boldsymbol{\theta}, \lambda) = (d/d\lambda)\ln(q(\boldsymbol{\theta}|\lambda))$, $\pi_\lambda(\lambda)$ is a prior density (completely known) for $\lambda \in [\lambda_1, \lambda_2]$, and the expectation is taken with respect to the joint density $\pi(\boldsymbol{\theta}, \lambda) = \pi(\boldsymbol{\theta}|\lambda)\pi_\lambda(\lambda)$, where $\pi(\boldsymbol{\theta}|\lambda) = q(\boldsymbol{\theta}|\lambda)/c(\lambda)$ for $\lambda = \lambda_1$ or λ_2. Let $\{(\boldsymbol{\theta}_i, \lambda_i), i = 1, 2, \ldots, n\}$, be a random sample from $\pi(\boldsymbol{\theta}, \lambda)$. Then, a PS estimator of ξ is given by

$$\hat{\xi}_{\text{PS}} = \frac{1}{n}\sum_{i=1}^{n}\frac{U(\boldsymbol{\theta}_i, \lambda_i)}{\pi_\lambda(\lambda_i)}. \tag{5.4.2}$$

It can be shown that $\hat{\xi}_{\text{PS}}$ is unbiased and consistent. The MC variance of $\hat{\xi}_{\text{PS}}$ is

$$\text{Var}(\hat{\xi}_{\text{PS}}) = \frac{1}{n}\left[\int_{\lambda_1}^{\lambda_2}\frac{E_\lambda\{U^2(\boldsymbol{\theta}, \lambda)\}}{\pi_\lambda(\lambda)}\,d\lambda - \xi^2\right], \tag{5.4.3}$$

where the expectation E_λ is taken with respect to $\pi(\boldsymbol{\theta}|\lambda)$.

In (5.4.2), the choice of $\pi_\lambda(\lambda)$ is somehow arbitrary. However, the following result gives the optimal choice of $\pi_\lambda(\lambda)$ in the sense of minimizing the MC variance $\text{Var}(\hat{\xi}_{\text{PS}})$.

Theorem 5.4.1 *The optimal prior density* $\pi_\lambda^{\text{opt}}(\lambda)$ *given by*

$$\pi_\lambda^{\text{opt}}(\lambda) = \frac{\sqrt{E_\lambda\{U^2(\boldsymbol{\theta}, \lambda)\}}}{\int_{\lambda_1}^{\lambda_2}\sqrt{E_\eta\{U^2(\boldsymbol{\theta}, \eta)\}}\,d\eta}, \tag{5.4.4}$$

minimizes the MC variance $\text{Var}(\hat{\xi}_{\text{PS}})$ *given in* (5.4.3). *The minimum value of* $\text{Var}(\hat{\xi})$ *is*

$$\text{Var}_{\text{opt}}(\hat{\xi}_{\text{PS}}) = \frac{1}{n}\left[\left(\int_{\lambda_1}^{\lambda_2}\sqrt{E_\lambda\{U^2(\boldsymbol{\theta}, \lambda)\}}\,d\lambda\right)^2 - \xi^2\right]. \tag{5.4.5}$$

The proof of Theorem 5.4.1 is analogous to the one of Theorem 5.3.1 by the Cauchy–Schwarz inequality, and thus is left as an exercise. Interestingly, when $c(\lambda)$ is independent of λ, the optimal density given in (5.4.4) is exactly the Jeffreys' prior density based on $\pi(\boldsymbol{\theta}|\lambda)$ restricted to $\lambda \in [\lambda_1, \lambda_2]$; see Gelman and Meng (1998) for further explanation of the optimal prior density in general cases.

Gelman and Meng (1998) conjecture that the optimal MC variance cannot be arbitrary small, and must be bounded below by a distance between $\pi(\boldsymbol{\theta}|\lambda_1)$ and $\pi(\boldsymbol{\theta}|\lambda_2)$. The following result confirms their conjecture:

Theorem 5.4.2 *Under certain regularity conditions, we have*

$$\mathrm{Var}(\hat{\xi}_{\mathrm{PS}}) \geq \frac{4}{n} \int_{\Omega} \left[\sqrt{\pi(\boldsymbol{\theta}|\lambda_1)} - \sqrt{\pi(\boldsymbol{\theta}|\lambda_2)} \right]^2 d\boldsymbol{\theta} \tag{5.4.6}$$

for any prior density $\pi_\lambda(\lambda)$ *with support* $[\lambda_1, \lambda_2]$.

The proof of Theorem 5.4.2 is given in the Appendix. It is interesting to see that the lower bound of $\mathrm{Var}(\hat{\xi}_{\mathrm{PS}})$ given in (5.4.6) indeed equals $(4/n)H^2(\pi_1, \pi_2)$, where

$$H(\pi_1, \pi_2) = \left\{ \int_{\Omega} \left[\sqrt{\pi_1(\boldsymbol{\theta})} - \sqrt{\pi_2(\boldsymbol{\theta})} \right]^2 d\boldsymbol{\theta} \right\}^{1/2} \tag{5.4.7}$$

is the Hellinger divergence between two densities π_1 and π_2, and $\pi_l(\boldsymbol{\theta}) = \pi(\boldsymbol{\theta}|\lambda_l)$ for $l = 1, 2$.

5.4.2 *Multivariate Path Sampling*

Now consider $\boldsymbol{\lambda}$ to be k-dimensional. Assume that a continuous path in the k-dimensional parameter space that links $q(\boldsymbol{\theta}|\boldsymbol{\lambda}_1)$ and $q(\boldsymbol{\theta}|\boldsymbol{\lambda}_2)$ is given by

$$\boldsymbol{\lambda}(t) = (\lambda_1(t), \ldots, \lambda_k(t)) \text{ for } t \in [0, 1]; \;\; \boldsymbol{\lambda}(0) = \boldsymbol{\lambda}_1 \text{ and } \boldsymbol{\lambda}(1) = \boldsymbol{\lambda}_2.$$

Under some regularity conditions, Gelman and Meng (1998) obtain the identity

$$\xi = -\ln \left\{ \frac{c(\boldsymbol{\lambda}_1)}{c(\boldsymbol{\lambda}_2)} \right\} = \int_0^1 E_{\boldsymbol{\lambda}(t)} \left[\sum_{j=1}^{k} \dot{\boldsymbol{\lambda}}_j(t) U_j(\boldsymbol{\theta}, \boldsymbol{\lambda}(t)) \right] dt,$$

where $\dot{\boldsymbol{\lambda}}_j(t) = d\boldsymbol{\lambda}_j(t)/dt$ and $U_j(\boldsymbol{\theta}, \boldsymbol{\lambda}(t)) = \partial \ln q(\boldsymbol{\theta}|\boldsymbol{\lambda})/\partial \boldsymbol{\lambda}_j$ for $j = 1, 2, \ldots, k$. Then, a corresponding PS estimator for ξ is given by

$$\hat{\xi}_{\mathrm{PS}} = \frac{1}{n} \sum_{i=1}^{n} \left[\sum_{j=1}^{k} \dot{\boldsymbol{\lambda}}_j(t_i) U_j(\boldsymbol{\theta}_i, \boldsymbol{\lambda}(t_i)) \right],$$

where the t_i's are sampled uniformly from $[0, 1]$ and $\boldsymbol{\theta}_i$ is a sample from $\pi(\boldsymbol{\theta}|\boldsymbol{\lambda}(t_i))$. The variance of $\hat{\xi}_{\mathrm{PS}}$ is

$$\mathrm{Var}(\hat{\xi}_{\mathrm{PS}}) = \frac{1}{n} \left[\int_0^1 \left(\sum_{i,j=1}^{k} g_{ij}(\boldsymbol{\lambda}(t)) \dot{\boldsymbol{\lambda}}_i(t) \dot{\boldsymbol{\lambda}}_j(t) \right) dt - \xi^2 \right], \tag{5.4.8}$$

where $g_{ij}(\boldsymbol{\lambda}(t)) = E_{\boldsymbol{\lambda}(t)}\{U_i(\boldsymbol{\theta}, \boldsymbol{\lambda}(t)) U_j(\boldsymbol{\theta}, \boldsymbol{\lambda}(t))\}$. The optimal path function $\boldsymbol{\lambda}(t)$ that minimizes the first term on the right side of (5.4.8) is the solution of the following Euler–Lagrange equations (e.g., see Atkinson and Mitchell 1981) with the boundary conditions $\boldsymbol{\lambda}(0) = \boldsymbol{\lambda}_1$ and $\boldsymbol{\lambda}(1) = \boldsymbol{\lambda}_2$:

$$\sum_{i=1}^{k} g_{ij}(\boldsymbol{\lambda}(t))\ddot{\boldsymbol{\lambda}}_i(t) + \sum_{i,j=1}^{k} [ij, l]\dot{\boldsymbol{\lambda}}_i(t)\dot{\boldsymbol{\lambda}}_j(t) = 0 \quad \text{for } l = 1, 2, \ldots, k, \tag{5.4.9}$$

where $\ddot{\boldsymbol{\lambda}}(t)$ denotes the second derivative with respect to t and $[ij,\ l]$ is the Christoffel symbol of the first kind:

$$[ij, l] = \frac{1}{2}\left[\frac{\partial g_{il}(\boldsymbol{\lambda})}{\partial \boldsymbol{\lambda}_j} + \frac{\partial g_{jl}(\boldsymbol{\lambda})}{\partial \boldsymbol{\lambda}_i} - \frac{\partial g_{ij}(\boldsymbol{\lambda})}{\partial \boldsymbol{\lambda}_l}\right], \quad i, j, l = 1, 2, \ldots, k.$$

5.4.3 Connection Between Path Sampling and Bridge Sampling

The fundamental idea underlying the BS approach is to take advantage of the "overlap" of the two densities. Indeed, a crucial (implicit) condition behind (5.3.2) is that $\Omega_1 \cap \Omega_2$ is nonempty: the more the overlap is, the more efficient the BS estimates are. To see this idea more clearly, Gelman and Meng (1998) consider a reexpression of (5.3.1) by taking $\alpha = q_{3/2}/(q_1 q_2)$ where $q_{3/2}$ is an arbitrary unnormalized density having support $\Omega_1 \cap \Omega_2$ while the subscript "3/2" indicates a density that is "between" π_1 and π_2. Substituting this α into (5.3.1) yields

$$r = \frac{c_1}{c_2} = \frac{E_2[q_{3/2}/q_2]}{E_1[q_{3/2}/q_1]}. \tag{5.4.10}$$

Comparing (5.4.10) to (5.2.4), we see that estimating r with (5.2.4) requires random samples from π_2 to "reach" π_1, whereas with (5.4.10) random samples from both q_1 and q_2 with $q_{3/2}$ as a connecting "bridge" can be used to estimate r. Thus, use of (5.4.10) effectively shortens the distance between the two densities. This idea essentially leads to extensions using multiple bridges, that is, by applying (5.4.10) in a "chain" fashion. Gelman and Meng (1998) show that the limit from using infinitely many bridges leads to the PS identity given in (5.4.1). Thus, BS is a natural extension of IS while PS is a further extension of BS.

5.5 Ratio Importance Sampling

5.5.1 The Method

In the same spirit as reducing the distance between two densities, Torrie and Valleau (1977) and Chen and Shao (1997a) propose another MC method for estimating a ratio of two normalizing constants. Their method is based on the following identity:

$$r = \frac{c_1}{c_2} = \frac{E_\pi\{q_1(\boldsymbol{\theta})/\pi(\boldsymbol{\theta})\}}{E_\pi\{q_2(\boldsymbol{\theta})/\pi(\boldsymbol{\theta})\}}, \tag{5.5.1}$$

where the expectation E_π is taken with respect to π and $\pi(\boldsymbol{\theta})$ is an arbitrary density with the support $\Omega = \Omega_1 \cup \Omega_2$. In (5.5.1), π serves as a "middle" density between π_1 and π_2. It is interesting to see that (5.5.1) is "opposite" to (5.4.10). With (5.4.10), we need random samples from both π_1 and π_2 while with (5.5.1), only one random sample from the "middle" density π is required for estimating r. This is advantageous in the context of computing posterior model probabilities since many normalizing constants need to be estimated simultaneously (see Chapters 8 and 9 for more details). It can also be observed that (5.5.1) is an extension of (5.2.4) since (5.5.1) reduces to (5.2.4) by taking $\pi = \pi_2$.

Torrie and Valleau (1977) call this method "umbrella sampling," conveying the intention of constructing a middle density that "covers" both ends. However, Chen and Shao (1997a) term this method RIS because:

(i) it is a natural extension of IS;

(ii) the identity given in (5.5.1) contains the "middle" density π in both numerator and denominator in a ratio fashion; and

(iii) most importantly, this method is used for estimating a ratio of two normalizing constants.

Although this method is initially proposed by Torrie and Valleau (1977), the theoretical properties of this method are explored by Chen and Shao (1997a) and extensions of this method to Bayesian variable selection are considered by Ibrahim, Chen, and MacEachern (1999) and Chen, Ibrahim, and Yiannoutsos (1999). Given a random sample $\{\boldsymbol{\theta}_1, \boldsymbol{\theta}_2, \ldots, \boldsymbol{\theta}_n\}$ from π, a RIS estimator of r is given by

$$\hat{r}_{\text{RIS}} = \hat{r}_{\text{RIS}}(\pi) = \frac{\sum_{i=1}^n q_1(\boldsymbol{\theta}_i)/\pi(\boldsymbol{\theta}_i)}{\sum_{i=1}^n q_2(\boldsymbol{\theta}_i)/\pi(\boldsymbol{\theta}_i)}. \tag{5.5.2}$$

For any π with the support Ω, $\hat{r}_{\text{RIS}}$ is a consistent estimator of r. To explore further properties of $\hat{r}_{\text{RIS}}$, we let

$$\text{RE}^2(\hat{r}_{\text{RIS}}) = \frac{E_\pi(\hat{r}_{\text{RIS}} - r)^2}{r^2} \tag{5.5.3}$$

denote the relative mean-square error which is similar to (5.2.2). The analytical calculation of (5.5.3) is typically intractable. However, under the assumption that the $\boldsymbol{\theta}_i$ are independent and identically distributed (i.i.d.) from π, we can obtain the asymptotic form of $\text{RE}^2(\hat{r}_{\text{RIS}})$. Let $f_1(\boldsymbol{\theta}) = q_1(\boldsymbol{\theta})/\pi(\boldsymbol{\theta})$ and $f_2(\boldsymbol{\theta}) = q_2(\boldsymbol{\theta})/\pi(\boldsymbol{\theta})$. Then, we have $E_\pi[f_1(\boldsymbol{\theta})] = c_1$ and $E_\pi[f_2(\boldsymbol{\theta})] = c_2$. We are led to the following theorem:

Theorem 5.5.1 *Let* $\{\boldsymbol{\theta}_i,\ i = 1, 2, \ldots\}$ *be* i.i.d. *random samples from* π. *Assume* $\int_\Omega |q_1(\boldsymbol{\theta}) - aq_2(\boldsymbol{\theta})|\, d\boldsymbol{\theta} > 0$ *for every* $a > 0$,

$$E_\pi \left(\frac{f_1(\boldsymbol{\theta})}{c_1} - \frac{f_2(\boldsymbol{\theta})}{c_2} \right)^2 < \infty, \ \ \textit{and}\ \ E_\pi \{f_1(\boldsymbol{\theta})/f_2(\boldsymbol{\theta})\}^2 < \infty.$$

Then

$$\lim_{n\to\infty} n\ \mathrm{RE}^2(\hat{r}_{\mathrm{RIS}}) = E_\pi \left\{ \frac{f_1(\boldsymbol{\theta})}{c_1} - \frac{f_2(\boldsymbol{\theta})}{c_2} \right\}^2, \tag{5.5.4}$$

and

$$\sqrt{n}(\hat{r}_{\mathrm{RIS}} - r) \xrightarrow{\mathcal{D}} N\left(0, r^2 E_\pi \left\{ \frac{f_1(\boldsymbol{\theta})}{c_1} - \frac{f_2(\boldsymbol{\theta})}{c_2} \right\}^2 \right) \quad \textit{as } n \to \infty. \tag{5.5.5}$$

If, in addition, $E_\pi(f_1(\boldsymbol{\theta})/c_1 - f_2(\boldsymbol{\theta})/c_2)^4 < \infty$ *and* $E_\pi f_2^4(\boldsymbol{\theta}) < \infty$, *then*

$$\mathrm{RE}^2(\hat{r}_{RIS}) = \frac{1}{n} E_\pi \left\{ \frac{f_1(\boldsymbol{\theta})}{c_1} - \frac{f_2(\boldsymbol{\theta})}{c_2} \right\}^2 + O\left(\frac{1}{n^2}\right) \quad \textit{as } n \to \infty. \tag{5.5.6}$$

The proof of Theorem 5.5.1 is given in the Appendix. By (5.5.4), we have the asymptotic form of $\mathrm{RE}^2(\hat{r}_{\mathrm{RIS}})$:

$$\mathrm{RE}^2(\hat{r}_{\mathrm{RIS}}) = \frac{1}{n} E_\pi \left[\frac{\{\pi_1(\boldsymbol{\theta}) - \pi_2(\boldsymbol{\theta})\}^2}{\pi^2(\boldsymbol{\theta})} \right] + o\Big(\frac{1}{n}\Big). \tag{5.5.7}$$

When $\Omega_1 \subset \Omega_2$ and $\pi(\boldsymbol{\theta}) = \pi_2(\boldsymbol{\theta}) = q_2(\boldsymbol{\theta})/c_2$, (5.5.2) becomes the importance sampling estimator (5.2.5) for r, and the corresponding relative mean-square error is

$$\mathrm{RE}^2(\hat{r}_{\mathrm{IS}_2}) = \frac{1}{n} \int_{\Omega_2} \frac{(\pi_1(\boldsymbol{\theta}) - \pi_2(\boldsymbol{\theta}))^2}{\pi_2(\boldsymbol{\theta})}\, d\boldsymbol{\theta}, \tag{5.5.8}$$

which is the χ^2-divergence, denoted by $\chi^2(\pi_2, \pi_1)$, between π_2 and π_1.

Since the RIS estimator $\hat{r}_\pi$ depends on π, it is of interest to determine the optimal RIS density π_{opt} of π. The result is given in the following theorem:

Theorem 5.5.2 *Assume* $\int_\Omega |q_1(\boldsymbol{\theta}) - aq_2(\boldsymbol{\theta})|\, d\boldsymbol{\theta} > 0$ *for every* $a > 0$. *The first term of the right side of* (5.5.7) *is minimized at*

$$\pi_{\mathrm{opt}}(\boldsymbol{\theta}) = \frac{|\pi_1(\boldsymbol{\theta}) - \pi_2(\boldsymbol{\theta})|}{\int_\Omega |\pi_1(\boldsymbol{\delta}) - \pi_2(\boldsymbol{\delta})|\, d\boldsymbol{\delta}} \tag{5.5.9}$$

with a minimal value

$$\frac{1}{n} \left[\int_\Omega |\pi_1(\boldsymbol{\theta}) - \pi_2(\boldsymbol{\theta})|\ d\boldsymbol{\theta} \right]^2. \tag{5.5.10}$$

The proof of Theorem 5.5.2 is given in the Appendix. It is interesting to note that (5.5.10) is $(1/n)L_1^2(\pi_1, \pi_2)$, where $L_1(\pi_1, \pi_2)$ is the L_1-divergence between π_1 and π_2. From Theorem 5.5.2, and (5.5.8) and (5.5.10), we also have $L_1^2(\pi_1, \pi_2) \le \chi^2(\pi_2, \pi_1)$.

Now, we compare the RIS method with the BS method. The following theorem states that the RIS estimator (5.5.2) with the optimal π_{opt} given in (5.5.9) has a smaller asymptotic relative mean-square error than the BS estimator (5.3.3) with the optimal choice α_{opt} given in (5.3.5).

Theorem 5.5.3 *For $0 < s_1, s_2 < 1$, and $s_1 + s_2 = 1$, we have*

$$\left[\int_\Omega |\pi_1(\boldsymbol{\theta}) - \pi_2(\boldsymbol{\theta})|\, d\boldsymbol{\theta}\right]^2 \le (s_1 s_2)^{-1} \left[\left\{\int_{\Omega_1 \cap \Omega_2} \frac{\pi_1(\boldsymbol{\theta})\pi_2(\boldsymbol{\theta})}{s_1\pi_1(\boldsymbol{\theta}) + s_2\pi_2(\boldsymbol{\theta})}\, d\boldsymbol{\theta}\right\}^{-1} - 1\right]. \quad (5.5.11)$$

The proof of the theorem given in the Appendix.

Next, we compare the RIS method with the PS method. Gelman and Meng (1998) point out that the asymptotic variance $\hat{\xi}_{\text{PS}}$ is the same as the asymptotic relative mean-square error of $\hat{r}$, i.e.,

$$\lim_{n\to\infty} n \operatorname{Var}(\hat{\xi}_{\text{PS}}) = \lim_{n\to\infty} nE(\hat{r}_{\text{PS}} - r)^2/r^2,$$

where $\hat{r}_{\text{PS}} = \exp(-\hat{\xi}_{\text{PS}})$. Thus, the next theorem shows that the asymptotic relative mean-square error of the RIS estimator (5.5.2) with the optimal π_{opt} is less than the lower bound, given on the right side of (5.4.6), of the variance of $\hat{\xi}_{\text{PS}}$ given in (5.4.3).

Theorem 5.5.4 *Defining $\pi_l(\boldsymbol{\theta}) = q_l(\boldsymbol{\theta})/c_l = \pi(\boldsymbol{\theta}|\boldsymbol{\lambda}_l)$ for $l = 1, 2$, we have*

$$\left[\int_\Omega |\pi_1(\boldsymbol{\theta}) - \pi_2(\boldsymbol{\theta})|\, d\boldsymbol{\theta}\right]^2 \le 4\int \left[\sqrt{\pi(\boldsymbol{\theta}|\boldsymbol{\lambda}_1)} - \sqrt{\pi(\boldsymbol{\theta}|\boldsymbol{\lambda}_2)}\right]^2 d\boldsymbol{\theta}. \quad (5.5.12)$$

The proof of Theorem 5.5.4 is given in the Appendix. From Theorem 5.5.4, we can see that $L_1^2(\pi_1, \pi_2) \le 4H^2(\pi_1, \pi_2)$ and that the optimal RIS estimator $\hat{r}_{\text{RIS}}(\pi_{\text{opt}})$ is always better than the BS estimator, and $\hat{r}_{\text{RIS}}(\pi_{\text{opt}})$ is also better than any PS estimator. However, π_{opt} depends on the unknown normalizing constants c_1 and c_2. Therefore, $\hat{r}_{\pi_{\text{opt}}}$ is not directly usable. We will address implementation issues in the next subsection.

5.5.2 Implementation

In this subsection, we present two approaches to implement the optimal RIS estimators. We also discuss other "nonoptimal" implementation schemes.

Exact Optimal Scheme

Let $\pi(\boldsymbol{\theta})$ be an arbitrary density over Ω such that $\pi(\boldsymbol{\theta}) > 0$ for $\boldsymbol{\theta} \in \Omega$.

Given a random sample $\{\boldsymbol{\theta}_i,\ i = 1, 2, \ldots, n\}$ from π, define

$$\tau_n = \frac{\sum_{i=1}^n q_1(\boldsymbol{\theta}_i)/\pi(\boldsymbol{\theta}_i)}{\sum_{i=1}^n q_2(\boldsymbol{\theta}_i)/\pi(\boldsymbol{\theta}_i)} \tag{5.5.13}$$

and let

$$\psi_n(\boldsymbol{\theta}) = \frac{|q_1(\boldsymbol{\theta}) - \tau_n q_2(\boldsymbol{\theta})|}{\int_\Omega |q_1(\boldsymbol{\delta}) - \tau_n q_2(\boldsymbol{\delta})|\, d\boldsymbol{\delta}}. \tag{5.5.14}$$

Then, take a random sample $\{\boldsymbol{\vartheta}_{n,1}, \boldsymbol{\vartheta}_{n,2}, \ldots, \vartheta_{n,n}\}$ from ψ_n and define the "optimal" estimator $\hat{r}_{\text{RIS},n}$ as follows:

$$\hat{r}_{\text{RIS},n} = \frac{\sum_{i=1}^n q_1(\boldsymbol{\vartheta}_{n,i})/\psi_n(\boldsymbol{\vartheta}_{n,i})}{\sum_{i=1}^n q_2(\boldsymbol{\vartheta}_{n,i})/\psi_n(\boldsymbol{\vartheta}_{n,i})}. \tag{5.5.15}$$

Then, we have the following result:

Theorem 5.5.5 *Suppose that there exists a neighborhood U_r of r such that the following conditions are satisfied:*

(i) $\displaystyle\inf_{a \in U_r} \int_\Omega |q_1(\boldsymbol{\theta}) - a q_2(\boldsymbol{\theta})|\, d\boldsymbol{\theta} > 0$;

(ii) $\displaystyle\int_\Omega \sup_{a \in U_r} \frac{q_1^2(\boldsymbol{\theta}) + q_2^2(\boldsymbol{\theta})}{|q_1(\boldsymbol{\theta}) - a q_2(\boldsymbol{\theta})|}\, d\boldsymbol{\theta} < \infty$; *and*

(iii) $\displaystyle\sup_{a \in U_r} \int_\Omega \frac{q_1^2(\boldsymbol{\theta})|q_1(\boldsymbol{\theta}) - a q_2(\boldsymbol{\theta})|}{q_2^2(\boldsymbol{\theta})}\, d\boldsymbol{\theta} < \infty.$

Then

$$\lim_{n \to \infty} nE\left(\frac{(\hat{r}_{\text{RIS},n} - r)^2}{r^2}\,\middle|\, \boldsymbol{\theta}_1, \boldsymbol{\theta}_2, \ldots, \boldsymbol{\theta}_n\right) = \left[\int_\Omega |\pi_1(\boldsymbol{\theta}) - \pi_2(\boldsymbol{\theta})|\, d\boldsymbol{\theta}\right]^2 \quad \text{a.s.} \tag{5.5.16}$$

The proof of Theorem 5.5.5 is given in the Appendix. Theorem 5.5.5 says that the "optimal" estimator $\hat{r}_{\text{RIS},n}$ obtained by the two-stage sampling scheme has the same optimal relative mean-square error as $\hat{r}_{\text{RIS}}(\pi_{\text{opt}})$. In the two-stage sampling scheme, sample sizes in stage 1 and stage 2 need not be the same. More specifically, we can use n_1 in (5.5.13) and (5.5.14) (the first-stage sample size) and n_2 in (5.5.15) (the second-stage sample size). Then, (5.5.16) still holds as long as $n_1 = o(n)$ and $n_1 \to \infty$, where $n = n_1 + n_2$.

Approximate Optimal Scheme

Let $\pi_l^{\text{I}}(\boldsymbol{\theta})$, $l = 1, 2$, be good importance sampling densities for $\pi_l(\boldsymbol{\theta})$, $l = 1, 2$, respectively. Then, the optimal RIS density, π_{opt}, can be approximated by

$$\pi_{\text{opt}}^{\text{I}}(\boldsymbol{\theta}) \propto \left|\pi_1^{\text{I}}(\boldsymbol{\theta}) - \pi_2^{\text{I}}(\boldsymbol{\theta})\right|.$$

Let $\{\boldsymbol{\theta}_i, \ i = 1, 2, \ldots, n\}$ be a random sample from $\pi^{\mathrm{I}}_{\mathrm{opt}}$. Then an approximate optimal RIS estimator is given by

$$\hat{r}_{\pi^{\mathrm{I}}_{\mathrm{opt}}} = \frac{\sum_{i=1}^n q_1(\boldsymbol{\theta}_i)/\left|\pi^{\mathrm{I}}_1(\boldsymbol{\theta}_i) - \pi^{\mathrm{I}}_2(\boldsymbol{\theta}_i)\right|}{\sum_{i=1}^n q_2(\boldsymbol{\theta}_i)/\left|\pi^{\mathrm{I}}_1(\boldsymbol{\theta}_i) - \pi^{\mathrm{I}}_2(\boldsymbol{\theta}_i)\right|}.$$

Note that when π_1 and π_2 do not overlap, we can choose $\pi^{\mathrm{I}}_{\mathrm{opt}}(\boldsymbol{\theta}) = \{\pi^{\mathrm{I}}_1(\boldsymbol{\theta}) + \pi^{\mathrm{I}}_2(\boldsymbol{\theta})\}/2$ because $\pi_{\mathrm{opt}}(\boldsymbol{\theta}) = \{\pi_1(\boldsymbol{\theta}) + \pi_2(\boldsymbol{\theta})\}/2$. For such cases, sampling from $\pi^{\mathrm{I}}_{\mathrm{opt}}$ is straightforward.

Other "Nonoptimal" Schemes

First, assume that π_1 and π_2 do not overlap, i.e., $\int_\Omega q_1(\boldsymbol{\theta})q_2(\boldsymbol{\theta})\, d\boldsymbol{\theta} = 0$. For this case, the IWMDE method of Chen (1994) will give a reasonably good estimator of r. Let $w_l(\boldsymbol{\theta})$ be a weighted density with a shape roughly similar to q_l, for $l = 1, 2$. Also let $\{\boldsymbol{\theta}_{l,i}, i = 1, 2, \ldots, n_l\}$, $l = 1, 2$, be independent random samples from π_l, $l = 1, 2$, respectively. Then, a consistent estimator of r is

$$\hat{r}_{\mathrm{IWMDE}} = \frac{(1/n_2)\sum_{i=1}^{n_2} w_2(\boldsymbol{\theta}_{2,i})/q_2(\boldsymbol{\theta}_{2,i})}{(1/n_1)\sum_{i=1}^{n_1} w_1(\boldsymbol{\theta}_{1,i})/q_1(\boldsymbol{\theta}_{1,i})}.$$

In this case, PS is also useful (if it is applicable).

Second, assume that $\int_\Omega p_1(\boldsymbol{\theta})p_2(\boldsymbol{\theta})\, d\boldsymbol{\theta} > 0$, i.e., π_1 and π_2 do overlap. We propose a BS type estimator as follows. Let $\{\boldsymbol{\theta}_i, i = 1, 2, \ldots, n\}$ be a random sample from a mixture density:

$$\pi_{\mathrm{mix}}(\boldsymbol{\theta}) = \psi\pi_1(\boldsymbol{\theta}) + (1-\psi)\pi_2(\boldsymbol{\theta}),$$

where $0 < \psi < 1$ is known (e.g., $\psi = \frac{1}{2}$). Note that we can straightforwardly sample from $\pi_{\mathrm{mix}}(\boldsymbol{\theta})$ by a composition method without knowing c_1 and c_2. Let

$$S_n(r) = \sum_{i=1}^n \frac{rq_2(\boldsymbol{\theta}_i)}{\psi q_1(\boldsymbol{\theta}_i) + r\cdot(1-\psi)q_2(\boldsymbol{\theta}_i)} - \sum_{i=1}^n \frac{q_1(\boldsymbol{\theta}_i)}{\psi q_1(\boldsymbol{\theta}_i) + r\cdot(1-\psi)q_2(\boldsymbol{\theta}_i)}.$$

Then, a BS type estimator $\hat{r}_{\mathrm{BS},n}$ of r is the solution of the following equation:

$$S_n(r) = 0. \tag{5.5.17}$$

Similar to (5.3.8), it can be shown that there exists a unique solution of (5.5.17). The asymptotic properties of $\hat{r}_{\mathrm{BS},n}$ are given in the next theorem.

Theorem 5.5.6 *Suppose that $\int_\Omega q_1(\boldsymbol{\theta})q_2(\boldsymbol{\theta})\, d\boldsymbol{\theta} > 0$. Then*

$$\hat{r}_{\mathrm{BS},n} \stackrel{\mathrm{a.s.}}{\longrightarrow} r \ \text{as } n \to \infty. \tag{5.5.18}$$

If, in addition, $E_{\pi_{\text{mix}}}(q_1(\boldsymbol{\theta})/q_2(\boldsymbol{\theta}))^2 < \infty$, *then*

$$\lim_{n\to\infty} n\, E_{\pi_{\text{mix}}} \frac{(\hat{r}_{\text{BS},n} - r)^2}{r^2} = \int_\Omega \frac{(\pi_1(\boldsymbol{\theta}) - \pi_2(\boldsymbol{\theta}))^2}{\psi\pi_1(\boldsymbol{\theta}) + (1-\psi)\pi_2(\boldsymbol{\theta})}\, d\boldsymbol{\theta} \cdot \left\{ \int_\Omega \frac{\pi_1(\boldsymbol{\theta}) \cdot \pi_2(\boldsymbol{\theta})}{\psi\pi_1(\boldsymbol{\theta}) + (1-\psi)\pi_2(\boldsymbol{\theta})}\, d\boldsymbol{\theta} \right\}^{-2}. \tag{5.5.19}$$

The proof of this theorem is given in the Appendix.

5.6 A Theoretical Illustration

To get a better understanding of IS, BS, PS, and RIS, we conduct two theoretical case studies based on two normal densities where we know the exact values of the two normalizing constants.

CASE 1. $N(0,1)$ *and* $N(\delta, 1)$
Let $q_1(\theta) = \exp(-\theta^2/2)$ and $q_2(\theta) = \exp(-(\theta-\delta)^2/2)$ with δ a known positive constant. In this case, $c_1 = c_2 = \sqrt{2\pi}$ and, therefore, $r = 1$ and $\xi = -\ln(r) = 0$. For PS, we consider q_1 and q_2 as two points in the family of unnormalized normal densities: $q(\theta|\boldsymbol{\lambda}) = \exp\{-(\theta-\mu)^2/2\sigma^2\}$, with $\boldsymbol{\lambda} = (\mu, \sigma)'$, $\boldsymbol{\lambda}_1 = (0,1)'$, and $\boldsymbol{\lambda}_2 = (\delta, 1)'$.

As discussed in Gelman and Meng (1998), in order to make fair comparisons, we assume that:

(i) with IS–version 2, we sample n i.i.d. observations from $N(\delta, 1)$;

(ii) with BS, we sample $n/2$ (assume n is even) i.i.d. observations from each of $N(0,1)$ and $N(\delta,1)$;

(iii) with PS, we first sample t_i, $i = 1, 2, \ldots, n$, uniformly from $(0,1)$ and then sample an observation from $N(\mu(t_i), \sigma^2(t_i))$ where $\boldsymbol{\lambda}(t) = (\mu(t), \sigma(t))'$ is a given path; and

(iv) with RIS, we sample n i.i.d. observations from the optimal RIS density:

$$\pi_{\text{opt}}(\theta) = \frac{|\phi(\theta) - \phi(\theta-\delta)|}{c_{\text{opt}}(\delta)}, \tag{5.6.1}$$

where

$$\begin{aligned} c_{\text{opt}}(\delta) &= \int_{-\infty}^{\infty} |\phi(\theta) - \phi(\theta-\delta)|\, d\theta \\ &= 2(\Phi(\delta/2) - \Phi(-\delta/2)) \\ &= 2(2\Phi(\delta/2) - 1), \end{aligned} \tag{5.6.2}$$

and ϕ and Φ are the $N(0,1)$ probability density function and cumulative distribution function, respectively.

Since the cumulative distribution function (cdf) for $\pi_{\text{opt}}(\theta)$ is

$$\Pi_{\text{opt}}(\theta) = \begin{cases} (\Phi(\theta) - \Phi(\theta-\delta))/2\,(2\Phi(\delta/2)-1) & \text{for } \theta \le \delta/2, \\ 1 - (\Phi(\theta) - \Phi(\theta-\delta))/2\,(2\Phi(\delta/2)-1) & \text{for } \theta > \delta/2, \end{cases} \tag{5.6.3}$$

then the generation from π_{opt} can be easily done by the inversion cdf method (see, e.g., Devroye (1986, pp. 27–35)).

Since the asymptotic variance of $\hat{\xi}_{\text{PS}}$ is the same as the asymptotic relative mean-square error of $\hat{r}_{\text{PS}} = \exp(-\hat{\xi}_{\text{PS}})$, that is,

$$\lim_{n\to\infty} n \operatorname{Var}(\hat{\xi}_{\text{PS}}) = \lim_{n\to\infty} nE(\hat{r}_{\text{PS}} - r)^2/r^2,$$

using (5.5.10), (5.6.2), and the results given by Gelman and Meng (1998), we obtain Table 5.1.

TABLE 5.1. Comparison of Asymptotic Relative Mean-Square Errors (I).

Index	Method	$\lim_{n\to\infty} \sqrt{nE(\hat{r}-r)^2/r^2}$
1	IS–version 2	$\left\{\exp(\delta^2)-1\right\}^{1/2}$
2	BS with $\alpha = (q_1q_2)^{-1/2}$	$2\left\{\exp\left(\frac{\delta^2}{4}\right)-1\right\}^{1/2}$
3	Optimal BS with α_{opt}	$2\left\{\frac{\delta\exp(\delta^2/8)}{\beta(\delta)\sqrt{2\pi}}-1\right\}^{1/2}$
4	Optimal PS in μ-space	δ
5	Optimal PS in $(\mu,\sigma)'$-space	$\sqrt{12}\left\{\ln\left(\frac{\delta}{\sqrt{12}}+\sqrt{1+\frac{\delta^2}{12}}\right)\right\}$
6	Lower bound of PS in (5.4.6)	$\sqrt{8}\left(1-\exp(-\delta^2/8)\right)^{1/2}$
7	Optimal RIS with π_{opt}	$2\,(2\Phi(\delta/2)-1)$

In Table 5.1, for optimal BS,

$$\beta(\delta) = \frac{1}{\pi}\int_0^\infty \exp(-\theta^2/2\delta^2)/\cosh(\theta/2)\,d\theta.$$

For the normal family $N(\mu(t), \sigma^2(t))$, the optimal path for PS in μ-space is the solution of the Euler–Lagrange equation given in (5.4.9) with $k=1$ and

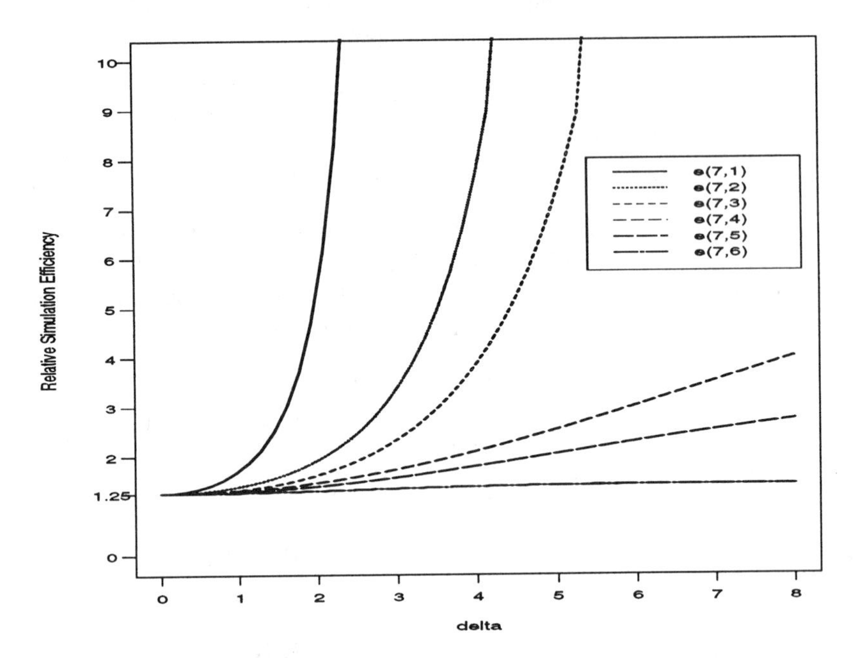

FIGURE 5.1. Relative simulation efficiency plot (I).

boundary conditions $\mu(0) = 0$ and $\mu(1) = \delta$ when we treat a fixed $\sigma^2(t) \equiv 1$, and the optimal path in $(\mu, \sigma)'$-space is the Euler–Lagrange equation with $k = 2$ while both $\mu(t)$ and $\sigma^2(t)$ are functions of t and boundary conditions are $(\mu(0), \sigma^2(0))' = (0,1)'$ and $(\mu(1), \sigma^2(1))' = (\delta, 1)'$. The derivation of Table 5.1 is left as an exercise.

We define the relative simulation efficiency as follows:

$$e(i,j) = \frac{\lim_{n\to\infty} \sqrt{nE(\hat{r}-r)^2/r^2} \text{ for method } j}{\lim_{n\to\infty} \sqrt{nE(\hat{r}-r)^2/r^2} \text{ for method } i} \quad \text{for } i,j = 1,2,\ldots,7, \tag{5.6.4}$$

where $\hat{r}$ is an estimator of r. Then, $e(7,j)$, $j = 1, \ldots, 6$, versus δ are plotted in Figure 5.1. Note that when $e(i,j) \geq 1$, method j has a greater asymptotic relative mean-square error than method i, and therefore, method i is more efficient than method j. It is easy to verify that $e(7,j) \geq \sqrt{2\pi}/2 = 1.2533$ for $j = 1, 2, \ldots, 6$, and

$$\lim_{\delta\to 0} e(7,j) = \sqrt{2\pi}/2 = 1.2533$$

for all $j = 1, 2, \ldots, 6$. Therefore, the lower bound of PS in (5.4.6) is quite close to the asymptotic relative mean-square error of the RIS method with the optimal π_{opt}. The RIS method is significantly better than the BS method, especially for $\delta > 3$, and it is also better than the PS method. In this case, both RIS and PS are much better than IS–version 2.

CASE 2. $N(0,1)$ *and* $N(0,\Delta^2)$
Without loss of generality, we consider $\Delta > 1$ only. Let $q_1(\theta) = \exp(-\theta^2/2)$ and $q_2(\theta) = \exp(-\theta^2/2\Delta^2)$ with Δ a known positive constant. In this case, $c_1 = \sqrt{2\pi}$, $c_2 = \sqrt{2\pi}\Delta$ and, therefore, the ratio $r = c_1/c_2 = 1/\Delta$. For PS, $\xi = \ln\Delta$. Let $q(\theta|\boldsymbol{\lambda}_1) = q_1(\theta)$ and $q(\theta|\boldsymbol{\lambda}_2) = q_2(\theta)$ with $\boldsymbol{\lambda}_1 = (0,1)'$ and $\boldsymbol{\lambda}_2 = (0,\Delta)'$.

For IS-version 2, BS, and PS, we use the sampling schemes similar to those in Case 1 by using $N(0,\Delta^2)$ to replace $N(\delta,1)$. For RIS, the optimal density is

$$\pi_{\text{opt}}(\theta) = \frac{|\phi(\theta) - (1/\Delta)\phi(\theta/\Delta)|}{c_{\text{opt}}(\Delta)},$$

where

$$\begin{aligned} c_{\text{opt}}(\Delta) &= \int_{-\infty}^{\infty} \left|\phi(\theta) - \frac{1}{\Delta}\phi\left(\frac{\theta}{\Delta}\right)\right| d\theta \\ &= 4\left[\Phi\left(\sqrt{\frac{2\ln\Delta}{1-1/\Delta^2}}\right) - \Phi\left(\frac{1}{\Delta}\sqrt{\frac{2\ln\Delta}{1-1/\Delta^2}}\right)\right]. \end{aligned} \tag{5.6.5}$$

The corresponding optimal cumulative distribution is

$$\Pi_{\text{opt}}(\theta) = \begin{cases} \dfrac{\Phi(\theta/\Delta) - \Phi(\theta)}{c_{\text{opt}}(\Delta)} & \text{for } \theta \le -\sqrt{\dfrac{2\ln\Delta}{1-1/\Delta^2}}, \\ \dfrac{1}{2} + \dfrac{\Phi(\theta) - \Phi(\dfrac{\theta}{\Delta})}{c_{\text{opt}}(\Delta)} & \text{for } -\sqrt{\dfrac{2\ln\Delta}{1-1/\Delta^2}} < \theta \le \sqrt{\dfrac{2\ln\Delta}{1-1/\Delta^2}}, \\ 1 - \dfrac{\Phi(\theta) - \Phi(\dfrac{\theta}{\Delta})}{c_{\text{opt}}(\Delta)} & \text{for } \theta < \sqrt{\dfrac{2\ln\Delta}{1-1/\Delta^2}}. \end{cases}$$

Thus, the inversion cdf method can be employed for generating a random variate θ from Π_{opt}.

In this case, the optimal path in $(\mu,\sigma)'$-space with boundary conditions $\mu(t) = 0$ and $\sigma(t) = \Delta^t$ for $0 \le t \le 1$ can be obtained using Problem 4.12 in the exercises. Then, using (5.3.6), (5.4.5), (5.4.8), (5.5.10), and (5.6.5), we derive the asymptotic relative mean-square errors (variances) for IS, BS, PS, and RIS, which are reported in Table 5.2. In Table 5.2,

$$b(\Delta) = \left[\frac{\sqrt{2\pi}}{2\int_{-\infty}^{\infty} \left(\exp(\theta^2/2) + \Delta\exp(\theta^2/2\Delta^2)\right)^{-1} d\theta} - 1\right]^{1/2}$$

and $h(\Delta) = (2\ln\Delta/(1-1/\Delta^2))^{1/2}$.

TABLE 5.2. Comparison of Asymptotic Relative Mean-Square Errors (II).

Index	Method	$\lim_{n\to\infty} \sqrt{nE(\hat{r}-r)^2/r^2}$
1	IS–version 2	$\sqrt{(\Delta^2/\sqrt{2\Delta^2-1})-1}$
2	BS with $\alpha = (q_1 q_2)^{-1/2}$	$\sqrt{2}(\Delta-1)/\sqrt{\Delta}$
3	Optimal BS α_{opt}	$2b(\Delta)$
4	Optimal PS in μ-space	$\sqrt{2}\ln\Delta$
5	Optimal PS in $(\mu,\sigma)'$-space	$\sqrt{2}\ln\Delta$
6	Lower bound of PS in (5.4.6)	$2\sqrt{2}\left(1-\sqrt{2\Delta/(1+\Delta^2)}\right)^{1/2}$
7	Optimal RIS with π_{opt}	$4\left[\Phi\left(h(\Delta)\right)-\Phi\left(\frac{1}{\Delta}h(\Delta)\right)\right]$

The relative simulation efficiencies defined in (5.6.4) are calculated and $e(7,j)$, $j = 1, 2, \ldots, 6$, versus Δ are also plotted in Figure 5.2. It can be shown that $\lim_{\Delta\to 1} e(7,j) = \sqrt{e\pi}/2 = 1.461$ and $e(7,j) > 1$ for all $j = 1, 2, \ldots, 6$. Therefore, the optimal RIS method is better than all five counterparts. Once again, the lower bound of PS and the asymptotic relative mean-square error of optimal RIS are very close. Note that it is not necessarily true that optimal BS is better than IS–version 2 because of our sampling scheme. However, it is true that

$$2\left[\frac{\sqrt{2\pi}}{2\int_{-\infty}^{\infty}\left(\exp(\theta^2/2)+\Delta\exp(\theta^2/2\Delta^2)\right)^{-1}\,d\theta}-1\right]^{1/2}$$
$$\leq \sqrt{2}\cdot\sqrt{(\Delta^2/\sqrt{2\Delta^2-1})-1}.$$

Thus, when one density has a heavier tail than another, taking samples from the heavier-tailed one is always more beneficial. For example, when one is a normal density and another is a Student t density, we recommend that a random sample be taken from the Student t distribution. Furthermore, for this case, we can see that even the simple IS method (version 2) is better than the optimal PS method. Therefore, PS is advantageous only for the cases where the two modes of π_1 and π_2 are far away from each other. Finally, we note that reverse logistic regression (see Section 5.10.2)

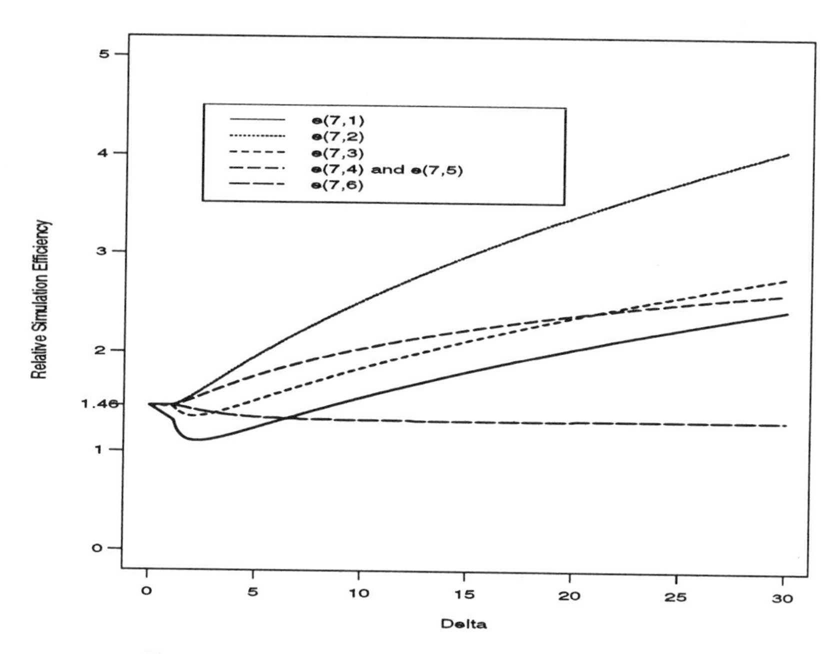

FIGURE 5.2. Relative simulation efficiency plot (II).

has the same $\lim_{n\to\infty} \sqrt{nE(\hat{r}-r)^2/r^2}$ as BS with optimal bridge α_{opt} for both cases.

5.7 Computing Simulation Standard Errors

In Sections 5.2–5.5, IS, BS, PS, and RIS are used to obtain MC estimates of the ratio of the two normalizing constants. In order to assess the simulation accuracy of each estimate, it is important to obtain its associated simulation standard error. In this section, we discuss how to use the asymptotic relative mean-square errors to obtain an approximation of the simulation standard error. Other methods for calculating the simulation standard errors can be found in Section 3.3.

We first start with the importance sampling estimates of r, which are given by (5.2.1) and (5.2.5), respectively. Using (5.2.3) and two independent random samples $\{\boldsymbol{\theta}_{l,1}, \boldsymbol{\theta}_{l,2}, \ldots, \boldsymbol{\theta}_{l,n_l}\}$, $l=1,2$, the simulation standard error of $\hat{r}_{\text{IS}_1}$ given in (5.2.1) can be approximated by

$$\text{se}(\hat{r}_{\text{IS}_1}) = \hat{r}_{\text{IS}_1} \left\{ \sum_{l=1}^{2} \frac{1}{n_l^2} \sum_{i=1}^{n_l} \left(\frac{q_l(\boldsymbol{\theta}_{l,i})/\hat{c}_l - \pi_l^{\text{I}}(\boldsymbol{\theta}_{l,i})}{\pi_l^{\text{I}}(\boldsymbol{\theta}_{l,i})} \right)^2 \right\}^{1/2}, \quad (5.7.1)$$

where $\hat{c}_l = (1/n_l)\sum_{i=1}^{n_l} q_l(\boldsymbol{\theta}_{l,i})/\pi_l^{\mathrm{I}}(\boldsymbol{\theta}_{l,i})$ for $l = 1, 2$. Similarly, using (5.2.6) and $\{\boldsymbol{\theta}_{2,1}, \boldsymbol{\theta}_{2,2}, \ldots, \boldsymbol{\theta}_{2,n}\}$, the simulation standard error of $\hat{r}_{\mathrm{IS}_2}$ is given by

$$\mathrm{se}(\hat{r}_{\mathrm{IS}_2}) = \frac{1}{\sqrt{n}}\left\{\frac{1}{n}\sum_{i=1}^{n}\left(\frac{q_1(\boldsymbol{\theta}_{2,i}) - \hat{r}_{\mathrm{IS}_2} q_2(\boldsymbol{\theta}_{2,i})}{q_2(\boldsymbol{\theta}_{2,i})}\right)^2\right\}^{1/2}. \tag{5.7.2}$$

Next, we consider the BS estimate $\hat{r}_{\mathrm{BS}}$. We have two approaches to compute $\mathrm{se}(\hat{r}_{\mathrm{BS}})$. Using $\{\boldsymbol{\theta}_{2,1}, \boldsymbol{\theta}_{2,2}, \ldots, \boldsymbol{\theta}_{2,n_2}\}$ and $\hat{r}_{\mathrm{BS}}$, an approximation of the simulation standard error is

$$\begin{aligned}\mathrm{se}(\hat{r}_{\mathrm{BS}}) = \frac{\hat{r}_{\mathrm{BS}}}{\sqrt{n s_1 s_2}}&\left\{\frac{1}{n_2}\sum_{i=1}^{n_2} q_1(\boldsymbol{\theta}_{2,i})(s_1 q_1(\boldsymbol{\theta}_{2,i}) + s_2 \hat{r}_{\mathrm{BS}} q_2(\boldsymbol{\theta}_{2,i}))\alpha^2(\boldsymbol{\theta}_{2,i})\right.\\ &\left.\times\left(\frac{1}{n_2}\sum_{i=1}^{n_2} q_1(\boldsymbol{\theta}_{2,i})\alpha(\boldsymbol{\theta}_{2,i})\right)^{-2} - 1\right\}^{1/2}. \end{aligned} \tag{5.7.3}$$

With $\{\boldsymbol{\theta}_{1,1}, \boldsymbol{\theta}_{1,2}, \ldots, \boldsymbol{\theta}_{1,n_1}\}$ and $\hat{r}_{\mathrm{BS}}$, we obtain

$$\begin{aligned}\mathrm{se}(\hat{r}_{\mathrm{BS}}) = \frac{\hat{r}_{\mathrm{BS}}}{\sqrt{n s_1 s_2}}&\left\{\frac{1}{n_1}\sum_{i=1}^{n_1} q_2(\boldsymbol{\theta}_{2,i})(s_1 q_1(\boldsymbol{\theta}_{1,i}) + s_2 \hat{r}_{\mathrm{BS}} q_2(\boldsymbol{\theta}_{1,i}))\alpha^2(\boldsymbol{\theta}_{1,i})\right.\\ &\left.\times\left[\hat{r}_{\mathrm{BS}}\left(\frac{1}{n_1}\sum_{i=1}^{n_1} q_2(\boldsymbol{\theta}_{1,i})\alpha(\boldsymbol{\theta}_{1,i})\right)^2\right]^{-1} - 1\right\}^{1/2}. \end{aligned} \tag{5.7.4}$$

In practice, we recommend that one may use (5.7.3) when $n_2 > n_1$ and (5.7.4) when $n_2 < n_1$. When $n_2 = n_1$, one can use either (5.7.3) or (5.7.4). Analogous to $\hat{r}_{\mathrm{BS}}$, using (5.3.6), an approximation of the simulation standard error for the optimal BS estimate $\hat{r}_{\mathrm{BS,opt}}$ can be written as

$$\mathrm{se}(\hat{r}_{\mathrm{BS,opt}}) = \frac{\hat{r}_{\mathrm{BS,opt}}}{\sqrt{n s_1 s_2}}\left[\left\{\frac{1}{n_2}\sum_{i=1}^{n_2}\frac{q_1(\boldsymbol{\theta}_{2,i})}{s_1 q_1(\boldsymbol{\theta}_{2,i}) + s_2 \hat{r}_{\mathrm{BS,opt}} q_2(\boldsymbol{\theta}_{2,i})}\right\}^{-1} - 1\right]^{1/2}. \tag{5.7.5}$$

For PS, since the variance of $\hat{\xi}_{\mathrm{PS}}$ has a closed form, a derivation of the formula for the simulation standard error of $\hat{\xi}_{\mathrm{PS}}$ is straightforward. In particular, the method for IS–version 2 can be exactly applied.

To compute the simulation standard error for a RIS estimate $\hat{r}_{\mathrm{RIS}}$, we write $\pi(\boldsymbol{\theta}) = q(\boldsymbol{\theta})/c_\pi$, where $q(\boldsymbol{\theta})$ is completely known, but c_π is an unknown quantity. Then, we can express the first-order term of $\mathrm{RE}^2(\hat{r}_{\mathrm{RIS}})$ in (5.5.7) as

$$\frac{1}{n}E_\pi\left[\frac{\{\pi_1(\boldsymbol{\theta}) - \pi_2(\boldsymbol{\theta})\}^2}{\pi^2(\boldsymbol{\theta})}\right] = \frac{1}{n}\left(\frac{c_\pi}{c_1}\right)^2 E_\pi\left[\left\{\frac{q_1(\boldsymbol{\theta}) - r q_2(\boldsymbol{\theta})}{q(\boldsymbol{\theta})}\right\}^2\right]. \tag{5.7.6}$$

Using (5.2.5), a consistent estimate of (c_1/c_π) in (5.7.6) is given by

$$\frac{1}{n}\sum_{i=1}^{n}\frac{q_1(\boldsymbol{\theta}_i)}{q(\boldsymbol{\theta}_i)}, \tag{5.7.7}$$

where $\{\boldsymbol{\theta}_i,\ i=1,2,\ldots,n\}$ is a random sample from $\pi(\boldsymbol{\theta})$. Also, we can use the same random sample from π to obtain a consistent estimate for $E_\pi[\{(q_1(\boldsymbol{\theta})-rq_2(\boldsymbol{\theta}))/q(\boldsymbol{\theta})\}^2]$, which is given by

$$\frac{1}{n}\sum_{i=1}^{n}\left\{\frac{q_1(\boldsymbol{\theta}_i)-\hat{r}_{\text{RIS}}q_2(\boldsymbol{\theta}_i)}{q(\boldsymbol{\theta}_i)}\right\}^2, \tag{5.7.8}$$

where $\hat{r}_{\text{RIS}}$ is defined by (5.5.2). Since q_1, q_2, and q are completely known, (5.7.7) and (5.7.7) are readily computed. Combining (5.7.6), (5.7.7), and (5.7.8) together gives a first-order approximation of the simulation standard error for $\hat{r}_{\text{RIS}}$ as follows:

$$\text{se}(\hat{r}_{\text{RIS}})=\frac{\hat{r}_{\text{RIS}}}{\sqrt{n}}\left[\frac{1}{n}\sum_{i=1}^{n}\left\{\frac{q_1(\boldsymbol{\theta}_i)-\hat{r}_{\text{RIS}}q_2(\boldsymbol{\theta}_i)}{q(\boldsymbol{\theta}_i)}\right\}^2\right]^{1/2}\left[\frac{1}{n}\sum_{i=1}^{n}\frac{q_1(\boldsymbol{\theta}_i)}{q(\boldsymbol{\theta}_i)}\right]^{-1}. \tag{5.7.9}$$

From the derivation of the approximation of the simulation standard error for an estimate of r, we observe an interesting feature. That is, the same random sample(s) can be used for computing both the estimate of r and its simulation standard error. This feature is important since it indicates that computing the simulation standard error does not require any additional random samples. On the other hand, we also observe that our derivation of the simulation standard error is based on a first-order asymptotic approximation. Hence, one may wonder how accurate this type of approximation is. To examine this, several simulation studies were conducted by Chen and Shao (1997b). Their simulation results indicate that the simulation standard error based on the first-order approximation is indeed quite accurate as long as the MCMC sample size is greater than 1000. However, a suggested MCMC sample size is 5000 or larger to ensure that a reliable approximation of the simulation standard error can be obtained.

5.8 Extensions to Densities with Different Dimensions

5.8.1 *Why Different Dimensions?*

Kass and Raftery (1995) illustrate a simple problem for testing the two hypotheses H_1 and H_2. Given data D, the Bayes factor is defined by

$$B=\frac{m(D|H_1)}{m(D|H_2)},$$

where the marginal likelihood function

$$m(D|H_l) = \int_{\Omega_l} L(\boldsymbol{\theta}_l|D, H_l)\pi(\boldsymbol{\theta}_l|H_l)\, d\boldsymbol{\theta}_l,$$

$\boldsymbol{\theta}_l$ is a $p_l \times 1$ parameter vector under H_l, $\pi(\boldsymbol{\theta}_l|H_l)$ is the prior density, $L(\boldsymbol{\theta}_l|D, H_l)$ is the likelihood function of $\boldsymbol{\theta}_l$, and Ω_l is the support of the posterior density that is proportional to $L(\boldsymbol{\theta}_l|D, H_l)\pi(\boldsymbol{\theta}_l|H_l)$ for $l = 1, 2$. (See Jeffreys (1961, Chap. 5) for several examples of this simple Bayesian hypothesis testing problem.) Clearly, the Bayes factor B is a ratio of two normalizing constants of two unnormalized densities $L(\boldsymbol{\theta}_l|D, H_l)\pi(\boldsymbol{\theta}_l|H_l)$, $l = 1, 2$, respectively. Note that when $p_1 \neq p_2$, we are dealing with a problem of two different dimensions.

Verdinelli and Wasserman (1996) also consider a similar problem for testing precise null hypotheses using the Bayes factors when nuisance parameters are present. Consider the parameter $(\boldsymbol{\theta}, \boldsymbol{\psi}) \in \Omega \times \boldsymbol{\psi}$, where $\boldsymbol{\psi}$ is a nuisance parameter, and suppose we wish to test the null hypothesis H_0: $\boldsymbol{\theta} = \boldsymbol{\theta}_0$ versus H_1: $\boldsymbol{\theta} \neq \boldsymbol{\theta}_0$. Then they obtain the Bayes factor $B = m_0/m$ where $m_0 = \int_{\Psi} L(\boldsymbol{\theta}_0, \boldsymbol{\psi}|D)\pi_0(\boldsymbol{\psi})\, d\boldsymbol{\psi}$ and $m = \int_{\Omega\times\Psi} L(\boldsymbol{\theta}, \boldsymbol{\psi}|D)\pi(\boldsymbol{\theta}, \boldsymbol{\psi})\, d\boldsymbol{\theta}\, d\boldsymbol{\psi}$ (Jeffreys 1961, Chap. 5). Here $L(\boldsymbol{\theta}, \boldsymbol{\psi}|D)$ is the likelihood function, and $\pi_0(\boldsymbol{\psi})$ and $\pi(\boldsymbol{\theta}, \boldsymbol{\psi})$ are the priors. Therefore, the Bayes factor B is a ratio of two normalizing constants again. In this case, one density is a function of $\boldsymbol{\psi}$ and the other density is a function of $\boldsymbol{\theta}$ and $\boldsymbol{\psi}$.

5.8.2 *General Formulation*

From the two illustrative examples given in Section 5.7.1, we can formulate the general problem of computing ratios of two normalizing constants with different dimensions. Let $\boldsymbol{\theta} = (\theta_1, \ldots, \theta_p)$ and $\boldsymbol{\psi} = (\psi_1, \ldots, \psi_k)$. Also let $\pi_1(\boldsymbol{\theta})$ be a density which is known up to a normalizing constant:

$$\pi_1(\boldsymbol{\theta}) = \frac{q_1(\boldsymbol{\theta})}{c_1}, \quad \boldsymbol{\theta} \in \Omega_1,$$

where $\Omega_1 \subset R^p$ is the support of π_1 and let $\pi_2(\boldsymbol{\theta}, \boldsymbol{\psi})$ be another density which is known up to a normalizing constant:

$$\pi_2(\boldsymbol{\theta}, \boldsymbol{\psi}) = \frac{q_2(\boldsymbol{\theta}, \boldsymbol{\psi})}{c_2}, \quad (\boldsymbol{\theta}, \boldsymbol{\psi}) \in \Theta_2,$$

where $\Theta_2 \subset R^{p+k}$ $(k \geq 1)$ is the support of π_2. We also denote

$$\Omega_2 = \{\boldsymbol{\theta} : \exists\, \boldsymbol{\psi} \in R^k \text{ such that } (\boldsymbol{\theta}, \boldsymbol{\psi}) \in \Theta_2\} \tag{5.8.1}$$

and $\Psi(\boldsymbol{\theta}) = \{\boldsymbol{\psi} : (\boldsymbol{\theta}, \boldsymbol{\psi}) \in \Theta_2\}$ for $\boldsymbol{\theta} \in \Omega_2$. Then the ratio of two normalizing constants is defined as $r = c_1/c_2$, which is (5.1.1).

Since the two densities of interest have different dimensions, the MC methods for estimating a ratio of two normalizing constants described in

Sections 5.2–5.5, which include IS, BS, PS, as well as RIS, cannot work directly here. To see this, we consider IS–version 2. The key identity for IS–version 2 is

$$r = \frac{c_1}{c_2} = E_{\pi_2}\left\{\frac{q_1(\boldsymbol{\theta})}{q_2(\boldsymbol{\theta}, \boldsymbol{\psi})}\right\},$$

which does not hold in general, unless under certain conditions such as $\int_{\Psi(\boldsymbol{\theta})} d\boldsymbol{\psi} = 1$ for all $\boldsymbol{\theta} \in \Omega_2$. Since IS–version 1 described in Section 5.2.1 depends highly on the choices of the two IS densities, we consider only IS–version 2 in this section. It is inconvenient here to construct a path to link π_1 and π_2 due to different dimensionality. Therefore, it is not feasible to apply PS for problems with different dimensions. On the other hand, if the conditional density of $\boldsymbol{\psi}$ given $\boldsymbol{\theta}$ is completely known, the problem of different dimensions disappears. This can be explained as follows. Let $\pi_2(\boldsymbol{\psi}|\boldsymbol{\theta})$ denote the conditional density of $\boldsymbol{\psi}$ given $\boldsymbol{\theta}$,

$$\pi_2(\boldsymbol{\psi}|\boldsymbol{\theta}) = \frac{q_2(\boldsymbol{\theta}, \boldsymbol{\psi})}{\int_{\Psi(\boldsymbol{\theta})} q_2(\boldsymbol{\theta}, \boldsymbol{\psi}^*)\, d\boldsymbol{\psi}^*}, \quad \boldsymbol{\psi} \in \Psi(\boldsymbol{\theta}) \text{ for } \boldsymbol{\theta} \in \Omega_2.$$

Then

$$\pi_2(\boldsymbol{\theta}, \boldsymbol{\psi}) = \frac{q_2(\boldsymbol{\theta}, \boldsymbol{\psi})}{c_2} = \frac{q_2(\boldsymbol{\theta})}{c_2} \cdot \pi_2(\boldsymbol{\psi}|\boldsymbol{\theta}),$$

where $q_2(\boldsymbol{\theta})$ is a completely known unnormalized marginal density of $\boldsymbol{\theta}$. Thus, one can directly apply the same-dimension identities to the problem that only involves $q_1(\boldsymbol{\theta})$ and $q_2(\boldsymbol{\theta})$. Therefore, we assume that $\pi_2(\boldsymbol{\psi}|\boldsymbol{\theta})$ is known only up to a normalizing constant

$$c(\boldsymbol{\theta}) = \int_{\Psi(\boldsymbol{\theta})} q_2(\boldsymbol{\theta}, \boldsymbol{\psi})\, d\boldsymbol{\psi}.$$

This assumption will be made throughout this section. Since $c(\boldsymbol{\theta})$ depends on $\boldsymbol{\theta}$, the different-dimension problem is challenging and difficult.

5.8.3 Extensions of the Previous Monte Carlo Methods

Although we cannot directly use IS, BS, and RIS for estimating r since $\pi(\boldsymbol{\theta})$ and $\pi(\boldsymbol{\theta}, \boldsymbol{\psi})$ are defined on two different dimensional parameter spaces, this different dimensions problem can be resolved by augmenting the lower-dimensional density into one that has the same dimension as the higher one by introducing a weight function. To illustrate the idea, let

$$q_1^*(\boldsymbol{\theta}, \boldsymbol{\psi}) = q_1(\boldsymbol{\theta}) w(\boldsymbol{\psi}|\boldsymbol{\theta})$$

and

$$\pi_1^*(\boldsymbol{\theta}, \boldsymbol{\psi}) = \frac{q_1^*(\boldsymbol{\theta}, \boldsymbol{\psi})}{c_1^*}, \tag{5.8.2}$$

where $w(\boldsymbol{\psi}|\boldsymbol{\theta})$ is a completely known weight density function so that

$$\int_{\boldsymbol{\psi}(\boldsymbol{\theta})} w(\boldsymbol{\psi}|\boldsymbol{\theta})\, d\boldsymbol{\psi} = 1,$$

and c_1^* is the normalizing constant of $\pi_1^*(\boldsymbol{\theta}, \boldsymbol{\psi})$. Then it is easy to show that $c_1^* = c_1$. Thus, we can view $r = c_1/c_2$ as the ratio of the two normalizing constants of $\pi_1^*(\boldsymbol{\theta}, \boldsymbol{\psi})$ and $\pi_2(\boldsymbol{\theta}, \boldsymbol{\psi})$. Therefore, we can directly apply the IS, BS, and RIS identities given in (5.2.4), (5.3.1), and (5.5.1) on the $(\boldsymbol{\theta}, \boldsymbol{\psi})$ space for estimating r. We summarize the IS, BS, and RIS estimators of r as follows.

First, we consider IS–version 2. Assume $\Omega_1 \subset \Omega_2$. Let $\{(\boldsymbol{\theta}_{2,1}, \boldsymbol{\psi}_{2,1}), \ldots, (\boldsymbol{\theta}_{2,n}, \boldsymbol{\psi}_{2,n})\}$ be a random sample from π_2. Then, on the $(\boldsymbol{\theta}, \boldsymbol{\psi})$ space, using the IS identity

$$r = \frac{c_1}{c_2} = E_{\pi_2}\left\{\frac{q_1(\boldsymbol{\theta})w(\boldsymbol{\psi}|\boldsymbol{\theta})}{q_2(\boldsymbol{\theta}, \boldsymbol{\psi})}\right\},$$

and r can be estimated by

$$\hat{r}_{\text{IS}}(w) = \frac{1}{n}\sum_{i=1}^{n} \frac{q_1(\boldsymbol{\theta}_{2,i})w(\boldsymbol{\psi}_{2,i}|\boldsymbol{\theta}_{2,i})}{q_2(\boldsymbol{\theta}_{2,i}, \boldsymbol{\psi}_{2,i})}. \tag{5.8.3}$$

Second, we extend BS. Using the BS identity given in (5.3.1) on the $(\boldsymbol{\theta}, \boldsymbol{\psi})$ space, we have

$$r = \frac{c_1}{c_2} = \frac{E_{\pi_2}\{q_1(\boldsymbol{\theta})w(\boldsymbol{\psi}|\boldsymbol{\theta})\alpha(\boldsymbol{\theta}, \boldsymbol{\psi})\}}{E_{\pi_1^*}\{q_2(\boldsymbol{\theta}, \boldsymbol{\psi})\alpha(\boldsymbol{\theta}, \boldsymbol{\psi})\}},$$

where $\pi_1^*(\boldsymbol{\theta}, \boldsymbol{\psi})$ is defined by (5.8.2) with the support of $\boldsymbol{\theta}_1 = \{(\boldsymbol{\theta}, \boldsymbol{\psi}) : \boldsymbol{\psi} \in \Psi_1(\boldsymbol{\theta}),\ \boldsymbol{\theta} \in \Omega_1\}$ and $\alpha(\boldsymbol{\theta}, \boldsymbol{\psi})$ is an arbitrary function defined on $\Theta_1 \cap \Theta_2$ such that

$$0 < \left|\int_{\Theta_1 \cap \Theta_2} \alpha(\boldsymbol{\theta}, \boldsymbol{\psi})q_1(\boldsymbol{\theta})w(\boldsymbol{\psi}|\boldsymbol{\theta})q_2(\boldsymbol{\theta}, \boldsymbol{\psi})\, d\boldsymbol{\theta}\, d\boldsymbol{\psi}\right| < \infty.$$

Then using two random samples $\{(\boldsymbol{\theta}_{l,1}), \boldsymbol{\psi}_{l,1}), \ldots, (\boldsymbol{\theta}_{l,n_l}, \boldsymbol{\psi}_{l,n_l})\}$, $l = 1, 2$, from π_1^* and π_2, respectively, we obtain a consistent estimator of r as

$$\hat{r}_{\text{BS}}(w, \alpha) = \frac{n_2^{-1}\sum_{i=1}^{n_2} q_1(\boldsymbol{\theta}_{2,i})w(\boldsymbol{\psi}_{2,i}|\boldsymbol{\theta}_{2,i})\alpha(\boldsymbol{\theta}_{2,i}, \boldsymbol{\psi}_{2,i})}{n_1^{-1}\sum_{i=1}^{n_1} q_2(\boldsymbol{\theta}_{1,i}, \boldsymbol{\psi}_{1,i})\alpha(\boldsymbol{\theta}_{1,i}, \boldsymbol{\psi}_{1,i})}. \tag{5.8.4}$$

Finally, we generalize RIS. Using the RIS identity given in (5.5.1) on the $(\boldsymbol{\theta}, \boldsymbol{\psi})$ space, we have

$$r = \frac{c_1}{c_2} = \frac{E_{\pi}\{q_1(\boldsymbol{\theta})w(\boldsymbol{\psi}|\boldsymbol{\theta})/\pi(\boldsymbol{\theta}, \boldsymbol{\psi})\}}{E_{\pi}\{q_2(\boldsymbol{\theta}, \boldsymbol{\psi})/\pi(\boldsymbol{\theta}, \boldsymbol{\psi})\}}, \tag{5.8.5}$$

where π is an arbitrary density over $\boldsymbol{\theta}$ such that $\pi(\boldsymbol{\theta}, \boldsymbol{\psi}) > 0$ for $(\boldsymbol{\theta}, \boldsymbol{\psi}) \in \boldsymbol{\theta} = \Theta_1 \cup \Theta_2$. We mention that in (5.8.5), it is not necessary for π to be completely known, i.e., π can be known up to an unknown normalizing constant:

$$\pi(\boldsymbol{\theta}, \boldsymbol{\psi}) = \frac{q(\boldsymbol{\theta}, \boldsymbol{\psi})}{c}.$$

Given a random sample $\{(\boldsymbol{\theta}_1, \boldsymbol{\psi}_1), \ldots, (\boldsymbol{\theta}_n, \boldsymbol{\psi}_n)\}$ from π, the RIS estimator of r is

$$\hat{r}_{\text{RIS}}(w, \pi) = \frac{\sum_{i=1}^n q_1(\boldsymbol{\theta}_i) w(\boldsymbol{\psi}_i|\boldsymbol{\theta}_i)/\pi(\boldsymbol{\theta}_i, \boldsymbol{\psi}_i)}{\sum_{i=1}^n q_2(\boldsymbol{\theta}_i, \boldsymbol{\psi}_i)/\pi(\boldsymbol{\theta}_i, \boldsymbol{\psi}_i)}. \tag{5.8.6}$$

5.8.4 Global Optimal Estimators

From (5.8.3), (5.8.4), and (5.8.5), it can be observed that all three estimators, namely, $\hat{r}_{\text{IS}}(w)$, $\hat{r}_{\text{BS}}(w, \alpha)$, and $\hat{r}_{\text{RIS}}(w, \pi)$, depend on w, while $\hat{r}_{\text{BS}}(w, \alpha)$ and $\hat{r}_{\text{RIS}}(w, \pi)$ further depend on α and π, respectively. Thus, a natural question is what are the optimal choices of these parameters? To address this question, we use a conventional criterion for optimality. An estimator is optimal if it minimizes the asymptotic relative mean-square error.

We first introduce some notation. Let $\pi_{21}(\boldsymbol{\theta})$ be the marginal density of $\boldsymbol{\theta}$ defined on Ω_2. Then

$$\pi_{21}(\boldsymbol{\theta}) = \int_{\Psi(\boldsymbol{\theta})} \frac{q_2(\boldsymbol{\theta}, \boldsymbol{\psi})}{c_2} \, d\boldsymbol{\psi} \ \text{ for } \boldsymbol{\theta} \in \Psi(\boldsymbol{\theta}),$$

where Ω_2 and $\Psi(\boldsymbol{\theta})$ are defined in (5.8.1). Let $\hat{r}$ denote the estimator of r. Then the asymptotic relative mean-square error (ARE) is defined as

$$\text{ARE}^2(\hat{r}) = \lim_{n \to \infty} n \, \text{RE}^2(\hat{r}),$$

where $\text{RE}^2(\hat{r})$ is defined in (5.2.2).

For a given weight density function $w(\boldsymbol{\psi}|\boldsymbol{\theta})$ on the $(\boldsymbol{\theta}, \boldsymbol{\psi})$ space, the generalized version of the REs and AREs for $\hat{r}_{\text{IS}}(w)$, $\hat{r}_{\text{BS}}(w, \alpha)$, and $\hat{r}_{\text{RIS}}(w, \pi)$ can be directly obtained from (5.2.6), (5.3.4), and (5.5.7). The results are summarized in the following three lemmas:

Lemma 5.8.1 *Assume* $\Omega_1 \subset \Omega_2$ *and*

$$\int_{\Theta_2} \{q_1^2(\boldsymbol{\theta}) w^2(\boldsymbol{\psi}|\boldsymbol{\theta})/q_2(\boldsymbol{\theta}, \boldsymbol{\psi})\} \, d\boldsymbol{\theta} \, d\boldsymbol{\psi} < \infty.$$

Then

$$\text{RE}^2(\hat{r}_{\text{IS}}(w)) = \frac{1}{r^2} \text{Var}(\hat{r}_{\text{IS}}(w)) = \frac{1}{n} \left[\int_{\Theta_2} \frac{\pi_1^2(\boldsymbol{\theta}) w^2(\boldsymbol{\psi}|\boldsymbol{\theta})}{\pi_2(\boldsymbol{\theta}, \boldsymbol{\psi})} \, d\boldsymbol{\theta} \, d\boldsymbol{\psi} - 1 \right]$$

and

$$\text{ARE}^2(\hat{r}_{\text{IS}}(w)) = \int_{\Theta_2} \frac{\pi_1^2(\boldsymbol{\theta}) w^2(\boldsymbol{\psi}|\boldsymbol{\theta})}{\pi_2(\boldsymbol{\theta}, \boldsymbol{\psi})} \, d\boldsymbol{\theta} \, d\boldsymbol{\psi} - 1.$$

Lemma 5.8.2 *Let $n = n_1 + n_2$ and $s_{l,n} = n_l/n$ for $l = 1, 2$. Assume that $s_l = \lim_{n\to\infty} s_{l,n} > 0$ $(l = 1, 2)$, $E_{\pi_2}\{q_1(\boldsymbol{\theta})w(\boldsymbol{\psi}|\boldsymbol{\theta})\alpha(\boldsymbol{\theta},\boldsymbol{\psi})\}^2 < \infty$, and*

$$E_{\pi_1^*}\{(q_2(\boldsymbol{\theta},\boldsymbol{\psi})\alpha(\boldsymbol{\theta},\boldsymbol{\psi}))^2 + 1/(q_2(\boldsymbol{\theta},\boldsymbol{\psi})\alpha(\boldsymbol{\theta},\boldsymbol{\psi}))^2\} < \infty.$$

Then

$$\begin{aligned}
&\mathrm{RE}^2(\hat{r}_{\mathrm{BS}}(w,\alpha))\\
&= \frac{1}{ns_{1,n}s_{2,n}}\Bigg\{\left(\int_{\Theta_1\cap\Theta_2}\pi_1(\boldsymbol{\theta})w(\boldsymbol{\psi}|\boldsymbol{\theta})\pi_2(\boldsymbol{\theta},\boldsymbol{\psi})\alpha(\boldsymbol{\theta},\boldsymbol{\psi})\,d\boldsymbol{\theta}\,d\boldsymbol{\psi}\right)^{-2}\\
&\quad\times\left(\int_{\Theta_1\cap\Theta_2}\pi_1(\boldsymbol{\theta})w(\boldsymbol{\psi}|\boldsymbol{\theta})\pi_2(\boldsymbol{\theta},\boldsymbol{\psi})(s_{1,n}\pi_1(\boldsymbol{\theta})w(\boldsymbol{\psi}|\boldsymbol{\theta})\right.\\
&\quad\left.+\, s_{2,n}\pi_2(\boldsymbol{\theta},\boldsymbol{\psi}))\alpha^2(\boldsymbol{\theta},\boldsymbol{\psi})\,d\boldsymbol{\theta}\,d\boldsymbol{\psi}\right) - 1\Bigg\} + o\left(\frac{1}{n}\right)
\end{aligned}$$

and

$$\begin{aligned}
&\mathrm{ARE}^2(\hat{r}_{\mathrm{BS}}(w,\alpha))\\
&= \frac{1}{s_1 s_2}\Bigg\{\left(\int_{\Theta_1\cap\Theta_2}\pi_1(\boldsymbol{\theta})w(\boldsymbol{\psi}|\boldsymbol{\theta})\pi_2(\boldsymbol{\theta},\boldsymbol{\psi})\alpha(\boldsymbol{\theta},\boldsymbol{\psi})\,d\boldsymbol{\theta}\,d\boldsymbol{\psi}\right)^{-2}\\
&\quad\times\left(\int_{\Theta_1\cap\Theta_2}\pi_1(\boldsymbol{\theta})w(\boldsymbol{\psi}|\boldsymbol{\theta})\pi_2(\boldsymbol{\theta},\boldsymbol{\psi})(s_1\pi_1(\boldsymbol{\theta})w(\boldsymbol{\psi}|\boldsymbol{\theta})\right.\\
&\quad\left.+\, s_2\pi_2(\boldsymbol{\theta},\boldsymbol{\psi}))\alpha^2(\boldsymbol{\theta},\boldsymbol{\psi})\,d\boldsymbol{\theta}\,d\boldsymbol{\psi}\right) - 1\Bigg\}.
\end{aligned}$$

Lemma 5.8.3 *Assume that $E_\pi\{(\pi_1(\boldsymbol{\theta})w(\boldsymbol{\psi}|\boldsymbol{\theta}) - \pi_2(\boldsymbol{\theta},\boldsymbol{\psi}))/\pi(\boldsymbol{\theta},\boldsymbol{\psi})\}^2 < \infty$ and*

$$E_\pi\{p_1(\boldsymbol{\theta})w(\boldsymbol{\psi}|\boldsymbol{\theta})/p_2(\boldsymbol{\theta},\boldsymbol{\psi})\}^2 < \infty.$$

Then

$$\mathrm{RE}^2(\hat{r}_{\mathrm{RIS}}(w,\pi)) = \frac{1}{n}E_\pi\left\{\frac{(\pi_1(\boldsymbol{\theta})w(\boldsymbol{\psi}|\boldsymbol{\theta}) - \pi_2(\boldsymbol{\theta},\boldsymbol{\psi}))^2}{\pi^2(\boldsymbol{\theta},\boldsymbol{\psi})}\right\} + o\left(\frac{1}{n}\right)$$

and

$$\mathrm{ARE}^2(\hat{r}_{\mathrm{RIS}}(w,\pi)) = \int_{\Theta_1\cup\Theta_2}\frac{(\pi_1(\boldsymbol{\theta})w(\boldsymbol{\psi}|\boldsymbol{\theta}) - \pi_2(\boldsymbol{\theta},\boldsymbol{\psi}))^2}{\pi(\boldsymbol{\theta},\boldsymbol{\psi})}\,d\boldsymbol{\theta}\,d\boldsymbol{\psi}. \quad (5.8.7)$$

The proofs of these three lemmas are left as exercises. Now, we present a general result that will be needed for deriving optimal choices of $w(\boldsymbol{\psi}|\boldsymbol{\theta})$, $\alpha(\boldsymbol{\theta},\boldsymbol{\psi})$, and $\pi(\boldsymbol{\theta},\boldsymbol{\psi})$ for IS, BS, and RIS.

Theorem 5.8.1 *Assume there exist functions h and g such that:*

(I) $\mathrm{ARE}^2(\hat{r}) \geq h\{E_{\pi_2}[g(\pi_1(\boldsymbol{\theta})w(\boldsymbol{\psi}|\boldsymbol{\theta})/\pi_2(\boldsymbol{\theta},\boldsymbol{\psi}))]\}$;

(II) *either* (i) *or* (ii) *holds:*

(i) h *is an increasing function and* g *is convex; and*
(ii) h *is a decreasing function and* g *is concave.*

Then for an arbitrary $w(\boldsymbol{\psi}|\boldsymbol{\theta})$ *defined on* $\Psi(\boldsymbol{\theta})$ *or* $\Psi_1(\boldsymbol{\theta})$,

$$\mathrm{ARE}^2(\hat{r}) \geq h\{E_{\pi_{21}}[g(\pi_1(\boldsymbol{\theta})/\pi_{21}(\boldsymbol{\theta}))]\}. \tag{5.8.8}$$

That is, the lower bound of $\mathrm{ARE}^2(\hat{r})$ *is* $h\{E_{\pi_{21}}[g(\pi_1(\boldsymbol{\theta})/\pi_{21}(\boldsymbol{\theta}))]\}$. *Furthermore, if the equality holds in* (I), *the lower bound of* $\mathrm{ARE}^2(\hat{r})$ *is achieved when* $w(\boldsymbol{\psi}|\boldsymbol{\theta}) = \pi_2(\boldsymbol{\psi}|\boldsymbol{\theta})$.

The proof of (5.8.8) follows from assumptions (i) and (ii) and Jensen's inequality and is thus left as an exercise.

Using the above theorem, we can easily obtain the optimal choices of $w(\boldsymbol{\psi}|\boldsymbol{\theta})$, $\alpha(\boldsymbol{\theta},\boldsymbol{\psi})$, and $\pi(\boldsymbol{\theta},\boldsymbol{\psi})$ for IS, BS, and RIS in the sense of minimizing their AREs. These optimal choices are denoted by $w_{\mathrm{opt}}^{\mathrm{IS}}$ for IS, $w_{\mathrm{opt}}^{\mathrm{BS}}$ and α_{opt} for BS, and $w_{\mathrm{opt}}^{\mathrm{RIS}}$ and π_{opt} for RIS. IS with $w(\boldsymbol{\psi}|\boldsymbol{\theta}) = w_{\mathrm{opt}}^{\mathrm{IS}}(\boldsymbol{\psi}|\boldsymbol{\theta})$, BS with $w = w_{\mathrm{opt}}^{\mathrm{BS}}$ and $\alpha = \alpha_{\mathrm{opt}}$, and RIS with $w = w_{\mathrm{opt}}^{\mathrm{RIS}}$ and $\pi = \pi_{\mathrm{opt}}$ are called optimal importance sampling (OIS), global optimal bridge sampling (GOBS), and global optimal ratio importance sampling (GORIS), respectively. We further denote

$$\hat{r}_{\mathrm{OIS}} = \hat{r}_{\mathrm{IS}}(w_{\mathrm{opt}}^{\mathrm{IS}}),\ \hat{r}_{\mathrm{GOBS}} = \hat{r}_{\mathrm{BS}}(w_{\mathrm{opt}}^{\mathrm{BS}}, \alpha_{\mathrm{opt}}) \text{ and } \hat{r}_{\mathrm{GORIS}} = \hat{r}_{\mathrm{RIS}}(w_{\mathrm{opt}}^{\mathrm{RIS}}, \pi_{\mathrm{opt}}).$$

We are led to the following theorem:

Theorem 5.8.2 *The optimal choices are*

$$w_{\mathrm{opt}}^{\mathrm{IS}} = w_{\mathrm{opt}}^{\mathrm{BS}} = w_{\mathrm{opt}}^{\mathrm{RIS}} = \pi_2(\boldsymbol{\psi}|\boldsymbol{\theta}),\quad \boldsymbol{\psi} \in \Psi(\boldsymbol{\theta}) \ \textit{for}\ \boldsymbol{\theta} \in \Omega_1 \cap \Omega_2$$

and $w_{\mathrm{opt}}^{\mathrm{BS}}$ *and* $w_{\mathrm{opt}}^{\mathrm{RIS}}$ *are arbitrary densities for* $\boldsymbol{\theta} \in \Omega_1 - \Omega_2$,

$$\alpha_{\mathrm{opt}}(\boldsymbol{\theta},\boldsymbol{\psi}) = \frac{c}{s_1\pi_1(\boldsymbol{\theta})w_{\mathrm{opt}}^{\mathrm{BS}}(\boldsymbol{\psi}|\boldsymbol{\theta}) + s_2\pi_2(\boldsymbol{\theta},\boldsymbol{\psi})},\quad (\boldsymbol{\theta},\boldsymbol{\psi}) \in \Theta_1 \cap \Theta_2,\ \forall c \neq 0,$$

and

$$\pi_{\mathrm{opt}}(\boldsymbol{\theta},\boldsymbol{\psi}) = \frac{|\pi_1(\boldsymbol{\theta})w_{\mathrm{opt}}^{\mathrm{RIS}}(\boldsymbol{\psi}|\boldsymbol{\theta}) - \pi_2(\boldsymbol{\theta},\boldsymbol{\psi})|}{\int_{\Theta_1\cup\Theta_2} |\pi_1(\boldsymbol{\theta}')w_{\mathrm{opt}}^{\mathrm{RIS}}(\boldsymbol{\psi}'|\boldsymbol{\theta}') - \pi_2(\boldsymbol{\theta}',\boldsymbol{\psi}')|\, d\boldsymbol{\theta}'\, d\boldsymbol{\psi}'}.$$

The optimal AREs *are*

$$\mathrm{ARE}^2(\hat{r}_{\mathrm{OIS}}) = \int_{\Omega_1} \frac{\pi_1^2(\boldsymbol{\theta})}{\pi_{21}(\boldsymbol{\theta})}\, d\boldsymbol{\theta} - 1, \tag{5.8.9}$$

$$\mathrm{ARE}^2(\hat{r}_{\mathrm{GOBS}}) = \frac{1}{s_1 s_2}\left\{\left(\int_{\Omega_1\cap\Omega_2} \frac{\pi_1(\boldsymbol{\theta})\pi_{21}(\boldsymbol{\theta})}{s_1\pi_1(\boldsymbol{\theta}) + s_2\pi_{21}(\boldsymbol{\theta})}\, d\boldsymbol{\theta}\right)^{-1} - 1\right\}, \tag{5.8.10}$$

and

$$\text{ARE}^2(\hat{r}_{\text{GORIS}}) = \left[\int_{\Omega_1 \cup \Omega_2} |\pi_1(\boldsymbol{\theta}) - \pi_{21}(\boldsymbol{\theta})| \, d\boldsymbol{\theta} \right]^2 . \tag{5.8.11}$$

The proof of Theorem 5.8.2 is given in the Appendix. It is interesting to mention that the optimal choices of w are the same for all three MC methods (IS, BS, and RIS). The optimal w is the conditional density $\pi_2(\boldsymbol{\psi}|\boldsymbol{\theta})$. These results are consistent with our intuitive guess. We also note that although IS is a special case of BS with $\alpha(\boldsymbol{\theta}, \boldsymbol{\psi}) = 1/\pi_2(\boldsymbol{\theta}, \boldsymbol{\psi})$, the proof for the optimal choice of w for IS cannot simply follow from that of BS because this α is not α_{opt}. With the global optimal choices of w, α, and π, the (asymptotic) relative mean-square errors (AREs) for all three methods depend only on $\pi_1(\boldsymbol{\theta})$ and $\pi_{21}(\boldsymbol{\theta})$, which implies that the extra parameter $\boldsymbol{\psi}$ does not add any extra simulation variation, i.e., we do not lose any simulation efficiency although the second unnormalized density π_2 has d extra dimensions. However, such conclusions are valid only if the optimal solutions can be implemented in practice, since $w(\boldsymbol{\psi}|\boldsymbol{\theta})$ is not completely known. We will discuss implementation issues in the next subsection.

5.8.5 Implementation Issues

In many practical problems, a closed-form of the conditional density $\pi_2(\boldsymbol{\psi}|\boldsymbol{\theta})$ is not available especially when $\Psi(\boldsymbol{\theta})$ is a constrained parameter space (see Chapter 4 for an explanation). Therefore, evaluating ratios of normalizing constants for densities with different dimensions is a challenging problem. Here we present detailed implementation schemes for obtaining $\hat{r}_{\text{OIS}}$, $\hat{r}_{\text{GOBS}}$, and $\hat{r}_{\text{GORIS}}$. We consider our implementation procedures for $k = 1$ and $k > 1$ separately.

First, we consider $k = 1$. In this case,

$$\pi_2(\psi|\boldsymbol{\theta}) = \frac{q(\boldsymbol{\theta}, \psi)}{c(\boldsymbol{\theta})},$$

where $c(\boldsymbol{\theta}) = \int_{\Psi(\boldsymbol{\theta})} q(\boldsymbol{\theta}, \psi') \, d\psi'$. Note that the integral in $c(\boldsymbol{\theta})$ is only one dimensional. Since one-dimensional numerical integration methods are well developed and computationally fast, one can use, for example, the IMSL subroutines QDAG or QDAGI; or as Verdinelli and Wasserman (1995) suggest, one can use a grid $\{\psi_1^*, \ldots, \psi_M^*\}$ that includes all sample points ψ_1, $\ldots$, ψ_n and then use the trapezoidal rule to approximate the integral. In the following three algorithms, we assume that $c(\boldsymbol{\theta})$ will be calculated or approximated by a numerical integration method. Detailed implementation schemes for obtaining $\hat{r}_{\text{OIS}}$, $\hat{r}_{\text{GOBS}}$ and $\hat{r}_{\text{GORIS}}$ are presented as follows.

For IS, $\hat{r}_{\text{OIS}}$ is available through the following two-step algorithm:

ALGORITHM OIS

Step 1. Generate a random sample $\{(\boldsymbol{\theta}_i, \psi_i),\ i = 1, 2, \ldots, n\}$ from $\pi_2(\boldsymbol{\theta}, \psi)$.

Step 2. Calculate $c(\boldsymbol{\theta}_i)$ and compute

$$\hat{r}_{\text{OIS}} = \frac{1}{n} \sum_{i=1}^{n} \frac{q_1(\boldsymbol{\theta}_i)}{c(\boldsymbol{\theta}_i)}. \tag{5.8.12}$$

If one uses a one-dimensional numerical integration subroutine, then one needs to sample the $\boldsymbol{\theta}_i$ from the marginal distribution of $\boldsymbol{\theta}$ in Step 1. However, sampling $\boldsymbol{\theta}_i$ and ψ_i together is often easier than sampling $\boldsymbol{\theta}_i$ alone from its marginal distribution. In such a case, ψ can be considered as an auxiliary variable or a latent variable. As Besag and Green (1993) and Polson (1996) point out, use of latent variables in MC sampling will greatly ease implementation difficulty and dramatically accelerate convergence. Furthermore, if one uses the aforementioned grid numerical integration method to approximate $c(\boldsymbol{\theta})$, the ψ_i can be used as part of the grid points.

For GOBS, similar to Algorithm OIS, we have the following algorithm:

ALGORITHM GOBS

Step 1. Generate random samples $\{(\boldsymbol{\theta}_{l,i}, \psi_{l,i}),\ i = 1, 2 \ldots, n_l\}$, $l = 1, 2$, $(n_1 + n_2 = n)$ as follows:

(i) Generate $\{\boldsymbol{\theta}_{1,i},\ i = 1, 2, \ldots, n_1\}$ from $\pi_1(\boldsymbol{\theta})$ and then generate $\{\boldsymbol{\theta}_{2,i},\ l = 1, 2, \ldots, n_2\}$ from the marginal distribution of $\boldsymbol{\theta}$ with respect to $\pi_2(\boldsymbol{\theta}, \psi)$.

(ii) Generate $\psi_{l,i}$ independently from $\pi_2(\psi|\boldsymbol{\theta}_{l,i})$ for $i = 1, 2, \ldots, n_l$ and $l = 1, 2$.

Step 2. Calculate $c(\boldsymbol{\theta}_{l,i})$ and set $\hat{r}_{\text{GOBS}}$ to be the unique zero root of the "score" function

$$\begin{aligned} S(r) = &\sum_{i=1}^{n_1} \frac{s_2 r}{s_1 q_1(\boldsymbol{\theta}_{1,i})/c(\boldsymbol{\theta}_{1,i}) + s_2 r} \\ &- \sum_{i=1}^{n_2} \frac{s_1 q_1(\boldsymbol{\theta}_{2,i})/c(\boldsymbol{\theta}_{2,i})}{s_1 q_1(\boldsymbol{\theta}_{2,i})/c(\boldsymbol{\theta}_{2,i}) + s_2 r}. \end{aligned} \tag{5.8.13}$$

In Step 1, generating the $\boldsymbol{\theta}_{ij}$ or the ψ_{ij} does not require knowing the normalizing constants since we can use, for example, a rejection/acceptance, Metropolis, or Gibbs sampler method. In Step 2, $\hat{r}_{\text{GOBS}}$ can also be obtained by using an iterative method described in Section 5.3. This method can be implemented as follows. Starting with an initial guess of r, $\hat{r}^{(0)}$, at the $(t+1)^{\text{th}}$ iteration, we compute

$$\hat{r}^{(t+1)} = \left\{ \frac{1}{n_2} \sum_{i=1}^{n_2} \frac{q_1(\boldsymbol{\theta}_{2,i})/c(\boldsymbol{\theta}_{2,i})}{s_1 q_1(\boldsymbol{\theta}_{2,i})/c(\boldsymbol{\theta}_{2,i}) + s_2 \hat{r}^{(t)}} \right\} \times \left\{ \frac{1}{n_1} \sum_{i=1}^{n_1} \frac{1/c(\boldsymbol{\theta}_{1,i})}{s_1 q_1(\boldsymbol{\theta}_{1,i})/c(\boldsymbol{\theta}_{1,i}) + s_2 \hat{r}^{(t)}} \right\}^{-1}.$$

Then the limit of $\hat{r}^{(t)}$ is $\hat{r}_{\text{GOBS}}$.

For RIS, we obtain an approximate $\hat{r}_{\text{GORIS}}$, denoted by $\hat{r}^*_{\text{GORIS}}$, by a two-stage procedure developed Section 5.5.2.

Algorithm GORIS

Step 1. Let $\pi(\boldsymbol{\theta}, \psi)$ be an arbitrary (known up to a normalizing constant) density over $\boldsymbol{\theta}$ such that $\pi(\boldsymbol{\theta}, \psi) > 0$ for $(\boldsymbol{\theta}, \psi) \in \boldsymbol{\theta}$. (For example, $\pi(\boldsymbol{\theta}, \psi) = \pi_2(\boldsymbol{\theta}, \psi)$.) Generate a random sample $\{(\boldsymbol{\theta}_i, \psi_i),\ i = 1, 2, \ldots, n\}$ from π. Calculate $c(\boldsymbol{\theta}_i)$ and compute

$$\tau_{n_1} = \frac{\sum_{i=1}^{n_1} q_1(\boldsymbol{\theta}_i) q_2(\boldsymbol{\theta}_i, \psi_i)/[c(\boldsymbol{\theta}_i)\pi(\boldsymbol{\theta}_i, \psi_i)]}{\sum_{i=1}^{n_1} q_2(\boldsymbol{\theta}_i, \psi_i)/\pi(\boldsymbol{\theta}_i, \psi_i)}. \tag{5.8.14}$$

Step 2. Let

$$\pi^*_{n_1}(\boldsymbol{\theta}, \psi) = \frac{|q_1(\boldsymbol{\theta})\pi_2(\psi|\boldsymbol{\theta}) - \tau_{n_1} q_2(\boldsymbol{\theta}, \psi)|}{\int_{\boldsymbol{\theta}} |q_1(\boldsymbol{\theta}')\pi_2(\psi'|\boldsymbol{\theta}') - \tau_{n_1} q_2(\boldsymbol{\theta}', \psi')|\, d\boldsymbol{\theta}'\, d\psi'}.$$

Then, take a random sample $\{(\boldsymbol{\vartheta}_i, \varphi_i),\ i = 1, 2, \ldots, n_2\}$ from $\pi^*_{n_1}$ $(n_1 + n_2 = n)$.

Step 3. Calculate $c(\boldsymbol{\vartheta}_i)$ and compute

$$\hat{r}^*_{\text{GORIS}} = \frac{\sum_{i=1}^{n_2} q_1(\boldsymbol{\vartheta}_i)/|q_1(\boldsymbol{\vartheta}_i) - \tau_{n_1} c(\boldsymbol{\vartheta}_i)|}{\sum_{i=1}^{n_2} c(\boldsymbol{\vartheta}_i)/|q_1(\boldsymbol{\vartheta}_i) - \tau_{n_1} c(\boldsymbol{\vartheta}_i)|}. \tag{5.8.15}$$

Similar to Theorem 5.5.5, we can prove that $\hat{r}^*_{\text{GORIS}}$ has the same asymptotic relative mean-square error as $\hat{r}_{\text{GORIS}}$ as long as $n_1 \to \infty$ and $n_2 \to \infty$. The most expensive/difficult part of Algorithm GORIS is Step 2. There are two possible approaches to sample $(\boldsymbol{\vartheta}_i, \varphi_i)$ from $\pi^*_{n_1}$. The first approach is the random-direction interior-point (RDIP) sampler given in Section 2.8. The RDIP sampler requires only that $|q_1(\boldsymbol{\theta})\pi_2(\psi|\boldsymbol{\theta}) - \tau_{n_1} q_2(\boldsymbol{\theta}, \psi)|$ can be computed at any point $(\boldsymbol{\theta}, \psi)$. Another approach is Metropolis sampling. In Metropolis sampling, one needs to choose a good proposal density that should be spread out enough (Tierney 1994). For example, if $\pi_2(\boldsymbol{\theta}, \psi)$ has a tail as heavy as the one of $q_1(\boldsymbol{\theta})\pi_2(\psi|\boldsymbol{\theta})$, then one can simply choose $\pi_2(\boldsymbol{\theta}, \psi)$ as a proposal density. Compared to Algorithms OIS and GOBS, Algorithm GORIS requires an evaluation of $c(\boldsymbol{\theta})$ in the sampling step; therefore, Algorithm GORIS is more expensive.

Second, we consider $k > 1$. In this case, the integral in $c(\boldsymbol{\theta})$ is multidimensional. Therefore, simple numerical integration methods might not be feasible. Instead of directly computing $c(\boldsymbol{\theta})$ in the case of $k = 1$, we develop MC schemes to estimate $\pi_2(\boldsymbol{\psi}|\boldsymbol{\theta})$. However, the basic structures of the implementation algorithms are similar to those for $k = 1$. Thus, in the following presentation, we mainly focus on how to estimate or approximate $\pi_2(\boldsymbol{\psi}|\boldsymbol{\theta})$. We propose "exact" and "approximate" approaches.

We start with an "exact" approach. Using the notation of Schervishand Carlin (1992), we let $\boldsymbol{\psi}^* = (\psi_1^*, \ldots, \psi_k^*)$, $\boldsymbol{\psi}^{*(j)} = (\psi_1, \ldots, \psi_j, \psi_{j+1}^*, \ldots, \psi_k^*)$, and $\boldsymbol{\psi}^{*(k)} = \boldsymbol{\psi}$. We denote a "one-step Gibbs transition" density as

$$\pi_2^{(j)}(\boldsymbol{\psi}|\boldsymbol{\theta}) = \pi_2(\psi_j|\psi_1, \ldots, \psi_{j-1}, \psi_{j+1}, \ldots, \psi_k, \boldsymbol{\theta})$$

and a "transition kernel" as

$$T(\boldsymbol{\psi}^*, \boldsymbol{\psi}|\boldsymbol{\theta}) = \prod_{j=1}^{k} \pi_2^{(j)}(\boldsymbol{\psi}^{*(j)}|\boldsymbol{\theta}).$$

Then we have the following key identity:

$$\pi_2(\boldsymbol{\psi}|\boldsymbol{\theta}) = \int_{\Psi(\boldsymbol{\theta})} T(\boldsymbol{\psi}', \boldsymbol{\psi}|\boldsymbol{\theta})\pi_2(\boldsymbol{\psi}'|\boldsymbol{\theta})\, d\boldsymbol{\psi}'.$$

Now we can obtain an MC estimator of $\pi_2(\boldsymbol{\psi}|\boldsymbol{\theta})$ by

$$\hat{\pi}_2(\boldsymbol{\psi}|\boldsymbol{\theta}) = \frac{1}{m}\sum_{l=1}^{m} T(\boldsymbol{\psi}_l, \boldsymbol{\psi}|\boldsymbol{\theta}), \tag{5.8.16}$$

where $\{\boldsymbol{\psi}_l,\ l = 1, 2, \ldots, m\}$ is a random sample from $\pi_2(\boldsymbol{\psi}|\boldsymbol{\theta})$. The above method is originally introduced by Ritter and Tanner (1992) for the Gibbs stopper. Here, we use this method for estimating conditional densities. Although the joint conditional density is not analytically available, one-dimensional conditional densities can be computed by the aforementioned numerical integration method, and sometimes some of the one-dimensional conditional densities are even analytically available or easy to compute. Therefore, (5.8.16) is advantageous. In (5.8.16), sampling from $\pi_2(\boldsymbol{\psi}|\boldsymbol{\theta})$ does not require knowing the normalizing constant $c(\boldsymbol{\theta})$ and convergence of $\hat{\pi}_2(\boldsymbol{\psi}|\boldsymbol{\theta})$ to $\pi_2(\boldsymbol{\psi}|\boldsymbol{\theta})$ is expected to be rapid. Algorithms OIS, GOBS, and GORIS for $k > 1$ are similar to the ones for $k = 1$. We only need the following minor adjustment. Generate $\boldsymbol{\psi}_l$, $l = 1, 2, \ldots, m$, from $\pi_2(\boldsymbol{\psi}|\boldsymbol{\theta}_i)$, $\pi_2(\boldsymbol{\psi}|\boldsymbol{\theta}_{ij})$, or $\pi_2(\boldsymbol{\psi}|\boldsymbol{\vartheta}_i)$ and compute $\hat{\pi}_2(\boldsymbol{\psi}_i|\boldsymbol{\theta}_i)$, $\hat{\pi}_2(\boldsymbol{\psi}_{ij}|\boldsymbol{\theta}_{ij})$, or $\hat{\pi}_2(\boldsymbol{\varphi}_i \mid \boldsymbol{\vartheta}_i)$ by using (5.8.16). Then, for OIS and GOBS, instead of (5.8.12) and (5.8.13), we use

$$\hat{r}_{\text{OIS}} = \frac{1}{n}\sum_{i=1}^{n} \frac{q_1(\boldsymbol{\theta}_i)\hat{\pi}_2(\boldsymbol{\psi}_i|\boldsymbol{\theta}_i)}{q_2(\boldsymbol{\theta}_i, \boldsymbol{\psi}_i)} \tag{5.8.17}$$

and

$$S(r) = \sum_{i=1}^{n_1} \frac{s_2 r q_2(\boldsymbol{\theta}_{1,i}, \boldsymbol{\psi}_{1,i})}{s_1 q_1(\boldsymbol{\theta}_{1,i}) \hat{\pi}_2(\boldsymbol{\psi}_{1,i}|\boldsymbol{\theta}_{1,i}) + s_2 r q_2(\boldsymbol{\theta}_{1,i}, \boldsymbol{\psi}_{1,i})} - \sum_{i=1}^{n_2} \frac{s_1 q_1(\boldsymbol{\theta}_{2,i}) \hat{\pi}_2(\boldsymbol{\psi}_{2,i}|\boldsymbol{\theta}_{2,i})}{s_1 q_1(\boldsymbol{\theta}_{2,i}) \hat{\pi}_2(\boldsymbol{\psi}_{2,i}|\boldsymbol{\theta}_{2,i}) + s_2 r q_2(\boldsymbol{\theta}_{2,i}, \boldsymbol{\psi}_{2,i})}. \tag{5.8.18}$$

For GORIS, instead of (5.8.14) and (5.8.15), we use

$$\tau_{n_1} = \frac{\sum_{i=1}^{n_1} q_1(\boldsymbol{\theta}_i) \hat{\pi}_2(\boldsymbol{\psi}_i|\boldsymbol{\theta}_i)/\pi(\boldsymbol{\theta}_i, \boldsymbol{\psi}_i)}{\sum_{i=1}^{n_1} q_2(\boldsymbol{\theta}_i, \boldsymbol{\psi}_i)/\pi(\boldsymbol{\theta}_i, \boldsymbol{\psi}_i)} \tag{5.8.19}$$

and

$$\hat{r}^*_{\text{GORIS}} = \frac{\sum_{i=1}^{n_2} q_1(\boldsymbol{\vartheta}_i) \hat{\pi}_2(\boldsymbol{\varphi}_i|\boldsymbol{\vartheta}_i)/|q_1(\boldsymbol{\vartheta}_i) \hat{\pi}_2(\boldsymbol{\varphi}_i|\boldsymbol{\vartheta}_i) - \tau_{n_1} q_2(\boldsymbol{\vartheta}_i, \boldsymbol{\varphi}_i)|}{\sum_{i=1}^{n_2} q_2(\boldsymbol{\vartheta}_i, \boldsymbol{\varphi}_i)/|q_1(\boldsymbol{\vartheta}_i) \hat{\pi}_2(\varphi_i|\boldsymbol{\vartheta}_i) - \tau_{n_1} q_2(\boldsymbol{\vartheta}_i, \boldsymbol{\varphi}_i)|}. \tag{5.8.20}$$

Although the above method involves extensive computation, it is quite simple especially for OIS and GOBS. More importantly, it achieves the optimal (relative) mean-square errors asymptotically as $m \to \infty$.

Finally, we briefly introduce an "approximate" approach that requires less computational effort. Mainly, one needs to find a completely known density $w^*(\boldsymbol{\psi}|\boldsymbol{\theta})$ that has a shape similar to $\pi_2(\boldsymbol{\psi}|\boldsymbol{\theta})$. The details of how to find a good $w^*(\boldsymbol{\psi}|\boldsymbol{\theta})$ are given in Section 4.3. When a good $w^*(\boldsymbol{\psi}|\boldsymbol{\theta})$ is chosen, we simply replace $\hat{\pi}_2$ by $w^*(\boldsymbol{\psi}|\boldsymbol{\theta})$ in (5.8.17), (5.8.18), (5.8.19), and (5.8.20) and then Algorithms OIS, GOBS, and GORIS give approximate $\hat{r}_{\text{OIS}}$, $\hat{r}_{\text{GOBS}}$, and $\hat{r}_{\text{GORIS}}$.

Chen and Shao (1997b) use two examples to illustrate the methodology as well as the implementation algorithms developed in this section. In their examples, they implement the asymptotically optimal versions of Algorithms OIS, GOBS, and GORIS, which are relatively computationally intensive. However, for higher-dimensional or more complex problems, "approximate" optimal approaches proposed in this section may be more attractive since they require much less computational effort. We note that the two-stage GORIS algorithm typically performs better when a small sample size n_1 in Step 1 is chosen. A rule of thumb of choosing n_1 and n_2 is that $n_1/n_2 \approx \frac{1}{4}$.

Next, we present an example for testing departures from normality to empirically examine the performance of the OIS, GOBS, and GORIS algorithms.

Example 5.1. Testing departures from normality. As an illustration of our implementation algorithms developed in Section 5.8.5 for $k = 1$, we consider an example given in Section 3.2 of Verdinelli and Wasserman (1995). Suppose that we have observations $y_1, \ldots, y_N$ and we want to test whether the sampling distribution is normal or heavier tailed. We use the Student t distribution with ν degrees of freedom for the data. Using the notation similar to that of Verdinelli and Wasserman (1995), we define $\psi = 1/\nu$ so that $\psi = 0$ corresponds to the null hypothesis of normality and larger values of ψ correspond to heavier-tailed distributions, with $\psi = 1$ corresponding to a Cauchy distribution ($0 \le \psi \le 1$). Let $\boldsymbol{\theta} = (\mu, \sigma)$, where μ and σ are location and scale parameters and denote $\bar{y}$ and s^2 to be the sample mean and the sample variance of $y_1, \dots, y_N$. Then using exactly the same choices of priors as in Verdinelli and Wasserman (1995), i.e., $\pi_0(\boldsymbol{\theta}) \propto 1/\sigma$, and independently $\pi_0(\psi) \propto 1$, we have the posteriors denoted by $\pi_1(\boldsymbol{\theta})$ under the null hypothesis and $\pi_2(\boldsymbol{\theta}, \psi)$ under the alternative hypothesis:

$$\pi_1(\boldsymbol{\theta}) = \frac{p_1(\boldsymbol{\theta})}{c_1} \quad \text{and} \quad \pi_2(\boldsymbol{\theta}, \psi) = \frac{p_2(\boldsymbol{\theta}, \psi)}{c_2},$$

where

$$\begin{aligned} p_1(\boldsymbol{\theta}) &= \left[\prod_{i=1}^{N} \frac{1}{\sqrt{2\pi}\sigma} \exp\left(-\frac{(y_i - \mu)^2}{2\sigma^2} \right) \right] \cdot \frac{1}{\sigma} \\ &= \frac{1}{(\sqrt{2\pi})^N \sigma^{N+1}} \exp\left(-\frac{(N-1)s^2 + N(\mu - \bar{y})^2}{2\sigma^2} \right) \end{aligned}$$

and

$$\begin{aligned} p_2(\boldsymbol{\theta}, \psi) &= \left[\prod_{i=1}^{N} \frac{\Gamma\left(\frac{1+\psi}{2\psi}\right)\sqrt{\psi}}{\sqrt{\pi}\sigma\Gamma\left(\frac{1}{2\psi}\right)} \frac{1}{\left(1 + \frac{\psi(y_i - \mu)^2}{\sigma^2}\right)^{(1+\psi)/2\psi}} \right] \cdot \frac{1}{\sigma} \\ &= \frac{\psi^{N/2}}{(\sqrt{\pi})^N \sigma^{N+1}} \left[\frac{\Gamma\left(\frac{1+\psi}{2\psi}\right)}{\Gamma\left(\frac{1}{2\psi}\right)} \right]^N \prod_{i=1}^{N} \left(1 + \frac{\psi(y_i - \mu)^2}{\sigma^2}\right)^{-(1+\psi)/2\psi}. \end{aligned}$$

Thus, the Bayes factor is $r = c_1/c_2$. It is easy to see that $\boldsymbol{\theta}$ is two dimensional ($p = 2$) and ψ is one dimensional ($k = 1$).

Now we apply Algorithms OIS, GOBS, and GORIS given in Section 5.8.5 to obtain estimates $\hat{r}_{\text{OIS}}$, $\hat{r}_{\text{GOBS}}$, and $\hat{r}_{\text{GORIS}}$ for the Bayes factor r when $k = 1$. To implement these three algorithms, we need to sample from π_1 and π_2. Sampling from π_1 is straightforward. To sample from π_2, instead of using an independence chain sampling scheme in Verdinelli and Wasserman (1995), we use the Gibbs sampler by introducing auxiliary variables (latent variables). Note that a Student t distribution is a scale mixture of normal distributions (e.g., see Albert and Chib 1993). Let $\boldsymbol{\lambda} = (\lambda_1, \dots, \lambda_N)$ and let the joint distribution of $(\boldsymbol{\theta}, \psi, \boldsymbol{\lambda})$ be

$$\pi_2^*(\boldsymbol{\theta}, \psi, \boldsymbol{\lambda}) \propto \left[\prod_{i=1}^{N} \left(\frac{\sqrt{\lambda_i}}{\sqrt{2\pi}\sigma} \exp\left(-\frac{\lambda_i (y_i - \mu)^2}{2\sigma^2} \right) \right) \right.$$
$$\left. \times \left(\frac{1}{\Gamma\left(\frac{1}{2\psi}\right)} \left(\frac{1}{2\psi}\right)^{1/2\psi} \lambda_i^{(1/2\psi)-1} \exp\left(-\frac{1}{2\psi} \lambda_i \right) \right) \right] \frac{1}{\sigma}.$$

Then the marginal distribution of $(\boldsymbol{\theta}, \psi)$ is $\pi_2(\boldsymbol{\theta}, \psi)$. We run the Gibbs sampler by taking

$$\lambda_i \sim \mathcal{G}\left(\frac{1+\psi}{\psi}, \frac{1}{2\psi} + \frac{(y_i - \mu)^2}{2\sigma^2} \right) \quad \text{for } i = 1, 2, \ldots, N,$$

$$\mu \sim N\left(\frac{\sum_{j=1}^N \lambda_j y_j}{\sum_{j=1}^N \lambda_j}, \frac{\sigma^2}{\sum_{j=1}^N \lambda_j} \right),$$

$$\frac{1}{\sigma^2} \sim \mathcal{G}\left(\frac{N}{2}, \frac{\sum_{j=1}^N \lambda_j (y_i - \mu)^2}{2} \right),$$

and

$$\frac{1}{2\psi} \sim \pi\left(\frac{1}{2\psi}\right) \propto \frac{1}{\left(\frac{1}{2\psi}\right)^2} \left[\frac{\left(\frac{1}{2\psi}\right)^{1/2\psi}}{\Gamma\left(\frac{1}{2\psi}\right)} \right]^N \left(\prod_{j=1}^N \lambda_j \right)^{1/2\psi}$$
$$\times \exp\left(-\left(\frac{1}{2\psi}\right) \sum_{j=1}^N \lambda_j \right),$$

where $\mathcal{G}(a, b)$ denotes a gamma distribution. Sampling λ_i, μ, and $1/\sigma^2$ from their corresponding conditional distributions is trivial and we use the adaptive rejection sampling algorithm of Gilks and Wild (1992) to generate $1/2\psi$ from $\pi(1/2\psi)$, since $\pi(1/2\psi)$ is log-concave when $N \geq 4$. Therefore, the Gibbs sampler can be exactly implemented. We believe that this Gibbs sampling scheme is superior to an independence chain Metropolis sampling scheme.

We implement the OIS, GOBS, and GORIS algorithms in double precision Fortran-77 using IMSL subroutines. We follow exactly the steps as the Algorithms OIS, GOBS, and GORIS presented in Section 5.8.5. We obtain a "random" sample $(\boldsymbol{\theta}_1, \psi_1)$, ..., $(\boldsymbol{\theta}_n, \psi_n)$ from π_2 by using the aforementioned Gibbs sampling scheme. First, we use several diagnostic methods to check convergence of the Gibbs sampler recommended by Cowles and Carlin (1996). Second, we take every Bth "stationary" Gibbs iterate so that the autocorrelations for the two components of $\boldsymbol{\theta}_i$ disappear. The autocorrelations are calculated by the IMSL subroutine DACF. We use another

IMSL subroutine DQDAG to calculate $c(\boldsymbol{\theta}_i)$. A random sample $\boldsymbol{\theta}_{11}, \ldots, \boldsymbol{\theta}_{1n_1}$ from π_1 can be obtained by using an exact sampling scheme. For Algorithm GORIS, we choose $\pi_2(\boldsymbol{\theta}, \psi)$ as π in Step 1 and take a "random" sample $\{(\boldsymbol{\theta}_i, \psi_i), i = 1, \ldots, n_1\}$ from π_2 to calculate τ_{n_1} given by (5.8.14). In Step 2, we adopt Metropolis sampling with $\pi_2(\boldsymbol{\theta}, \psi)$ as a proposal density. Let $(\boldsymbol{\theta}_j, \psi_j)$ denote the current values of the parameters. We take candidate values $(\boldsymbol{\theta}_c, \psi_c)$ from every Bth "stationary" Gibbs iterate with the target distribution $\pi_2(\boldsymbol{\theta}, \psi)$. We compute

$$a = \min\left\{\frac{\omega(\boldsymbol{\theta}_c)}{\omega(\boldsymbol{\theta}_j)}, 1\right\},$$

where $\omega(\boldsymbol{\theta}) = |p_1(\boldsymbol{\theta})/c(\boldsymbol{\theta}) - \tau_{n_1}|$. We set $(\boldsymbol{\theta}_{j+1}, \psi_{j+1})$ equal to (θ_c, ψ_c) with acceptance probability a and to $(\boldsymbol{\theta}_j, \psi_j)$ with probability $1-a$. We then take every (B')th Metropolis iteration to obtain a "random" sample $(\boldsymbol{\vartheta}_1, \varphi_1)$, $\ldots$, $(\boldsymbol{\vartheta}_{n_2}, \varphi_{n_2})$. The above sampling schemes may not be the most efficient ones, but they do provide roughly independent samples and they are also straightforward to implement.

In order to obtain informative empirical evidence of the performance of OIS, GOBS, and GORIS, we conduct a small-scale simulation study. We take a dataset of $N = 100$ random numbers from $N(0, 1)$. Using this dataset, first we implement GOBS with $n_1 = n_2 = 50000$ to obtain an approximate "true" value of the Bayes factor r, which gives $r = 6.958$. In our implementation, we took $B = 30$ for Gibbs sampling and $B' = 10$ for Metropolis sampling to ensure an approximately "independent" MC sample obtained. (Note that the Gibbs sampler converges earlier than 500 iterations.) Second, we use $n = 1000$ for Algorithm OIS, $n_1 = n_2 = 500$ for Algorithm GOBS, and $n_1 = 200$ and $n_2 = 800$ for Algorithm GORIS. As discussed in Section 5.7, we compute the simulation standard errors based on the estimated first-order approximation of $\mathrm{RE}(\hat{r})$ using the available random samples. (No extra random samples are required for this stage of the computation.) For example, the standard error for $\hat{r}_{\text{GOBS}}$ is given by

$$\begin{aligned} &\mathrm{se}(\hat{r}_{\text{GOBS}}) \\ &= \hat{r}_{\text{GOBS}} \left(\frac{1}{ns_1 s_2} \left[\left(\frac{1}{n_2} \sum_{i=1}^{n_2} \frac{p_1(\theta_{2i})}{s_1 p_1(\theta_{2i}) + s_2 \hat{r}_{\text{GOBS}} c(\theta_{2i})} \right)^{-1} - 1 \right] \right)^{-1/2}, \end{aligned}$$

where $n = n_1 + n_2 = 1000$. Third, using the above implementation scheme with the same simulated dataset, we independently replicate the three estimation procedures 500 times. Then, we calculate the averages of $\hat{r}_{\text{OIS}}$, $\hat{r}_{\text{GOBS}}$, and $\hat{r}_{\text{GORIS}}$, simulation standard errors (simulation se), estimated biases $(E(\hat{r}) - r)$, mean-square errors (mse), averages of the approximate standard errors (approx. se), and the average CPU time. (Note that our computation was performed on the DEC-station 5000-260.) The results are summarized in Table 5.3.

TABLE 5.3. Results of Simulation Study.

	Method		
	OIS	GOBS	GORIS
Average of $\hat{r}$'s	6.995	6.971	6.933
Bias	0.037	0.013	−0.025
Mse	0.066	0.063	0.054
Simulation se	0.254	0.250	0.231
Approx. se	0.187	0.193	0.184
Average CPU (in minutes)	1.52	1.22	2.10

From Table 5.3, we see that:

(i) all three averages are close to the "true" value and the biases are relatively small;

(ii) GORIS produces a slightly smaller simulation standard error than the other two;

(iii) all three approximate standard errors are slightly understated, which is intuitively appealing since we use the estimated first-order approximation of RE($\hat{r}$); and

(iv) GOBS uses the least CPU time since sampling from $\pi_2(\boldsymbol{\theta}, \psi)$ is much more expensive than sampling from $\pi_1(\boldsymbol{\theta})$, and GORIS uses the most CPU time since sampling from $\pi^*_{n_1}(\boldsymbol{\theta}, \psi)$ in Step 2 of Algorithm GORIS is relatively more expensive.

Finally, we mention that based on the above-estimated value of r, the normal data results in a posterior marginal that is concentrated near $\psi = 0$, leading to a Bayes factor strongly favoring the null hypothesis of normality.

5.9 Estimation of Normalizing Constants After Transformation

When the "distance" between the two densities π_1 and π_2 gets large, the MC methods such as IS, BS, PS, and RIS will become less efficient. See Section 5.6 for illustrative examples. To remedy this problem, we can use a random variable transformation technique, which can help shorten the distance between the two densities π_1 and π_2, before applying the aforementioned MC methods.

Voter (1985) suggests applying a location shift before using the method of Bennett (1976) (see Section 5.3) to calculate free-energy differences between systems that are highly separated in configuration space. Meng and Schilling (1996a) extend Voter's idea by considering a general transformation before applying bridge sampling. To illustrate this idea, consider the following one-to-one transformation:

$$u = T_l(\boldsymbol{\theta}).$$

After the transformation, $\pi_l(\boldsymbol{\theta})$ can be rewritten as

$$\pi_l^*(u) \equiv \pi_l(T_l^{-1}(u))J_l(u) = \frac{q_l^*(u)}{c_l},$$

where $q_l^*(u) = q_l(T_l^{-1}(u))J_l(u)$ and $J_l(u)$ denotes the Jacobian, that is,

$$J_l(u) = \left|\frac{\partial T_l^{-1}(u)}{\partial u}\right|$$

for $l = 1, 2$. Now it is easy to see that c_i serves as the common normalizing constant for both π_l and π_l^*. Instead of directly working with the π_l, we can apply IS, BS, PS, and RIS to the π_l^*. Thus, the theory developed in Sections 5.2–5.4 remains the same. However, the transformation can greatly improve the simulation precision of an MC estimator of r. To see this, we revisit the two illustrative examples given in Section 5.6. For the case involving two densities from $N(0,1)$ and $N(\delta, 1)$, we let $u = T_1(\boldsymbol{\theta}) = \boldsymbol{\theta}$ for $N(0,1)$ and $u = T_2(\boldsymbol{\theta}) = \boldsymbol{\theta} - \delta$ for $N(\delta, 1)$. After the transformation, the two densities π_i^* are the same and both are $N(0,1)$. Thus all MC methods discussed in Section 5.6 give a precise estimate of r, yielding a zero simulation error. This is also true for the second case where we consider $N(0,1)$ and $N(0,\Delta^2)$ and we take $T_1(\boldsymbol{\theta}) = \boldsymbol{\theta}$ and $T_2(\boldsymbol{\theta}) = (\Delta^{-1})\boldsymbol{\theta}$. In these two illustrative examples, we indeed use two useful transformations, that is, recentering and rescaling. In general, the standardization, which is the combination of recentering and rescaling, may be a natural choice for T_l. More specifically, for $l = 1, 2$, we let

$$T_l(\boldsymbol{\theta}) = \Sigma_l^{-1/2}(\boldsymbol{\theta} - \mu_l),$$

where μ_l and Σ_l are the mean and covariance matrix for $\boldsymbol{\theta} \sim \pi_l$. If the analytical evaluation of μ_l and Σ_l does not appear possible, the MC approximation of μ_l and Σ_l can be easily obtained using the techniques described in Section 3.2.

Meng and Schilling (1996b) use a full information item factor model to empirically demonstrate the gain in simulation precision of BS after transformation. We conclude this section with a recommendation from Meng and Schilling (1996b), that one should apply transformations whenever feasible and appropriate.

5.10 Other Methods

In addition to IS, BS, PS, and RIS, several other MC methods have been developed recently. In this section, we briefly summarize some of these.

5.10.1 *Marginal Likelihood Approach*

In the context of Bayesian inference, the posterior is typically of the form

$$\pi(\boldsymbol{\theta}|D) = L(\boldsymbol{\theta}|D)\pi(\boldsymbol{\theta})/m(D),$$

where $L(\boldsymbol{\theta}|D)$ is the likelihood function, D is the data, $\boldsymbol{\theta}$ is the parameter vector, $\pi(\boldsymbol{\theta})$ is the prior, and $m(D)$ is the marginal density (marginal likelihood). Clearly, $m(D)$ is the normalizing constant of the posterior distribution $\pi(\boldsymbol{\theta}|D)$. Calculating the marginal likelihood, $m(D)$, plays an important role in the computation of Bayes factors.

Consider the following identity:

$$m(D) = \frac{L(\boldsymbol{\theta}|D)\pi(\boldsymbol{\theta})}{\pi(\boldsymbol{\theta}|D)}. \tag{5.10.1}$$

Let $\boldsymbol{\theta}^*$ be the posterior mean or the posterior mode and let $\hat{\pi}(\boldsymbol{\theta}^*|D)$ be an estimator of the joint posterior density evaluated at $\boldsymbol{\theta}^*$. Chib (1995) obtains the following estimator for $m(D)$:

$$\hat{m}(D) = \frac{L(\boldsymbol{\theta}^*|D)\pi(\boldsymbol{\theta}^*)}{\hat{\pi}(\boldsymbol{\theta}^*|D)}.$$

He also develops a data augmentation technique of Tanner and Wong (1987) to estimate $\hat{\pi}(\boldsymbol{\theta}^*|D)$ by introducing latent variables. Chib's method is particularly useful for multivariate problems when the full conditional densities are completely known. The technical details and applications of this method are presented in Chapter 8. Another approach to estimating $\hat{\pi}(\boldsymbol{\theta}^*|D)$ is the importance-weighted marginal density estimation (IWMDE) method of Chen (1994), which has been extensively discussed in Chapter 4. Furthermore, the IWMDE method can be used to estimate $m(D)$ directly. Let $\boldsymbol{\theta}_i$, $i = 1, 2, \ldots, n$, be a random sample from $\pi(\boldsymbol{\theta}|D)$. Then, IWMDE yields a consistent estimator for $m(D)$:

$$\hat{m}_{\text{IWMDE}}(D) = \left[\frac{1}{n}\sum_{i=1}^{n}\frac{w(\boldsymbol{\theta}_i)}{L(\boldsymbol{\theta}_i|D)\pi(\boldsymbol{\theta}_i)}\right]^{-1},$$

where $w(\boldsymbol{\theta})$ is a weighted density function (completely known) with support $\Omega_w \subset \Omega_{\pi(\cdot|D)}$ (the support of the posterior distribution $\pi(\cdot|D)$).

DiCiccio, Kass, Raftery, and Wasserman (1997) obtain the Laplace approximation to the normalizing constant $m(D)$ by approximating the posterior with a normal distribution, which is easy to sample from. Let $\boldsymbol{\theta}^*$ be the posterior mode and let Σ^* be minus the inverse of the Hessian of the log-posterior evaluated at $\boldsymbol{\theta}^*$. Then the Laplace approximation to $m(D)$ is given by

$$\hat{m}_L(D) = \frac{L(\boldsymbol{\theta}^*|D)\pi(\boldsymbol{\theta}^*)}{\phi(\boldsymbol{\theta}^*;\boldsymbol{\theta}^*,\Sigma^*)} = (2\pi)^{p/2}|\Sigma^*|^{1/2}L(\boldsymbol{\theta}^*|D)\pi(\boldsymbol{\theta}^*),$$

where p is the dimension of $\boldsymbol{\theta}$ and $\phi(\cdot|\boldsymbol{\theta}^*, \Sigma^*)$ denotes a normal density with mean vector $\boldsymbol{\theta}^*$ and covariance matrix Σ^*. This approximation has error of order $O(1/n)$; that is, $m(D) = \hat{m}_L(D)(1 + O(1/n))$. By (5.10.1), we have

$$m(D) = \frac{L(\boldsymbol{\theta}^*|D)\pi(\boldsymbol{\theta}^*)}{\phi(\boldsymbol{\theta}^*|\boldsymbol{\theta}^*, \Sigma^*)} \frac{\phi(\boldsymbol{\theta}^*|\boldsymbol{\theta}^*, \Sigma^*)}{\pi(\boldsymbol{\theta}^*|D)} \approx \frac{L(\boldsymbol{\theta}^*|D)\pi(\boldsymbol{\theta}^*)}{\phi(\boldsymbol{\theta}^*|\boldsymbol{\theta}^*, \Sigma^*)} \frac{\alpha}{P(B)},$$

where $\alpha = \Phi(B) = \int_B \phi(\boldsymbol{\theta}|\boldsymbol{\theta}^*, \Sigma^*)\, d\boldsymbol{\theta}$, $P(B) = \int_B (\pi(\boldsymbol{\theta}|D)\, d\boldsymbol{\theta}$, and $B = \{\boldsymbol{\theta} : \ ||(\boldsymbol{\theta} - \boldsymbol{\theta}^*)'(\Sigma^*)^{-1}(\boldsymbol{\theta} - \boldsymbol{\theta}^*)|| \le \delta\}$. DiCiccio, Kass, Raftery, and Wasserman (1997) suggest the following volume-corrected Laplace approximation estimator for $m(D)$:

$$\hat{m}_L^*(D) = \frac{L(\boldsymbol{\theta}^*|D)\pi(\boldsymbol{\theta}^*)}{\phi(\boldsymbol{\theta}^*|\boldsymbol{\theta}^*, \Sigma^*)} \frac{\alpha}{P(B)}.$$

To improve first-order approximations, they also suggest the Bartlett-adjusted Laplace estimator for $m(D)$, which is given by

$$\hat{m}_B^*(D) = \hat{m}_L(D) \cdot \left\{ \frac{E(W(\boldsymbol{\theta})|D)}{d} \right\}^{d/2},$$

where $W(\boldsymbol{\theta}) = 2\ln[L(\boldsymbol{\theta}^*|D)\pi(\boldsymbol{\theta}^*)/(L(\boldsymbol{\theta}|D)\pi(\boldsymbol{\theta}))]$ and the expectation is taken with respect to $\pi(\boldsymbol{\theta}|D)$. They further show that this adjusted estimator has error of order $O(n^{-2})$. To completely determine $\hat{m}_L^*(D)$ and $\hat{m}_B^*(D)$, we must compute α, $P(B)$, and $E(W(\boldsymbol{\theta})|D)$. As long as a sample from the posterior distribution $\pi(\boldsymbol{\theta}|D)$ is available, $P(B)$ and $E(W(\boldsymbol{\theta})|D)$ are easy to calculate; see Section 3.2 for details. To compute α, one can use a numerical integration approach or an MC method since the normal distribution is easy to generate.

5.10.2 Reverse Logistic Regression

In this subsection, we discuss how reverse logistic regression (Geyer 1994) can be adapted for estimating ratios of normalizing constants.

Let $\{\boldsymbol{\theta}_{l,i}, i = 1, \ldots, n_l\}$, $l = 1, 2$, be independent random samples from π_i, $l = 1, 2$, respectively. Also let $n = n_1 + n_2$, $s_{l,n} = n_l/n$, and $s_l = \lim_{n\to\infty} s_{l,n}$ for $l = 1, 2$. Consider a mixture distribution with density

$$\pi_{\text{mix}}(\boldsymbol{\theta}) = s_1 \frac{q_1(\boldsymbol{\theta})}{c_1} + s_2 \frac{q_2(\boldsymbol{\theta})}{c_2}.$$

Define

$$q_1^*(\boldsymbol{\theta}, r) = \frac{s_1 q_1(\boldsymbol{\theta})/c_1}{s_1 q_1(\boldsymbol{\theta})/c_1 + s_2 q_2(\boldsymbol{\theta})/c_2} = \frac{s_1 q_1(\boldsymbol{\theta})}{s_1 q_1(\boldsymbol{\theta}) + r \cdot s_2 q_2(\boldsymbol{\theta})},$$

$$q_2^*(\boldsymbol{\theta}, r) = \frac{s_2 q_2(\boldsymbol{\theta})/c_2}{s_1 q_1(\boldsymbol{\theta})/c_1 + s_2 q_2(\boldsymbol{\theta})/c_2} = \frac{r s_2 q_2(\boldsymbol{\theta})}{s_1 q_1(\boldsymbol{\theta}) + r \cdot s_2 q_2(\boldsymbol{\theta})},$$

and also define the log quasi-likelihood as

$$l_n(r) = \sum_{l=1}^{2} \sum_{i=1}^{n_l} \ln q_l^*(\boldsymbol{\theta}_{l,i}, r). \tag{5.10.2}$$

Then the reverse logistic regression (RLR) estimator, $\hat{r}_{\text{RLR}}$, of r is obtained by maximizing the log quasi-likelihood $l_n(r)$ in (5.10.2). Clearly, $\hat{r}_{\text{RLR}}$ satisfies the following equation:

$$\sum_{i=1}^{n_2} \frac{s_1 q_1(\boldsymbol{\theta}_{2,i})}{\hat{r}_{\text{RLR}}(s_1 q_1(\boldsymbol{\theta}_{2,i}) + \hat{r}_{\text{RLR}} \cdot s_2 q_2(\boldsymbol{\theta}_{2,i}))} - \sum_{i=1}^{n_1} \frac{s_2 q_2(\boldsymbol{\theta}_{1,i})}{s_1 q_1(\boldsymbol{\theta}_{1,i}) + \hat{r}_{\text{RLR}} \cdot s_2 q_2(\boldsymbol{\theta}_{1,i})} = 0. \tag{5.10.3}$$

Therefore, when π_1 and π_2 overlap, i.e.,

$$\int_{\Omega} \pi_1(\boldsymbol{\theta}) \pi_2(\boldsymbol{\theta}) \, d\boldsymbol{\theta} > 0,$$

and under some regularity conditions, we have

$$\hat{r}_{\text{RLR}} \xrightarrow{\text{a.s.}} r \text{ as } n \to \infty.$$

The asymptotic value of $E\left((\hat{r}_{\text{RLR}} - r)^2 / r^2\right)$ is

$$\frac{1}{n s_1 s_2} \left[\left\{ \int_{\Omega} \frac{\pi_1(\boldsymbol{\theta}) \pi_2(\boldsymbol{\theta})}{s_1 \pi_1(\boldsymbol{\theta}) + s_2 \pi_2(\boldsymbol{\theta})} \, d\boldsymbol{\theta} \right\}^{-1} - 1 \right]. \tag{5.10.4}$$

From (5.10.3) and (5.10.4), we can see that the reverse logistic regression estimator, $\hat{r}_{\text{RLR}}$, is exactly the same as the optimal BS estimator, $\hat{r}_{\text{BS,opt}}$, given by (5.3.3) and (5.3.5) because (5.10.3) is identical to $S(r) = 0$, where $S(r)$ is given in (5.3.8). When π_1 and π_2 do not overlap, the reverse logistic regression method does not work directly.

5.10.3 The Savage–Dickey Density Ratio

In Section 5.8.1, we introduce a hypothesis testing problem considered by Verdinelli and Wasserman (1996). Suppose that the posterior $\pi(\boldsymbol{\theta}, \boldsymbol{\psi}|D)$ is proportional to $L(\boldsymbol{\theta}, \boldsymbol{\psi}|D) \times \pi(\boldsymbol{\theta}, \boldsymbol{\psi})$, where $(\boldsymbol{\theta}, \boldsymbol{\psi}) \in \Omega \times \boldsymbol{\psi}$, $L(\boldsymbol{\theta}, \boldsymbol{\psi}|D)$ is the likelihood function given data D, and $\pi(\boldsymbol{\theta}, \boldsymbol{\psi})$ is the prior. We wish to test H_0: $\boldsymbol{\theta} = \boldsymbol{\theta}_0$ versus H_1: $\boldsymbol{\theta} \neq \boldsymbol{\theta}_0$. The Bayes factor is

$$B = m_0 / m,$$

where $m_0 = \int_{\Psi} L(\boldsymbol{\theta}_0, \boldsymbol{\psi}|D) \pi_0(\boldsymbol{\psi}) \, d\boldsymbol{\psi}$, $m = \int_{\Omega \times \Psi} L(\boldsymbol{\theta}, \boldsymbol{\psi}|D) \pi(\boldsymbol{\theta}, \boldsymbol{\psi}) \, d\boldsymbol{\theta} \, d\boldsymbol{\psi}$, and $\pi_0(\boldsymbol{\psi})$ is the prior under H_0. As discussed in Section 5.8, B is a ratio of two normalizing constants with different dimensions. In contrast to the MC methods presented in Section 5.8, Verdinelli and Wasserman (1995) suggest a generalization of the Savage–Dickey density ratio for estimating B. Dickey (1971) shows that if

$$\pi(\boldsymbol{\psi}|\boldsymbol{\theta}_0) = \pi_0(\boldsymbol{\psi}),$$

then

$$B = \frac{\pi(\boldsymbol{\theta}_0|D)}{\pi(\boldsymbol{\theta}_0)}, \tag{5.10.5}$$

where $\pi(\boldsymbol{\theta}_0|D) = \int_\Psi \pi(\boldsymbol{\theta}, \boldsymbol{\psi}|D)\, d\boldsymbol{\psi}$ and $\pi(\boldsymbol{\theta}) = \int_\Psi \pi(\boldsymbol{\theta}, \boldsymbol{\psi})\, d\boldsymbol{\psi}$. The reduced form of the Bayes factor B given in (5.10.5) is called the "Savage–Dickey density ratio."

In the cases where $\pi(\boldsymbol{\psi}|\boldsymbol{\theta}_0)$ depends on $\boldsymbol{\theta}_0$, Verdinelli and Wasserman (1995) obtain a generalized version of the Savage–Dickey density ratio. Assume that $0 < \pi(\boldsymbol{\theta}_0|D) < \infty$ and $0 < \pi(\boldsymbol{\theta}_0, \boldsymbol{\psi}) < \infty$ for almost all $\boldsymbol{\psi}$. Then the generalized Savage–Dickey density ratio is given by

$$B = \pi(\boldsymbol{\theta}_0|D) E\left[\frac{\pi_0(\boldsymbol{\psi})}{\pi(\boldsymbol{\theta}_0, \boldsymbol{\psi})}\right] = \frac{\pi(\boldsymbol{\theta}_0|D)}{\pi(\boldsymbol{\theta}_0)} E\left[\frac{\pi_0(\boldsymbol{\psi})}{\pi(\boldsymbol{\psi}|\boldsymbol{\theta}_0)}\right], \tag{5.10.6}$$

where the expectation is taken with respect to $\pi(\boldsymbol{\psi}|\boldsymbol{\theta}_0, D)$ (the conditional posterior density of $\boldsymbol{\psi}$ given $\boldsymbol{\theta} = \boldsymbol{\theta}_0$). To evaluate the generalized density ratio, we must compute $\pi(\boldsymbol{\theta}_0|D)$ and $E[\pi_0(\boldsymbol{\psi})/\pi(\boldsymbol{\theta}_0, \boldsymbol{\psi})]$. If a sample from the posterior $\pi(\boldsymbol{\theta}, \boldsymbol{\psi}|D)$ is available, and closed forms of $\pi_0(\boldsymbol{\psi})$ and $\pi(\boldsymbol{\theta}_0, \boldsymbol{\psi})$ are also available (see Section 3.2 for details), computing $E[\pi_0(\boldsymbol{\psi})/\pi(\boldsymbol{\theta}_0, \boldsymbol{\psi})]$ is trivial. If closed forms for $\pi_0(\boldsymbol{\psi})$ and $\pi(\boldsymbol{\theta}_0, \boldsymbol{\psi})$ are not available, $\pi(\boldsymbol{\theta}_0|D)$ can be estimated by, for example, the IWMDE method discussed in Section 4.3. The application of the Savage–Dickey density ratio to the computation involving Bayesian model comparisons and Bayesian variable selection will be discussed in detail in Chapters 8 and 9.

5.11 An Application of Weighted Monte Carlo Estimators

In this section, we illustrate how the new weighted MC estimator given by (3.4.15) can be used for computing the ratio of normalizing constants. For illustrative purposes, we only consider the development of the weighted version of the importance sampling estimator $\hat{r}_{\mathrm{IS}_2}$ given by (5.2.5).

Let $\pi_j(\boldsymbol{\theta})$, $j = 1, 2$, be two densities, each of which is known up to a normalizing constant:

$$\pi_j(\boldsymbol{\theta}) = \frac{q_j(\boldsymbol{\theta})}{c_j}, \quad \boldsymbol{\theta} \in \Omega_j, \tag{5.11.1}$$

where $\Omega_j \subset R^p$ is the support of π_j, and the unnormalized density $q_j(\boldsymbol{\theta})$ can be evaluated at any $\boldsymbol{\theta} \in \Omega_j$ for $j = 1, 2$. Our objective is to estimate the ratio of two normalizing constants defined as

$$r = \frac{c_1}{c_2}. \tag{5.11.2}$$

Let $\{\boldsymbol{\theta}_{2,1}, \boldsymbol{\theta}_{2,2}, \ldots, \boldsymbol{\theta}_{2,n}\}$ be a random sample from π_2. Then the IS estimator of r denoted by $\hat{r}_{\text{IS}_2}$ and its variance, $\text{Var}(\hat{r}_{\text{IS}_2})$, are given by (5.2.5) and (5.2.6), respectively. As discussed in Sections 5.2.2 and 5.6, $\hat{r}_{\text{IS}_2}$ is efficient when $\pi_2(\boldsymbol{\theta})$ has tails that are heavier than those of $\pi_1(\boldsymbol{\theta})$. However, when the two densities π_1 and π_2 have very little overlap (i.e., $E_2(\pi_1(\boldsymbol{\theta}))$ is very small), this method will work poorly.

To improve the simulation efficiency of $\hat{r}_{\text{IS}_2}$, we use the weighted estimator defined by (3.4.15) with the optimal weight $a_{\text{opt},l}$ given in (3.4.18). Let $\{A_l,\ l = 1, 2, \ldots, \kappa\}$ denote a partition of Ω_2. Using (3.4.14), we have

$$\mu_l = E_2\left[\frac{q_1(\boldsymbol{\theta})}{q_2(\boldsymbol{\theta})} 1\{\boldsymbol{\theta} \in A_l\}\right] = r \int_{A_l} \pi_1(\boldsymbol{\theta}|D)\, d\boldsymbol{\theta} = r\pi_1(A_l|D),$$

where $\pi_1(A_l|D)$ is the probability of set A_l with respect to π_1. Let $p_l = \pi_1(A_l)$ for $l = 1, 2, \ldots, \kappa$. The constraint given in (3.4.16) becomes

$$\sum_{l=1}^{\kappa} a_l p_l = 1. \tag{5.11.3}$$

The weighted estimator defined by (3.4.15) with the optimal weight a_{opt} reduces to

$$\hat{r}(a_{\text{opt}}) = \frac{1}{n} \sum_{i=1}^{n} \sum_{l=1}^{k} a_{\text{opt},l} \left[\frac{q_1(\boldsymbol{\theta}_{2,i})}{q_2(\boldsymbol{\theta}_{2,i})}\right] 1\{\boldsymbol{\theta}_{2,i} \in A_l\}, \tag{5.11.4}$$

where

$$a_{\text{opt},l} = \frac{p_l}{b_l} \frac{1}{\sum_{j=1}^{\kappa} p_j^2/b_j}, \tag{5.11.5}$$

and

$$b_l = E_2\left[\left(\frac{q_1(\boldsymbol{\theta})}{q_2(\boldsymbol{\theta})}\right)^2 1\{\boldsymbol{\theta} \in A_l\}\right]. \tag{5.11.6}$$

The variance given by (3.4.19) can be simplified to

$$\text{Var}(\hat{r}(a_{\text{opt}})) = \frac{1}{n}\left(\frac{1}{\sum_{l=1}^{\kappa} p_l^2/b_l} - r^2\right). \tag{5.11.7}$$

It is easy to see that $\hat{r}(a_{\text{opt}})$ is an unbiased estimator of r. Also, it directly follows from Theorem 3.4.2 that $\hat{r}(a_{\text{opt}})$ is always better than $\hat{r}_{\text{IS}_2}$. We also note that in the weighted estimator $\hat{r}(a_{\text{opt}})$, the observations with larger probabilities, p_l's, and smaller second moments are assigned more weight. In contrast, the same weight is assigned to each observation in the estimator $\hat{r}_{\text{IS}_2}$. In addition, the weighted estimator $\hat{r}(a_{\text{opt}})$ combines information from both densities.

In practice, p_l and b_l are unknown. However, the computation of p_l is relatively easy if a random sample from $\pi_1(\boldsymbol{\theta})$ is available. More specifically, if $\{\boldsymbol{\theta}_{1,i},\ i = 1, 2, \ldots, m\}$ is a random sample from π_1, an estimator of p_l is given by

$$\hat{p}_l = \frac{1}{m} \sum_{i=1}^{m} 1\{\boldsymbol{\theta}_{1,i} \in A_l\}.$$

For b_l, we can simply use the random sample $\{\boldsymbol{\theta}_{2,i},\ i = 1, 2, \ldots, n\}$ to obtain an estimated value. That is,

$$\hat{b}_l = \frac{1}{n} \sum_{i=1}^{n} \left[\frac{q_1(\boldsymbol{\theta}_{2,i})}{q_2(\boldsymbol{\theta}_{2,i})} \right]^2 1\{\boldsymbol{\theta}_{2,i} \in A_l\}. \tag{5.11.8}$$

Replacing p_l and b_l by $\hat{p}_l$ and $\hat{b}_l$ in (5.11.5), an estimate of $a_{\text{opt},l}$ is given by

$$\hat{a}_{\text{opt},l} = \frac{\hat{p}_l}{\hat{b}_l} \frac{1}{\sum_{j=1}^{\kappa} \hat{p}_j^2 / \hat{b}_j}. \tag{5.11.9}$$

Plugging $\hat{a}_{\text{opt},l}$ into (5.11.4) yields

$$\hat{r}(\hat{a}_{\text{opt}}) = \frac{1}{n} \sum_{i=1}^{n} \sum_{l=1}^{\kappa} \hat{a}_{\text{opt},l} \left[\frac{q_1(\boldsymbol{\theta}_{2,i})}{q_2(\boldsymbol{\theta}_{2,i})} \right] 1\{\boldsymbol{\theta}_{2,i} \in A_l\}. \tag{5.11.10}$$

It is easy to show that $\hat{r}(\hat{a}_{\text{opt}})$ is a consistent estimator as $n \to \infty$ and $m \to \infty$. Moreover, the next theorem shows that $\hat{r}(\hat{a}_{\text{opt}})$ achieves the same variance as that of $\hat{r}(a_{\text{opt}})$ given in (5.11.7) asymptotically.

Theorem 5.11.1 *Assume that $\{\boldsymbol{\theta}_{1,i},\ i = 1, 2, \ldots, m\}$ and $\{\boldsymbol{\theta}_{2,i},\ i = 1, 2, \ldots, n\}$ are two independent random samples. If $n = o(m)$, then*

$$\lim_{n\to\infty} nE\left(\hat{r}(\hat{a}_{\text{opt}}) - r\right)^2 = \frac{1}{\sum_{l=1}^{\kappa} p_l^2 / b_l} - r^2. \tag{5.11.11}$$

The proof of this theorem is given in the Appendix. The weighted estimator $\hat{r}(\hat{a}_{\text{opt}})$ is always better than $\hat{r}$. However, the trade-off here is that we have to pay a price to obtain an additional sample from π_1. Since it is relatively easy to compute $\hat{p}_l$ and $\hat{r}(\hat{a}_{\text{opt}})$, the weighted estimator is potentially useful, if $\hat{r}(\hat{a}_{\text{opt}})$ leads to a substantial gain in simulation efficiency. The following two examples demonstrate how the weighted estimator $\hat{r}(a_{\text{opt}})$ performs.

Example 5.2. A theoretical case study. To get a better understanding of the weighted estimators developed in this section, we conduct a theoretical case study based on two normal densities considered in Section 5.6. Let $q_1(\theta) = \exp(-\theta^2/2)$ and $q_2(\theta) = \exp(-(\theta - \delta)^2/2)$ with δ a known positive constant. In this case, $c_1 = c_2 = \sqrt{2\pi}$ and, therefore, $r = 1$.

TABLE 5.4. Comparison of Variances.

δ	n Var $(\hat{r}_{\mathrm{IS}_2})$	κ	n Var$(\hat{r}(a_{\mathrm{opt}}))$
1	1.718	2	0.451
		5	0.116
		10	0.105
		20	0.103
2	53.598	2	3.855
		5	0.343
		10	0.107
		20	0.073
3	8102.084	2	42.694
		5	1.250
		10	0.242
		20	0.069

For the optimal weighted estimator $\hat{r}(a_{\mathrm{opt}})$ given by (5.11.4), we consider the following partitions:

(i) $\kappa = 2$, $A_1 = (-\infty, 0]$, and $A_2 = (0, \infty)$; and

(ii) $\kappa > 2$, $A_1 = (-\infty, 0]$, $A_l = ((l-2)/(\kappa-2) \times 1.5\delta, (l-1)/(\kappa-2) \times 1.5\delta]$, $l = 2, 3, \ldots, \kappa - 1$, and $A_\kappa = (1.5\delta, \infty)$.

For (i), it can be shown that

$$\mathrm{Var}(\hat{r}(a_{\mathrm{opt}})) = \frac{1}{n}[\exp(\delta^2) 4\Phi(\delta)(1 - \Phi(\delta)) - 1],$$

where Φ is the standard normal ($N(0,1)$) cumulative distribution function (cdf). From Table 5.1, the variance of $\hat{r}_{\mathrm{IS}_2}$ is given by

$$\mathrm{Var}(\hat{r}_{\mathrm{IS}_2}) = \frac{1}{n}\left[\exp(\delta^2) - 1\right].$$

Table 5.4 shows the values of n Var$(\hat{r}(a_{\mathrm{opt}}))$ and n Var $(\hat{r}_{\mathrm{IS}_2})$ for several different choices of δ and κ. From Table 5.4, it is easy to see that the weighted estimator $\hat{r}(a_{\mathrm{opt}})$ dramatically improves the simulation efficiency compared to the importance sampling estimator $\hat{r}_{\mathrm{IS}_2}$. For example, when $\delta = 3$ and $\kappa = 20$,

$$\mathrm{Var}(\hat{r}_{\mathrm{IS}_2})/\mathrm{Var}(\hat{r}(a_{\mathrm{opt}})) = 117,421.51,$$

i.e., $\hat{r}(a_{\mathrm{opt}})$ is about 117,421 times better than $\hat{r}_{\mathrm{IS}_2}$. Also, it is interesting to see that a finer partition yields a smaller variance. When the two densities are not far apart from each other, the variances of the weighted estimators are quite robust for $\kappa \geq 5$. However, when the two densities do not have much overlap, which is the case when $\delta = 3$, a substantial gain in simulation efficiency can be achieved by a finer partition.

In Section 5.6, we have shown that the ratio importance sampling estimator $\hat{r}_{\text{RIS}}$ given by (5.5.2) with the optimal π_{opt} given by (5.5.9) achieves the smallest asymptotic relative mean-square error, while the importance sampling estimator $\hat{r}_{\text{IS}_2}$ leads to the worst simulation efficiency. With the optimal density π_{opt}, Table 5.1 gives

$$\lim_{n\to\infty} n \,\text{RE}^2(\hat{r}_{\text{RIS}}(\pi_{\text{opt}})) = \left[2(2\Phi(\delta/2)-1)\right]^2,$$

where $\text{RE}^2(\hat{r}_{\text{RIS}}(\pi_{\text{opt}}))$ is defined by (5.5.3). It is easy to verify that

$$\lim_{n\to\infty} n \,\text{RE}^2(\hat{r}_{\text{RIS}}(\pi_{\text{opt}})) = 0.587, \ 1.864, \ \text{and } 3.002$$

for $\delta = 1, 2, 3$, respectively. Thus, from Table 5.4, it can be observed that $\hat{r}(a_{\text{opt}})$ is better than the optimal RIS estimator when $\kappa \geq 5$. This theoretical illustration is quite interesting, and demonstrates that the weighted version of the worst estimator can be better than the best estimator.

Example 5.3. ACTG036 data. In this example, we consider a data set from the AIDS study ACTG036. A detailed description of the ACTG036 study is given in Example 1.4. The sample size in this study, excluding cases with missing data, was 183. The response variable (y) for these data is binary with a 1 indicating death, development of AIDS, or AIDS related complex (ARC), and a 0 indicates otherwise. Several covariates were measured for these data. The ones we use here are CD4 count (x_1), age (x_2), treatment (x_3), and race (x_4). Chen, Ibrahim, and Yiannoutsos (1999) analyze the ACTG036 data using a logistic regression model.

Here we use the Bayes factor approach (see, e.g., Kass and Raftery 1995) to compare the logit model to the complementary log–log link model. This comparison is of practical interest, since it is not clear whether a symmetric link model is adequate for these data. Let $F_1(t) = \exp(t)/(1+\exp(t))$ and $F_2(t) = 1 - \exp(-\exp(t))$. Also, let $D = (\boldsymbol{y}, X)$ denote the observed data, where $\boldsymbol{y} = (y_1, y_2, \ldots, y_{183})'$ and X is the design matrix with the ith row $\boldsymbol{x}_i' = (1, x_{i1}, x_{i2}, x_{i3}, x_{i4})$. The likelihood functions corresponding to these two links can be written as

$$L_j(\boldsymbol{\theta}|D) = \prod_{i=1}^{183} F_j^{y_i}(x_i'\boldsymbol{\theta})[1 - F_j(x_i'\boldsymbol{\theta})]^{1-y_i},$$

for $j = 1, 2$, where $\boldsymbol{\theta} = (\theta_0, \theta_1, \ldots, \theta_4)'$ denotes a 5×1 vector of regression coefficients. We take the same improper uniform prior for $\boldsymbol{\theta}$ under both models. Then the Bayes factor for comparing F_1 to F_2 can be calculated as follows:

$$B = \frac{\int_{R^5} L_1(\boldsymbol{\theta}|D)\, d\boldsymbol{\theta}}{\int_{R^5} L_2(\boldsymbol{\theta}|D)\, d\boldsymbol{\theta}} \equiv \frac{c_1}{c_2}, \tag{5.11.12}$$

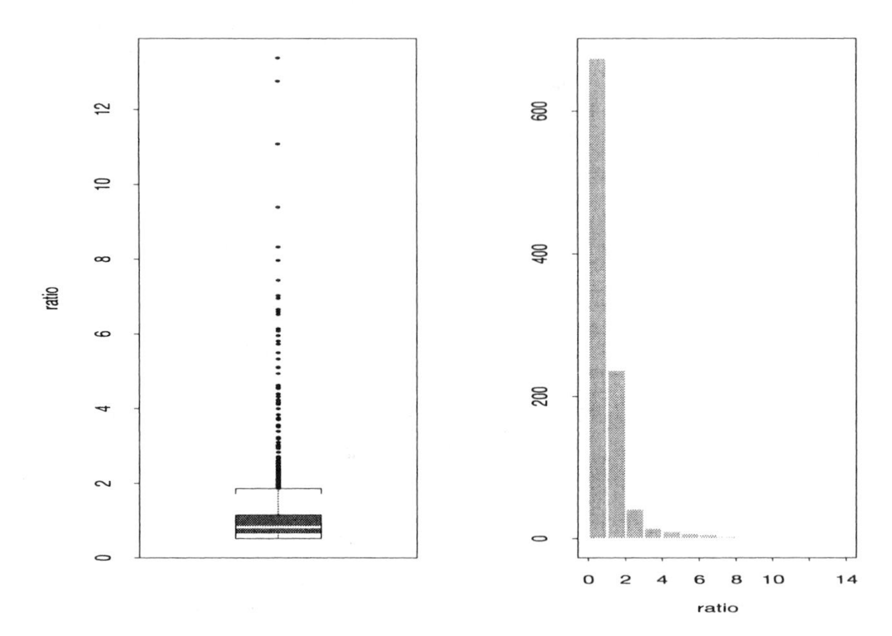

FIGURE 5.3. The box plot and histogram of the ratio $h(\boldsymbol{\theta}_i)$.

where c_j is the normalizing constant of the posterior distribution under F_j for $j = 1, 2$. Clearly, the Bayes factor B is a ratio of two normalizing constants.

We use the Gibbs sampler to sample from the posterior distribution $\pi_2(\boldsymbol{\theta}|D) \propto L_2(\boldsymbol{\theta}|D)$. The autocorrelations for all the parameters disappear after lag 5. We obtain a sample of size $n = 1000$ by taking every 10th Gibbs iterate. Then, using (5.2.5) and (5.2.6), we obtain $\hat{B} = 1.161$ and $n\,\widehat{\text{Var}}(\hat{B}) = 1.331$. In addition, we compute the ratio

$$h(\boldsymbol{\theta}_i) = L_1(\boldsymbol{\theta}_i|D)/L_2(\boldsymbol{\theta}_i|D)$$

for each observation. The box plot and histogram of these 1000 ratios are displayed in Figure 5.3.

Figure 5.3 clearly indicates that the posterior distribution of $h(\boldsymbol{\theta})$ is very skewed to the right. This suggests that the importance sampling estimator $\hat{B}$ cannot be reliable or accurate. To obtain a better estimate of B, we use the weighted estimators. We consider the following two partitions:

(i) $\kappa = 5$, $A_1 = \{\boldsymbol{\theta} : 0 < h(\boldsymbol{\theta}) \le 0.75\}$, $A_2 = \{\boldsymbol{\theta} : 0.75 < h(\boldsymbol{\theta}) \le 1.5\}$, $A_3 = \{\boldsymbol{\theta} : 1.5 < h(\boldsymbol{\theta}) \le 2.5\}$, $A_4 = \{\boldsymbol{\theta} : 2.5 < h(\boldsymbol{\theta}) \le 3.5\}$, and $A_5 = \{\boldsymbol{\theta} : 3.5 < h(\boldsymbol{\theta})\}$; and

(ii) $\kappa = 10$, $A_1 = \{\boldsymbol{\theta} : 0 < h(\boldsymbol{\theta}) \le 0.75\}$, $A_2 = \{\boldsymbol{\theta} : 0.75 < h(\boldsymbol{\theta}) \le 1.0\}$, $A_3 = \{\boldsymbol{\theta} : 1.0 < h(\boldsymbol{\theta}) \le 1.25\}$, $A_4 = \{\boldsymbol{\theta} : 1.25 < h(\boldsymbol{\theta}) \le 1.5\}$,

$A_5 = \{\boldsymbol{\theta} : 1.5 < h(\boldsymbol{\theta}) \leq 2.0\}$, $A_6 = \{\boldsymbol{\theta} : 2.0 < h(\boldsymbol{\theta}) \leq 2.5\}$, $A_7 = \{\boldsymbol{\theta} : 2.5 < h(\boldsymbol{\theta}) \leq 3.0\}$, $A_8 = \{\boldsymbol{\theta} : 3.0 < h(\boldsymbol{\theta}) \leq 3.5\}$, $A_9 = \{\boldsymbol{\theta} : 3.5 < h(\boldsymbol{\theta}) \leq 4.0\}$, and $A_{10} = \{\boldsymbol{\theta} : 4.0 < h(\boldsymbol{\theta})\}$.

We generate a sample of size $m = 50000$ from the posterior distribution $\pi_1(\boldsymbol{\theta}|D) \propto L_1(\boldsymbol{\theta}|D)$ to estimate the probability p_j under each partition. Using (5.11.8), (5.11.9), (5.11.10), and (5.11.7), we obtain that $\hat{B}(\hat{a}_{\text{opt}})$ and $n\,\widehat{\text{Var}}(\hat{B}(\hat{a}_{\text{opt}}))$ are 1.099 and 0.050 for $\kappa = 5$, and 1.100 and 0.030 for $\kappa = 10$. For each observation, we also compute $w_i h(\boldsymbol{\theta}_i)$ (weight-times-ratio) for $\kappa = 10$, where $w_i = \sum_{l=1}^{\kappa} \hat{a}_l 1\{\boldsymbol{\theta}_i \in A_l\}$, and the box plot and the histogram of these 1000 values are displayed in Figure 5.4. From Figure 5.4, the reweighted observations are quite symmetric around the mean value. This result partially explains the reason why the weighted estimate works better. We also record the computing times for $\hat{B}$ and $\hat{B}(\hat{a}_{\text{opt}})$. The computing time for $\hat{B}$ is 137 seconds, and the computing time for $\hat{B}(\hat{a}_{\text{opt}})$ takes an additional 150 seconds on a digital alpha machine. In addition, we run the simulation with a very large number of iterations ($n = 500,000$), and we find that the "golden value" of B is around 1.102, which confirms that the weighted estimate is quite accurate, even when $n = 1000$. Based on the estimated Bayes factor, we can conclude that the logit model is slightly better than the complementary log–log link model.

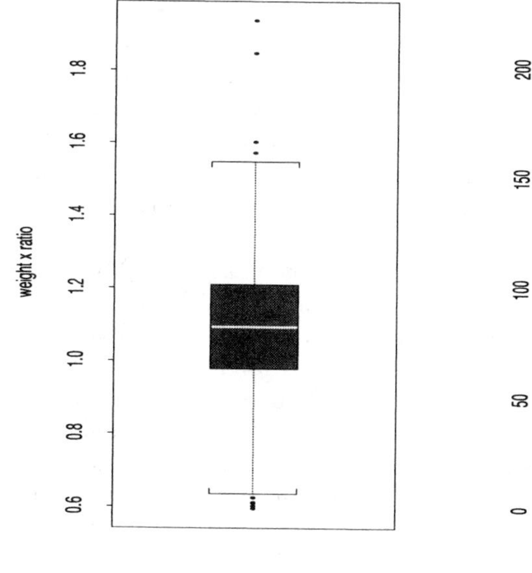

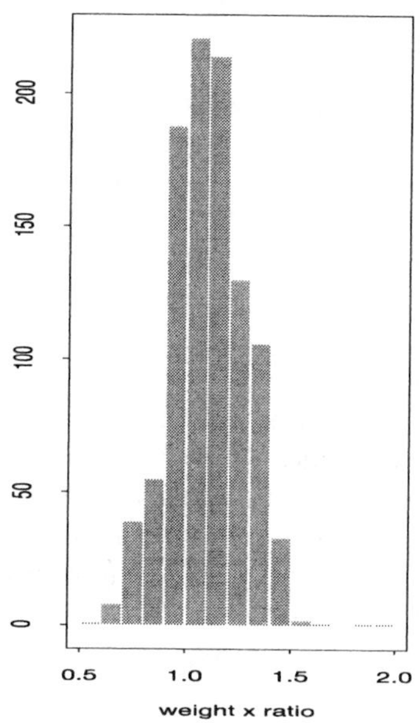

FIGURE 5.4. The box plot and histogram of the weight-times-ratio.

Finally, we note that the weighted estimators for the other MC methods such as BS and RIS can also be developed. The weighted versions of the BS estimator $\hat{r}_{\text{BS}}$ defined in (5.3.3) and the RIS estimator $\hat{r}_{\text{RIS}}$ given by (5.5.2) are analogous to the one for the IS estimator $\hat{r}_{\text{IS}_2}$. The detailed formulations are left as an exercise. We also note that Peng (1998) develops an efficient weighted MC method for computing the normalizing constants, which are essentially the posterior model probabilities obtained from the Stochastic Search Variable Selection method of George and McCulloch (1993). She obtains the fixed weight and data-dependent weight estimators of the normalizing constants. However, the support of the posterior distribution considered in Peng (1998) is discrete and finite. The main idea of her method is to "partition" an MC sample (not the support of the posterior distribution) into several subsets, and then she assigns a fixed or random weight to each subset. The noticeable difference between her method and the one presented in this section is that she partitions the sample, and the subsets in her partition must not be mutually exclusive. Therefore, her method is useful for computing the normalizing constant of a discrete posterior distribution.

5.12 Discussion

In this chapter, we have assumed independence among samples when deriving all theoretical results. However, the samples from a desired distribution using MCMC sampling as described in Chapter 2 are typically dependent. Under certain regularity assumptions, such as ergodicity and weak dependence, the consistency and the central limit theorem of an estimator of r still hold. The only problem is the derivation of the relative mean-square error. One simple remedy is to obtain an approximately random sample by taking every Bth iterate in MCMC sampling, where B is selected so that the autocorrelations are negligible with respect to their standard errors; see, for example, Gelfand and Smith (1990). Other possible approaches are to use the expensive regeneration technique in Markov chain sampling (Mykland, Tierney, and Yu 1995) to obtain a random sample from different regeneration tours, *effective sample sizes* (Meng and Wong 1996) to derive the relative mean-square error, and a coupling-regeneration scheme of Johnson (1998). In addition, Meng and Wong (1996) comment that empirical studies, as reported in DiCiccio, Kass, Raftery, and Wasserman (1997) and in Meng and Schilling (1996a), suggest that the optimal or near-optimal procedures constructed under the independence assumption can work remarkably well in general, providing orders of magnitude improvement over other methods with similar computational effort.

We have shown that RIS with an optimal "middle" density π_{opt} works better than IS, BS, and PS. However, the implementation of the optimal

RIS estimator is expensive, which can be seen from Sections 5.5.2 and 5.8.5. As we discuss in Section 5.5.1, the idea of RIS is useful particularly when one deals with a Bayesian computational problem involving many ratios of normalizing constants. The idea of RIS will be extended to solve computationally intensive problems arising from Bayesian constrained parameter problems in Chapter 6 and Bayesian model comparisons in Chapters 8 and 9.

The different dimensions problems presented in Section 5.8 are important as they often arise in Bayesian model comparison and Bayesian variable selection. The algorithms presented in Section 5.8.5 can asymptotically or approximately achieve the optimal simulation errors, and they can be programmed in a routine manner. The methodology presented in this chapter will also be useful in the computation of Bayes factors (Kass and Raftery 1995), intrinsic Bayes factors (Berger and Pericchi 1996), Bayesian model comparisons (Geweke 1994), and model selection. In particular, the methods developed in this chapter can be directly applied to Bayesian model comparisons, which will be discussed in detail in Chapters 8 and 9.

Appendix

Proof of Theorem 5.3.1. By the Cauchy–Schwarz inequality, we have

$$\begin{aligned}\left\{\int_{\Omega_1\cap\Omega_2}\pi_1(\boldsymbol{\theta})\pi_2(\boldsymbol{\theta})\alpha(\boldsymbol{\theta})\,d\boldsymbol{\theta}\right\}^2 &\le \left\{\int_{\Omega_1\cap\Omega_2}\sqrt{\frac{\pi_1(\boldsymbol{\theta})\pi_2(\boldsymbol{\theta})}{s_1\pi_1(\boldsymbol{\theta})+s_2\pi_2(\boldsymbol{\theta})}}\right.\\ &\quad\left.\times\left[\sqrt{\pi_1(\boldsymbol{\theta})\pi_2(\boldsymbol{\theta})(s_1\pi_1(\boldsymbol{\theta})+s_2\pi_2(\boldsymbol{\theta}))}|\alpha(\boldsymbol{\theta})|\right]d\boldsymbol{\theta}\right\}^2\\ &\le \int_{\Omega_1\cap\Omega_2}\frac{\pi_1(\boldsymbol{\theta})\pi_2(\boldsymbol{\theta})}{s_1\pi_1(\boldsymbol{\theta})+s_2\pi_2(\boldsymbol{\theta})}\,d\boldsymbol{\theta}\\ &\quad\times\int_{\Omega_1\cap\Omega_2}\pi_1(\boldsymbol{\theta})\pi_2(\boldsymbol{\theta})(s_1\pi_1(\boldsymbol{\theta})+s_2\pi_2(\boldsymbol{\theta}))\alpha^2(\boldsymbol{\theta})\,d\boldsymbol{\theta}.\end{aligned}$$

Thus,

$$\begin{aligned}&\frac{\int_{\Omega_1\cap\Omega_2}\pi_1(\boldsymbol{\theta})\pi_2(\boldsymbol{\theta})(s_1\pi_1(\boldsymbol{\theta})+s_2\pi_2(\boldsymbol{\theta}))\alpha^2(\boldsymbol{\theta})\,d\boldsymbol{\theta}}{\{\int_{\Omega_1\cap\Omega_2}\pi_1(\boldsymbol{\theta})\pi_2(\boldsymbol{\theta})\alpha(\boldsymbol{\theta})\,d\boldsymbol{\theta}\}^2}\\ &\qquad\ge\left[\int_{\Omega_1\cap\Omega_2}\frac{\pi_1(\boldsymbol{\theta})\pi_2(\boldsymbol{\theta})}{s_1\pi_1(\boldsymbol{\theta})+s_2\pi_2(\boldsymbol{\theta})}\,d\boldsymbol{\theta}\right]^{-1},\end{aligned}$$

where equality holds if and only if (up to a zero-measure set)

$$[\sqrt{\pi_1(\boldsymbol{\theta})\pi_2(\boldsymbol{\theta})(s_1\pi_1(\boldsymbol{\theta})+s_2\pi_2(\boldsymbol{\theta}))}]\alpha(\boldsymbol{\theta}) \propto \sqrt{\frac{\pi_1(\boldsymbol{\theta})\pi_2(\boldsymbol{\theta})}{s_1\pi_1(\boldsymbol{\theta})+s_2\pi_2(\boldsymbol{\theta})}},$$

which yields (5.3.5). □

Proof of Theorem 5.4.2. Letting $c(\lambda)=\int_\Omega q(\boldsymbol{\theta}|\lambda)\,d\boldsymbol{\theta}$, we have

$$\xi = \int_{\lambda_1}^{\lambda_2}\left[\frac{d}{d\lambda}\ln c(\lambda)\right]\,d\lambda$$

and

$$E_\lambda\{U^2(\boldsymbol{\theta},\lambda)\} = \int_\Omega\left[\frac{d}{d\lambda}\ln\pi(\boldsymbol{\theta}|\lambda)\right]^2\pi(\boldsymbol{\theta}|\lambda)\,d\boldsymbol{\theta} + \left[\frac{d}{d\lambda}\ln c(\lambda)\right]^2. \tag{5.A.1}$$

Equations (5.4.3) and (5.A.1) lead to

$$\begin{aligned} n\,\mathrm{Var}(\hat{\xi}_{\mathrm{PS}}) &= \int_{\lambda_1}^{\lambda_2}\int_\Omega\left[\frac{d}{d\lambda}\ln\pi(\boldsymbol{\theta}|\lambda)\right]^2\frac{\pi(\boldsymbol{\theta}|\lambda)}{\pi_\lambda(\lambda)}\,d\boldsymbol{\theta}\,d\lambda \\ &\quad + \left[\int_{\lambda_1}^{\lambda_2}\left[\frac{d}{d\lambda}\ln c(\lambda)\right]^2\frac{1}{\pi_\lambda(\lambda)}\,d\lambda - \xi^2\right]. \end{aligned} \tag{5.A.2}$$

Using the Cauchy–Schwarz inequality and $\int_{\lambda_1}^{\lambda_2}\pi_\lambda(\lambda)\,d\lambda=1$, we have

$$\begin{aligned} &\int_{\lambda_1}^{\lambda_2}\left[\frac{d}{d\lambda}\ln c(\lambda)\right]^2\frac{1}{\pi_\lambda(\lambda)}\,d\lambda - \xi^2 \\ &\qquad \geq \left[\int_{\lambda_1}^{\lambda_2}\frac{(d/d\lambda)\ln c(\lambda)}{\sqrt{\pi_\lambda(\lambda)}}\sqrt{\pi_\lambda(\lambda)}\,d\lambda\right]^2 - \xi^2 = 0. \end{aligned} \tag{5.A.3}$$

Similarly,

$$\begin{aligned} &\int_{\lambda_1}^{\lambda_2}\int_\Omega\left[\frac{d}{d\lambda}\ln\pi(\boldsymbol{\theta}|\lambda)\right]^2\frac{\pi(\boldsymbol{\theta}|\lambda)}{\pi_\lambda(\lambda)}\,d\boldsymbol{\theta}\,d\lambda \\ &\qquad = \int_{\lambda_1}^{\lambda_2}\int_\Omega 4\left[\frac{d}{d\lambda}\sqrt{\pi(\boldsymbol{\theta}|\lambda)}\right]^2\frac{1}{\pi_\lambda(\lambda)}\,d\boldsymbol{\theta}\,d\lambda \\ &\qquad \geq 4\int_\Omega\left[\int_{\lambda_1}^{\lambda_2}\frac{(d/d\lambda)\sqrt{\pi(\boldsymbol{\theta}|\lambda)}}{\sqrt{\pi_\lambda(\lambda)}}\sqrt{\pi_\lambda(\lambda)}\,d\lambda\right]^2\,d\boldsymbol{\theta} \\ &\qquad = 4\int_\Omega\left[\int_{\lambda_1}^{\lambda_2}\frac{d}{d\lambda}\sqrt{\pi(\boldsymbol{\theta}|\lambda)}\,d\lambda\right]^2\,d\boldsymbol{\theta} \\ &\qquad = 4\int_\Omega\left[\sqrt{\pi(\boldsymbol{\theta}|\lambda_2)}-\sqrt{\pi(\boldsymbol{\theta}|\lambda_1)}\right]^2\,d\boldsymbol{\theta}. \end{aligned} \tag{5.A.4}$$

Thus, the theorem follows from (5.A.2), (5.A.3), and (5.A.4). □

Proof of Theorem 5.5.1. Write

$$\sqrt{n}(\hat{r}_{\text{RIS}} - r) = \frac{c_1 n^{-1/2} \sum_{i=1}^{n} \{f_1(\boldsymbol{\theta}_i)/c_1 - f_2(\boldsymbol{\theta}_i)/c_2\}}{(1/n)\sum_{i=1}^{n} f_2(\boldsymbol{\theta}_i)}. \tag{5.A.5}$$

It follows from the central limit theorem that

$$n^{-1/2}\sum_{i=1}^{n}\{f_1(\boldsymbol{\theta}_i)/c_1 - f_2(\boldsymbol{\theta}_i)/c_2\} \xrightarrow{\mathcal{D}} N\left(0, E_\pi\left\{\frac{f_1(\boldsymbol{\theta})}{c_1} - \frac{f_2(\boldsymbol{\theta})}{c_2}\right\}^2\right) \quad \text{as } n \to \infty \tag{5.A.6}$$

and from the law of large numbers that

$$(1/n)\sum_{i=1}^{n} f_2(\boldsymbol{\theta}_i) \xrightarrow{\text{a.s.}} c_2 \quad \text{as } n \to \infty. \tag{5.A.7}$$

Now (5.5.5) is an immediate consequence of (5.A.6) and (5.A.7). To prove (5.5.4), it suffices to show that $\{n(\hat{r}_{\text{RIS}} - r)^2,\ n \geq 1\}$ is uniformly integrable. In this case, by (5.5.5), we shall have $E\{\sqrt{n}(\hat{r}_{\text{RIS}} - r)\} = o(1)$ as $n \to \infty$. Thus

$$\frac{1}{r^2}E\left\{n(\hat{r}_{\text{RIS}} - r)^2\right\} \to E\left\{\frac{f_1(\boldsymbol{\theta})}{c_1} - \frac{f_2(\boldsymbol{\theta})}{c_2}\right\}^2 \quad \text{as } n \to \infty,$$

which gives (5.5.4). We show below the uniform integrability of $\{n(\hat{r}_{\text{RIS}} - r)^2,\ n \geq 1\}$. Rewrite

$$\sqrt{n}(\hat{r}_{\text{RIS}} - r) = \frac{n^{-1/2}\sum_{i=1}^{n}\{c_2 f_1(\boldsymbol{\theta}_i) - c_1 f_2(\boldsymbol{\theta}_i)\}}{c_2(1/n)\sum_{i=1}^{n} f_2(\boldsymbol{\theta}_i)} \tag{5.A.8}$$

and let $U_n = n^{-1/2}\sum_{i=1}^{n}\{c_2 f_1(\boldsymbol{\theta}_i) - c_1 f_2(\boldsymbol{\theta}_i)\}$ and $V_n = n^{-1}\sum_{i=1}^{n} f_2(\boldsymbol{\theta}_i)$. By (5.A.8), for every $A \geq 2$,

$$\begin{aligned}
&E[n(\hat{r}_{\text{RIS}} - r)^2 1\{n(\hat{r}_{\text{RIS}} - r)^2 \geq A^2\}] \\
&= E\left[\frac{U_n^2}{c_2^2 V_n^2} 1\{|U_n| \geq c_2 A V_n\}\right] \\
&= E\left[\frac{U_n^2}{c_2^2 V_n^2} 1\{|U_n| \geq A c_2 V_n, V_n \geq c_2/2\}\right] \\
&\quad + E\left[\frac{U_n^2}{c_2 V_n^2} 1\{|U_n| \geq A c_2 V_n, V_n < c_2/2\}\right] \\
&\leq 4c_2^{-4} E[U_n^2 1\{|U_n| \geq A c_2^2/2\}] \\
&\quad + E[n(\hat{r}_{\text{RIS}} - r)^2 1\{V_n < c_2/2\}],
\end{aligned} \tag{5.A.9}$$

where $1\{n(\hat{r}_{\text{RIS}} - r)^2 \geq A^2\}$ is an indicator function. It is known that $\{U_n^2,\ n \geq 1\}$ is uniformly integrable. Hence

$$\lim_{A\to\infty} \sup_n E[U_n^2 1\{|U_n| \geq Ac_2^2/2\}] = 0. \tag{5.A.10}$$

Noting that $\hat{r}_{\text{RIS}} \leq \sum_{i=1}^n f_1(\boldsymbol{\theta}_i)/f_2(\boldsymbol{\theta}_i)$, we have

$$\begin{aligned}
E[n(\hat{r}_{\text{RIS}} &- r)^2 1\{V_n < c_2/2\}] \\
&\leq nE_\pi\left[(\hat{r}_{\text{RIS}}^2 + r^2)1\{V_n < c_2/2\}\right] \\
&\leq nE\left[\left\{r^2 + n\sum_{i=1}^n (f_1(\boldsymbol{\theta}_i)/f_2(\boldsymbol{\theta}_i))^2\right\} 1\{V_n < c_2/2\}\right] \\
&\leq n\Bigg[r^2 P(V_n < c_2/2) \\
&\qquad + n\sum_{i=1}^n E\left\{(f_1(\boldsymbol{\theta}_i)/f_2(\boldsymbol{\theta}_i))^2 1\Big\{\sum_{j\neq i} f_2(\boldsymbol{\theta}_j) < nc_2/2\Big\}\right\}\Bigg] \\
&= n\Bigg[r^2 P(V_n < c_2/2) \\
&\qquad + n^2 E\left(f_1(\boldsymbol{\theta})/f_2(\boldsymbol{\theta})\right)^2 P\left(\sum_{j=1}^{n-1} f_2(\boldsymbol{\theta}_j) < nc_2/2\right)\Bigg].
\end{aligned} \tag{5.A.11}$$

Using the Chebyshev inequality, we get

$$\begin{aligned}
P(V_n < c_2/2) &= P\left(\sum_{i=1}^n \{Ef_2(\boldsymbol{\theta}_i) - f_2(\boldsymbol{\theta}_i)\} > nc_2/2\right) \\
&\leq \inf_{t\geq 0} \exp(-tc_2 n/2) E\left[\exp\left(\sum_{i=1}^n \{Ef_2(\boldsymbol{\theta}_i) - f_2(\boldsymbol{\theta}_i)\}\right)\right] \\
&= \left(\inf_{t\geq 0} \exp(-tc_2/2) E\exp[t(c_2 - f_2(\boldsymbol{\theta}))]\right)^n.
\end{aligned} \tag{5.A.12}$$

From $E(c_2 - f_2(\boldsymbol{\theta})) = 0$, it follows that

$$\varepsilon = \inf_{t\geq 0} \exp(-tc_2/4) E\exp\{t(c_2 - f_2(\boldsymbol{\theta}))\} < 1.$$

Thus, $P(V_n < c_2/2) \leq \varepsilon^n$. Similarly, for $n \geq 3$, we have

$$\begin{aligned}
P\left(\sum_{j=1}^{n-1} f_2(\boldsymbol{\theta}_j) < nc_2/2\right) \\
&= P\left(\sum_{j=1}^{n-1}\{Ef_2(\boldsymbol{\theta}_j) - f_2(\boldsymbol{\theta}_j)\} > (n-2)c_2/2\right) \\
&\leq \left(\inf_{t\geq 0} \exp[-(n-2)tc_2/2(n-1)]E\exp\{t(c_2 - f_2(\boldsymbol{\theta}))\}\right)^{n-1} \\
&\leq \varepsilon^{n-1}. \qquad (5.A.13)
\end{aligned}$$

Putting together the above inequalities yields

$$E[n(\hat{r}_{\text{RIS}} - r)^2 1\{V_n < c_2/2\}] = O(n^3\varepsilon^n) = o(1). \qquad (5.A.14)$$

Therefore, (5.5.4) follows from (5.A.9), (5.A.10), and (5.A.14).

Next, we prove (5.5.6). Observe that

$$\begin{aligned}
nE(\hat{r}_{\text{RIS}} - r)^2 &- c_2^{-4}E\{c_2 f_1(\boldsymbol{\theta}) - c_1 f_2(\boldsymbol{\theta})\}^2 \\
&= c_2^{-2} n \left[E\left\{\frac{\sum_{i=1}^n (c_2 f_1(\boldsymbol{\theta}_i) - c_1 f_2(\boldsymbol{\theta}_i))}{\sum_{i=1}^n f_2(\boldsymbol{\theta}_i)}\right\}^2\right. \\
&\qquad \left. - E\left\{\frac{\sum_{i=1}^n (c_2 f_1(\boldsymbol{\theta}_i) - c_1 f_2(\boldsymbol{\theta}_i))}{nc_2}\right\}^2\right] \\
&= \frac{c_2^{-4}}{n}\left[E\left\{\frac{(\sum_{i=1}^n (c_2 f_1(\boldsymbol{\theta}_i) - c_1 f_2(\boldsymbol{\theta}_i)))^2}{(\sum_{i=1}^n f_2(\boldsymbol{\theta}_i))^2}\right.\right. \\
&\qquad \left.\left. \times \sum_{i=1}^n (c_2 - f_2(\boldsymbol{\theta}_i)) \cdot \sum_{i=1}^n (c_2 + f_2(\boldsymbol{\theta}_i))\right\}\right] \\
&\stackrel{\text{def}}{=} \frac{c_2^{-4}}{n}\varepsilon_n, \qquad (5.A.15)
\end{aligned}$$

where

$$\begin{aligned}
\varepsilon_n &= E\left\{\frac{(\sum_{i=1}^n (c_2 f_1(\boldsymbol{\theta}_i) - c_1 f_2(\boldsymbol{\theta}_i)))^2 \cdot \sum_{i=1}^n (c_2 - f_2(\boldsymbol{\theta}_i)) \cdot 2nc_2}{(\sum_{i=1}^n f_2(\boldsymbol{\theta}_i))^2}\right\} \\
&\quad - E\left\{\frac{(\sum_{i=1}^n (c_2 f_1(\boldsymbol{\theta}_i) - c_1 f_2(\boldsymbol{\theta}_i)))^2 \cdot (\sum_{i=1}^n (c_2 - f_2(\boldsymbol{\theta}_i)))^2}{(\sum_{i=1}^n f_2(\boldsymbol{\theta}_i))^2}\right\}.
\end{aligned}$$

After some algebra, we have

$$\begin{aligned}
\varepsilon_n &= 2E\left\{\frac{\left(\sum_{i=1}^n (c_2 f_1(\boldsymbol{\theta}_i) - c_1 f_2(\boldsymbol{\theta}_i))\right)^2 \cdot \sum_{i=1}^n (c_2 - f_2(\boldsymbol{\theta}_i))}{(n\,c_2)}\right\} \\
&\quad + 2E\left\{\frac{\left(\sum_{i=1}^n (c_2 f_1(\boldsymbol{\theta}_i) - c_1 f_2(\boldsymbol{\theta}_i))\right)^2 \cdot \sum_{i=1}^n (c_2 - f_2(\boldsymbol{\theta}_i))}{nc_2(\sum_{i=1}^n f_2(\boldsymbol{\theta}_i))^2}\right. \\
&\quad \times \left.\left((nc_2)^2 - \left(\sum_{i=1}^n f_2(\boldsymbol{\theta}_i)\right)^2\right)\right\} \\
&\quad - E\left\{\frac{\left(\sum_{i=1}^n (c_2 f_1(\boldsymbol{\theta}_i) - c_1 f_2(\boldsymbol{\theta}_i))\right)^2 \cdot \left(\sum_{i=1}^n (c_2 - f_2(\boldsymbol{\theta}_i))\right)^2}{(\sum_{i=1}^n f_2(\boldsymbol{\theta}_i))^2}\right\} \\
&\overset{\text{def}}{=} \varepsilon_{n,1} + \varepsilon_{n,2} + \varepsilon_{n,3}.
\end{aligned}$$

It is easy to see that

$$\begin{aligned}
\varepsilon_{n,1} &= 2(nc_2)^{-1}E\left\{\left(\sum_{i=1}^n (c_2 f_1(\boldsymbol{\theta}_i) - c_1 f_2(\boldsymbol{\theta}_i))^2\right.\right. \\
&\quad \left. + 2\sum_{1\le i<j\le n} (c_2 f_1(\boldsymbol{\theta}_i) - c_1 f_2(\boldsymbol{\theta}_i))(c_2 f_1(\boldsymbol{\theta}_j) - c_1 f_2(\boldsymbol{\theta}_j))\right) \\
&\quad \left.\times \sum_{i=1}^n (c_2 - f_2(\boldsymbol{\theta}_i))\right\} \\
&= 2(nc_2)^{-1}E\left\{\left(\sum_{i=1}^n (c_2 f_1(\boldsymbol{\theta}_i) - c_1 f_2(\boldsymbol{\theta}_i))^2\right) \cdot \sum_{i=1}^n (c_2 - f_2(\boldsymbol{\theta}_i))\right\} \\
&= 2(nc_2)^{-1}E\left\{\left(\sum_{i=1}^n \{(c_2 f_1(\boldsymbol{\theta}_i) - c_1 f_2(\boldsymbol{\theta}_i))^2 - E(c_2 f_1(\boldsymbol{\theta}_i) - c_1 f_2(\boldsymbol{\theta}_i))^2\}\right)\right. \\
&\qquad \left.\times \sum_{i=1}^n (c_2 - f_2(\boldsymbol{\theta}_i))\right\} \\
&\le (nc_2)^{-1}\left[\mathrm{Var}\left(\sum_{i=1}^n (c_2 f_1(\boldsymbol{\theta}_i) - c_1 f_2(\boldsymbol{\theta}_i))^2\right)\right]^{1/2} \\
&\quad \times \left[\mathrm{Var}\left(\sum_{i=1}^n (c_2 - f_2(\boldsymbol{\theta}_i))\right)\right]^{1/2} \\
&= O(1).
\end{aligned}$$

As for $\varepsilon_{n,2}$, we have

$$
\begin{aligned}
|\varepsilon_{n,2}| &= 2\left|E\left\{\frac{\left(\sum_{i=1}^n (c_2 f_1(\boldsymbol{\theta}_i) - c_1 f_2(\boldsymbol{\theta}_i))\right)^2 \cdot \left(\sum_{i=1}^n (c_2 - f_2(\boldsymbol{\theta}_i))\right)^2}{n c_2 (\sum_{i=1}^n f_2(\boldsymbol{\theta}_i))^2}\right.\right. \\
&\qquad \left.\left. \times \left(n c_2 + \sum_{i=1}^n f_2(\boldsymbol{\theta}_i)\right)\right\}\right| \\
&\le 12(n c_2)^{-2} E\left\{\left(\sum_{i=1}^n (c_2 f_1(\boldsymbol{\theta}_i) - c_1 f_2(\boldsymbol{\theta}_i))\right)^2 \cdot \left(\sum_{i=1}^n (c_2 - f_2(\boldsymbol{\theta}_i))\right)^2\right\} \\
&\quad + 2\left|E\left\{\frac{\left(\sum_{i=1}^n (c_2 f_1(\boldsymbol{\theta}_i) - c_1 f_2(\boldsymbol{\theta}_i))\right)^2 \cdot \left(\sum_{i=1}^n (c_2 - f_2(\boldsymbol{\theta}_i))\right)^2}{n c_2 (\sum_{i=1}^n f_2(\boldsymbol{\theta}_i))^2}\right.\right. \\
&\qquad \left.\left. \times \left(n c_2 + \sum_{i=1}^n f_2(\boldsymbol{\theta}_i)\right) 1\{V_n < c_2/2\}\right\}\right| \\
&\le 12(n c_2)^{-2}\left[E\left\{\sum_{i=1}^n (c_2 f_1(\boldsymbol{\theta}_i) - c_1 f_2(\boldsymbol{\theta}_i))\right\}^4\right. \\
&\qquad \left. \times E_\pi\left\{\sum_{i=1}^n (c_2 - f_2(\boldsymbol{\theta}_i))\right\}^4\right]^{1/2} \\
&\quad + 4(n c_2)^3 E\left\{\left(c_1 + c_2 \sum_{i=1}^n f_1(\boldsymbol{\theta}_i)/f_2(\boldsymbol{\theta}_i)\right)^2 1\{V_n < c_2/2\}\right\} \\
&= O(1) + O(n^5 \varepsilon^n) = O(1),
\end{aligned}
$$

where the last inequality is from (5.A.12) and the proof of (5.A.11). Similarly, we have

$$
\varepsilon_{n,3} = O(1).
$$

Now (5.5.6) follows from the above inequalities. This proves the theorem. □

<u>**Proof of Theorem 5.5.2.**</u> By the Cauchy–Schwarz inequality, for an arbitrary density $\pi(\cdot)$,

$$
\left[\int_\Omega |\pi_1(\boldsymbol{\theta}) - \pi_2(\boldsymbol{\theta})|\ d\boldsymbol{\theta}\right]^2 \le \int_\Omega \frac{[\pi_1(\boldsymbol{\theta}) - \pi_2(\boldsymbol{\theta})]^2}{\pi(\boldsymbol{\theta})}\ d\boldsymbol{\theta} \cdot \int_\Omega \pi(\boldsymbol{\theta})\ d\boldsymbol{\theta}.
$$

Thus,

$$
E\left[\frac{\{\pi_1(\boldsymbol{\theta}) - \pi_2(\boldsymbol{\theta})\}^2}{\pi^2(\boldsymbol{\theta})}\right] \ge \left[\int_\Omega |\pi_1(\boldsymbol{\theta}) - \pi_2(\boldsymbol{\theta})|\ d\boldsymbol{\theta}\right]^2
$$

with equality holding if and only if (up to a zero-measure set)

$$\pi(\boldsymbol{\theta}) \propto |\pi_1(\boldsymbol{\theta}) - \pi_2(\boldsymbol{\theta})|,$$

that is, $\pi(\boldsymbol{\theta}) = \pi_{\text{opt}}(\boldsymbol{\theta})$. This proves (5.5.9). Replacing π by π_{opt} in (5.5.7) gives (5.5.10). □

Proof of Theorem 5.5.3. Since

$$\begin{aligned}
1 - \int_{\Omega_1 \cap \Omega_2} & \frac{\pi_1(\boldsymbol{\theta})\pi_2(\boldsymbol{\theta})}{s_1\pi_1(\boldsymbol{\theta}) + s_2\pi_2(\boldsymbol{\theta})}\, d\boldsymbol{\theta} \\
&= \int_{\Omega} \frac{(s_2\pi_1(\boldsymbol{\theta}) + s_1\pi_2(\boldsymbol{\theta}))(s_1\pi_1(\boldsymbol{\theta}) + s_2\pi_2(\boldsymbol{\theta})) - \pi_1(\boldsymbol{\theta})\pi_2(\boldsymbol{\theta})}{s_1\pi_1(\boldsymbol{\theta}) + s_2\pi_2(\boldsymbol{\theta})}\, d\boldsymbol{\theta} \\
&= \int_{\Omega} \frac{(s_1\, s_2\pi_1^2(\boldsymbol{\theta}) + s_1 s_2 \pi_2^2(\boldsymbol{\theta}) + (s_1^2 + s_2^2 - 1)\pi_1(\boldsymbol{\theta})\pi_2(\boldsymbol{\theta})}{s_1\pi_1(\boldsymbol{\theta}) + s_2\pi_2(\boldsymbol{\theta})}\, d\boldsymbol{\theta} \\
&= s_1 s_2 \int_{\Omega} \frac{(\pi_1(\boldsymbol{\theta}) - \pi_2(\boldsymbol{\theta}))^2}{s_1\pi_1(\boldsymbol{\theta}) + s_2\pi_2(\boldsymbol{\theta})}\, d\boldsymbol{\theta}, \qquad (5.A.16)
\end{aligned}$$

the right-hand side of (5.5.11)

$$\begin{aligned}
&= \int_{\Omega} \frac{(\pi_1(\boldsymbol{\theta}) - \pi_2(\boldsymbol{\theta}))^2}{s_1\pi_1(\boldsymbol{\theta}) + s_2\pi_2(\boldsymbol{\theta})}\, d\boldsymbol{\theta} \cdot \left[\int_{\Omega} \frac{\pi_1(\boldsymbol{\theta})\pi_2(\boldsymbol{\theta})}{s_1\pi_1(\boldsymbol{\theta}) + s_2\pi_2(\boldsymbol{\theta})}\, d\boldsymbol{\theta}\right]^{-1} \\
&= \int_{\Omega} \frac{(\pi_1(\boldsymbol{\theta}) - \pi_2(\boldsymbol{\theta}))^2}{s_1\pi_1(\boldsymbol{\theta}) + s_2\pi_2(\boldsymbol{\theta})}\, d\boldsymbol{\theta} \cdot \int_{\Omega} (s_1\pi_1(\boldsymbol{\theta}) + s_2\pi_2(\boldsymbol{\theta}))\, d\boldsymbol{\theta} \\
&\quad \times \left[\int_{\Omega} \frac{\pi_1(\boldsymbol{\theta})\pi_2(\boldsymbol{\theta})}{s_1\pi_1(\boldsymbol{\theta}) + s_2\pi_2(\boldsymbol{\theta})}\, d\boldsymbol{\theta}\right]^{-1} \\
&\geq \left[\int_{\Omega} \frac{|\pi_1(\boldsymbol{\theta}) - \pi_2(\boldsymbol{\theta})|}{\sqrt{s_1\pi_1(\boldsymbol{\theta}) + s_2\pi_2(\boldsymbol{\theta})}} \cdot \sqrt{s_1\pi_1(\boldsymbol{\theta}) + s_2\pi_2(\boldsymbol{\theta})}\, d\boldsymbol{\theta}\right]^2 \\
&\quad \times \left[\int_{\Omega} \frac{\pi_1(\boldsymbol{\theta})\pi_2(\boldsymbol{\theta})}{s_1\pi_1(\boldsymbol{\theta}) + s_2\pi_2(\boldsymbol{\theta})}\, d\boldsymbol{\theta}\right]^{-1} \qquad (5.A.17) \\
&= \left[\int_{\Omega} |\pi_1(\boldsymbol{\theta}) - \pi_2(\boldsymbol{\theta})|\, d\boldsymbol{\theta}\right]^2 \cdot \left[\int_{\Omega} \frac{\pi_1(\boldsymbol{\theta})\pi_2(\boldsymbol{\theta})}{s_1\pi_1(\boldsymbol{\theta}) + s_2\pi_2(\boldsymbol{\theta})}\, d\boldsymbol{\theta}\right]^{-1}, \\
&\qquad (5.A.18)
\end{aligned}$$

where (5.A.17) is obtained by the Cauchy–Schwarz inequality. From (5.A.16) it can be shown that

$$\int_{\Omega_1 \cap \Omega_2} \frac{\pi_1(\boldsymbol{\theta})\pi_2(\boldsymbol{\theta})}{s_1\pi_1(\boldsymbol{\theta}) + s_2\pi_2(\boldsymbol{\theta})}\, d\boldsymbol{\theta} \leq 1. \qquad (5.A.19)$$

Now (5.5.11) follows from (5.A.18) and (5.A.19). This proves the theorem. □

Proof of Theorem 5.5.4. By the Cauchy–Schwarz inequality, the left side of (5.5.12) equals

$$\left[\int_\Omega \left|\sqrt{\pi_1(\boldsymbol{\theta})} - \sqrt{\pi_2(\boldsymbol{\theta})}\right| \left(\sqrt{\pi_1(\boldsymbol{\theta})} + \sqrt{\pi_2(\boldsymbol{\theta})}\right) d\boldsymbol{\theta}\right]^2$$

$$\leq \int_\Omega \left[\sqrt{\pi_1(\boldsymbol{\theta})} - \sqrt{\pi_2(\boldsymbol{\theta})}\right]^2 d\boldsymbol{\theta} \cdot \int_\Omega \left[\sqrt{\pi_1(\boldsymbol{\theta})} + \sqrt{\pi_2(\boldsymbol{\theta})}\right]^2 d\boldsymbol{\theta}. \tag{5.A.20}$$

It is easy to see that

$$\int_\Omega \left[\sqrt{\pi_1(\boldsymbol{\theta})} + \sqrt{\pi_2(\boldsymbol{\theta})}\right]^2 d\boldsymbol{\theta} \leq 2\int_\Omega [\pi_1(\boldsymbol{\theta}) + \pi_2(\boldsymbol{\theta})]\ d\boldsymbol{\theta} = 4. \tag{5.A.21}$$

Thus, (5.5.12) follows from (5.A.20) and (5.A.21). □

Proof of Theorem 5.5.5. Write $f_n(\boldsymbol{\theta}) = p_1(\boldsymbol{\theta})/\psi_n(\boldsymbol{\theta})$ and $g_n(\boldsymbol{\theta}) = p_2(\boldsymbol{\theta})/\psi_n(\boldsymbol{\theta})$. By (5.A.15), we have

$$\begin{aligned} & nE\left(\frac{(\hat{r}_{\mathrm{RIS},n} - r)^2}{r^2}\,\middle|\, \boldsymbol{\theta}_1, \boldsymbol{\theta}_2, \ldots, \boldsymbol{\theta}_n\right) \\ &\quad - r^{-2}c_2^{-4}\int_\Omega \{c_2 f_n(\boldsymbol{\theta}) - c_1 g_n(\boldsymbol{\theta})\}^2 \psi_n(\boldsymbol{\theta})\ d\boldsymbol{\theta} \\ &= c_2^{-4} r^{-2} n^{-1} E\left\{\frac{\left(\sum_{i=1}^n (c_2 f_n(\boldsymbol{\vartheta}_{n,i}) - c_1 g_n(\boldsymbol{\vartheta}_{n,i}))\right)^2}{(\sum_{i=1}^n g_n(\boldsymbol{\vartheta}_{n,i}))^2}\right. \\ &\quad \left.\times \sum_{i=1}^n (c_2 - g_n(\boldsymbol{\vartheta}_{n,i})) \cdot \sum_{i=1}^n (c_2 + g_n(\boldsymbol{\vartheta}_{n,i}))\,\middle|\, \tau_n\right\} \\ &\stackrel{\text{def}}{=} c_2^{-4} r^{-2} \eta_n. \end{aligned}$$

By the law of large numbers, we have

$$\tau_n \rightarrow r \text{ a.s. as } n \rightarrow \infty, \tag{5.A.22}$$

and hence

$$\begin{aligned} &\lim_{n\rightarrow\infty} r^{-2} c_2^{-4} \int_\Omega \{c_2 f_n(\boldsymbol{\theta}) - c_1 g_n(\boldsymbol{\theta})\}^2 \psi_n(\boldsymbol{\theta})\ d\boldsymbol{\theta} \\ &\quad = \left[\int_\Omega \left|\frac{p_1(\boldsymbol{\theta})}{c_1} - \frac{p_2(\boldsymbol{\theta})}{c_2}\right| d\boldsymbol{\theta}\right]^2 \text{ a.s.} \end{aligned}$$

To finish the proof of the theorem, it suffices to show that

$$\eta_n \rightarrow 0 \text{ a.s. as } n \rightarrow \infty. \tag{5.A.23}$$

Let

$$G_n = \sum_{i=1}^{n} g_n(\boldsymbol{\vartheta}_{n,i}) \text{ and } T_n = \sum_{i=1}^{n} (c_2 f_n(\boldsymbol{\vartheta}_{n,i}) - c_1 g_n(\boldsymbol{\vartheta}_{n,i})).$$

Note that

$$\begin{aligned}
|\eta_n| &= \left| E\left\{ \frac{T_n^2 \cdot (nc_2 - G_n)\cdot(nc_2 + G_n)}{nG_n^2} \middle| \tau_n \right\} \right| \\
&\le 6n^{-1}E\{T_n^2 1\{|T_n| \ge n^{2/3}\}|\tau_n\} \\
&\quad + 6(nc_2)^{-1}n^{-1}E\{T_n^2|nc_2 - G_n| 1\{G_n \ge nc_2/2\}\, 1\{|T_n| \ge n^{2/3}\}|\tau_n\} \\
&\quad + 2(nc_2)^2 n^{-1} E\{(T_n/G_n)^2 1\{G_n \le nc_2/2\}|\tau_n\} \\
&\le n^{-1}E\{T_n^2 1\{|T_n| \ge n^{2/3}\}|\tau_n\} + 6c_2^{-1}n^{-2/3}E\{|nc_2 - G_n||\tau_n\} \\
&\quad + 2(nc_2)^2 n^{-1} E\{(T_n/G_n)^2 1\{G_n \le nc_2/2\}|\tau_n\} \\
&\stackrel{\text{def}}{=} \eta_{n,1} + \eta_{n,2} + \eta_{n,3}.
\end{aligned} \tag{5.A.24}$$

Since T_n is a partial sum of i.i.d random variables under the given τ_n, by (5.A.22) and (ii), we have

$$\begin{aligned}
\eta_{n,1} &\le K(n^{-1/15}) + E\{(c_2 f_n(\boldsymbol{\vartheta}_{n,1}) - c_1 g_n(\boldsymbol{\vartheta}_{n,1}))^2 \\
&\quad \times 1\{|c_2 f_n(\boldsymbol{\vartheta}_{n,1}) - c_1 g_n(\boldsymbol{\vartheta}_{n,1})| \ge n^{1/15}\}|\tau_n\} \\
&\le K(n^{-1/15}) + \int_{\{\boldsymbol{\theta}: |c_2 p_1(\boldsymbol{\theta}) - c_1 p_2(\boldsymbol{\theta})| \ge n^{1/15}\psi_n(\boldsymbol{\theta})\}} \frac{|c_2 p_1(\boldsymbol{\theta}) - c_1 p_2(\boldsymbol{\theta})|^2}{\psi_n(\boldsymbol{\theta})}\, d\boldsymbol{\theta} \\
&\stackrel{\text{a.s.}}{\to} 0 \text{ as } n \to \infty,
\end{aligned}$$

where K denotes a positive constant not depending on n. Similarly, one has

$$\lim_{n\to\infty} \eta_{n,2} = 0 \text{ a.s.}$$

Note that for any positive random variable X with $EX = \mu$ and $EX^2 = \sigma^2$, and for any $0 < t < 1$,

$$\begin{aligned}
&E[\exp[t(\mu - X)] \\
&\le E\left\{ 1 + t(\mu - X) + (t(\mu - X))^2/2 + \sum_{k=3}^{\infty} \frac{(t(\mu - X))^k}{k!} 1\{\mu - X \ge 0\} \right\} \\
&\le 1 + t^2 EX^2 + (\mu t)^3 \exp(t\mu) \le \exp(t^2(EX^2 + e^{4\mu})).
\end{aligned}$$

Hence, for $0 < a < EX^2 + e^{4\mu}$,

$$\inf_{t>0} e^{-ta} E[\exp(t(\mu - X))] \le \exp(-\frac{a^2}{4(EX^2 + e^{4\mu})}). \tag{5.A.25}$$

By (5.A.25) and similar to (5.A.13), we have

$$P\left(\sum_{j=1}^{n-1} g_n(\boldsymbol{\vartheta}_{n,j}) \le nc_2/2 \middle| \tau_n\right) \le \left(\inf_{t>0} e^{-tc_2/4} E\{\exp[c_2 - g_n(\boldsymbol{\vartheta}_{n,1})] | \tau_n\}\right)^{n-1}$$
$$\le \exp\left(-\frac{(n-1)c_2^2}{64(e^{4c_2} + E\left\{g_n^2(\boldsymbol{\vartheta}_{n,1}) \middle| \tau_n\right\})}\right).$$

Thus, in terms of (5.A.22) and the conditions (ii) and (iii),

$$\limsup_{n\to\infty} \eta_{n,3} \le K \limsup_{n\to\infty} n^3 E\{(f_n(\boldsymbol{\vartheta}_{n,1})/g_n(\boldsymbol{\vartheta}_{n,1}))^2 | \tau_n\}$$
$$\times \exp\left(-\frac{(n-1)c_2^2}{64(e^{4c_2} + E\{g_n^2(\boldsymbol{\vartheta}_{n,1}) \middle| \tau_n\})}\right) = 0 \text{ a.s.}$$

Putting the above inequalities together yields (5.A.23). This proves the theorem. □

Proof of Theorem 5.5.6. Let

$$\zeta(x,t) = \frac{q_1(x)}{\psi q_1(x) + (1-\psi) t q_2(x)}.$$

Since $S_n(\hat{r}_{\text{BS}}, n) = 0$, we have

$$\sum_{i=1}^{n} \zeta(\boldsymbol{\theta}_i, \hat{r}_{\text{BS},n}) = n.$$

Note that for each fixed x, $\zeta(x,\cdot)$ is decreasing. Hence, $\forall\, x > 0$,

$$\{\hat{r}_{\text{BS},n} \ge x\} = \left\{\sum_{i=1}^{n} \zeta(\boldsymbol{\theta}_i, x) \ge n\right\}. \tag{5.A.26}$$

In particular, $\forall\ 0 < \varepsilon < r$,

$$P(\hat{r}_{\text{BS},n} \ge r + \varepsilon, \text{i.o.}) = P\left(\sum_{i=1}^{n} \zeta(\boldsymbol{\theta}_i, r+\varepsilon) \ge n, \text{i.o.}\right)$$

and

$$P(\hat{r}_{\text{BS},n} \le r - \varepsilon, \text{i.o.}) = P\left(\sum_{i=1}^{n} \zeta(\boldsymbol{\theta}_i, r-\varepsilon) \le n, \text{i.o.}\right).$$

Noting that for $x > 0$

$$E_{\pi_{\text{mix}}}\zeta(\boldsymbol{\theta},x) = \int_\Omega \frac{q_1(\boldsymbol{\theta})(\psi\pi_1(\boldsymbol{\theta}) + (1-\psi)\pi_2(\boldsymbol{\theta}))}{\psi q_1(\boldsymbol{\theta}) + (1-\psi)x\, q_2(\boldsymbol{\theta})}\, d\boldsymbol{\theta}$$

$$\begin{cases} < 1 & \text{if } x > r, \\ = 1 & \text{if } x = r, \\ > 1 & \text{if } x < r, \end{cases} \tag{5.A.27}$$

and by the strong law of large numbers, we have

$$P\left(\sum_{i=1}^n \zeta(\boldsymbol{\theta}_i, r+\varepsilon) \geq n, \text{i.o.}\right) = 0$$

and

$$P\left(\sum_{i=1}^n \zeta(\boldsymbol{\theta}_i, r-\varepsilon) \leq n, \text{i.o.}\right) = 0.$$

This proves (5.5.18). Write $\lambda(x) = E_{\pi_{\text{mix}}}(\zeta(\boldsymbol{\theta},x)-1)$. Then, by (5.A.27), $\lambda(r) = 0$ and

$$\dot{\lambda}(x) = \frac{d\lambda(x)}{dx} = -(1-\psi)\int_\Omega \frac{q_1(\boldsymbol{\theta})q_2(\boldsymbol{\theta})(\psi\pi_1(\boldsymbol{\theta}) + (1-\psi)\pi_2(\boldsymbol{\theta}))}{(\psi q_1(\boldsymbol{\theta}) + (1-\psi)xq_2(\boldsymbol{\theta}))^2}\, d\boldsymbol{\theta}.$$

In particular,

$$\dot{\lambda}(r) = -(1-\psi)(c_2/c_1)\int_\Omega \frac{\pi_1(\boldsymbol{\theta})\cdot\pi_2(\boldsymbol{\theta})}{\psi\pi_1(\boldsymbol{\theta}) + (1-\psi)\pi_2(\boldsymbol{\theta})}\, d\boldsymbol{\theta}.$$

By a strong Bahadur representation of He and Shao (1996) or Janssen, Jureckova, and Veraverbeke (1985),

$$\hat{r}_{\text{BS},n} - r = -\frac{1}{n}\sum_{i=1}^n (\zeta(\boldsymbol{\theta}_i, r) - 1)/\dot{\lambda}(r) + o(n^{-1}(\ln n)^3) \text{ a.s.},$$

which implies immediately, by the central limit theorem,

$$\sqrt{n}(\hat{r}_{\text{BS},n} - r) \xrightarrow{\mathcal{D}} N(0,\sigma^2), \tag{5.A.28}$$

where

$$\begin{aligned}\sigma^2 &= \text{Var}(\zeta(\boldsymbol{\theta}_1, r))/(\dot{\lambda}(r))^2 \\ &= r^2\left[\int_\Omega \frac{(\pi_1(\boldsymbol{\theta}) - \pi_2(\boldsymbol{\theta}))^2}{\psi\pi_1(\boldsymbol{\theta}) + (1-\psi)\pi_2(\boldsymbol{\theta})}\, d\boldsymbol{\theta}\right. \\ &\quad \left.\times\left\{\int_\Omega \frac{\pi_1(\boldsymbol{\theta})\cdot\pi_2(\boldsymbol{\theta})}{\psi\pi_1(\boldsymbol{\theta}) + (1-\psi)\pi_2(\boldsymbol{\theta})}\, d\boldsymbol{\theta}\right\}^{-2}\right].\end{aligned}$$

In terms of (5.A.26), as in the proof of Theorem 5.5.1, one can show that $\{n(\hat{r}_{\text{BS},n} - r)^2, n \geq 1\}$ is uniformly integrable. Thus, (5.5.19) follows from

(5.A.28). □

Proof of Theorem 5.8.2. We prove the theorem in turn for IS, BS, and RIS.

For IS, from Lemma 5.8.1, we take $h(y) = y - 1$, which is an increasing function of y, and $g(x) = x^2$, which is convex. Therefore, Theorem 5.8.1 implies that the lower bound of $\text{ARE}^2(\hat{r}_{\text{IS}}(w))$ is $\int_{\Omega_1} \pi_1^2(\boldsymbol{\theta})/\pi_{21}(\boldsymbol{\theta})\, d\boldsymbol{\theta} - 1$. Since the equality holds in (I) of Theorem 5.8.1, this lower bound is attained at $w = \pi_2(\psi|\boldsymbol{\theta})$. This proves the optimality result for IS.

For BS, analogous to the proof of Theorem 5.3.1, by Lemma 5.8.2 and the Cauchy–Schwarz inequality, for all $\alpha(\boldsymbol{\theta}, \psi)$,

$$\text{ARE}^2(\hat{r}_{\text{BS}}(w, \alpha)) \geq \frac{1}{s_1 s_2} \left\{ \left(\int_{\Theta_1 \cap \Theta_2} \frac{\pi_1(\boldsymbol{\theta}) w(\psi|\boldsymbol{\theta}) \pi_2(\boldsymbol{\theta}, \psi)}{s_1 \pi_1(\boldsymbol{\theta}) w(\psi|\boldsymbol{\theta}) + s_2 \pi_2(\boldsymbol{\theta}, \psi)}\, d\boldsymbol{\theta}\, d\psi \right)^{-1} - 1 \right\}.$$

We take $h(y) = (1/s_1 s_2)(1/y - 1)$ and $g(x) = x/(s_1 x + s_2)$. Then $h(y)$ is a decreasing function of y and $g''(x) = -2 s_1 s_2/(s_1 x + s_2)^3 < 0$ which implies that g is concave. Therefore, Theorem 5.8.1 yields that the lower bound of $\text{ARE}^2(\hat{r}_{\text{BS}}(w, \alpha))$ is

$$\frac{1}{s_1 s_2} \left\{ \left(\int_{\Omega_1 \cap \Omega_2} \frac{\pi_1(\boldsymbol{\theta}) \pi_{21}(\boldsymbol{\theta})}{s_1 \pi_1(\boldsymbol{\theta}) + s_2 \pi_{21}(\boldsymbol{\theta})}\, d\boldsymbol{\theta} \right)^{-1} - 1 \right\}. \tag{5.A.29}$$

Although the equality does not hold in (I) of Theorem 5.8.1, it can be easily verified that the lower bound (5.A.29) is attained at $w = w_{\text{opt}}^{\text{BS}}$ and $\alpha = \alpha_{\text{opt}}$. This proves Theorem 5.8.2 for BS.

Finally, for RIS, by Lemma 5.8.3 and the Cauchy–Schwarz inequality, for an arbitrary density π,

$$\text{ARE}^2(\hat{r}_{\text{RIS}}(w, \pi)) \geq \left[\int_{\Theta_1 \cup \Theta_2} |\pi_1(\boldsymbol{\theta}) w(\psi|\boldsymbol{\theta}) - \pi_2(\boldsymbol{\theta}, \psi)|\, d\boldsymbol{\theta}\, d\psi \right]^2. \tag{5.A.30}$$

Now we take $h(y) = y^2$ and $g(x) = |x - 1|$. Obviously, $h(y)$ is an increasing function of y for $y > 0$ and $g(x)$ is convex. Therefore, from Theorem 5.8.1 the lower bound of $\text{ARE}^2(\hat{r}_{\text{RIS}}(w, \pi))$ is

$$\left[\int_{\Omega_1 \cup \Omega_2} |\pi_1(\boldsymbol{\theta}) - \pi_{21}(\boldsymbol{\theta})|\, d\boldsymbol{\theta} \right]^2.$$

Note that since the region of integration on the right side of inequality (5.A.30) is bigger than the support of π_2, Theorem 5.8.1 needs an obvious adjustment. Plugging $w = w_{\text{opt}}^{\text{RIS}}$ and $\pi = \pi_{\text{opt}}$ into (5.8.7) leads to (5.8.11). This completes the proof of Theorem 5.8.2. □

Proof of Theorem 5.11.1. Write

$$
\begin{aligned}
&\hat{r}(\hat{a}_{\text{opt}}) - r \\
&\quad = \frac{1}{c_2 \sum_{j=1}^{\kappa} \hat{p}_j^2/\hat{b}_j} \sum_{l=1}^{\kappa} \frac{\hat{p}_l}{\hat{b}_l} \left(\frac{1}{n} \sum_{i=1}^{n} c_2 \hat{a}_{\text{opt},l} \left[\frac{q_1(\boldsymbol{\theta}_{2,i})}{q_2(\boldsymbol{\theta}_{2,i})} \right] 1\{\boldsymbol{\theta}_{2,i} \in A_l\} - c_1 \hat{p}_l \right) \\
&\quad := \frac{1}{c_2 \sum_{j=1}^{\kappa} \hat{p}_j^2/\hat{b}_j} \times R
\end{aligned}
$$

and

$$
\begin{aligned}
R &= \sum_{l=1}^{\kappa} \frac{\hat{p}_l}{\hat{b}_l} \left(\frac{1}{n} \sum_{i=1}^{n} c_2 \hat{a}_{\text{opt},l} \left[\frac{q_1(\boldsymbol{\theta}_{2,i})}{q_2(\boldsymbol{\theta}_{2,i})} \right] 1\{\boldsymbol{\theta}_{2,i} \in A_l\} - c_1 p_l \right) \\
&\quad + c_1 \sum_{l=1}^{\kappa} \frac{\hat{p}_l}{\hat{b}_l} (p_l - \hat{p}_l) \\
&= \sum_{l=1}^{\kappa} \frac{p_l}{\hat{b}_l} \left(\frac{1}{n} \sum_{i=1}^{n} c_2 \hat{a}_{\text{opt},l} \left[\frac{q_1(\boldsymbol{\theta}_{2,i})}{q_2(\boldsymbol{\theta}_{2,i})} \right] 1\{\boldsymbol{\theta}_{2,i} \in A_l\} - c_1 p_l \right) \\
&\quad + \sum_{l=1}^{\kappa} \frac{\hat{p}_l - p_l}{\hat{b}_l} \left(\frac{1}{n} \sum_{i=1}^{n} c_2 \hat{a}_{\text{opt},l} \left[\frac{q_1(\boldsymbol{\theta}_{2,i})}{q_2(\theta_{2,i})} \right] 1\{\boldsymbol{\theta}_{2,i} \in A_l\} - c_1 p_l \right) \\
&\quad + c_1 \sum_{l=1}^{\kappa} \frac{\hat{p}_l}{\hat{b}_l} (p_l - \hat{p}_l) \\
&= \sum_{l=1}^{\kappa} \frac{p_l}{b_l} \left(\frac{1}{n} \sum_{i=1}^{n} c_2 \hat{a}_{\text{opt},l} \left[\frac{q_1(\boldsymbol{\theta}_{2,i})}{q_2(\theta_{2,i})} \right] 1\{\boldsymbol{\theta}_{2,i} \in A_l\} - c_1 p_l \right) \\
&\quad + \sum_{l=1}^{\kappa} \left(\frac{p_l}{\hat{b}_l} - \frac{p_l}{b_l} \right) \left(\frac{1}{n} \sum_{i=1}^{n} c_2 \hat{a}_{\text{opt},l} \left[\frac{q_1(\boldsymbol{\theta}_{2,i})}{q_2(\boldsymbol{\theta}_{2,i})} \right] 1\{\boldsymbol{\theta}_{2,i} \in A_l\} - c_1 p_l \right) \\
&\quad + \sum_{l=1}^{\kappa} \frac{\hat{p}_l - p_l}{\hat{b}_l} \left(\frac{1}{n} \sum_{i=1}^{n} c_2 \hat{a}_{\text{opt},l} \left[\frac{q_1(\boldsymbol{\theta}_{2,i})}{q_2(\boldsymbol{\theta}_{2,i})} \right] 1\{\boldsymbol{\theta}_{2,i} \in A_l\} - c_1 p_l \right) \\
&\quad + c_1 \sum_{l=1}^{\kappa} \frac{\hat{p}_l}{\hat{b}_l} (p_l - \hat{p}_l) \\
&:= R_1 + R_2 + R_3 + R_4.
\end{aligned}
$$

It follows from the law of large numbers that

$$
\frac{1}{c_2 \sum_{j=1}^{\kappa} \hat{p}_j^2/\hat{b}_j} \to \frac{1}{c_2 \sum_{j=1}^{\kappa} p_j^2/b_j} \text{ a.s.}
$$

By the assumption that $n = o(m)$, we have

$$
E(R_2^2) + E(R_3^2) + E(R_4^2) = o(1/n)
$$

and

$$\frac{E(R_1^2)}{(c_2\sum_{j=1}^{\kappa} p_j^2/b_j)^2} = \frac{1}{n}\left(\frac{1}{\sum_{l=1}^{\kappa} p_l^2/b_l} - r^2\right)$$

by (5.11.7). This proves (5.11.11) by the above inequalities. □

Exercises

5.1 For $\hat{r}_{\text{IS}_2}$ given in (5.2.5), show that

$$nr^{-2}\operatorname{Var}(\hat{r}_{\text{IS}_2}) = E_2\left(\frac{\pi_1(\boldsymbol{\theta}) - \pi_2(\boldsymbol{\theta})}{\pi_2(\boldsymbol{\theta})}\right)^2 \geq \frac{\left[E_1(\sqrt{\pi_1(\boldsymbol{\theta})})\right]^2}{E_2(\pi_1(\boldsymbol{\theta}))} - 1.$$

[*Hint*: Use the Cauchy–Schwartz inequality.]
This result implies that if the two densities π_1 and π_2 have very little overlap, i.e., $E_2(\pi_1(\boldsymbol{\theta}))$ is small, then the variance, $\operatorname{Var}(\hat{r}_{\text{IS}_2})$, of $\hat{r}_{\text{IS}_2}$ is large, and therefore, this importance sampling-based method works poorly.

5.2 Prove the identity given in (5.3.1).

5.3 Geometric Bridge
Let $\alpha_G(\boldsymbol{\theta}) = [q_1(\boldsymbol{\theta})q_2(\boldsymbol{\theta})]^{-1/2}$. With $\alpha(\boldsymbol{\theta}) = \alpha_G(\boldsymbol{\theta})$, the resulting BS estimator $\hat{r}_{\text{BS}}$ given in (5.3.3) is called a geometric bridge sampling (GBS) estimator of r. Show that $\text{RE}^2(\hat{r}_{\text{BS}})$ given in (5.3.4) reduces to

$$\text{RE}_G^2 = \frac{1}{ns_1s_2}\left\{\frac{\int_{\Omega_1\cap\Omega_2}[s_1\pi_1(\boldsymbol{\theta}) + s_2\pi_2(\boldsymbol{\theta})]\,d\boldsymbol{\theta}}{(\int_{\Omega_1\cap\Omega_2}[\pi_1(\boldsymbol{\theta})\pi_2(\boldsymbol{\theta})]^{1/2}\,d\boldsymbol{\theta})^2} - 1\right\} + o\left(\frac{1}{n}\right). \tag{5.E.1}$$

Further show that the first term on the right side of (5.E.1) is equal to

$$\frac{1}{ns_1s_2}\left\{\frac{\int_{\Omega_1\cap\Omega_2}[s_1\pi_1(\boldsymbol{\theta}) + s_2\pi_2(\boldsymbol{\theta})]\,d\boldsymbol{\theta}}{(1 - \frac{1}{2}H^2(\pi_1,\pi_2))^2} - 1\right\},$$

where $H(\pi_1,\pi_2)$ is the Hellinger divergence defined in (5.4.7).

5.4 Power Family Bridge
Let

$$\alpha_{k,A}(\boldsymbol{\theta}) = [q_1^{1/k}(\boldsymbol{\theta}) + (Aq_2(\boldsymbol{\theta}))^{1/k}]^{-k}.$$

With $\alpha(\boldsymbol{\theta}) = \alpha_{k,A}(\boldsymbol{\theta})$, the resulting BS estimator $\hat{r}_{\text{BS}}$ given in (5.3.3) is called a power family bridge sampling (PFBS) estimator of r. Show that:

(i) $\lim_{k\to\infty} 2^k \alpha_{k,A}(\boldsymbol{\theta}) = [Aq_1(\boldsymbol{\theta})q_2(\boldsymbol{\theta})]^{-1/2}$, which implies that when k approaches infinity, the PFBS estimator approaches the GBS estimator.

(ii) $\lim_{k\to 0} \alpha_{k,A}(\boldsymbol{\theta}) = 1/\max\{q_1(\boldsymbol{\theta}), Aq_2(\boldsymbol{\theta})\}$.

5.5 Prove the identity given by (5.4.1).

5.6 Prove Theorem 5.4.1.

5.7 A family of random variables $\{X_t,\ t \in T\}$ is said to be uniformly integrable if

$$\lim_{A\to\infty} \sup_{t\in T} E|X_t| 1\{|X_t| > A\} = 0.$$

Prove that $\{X_t,\ t \in T\}$ is uniformly integrable if $\sup_{t\in T} E|X_t|^q < \infty$ for some $q > 1$.

5.8 Prove that if $\{T_n, n \geq 1\}$ and $\{S_n, n \geq 1\}$ are uniformly integrable, so is $\{T_n + S_n,\ n \geq 1\}$.

5.9 Let $X_1, X_2, \ldots$ be i.i.d. random variables with $EX_i = 0$ and $EX_i^2 = 1$. Prove that $\{n^{-1}S_n^2,\ n \geq 1\}$ is uniformly integrable where $S_n = \sum_{i=1}^n X_i$.

5.10 Verify (5.A.26).

5.11 Consider the normal family $N(\mu(t), \sigma^2(t))$.

(i) Show that the Euler–Lagrange equation given in (5.4.9) with $k = 1$ reduces to

$$\ddot{\mu}(t) = 0. \tag{5.E.2}$$

(ii) Given $\sigma^2 = 1$, and the boundary conditions $\mu(0) = 0$ and $\mu(t) = \delta$, find the solution of the Euler–Lagrange equation given in (5.E.2).

(iii) Show that the Euler–Lagrange equation given in (5.4.9) with $k = 2$ becomes

$$\begin{cases} \dot{\mu}(t) - c_0\sigma^2(t) = 0, \\ 3\ddot{\sigma}(t)\sigma(t) - 3\dot{\sigma}^2(t) + \dot{\mu}^2(t) = 0, \end{cases} \tag{5.E.3}$$

where c_0 is a constant to be determined from the boundary conditions.

(iv) Given the boundary conditions:

$$(\mu(0), \sigma^2(0))' = (0, 1)' \text{ and } (\mu(1), \sigma^2(1))' = (\delta, 1)',$$

find the solution of the differential equation (5.E.3).

5.12 Derive Table 5.1.

5.13 A Simulation Study

Consider Case 1 of Section 5.6.

(i) Use the inverse cdf method of Devroye (1986, pp. 27–35) to generate a random sample of size n from the optimal RIS cumulative distribution function $\Pi_{\text{opt}}(\boldsymbol{\theta})$ given in (5.6.3) and compute $\hat{r}_{\text{RIS}}$ given in (5.5.2) with the optimal $\pi_{\text{opt}}(\boldsymbol{\theta})$ given in (5.6.1).

(ii) Repeat (i) m times and then use the standard macro-repetition simulation technique to obtain an estimate of $nE(\hat{r}-r)^2/r^2$. (*Hint*: Here $r=1$.)

(iii) Compare your estimates to the theoretical result given in Table 5.1 for different values of n and m. Discuss your findings from this simulation study.

5.14 Derive Table 5.2.

5.15 Prove Lemmas 5.8.1, 5.8.2, and 5.8.3.

5.16 Prove Theorem 5.8.1.

5.17 Assuming that $\Psi(\boldsymbol{\theta}) = \Psi \subset R^m$ for all $\boldsymbol{\theta} \in \Omega_2$ and $\Omega_1 \subset \Omega_2$, we have the identity

$$r = E_{\pi_2}\{q_2(\boldsymbol{\theta}^*, \boldsymbol{\psi}) q_1(\boldsymbol{\theta}) / q_2(\boldsymbol{\theta}, \boldsymbol{\psi})\} / c(\boldsymbol{\theta}^*),$$

where $\pi_2(\boldsymbol{\theta}, \boldsymbol{\psi}) \propto q_2(\boldsymbol{\theta}, \boldsymbol{\psi})$, $c(\boldsymbol{\theta}^*) = \int_\Psi q_2(\boldsymbol{\theta}^*, \boldsymbol{\psi})\, d\boldsymbol{\psi}$, and $\boldsymbol{\theta}^* \in \Omega_2$ is a fixed point. Thus, a marginal-likelihood estimator of r can be defined by

$$\hat{r}_{\text{ML}} = \left\{ \frac{1}{n} \sum_{i=1}^n \frac{q_2(\boldsymbol{\theta}^*, \boldsymbol{\psi}_i) q_1(\boldsymbol{\theta}_i)}{q_2(\boldsymbol{\theta}_i, \boldsymbol{\psi}_i)} \right\} \cdot \left\{ \frac{1}{n} \sum_{i=1}^n \frac{w^*(\boldsymbol{\psi}_i^* | \boldsymbol{\theta}^*)}{p_2(\boldsymbol{\theta}^*, \boldsymbol{\psi}_i^*)} \right\},$$

where $\{(\boldsymbol{\theta}_i, \boldsymbol{\psi}_i),\ i = 1, 2, \dots, n\}$ and $\{\boldsymbol{\psi}_i^*,\ i = 1, 2, \dots, n\}$ are two independent random samples from $\pi_2(\boldsymbol{\theta}, \boldsymbol{\psi})$ and $\pi_2(\boldsymbol{\psi}|\boldsymbol{\theta}^*)$ (the conditional density of $\boldsymbol{\psi}$ given $\boldsymbol{\theta}^*$), respectively, and $w^*(\boldsymbol{\psi}|\boldsymbol{\theta}^*)$ is an arbitrary (completely known) density defined on Ψ.

(a) Verify that

$$\begin{aligned} \text{Var}(\hat{r}_{\text{ML}}) = r^2 & \left[\frac{1}{n} \left\{ \int_{\Omega_1} \frac{\pi_1^2(\boldsymbol{\theta})}{\pi_{21}(\boldsymbol{\theta})} \left(\int_\Psi \frac{\pi_2^2(\boldsymbol{\psi}|\boldsymbol{\theta}^*)}{\pi_2(\boldsymbol{\psi}|\boldsymbol{\theta})}\, d\boldsymbol{\psi} \right) d\boldsymbol{\theta} - 1 \right\} + 1 \right] \\ & \times \left[\frac{1}{n} \left\{ \int_\Psi \frac{w^{*2}(\boldsymbol{\psi}|\boldsymbol{\theta}^*)}{\pi_2(\boldsymbol{\psi}|\boldsymbol{\theta}^*)}\, d\boldsymbol{\psi} - 1 \right\} + 1 \right] - r^2. \end{aligned}$$

(b) Further show that for all $w^*(\boldsymbol{\psi}|\boldsymbol{\theta}^*)$

$$\text{Var}(\hat{r}_{\text{ML}}) \geq \text{Var}(\hat{r}_{\text{OIS}}),$$

where $\text{Var}(\hat{r}_{\text{OIS}}) = (r^2/n)\text{ARE}^2(\hat{r}_{\text{OIS}})$ given in (5.8.9). Hence, $\hat{r}_{\text{ML}}$ is not as good as $\hat{r}_{\text{OIS}}$.

5.18 Prove the Savage–Dickey density ratio given in (5.10.5) and the generalized Savage–Dickey density ratio given in (5.10.6). Also show that (5.10.5) is a special case of (5.10.6).

5.19 Similar to the IS estimator $\hat{r}_{\text{IS}_2}$, derive the weighted versions of the BS estimator $\hat{r}_{\text{BS}}$ and the RIS estimator $\hat{r}_{\text{RIS}}$ given by (5.3.3) and (5.5.2), respectively.

6

Monte Carlo Methods for Constrained Parameter Problems

Constraints on the parameters in Bayesian hierarchical models typically make Bayesian computation and analysis complicated. Posterior densities that contain analytically intractable integrals as normalizing constants that depend on the hyperparameters often lead to implementation of Gibbs sampling or Metropolis–Hastings algorithms difficult. In this chapter, we use simulation-based methods via the "reweighting mixtures" of Geyer (1994) to compute posterior quantities of the desired Bayesian posterior distribution.

6.1 Constrained Parameter Problems

As discussed in Gelfand, Smith, and Lee (1992), constrained parameter problems arise in a wide variety of applications, including bioassay, actuarial graduation, ordinal categorical data, response surfaces, reliability development testing, and variance component models. Truncated data problems, to be understood as encompassing both censoring and scoring or grouping mechanisms, arise naturally in survival and failure time studies, ordinal data models, and categorical data studies aimed at uncovering underlying continuous distributions. In many applications, parameter constraints and data truncation occur. Gelfand, Smith, and Lee (1992) show that Bayesian calculations can be implemented routinely for such constrained parameter and truncated data problems by means of Markov chain Monte Carlo (MCMC) sampling. However, Bayesian computation can become extremely challenging when constraints are imposed on lower-level parameters while higher-level parameters are random in a Bayesian hierarchical model. This typically leads to a posterior density which contains analytically intractable normalizing constants that depend on higher-level parameters or hyperparameters. We note that such containing constrained parameter problems also arise in Bayesian inference using weighted distributions; see, for example, Larose and Dey (1996). As a result of the computational difficulties, one often avoids these problems either by specifying the values of the hyperparameters or by simply ignoring the normalizing constants. This, however, leads to an incorrect Bayesian formulation of the model. Due to recent developments on computing normalizing constants (see Chapter 5 for details), it is now possible to carry out this difficult computational problem using Monte Carlo (MC) methods.

Throughout this chapter, we assume that $\boldsymbol{\theta}$ is a p-dimensional parameter vector and $\boldsymbol{\lambda}$ denotes a k-dimensional parameter vector. Typically, $\boldsymbol{\theta}$ contains the parameters of interest and $\boldsymbol{\lambda}$ is a vector of hyper- or nuisance parameters. Let the posterior distribution be of the form

$$\pi(\boldsymbol{\theta},\boldsymbol{\lambda}|D) = \frac{1}{c_w} L(\boldsymbol{\theta}|D) \times \frac{\pi(\boldsymbol{\theta}|\boldsymbol{\lambda})}{c(\boldsymbol{\lambda})} 1\{\boldsymbol{\theta} \in \Theta\} \times \pi(\boldsymbol{\lambda}) 1\{\boldsymbol{\lambda} \in \Lambda\}, \tag{6.1.1}$$

where D denotes *data*, $L(\boldsymbol{\theta}|D)$ is the likelihood function, $\pi(\boldsymbol{\theta}|\boldsymbol{\lambda})$ and $\pi(\boldsymbol{\lambda})$ are priors, and

$$c(\boldsymbol{\lambda}) = \int_{\Theta} \pi(\boldsymbol{\theta}|\boldsymbol{\lambda})\, d\boldsymbol{\theta}. \tag{6.1.2}$$

Here, the constrained space Θ is a subset of R^p that may or may not depend on the data according to the nature of the problem, and $\Lambda \subset R^k$ is the support of $\pi(\boldsymbol{\lambda})$. In (6.1.1), the support of $\pi(\boldsymbol{\theta},\boldsymbol{\lambda}|D)$ is

$$\Omega = \Theta \otimes \Lambda = \{(\boldsymbol{\theta},\boldsymbol{\lambda}):\ \boldsymbol{\theta} \in \Theta \ \text{ and } \ \boldsymbol{\lambda} \in \Lambda\},$$

$$c_w = \int_{\Omega} L(\boldsymbol{\theta}|D)\{\pi(\boldsymbol{\theta}|\boldsymbol{\lambda})/c(\boldsymbol{\lambda})\}\pi(\boldsymbol{\lambda})\, d\boldsymbol{\theta}\, d\boldsymbol{\lambda},$$

and the indicator function $1\{\boldsymbol{\theta} \in \Theta\} = 1$ if $\boldsymbol{\theta} \in \Theta$ and 0 otherwise. We also define a pseudo-posterior density by

$$\pi^*(\boldsymbol{\theta},\boldsymbol{\lambda}|D) = \frac{1}{c^*} L(\boldsymbol{\theta}|D)\pi(\boldsymbol{\theta}|\boldsymbol{\lambda}) 1\{\boldsymbol{\theta} \in \Theta\}\pi(\boldsymbol{\lambda}) 1\{\boldsymbol{\lambda} \in \Lambda\}, \tag{6.1.3}$$

where

$$c^* = \int_{\Omega} L(\boldsymbol{\theta}|D)\pi(\boldsymbol{\theta}|\boldsymbol{\lambda})\pi(\boldsymbol{\lambda})\, d\boldsymbol{\theta}\, d\boldsymbol{\lambda}.$$

It can be shown that $c_w = c^* E_{\pi^*}\{1/c(\boldsymbol{\lambda})\}$, where the expectation E_{π^*} is taken with respect to $\pi^*(\boldsymbol{\theta},\boldsymbol{\lambda}|D)$. This convention will be used throughout this chapter.

Without the constraints, $\pi(\boldsymbol{\theta}|\boldsymbol{\lambda})$ is a completely known density function, i.e., $\int_{R^p} \pi(\boldsymbol{\theta}|\boldsymbol{\lambda})\, d\boldsymbol{\theta} = 1$. Note that $c(\boldsymbol{\lambda})$ is a normalizing constant of the density function $\pi(\boldsymbol{\theta}|\boldsymbol{\lambda})1\{\boldsymbol{\theta} \in \Theta\}$ or the conditional probability, $P(\boldsymbol{\theta} \in \Theta|\boldsymbol{\lambda})$, with respect to $\pi(\boldsymbol{\theta}|\boldsymbol{\lambda})$. Therefore, $0 < c(\boldsymbol{\lambda}) \leq 1$. As a result of the complexity of the constrained parameter space, Θ, analytical evaluation of $c(\boldsymbol{\lambda})$ is typically not available and $c(\boldsymbol{\lambda})$ often depends on the hyperparameter vector $\boldsymbol{\lambda}$, which makes Bayesian analysis very difficult. As Gelfand, Smith, and Lee (1992) note, directly sampling from $\pi(\boldsymbol{\theta}, \boldsymbol{\lambda}|D)$ is nearly impossible. Therefore, the Gibbs sampler (Geman and Geman 1984; Gelfand and Smith 1990) and the Metropolis–Hastings algorithm (Metropolis et al. 1953; Hastings 1970) either cannot be directly applied or are too expensive.

Borrowing the idea of reweighting mixtures from Geyer (1994, 1995b), we consider MC based methods to solve these difficult Bayesian computational problems. Since the pseudo-posterior density $\pi^*(\boldsymbol{\theta}, \boldsymbol{\lambda}|D)$ does not contain $c(\boldsymbol{\lambda})$, a natural choice of a proposal density for $\pi(\boldsymbol{\theta}, \boldsymbol{\lambda}|D)$ is $\pi^*(\boldsymbol{\theta}, \boldsymbol{\lambda}|D)$. For many Bayesian hierarchical models, it is possible to simulate from $\pi^*(\boldsymbol{\theta}, \boldsymbol{\lambda}|D)$ by using an MCMC sampling algorithm as in Section 6.4. Further, note that $\pi^*(\boldsymbol{\theta}, \boldsymbol{\lambda}|D)$ will serve as a good proposal density if $c(\boldsymbol{\lambda})$ is bounded away from 0. If the constraints naturally arise from a practical problem and the data support the constraints, the probability of the constrained parameter space should not be too small; see Chen and Deely (1996) for an example.

Using a random sample from $\pi^*(\boldsymbol{\theta}, \boldsymbol{\lambda}|D)$, we consider MC methods to compute the posterior quantities of interest in $\pi(\boldsymbol{\theta}, \boldsymbol{\lambda}|D)$. Thus, essentially as in Geyer (1994, 1995b), one obtains samples from one distribution but wants to do integration with respect to another distribution. In the next two sections, we illustrate how to estimate posterior quantities of $\pi(\boldsymbol{\theta}, \boldsymbol{\lambda}|D)$ based on a sample from $\pi^*(\boldsymbol{\theta}, \boldsymbol{\lambda}|D)$.

6.2 Posterior Moments and Marginal Posterior Densities

Throughout this section, we let $\{(\boldsymbol{\theta}_i, \boldsymbol{\lambda}_i), i = 1, 2, \ldots, n\}$ be a random sample from $\pi^*(\boldsymbol{\theta}, \boldsymbol{\lambda}|D)$ and we temporarily assume that $c(\boldsymbol{\lambda})$ is known.

First, we consider how to compute posterior moments. Let $h(\boldsymbol{\theta}, \boldsymbol{\lambda})$ be a function of $\boldsymbol{\theta}$ and $\boldsymbol{\lambda}$, and assume that $E_\pi\,|h(\boldsymbol{\theta}, \boldsymbol{\lambda})| < \infty$. Then

$$E_\pi\{h(\boldsymbol{\theta}, \boldsymbol{\lambda})\} = \frac{\displaystyle\int_\Omega \frac{h(\boldsymbol{\theta}, \boldsymbol{\lambda})}{c(\boldsymbol{\lambda})} \pi^*(\boldsymbol{\theta}, \boldsymbol{\lambda}|D)\, d\boldsymbol{\theta}\, d\boldsymbol{\lambda}}{\displaystyle\int_\Omega \frac{1}{c(\boldsymbol{\lambda})} \pi^*(\boldsymbol{\theta}, \boldsymbol{\lambda}|D)\, d\boldsymbol{\theta}\, d\boldsymbol{\lambda}}. \tag{6.2.1}$$

Typical forms of $h(\boldsymbol{\theta}, \boldsymbol{\lambda})$ are listed in Section 3.1. Using the sample $\{(\boldsymbol{\theta}_i, \boldsymbol{\lambda}_i), i = 1, 2, \ldots, n\}$, we estimate $E_\pi \{h(\boldsymbol{\theta}, \boldsymbol{\lambda})\}$ by

$$\hat{h} = \left\{ \sum_{i=1}^{n} \frac{h(\boldsymbol{\theta}_i, \boldsymbol{\lambda}_i)}{c(\boldsymbol{\lambda}_i)} \right\} \left\{ \sum_{i=1}^{n} \frac{1}{c(\boldsymbol{\lambda}_i)} \right\}^{-1} = \sum_{i=1}^{n} w_i h(\boldsymbol{\theta}_i, \boldsymbol{\lambda}_i), \quad (6.2.2)$$

where the weight w_i is defined as

$$\begin{aligned} w_i &= \frac{1}{c(\boldsymbol{\lambda}_i)} \left\{ \sum_{j=1}^{n} \frac{1}{c(\boldsymbol{\lambda}_j)} \right\}^{-1} = \left\{ \sum_{j=1}^{n} \frac{c(\boldsymbol{\lambda}_i)}{c(\boldsymbol{\lambda}_j)} \right\}^{-1} \\ &= \left\{ 1 + \sum_{j \neq i} \frac{c(\boldsymbol{\lambda}_i)}{c(\boldsymbol{\lambda}_j)} \right\}^{-1}. \end{aligned} \quad (6.2.3)$$

Thus w_i is a function of the normalizing constants $c(\boldsymbol{\lambda}_1)$, $c(\boldsymbol{\lambda}_2)$, $\ldots$, $c(\boldsymbol{\lambda}_n)$ with $0 \leq w_i \leq 1$.

A nice feature of (6.2.2) is that, whenever a random sample $\{(\boldsymbol{\theta}_i, \boldsymbol{\lambda}_i), i = 1, 2, \ldots, n\}$ is taken and w_i is computed, the same w_i can be used for calculating $\hat{h}$ for all h as long as $E_\pi |h(\boldsymbol{\theta}, \boldsymbol{\lambda})| < \infty$. For example, one obtains $\hat{h}$ and its posterior standard deviation using the same w_i. Finally, it is easy to observe that $\hat{h}$ is a consistent estimator of $E_\pi\{h(\boldsymbol{\theta}, \boldsymbol{\lambda})\}$, i.e.,

$$\hat{h} \longrightarrow E_\pi[h(\boldsymbol{\theta}, \boldsymbol{\lambda})] \text{ a.s. as } n \to \infty. \quad (6.2.4)$$

Next, we consider the computation of marginal posterior densities. If we use the IWMDE method discussed in Section 4.3, it can be observed that a marginal posterior density is indeed an integral-type posterior quantity if we choose an appropriate h.

Write $\boldsymbol{\theta} = (\boldsymbol{\theta}^{(p_0)}, \boldsymbol{\theta}^{(-p_0)})$, where $1 \leq p_0 \leq p$, $\boldsymbol{\theta}^{(p_0)}$ is the vector of p_0 components of $\boldsymbol{\theta}$, and $\boldsymbol{\theta}^{(-p_0)}$ is the vector of the remaining p - p_0 components. Let $\pi(\boldsymbol{\theta}^{*(p_0)}|D)$ be the joint marginal posterior density at a fixed point $\boldsymbol{\theta}^{*(p_0)}$. The support of the conditional posterior density of $\boldsymbol{\theta}^{(p_0)}$ given $\boldsymbol{\theta}^{(-p_0)}$ and $\boldsymbol{\lambda}$ is denoted by $\Theta_{p_0}(\boldsymbol{\theta}^{(-p_0)}, \boldsymbol{\lambda}) = \{\boldsymbol{\theta}^{(p_0)} : (\boldsymbol{\theta}^{(p_0)}, \boldsymbol{\theta}^{(-p_0)}, \boldsymbol{\lambda}) \in \Theta \times \Lambda\}$. We take

$$\begin{aligned} h(\boldsymbol{\theta}, \boldsymbol{\lambda}) &= \omega^*(\boldsymbol{\theta}^{(p_0)}|\boldsymbol{\theta}^{(-p_0)}, \boldsymbol{\lambda}) \\ &\quad \times \frac{L(\boldsymbol{\theta}^{*(p_0)}, \boldsymbol{\theta}^{(-p_0)}|D)\pi(\boldsymbol{\theta}^{*(p_0)}, \boldsymbol{\theta}^{(-p_0)}|\boldsymbol{\lambda})}{L(\boldsymbol{\theta}|D)\pi(\boldsymbol{\theta}|\boldsymbol{\lambda})}, \end{aligned} \quad (6.2.5)$$

where $\pi^*(\boldsymbol{\theta}, \boldsymbol{\lambda}|D)$ is given in (6.1.3) and $w^*(\boldsymbol{\theta}^{(p_0)}|\boldsymbol{\theta}^{(-p_0)}, \boldsymbol{\lambda})$ is a weight conditional density given $\boldsymbol{\theta}^{(-p_0)}$ and $\boldsymbol{\lambda}$, with support $\Theta_{p_0}(\boldsymbol{\theta}^{(-p_0)}, \boldsymbol{\lambda})$. It is then straightforward to show that (6.2.1) reduces to $\pi(\boldsymbol{\theta}^{*(p_0)}|D)$. Using the random sample $\{(\boldsymbol{\theta}_i, \boldsymbol{\lambda}_i), i = 1, 2, \ldots, n\}$, $\hat{h}$ defined by (6.2.2) gives an estimate, denoted by $\hat{\pi}(\boldsymbol{\theta}^{*(p_0)}|D)$, of $\pi(\boldsymbol{\theta}^{*(p_0)}|D)$. Section 4.3 shows that the optimal choice of w^* in (6.2.5), in the sense of minimizing the asymptotic variance, is the conditional posterior density of $\boldsymbol{\theta}^{(p_0)}$ given $\boldsymbol{\theta}^{(-p_0)}$ and $\boldsymbol{\lambda}$ with respect to the desired full posterior distribution $\pi(\boldsymbol{\theta}, \boldsymbol{\lambda}|D)$. Therefore, following the guidelines given in Section 4.3, we can choose a good conditional density $w^*(\boldsymbol{\theta}^{(p_0)}|\boldsymbol{\theta}^{(-p_0)}, \boldsymbol{\lambda})$ that has a shape roughly similar to that of the conditional posterior density of $\boldsymbol{\theta}^{(p_0)}$ given $\boldsymbol{\theta}^{(-p_0)}$ and $\boldsymbol{\lambda}$. Note that the same weights, $w_1, w_2, \ldots, w_n$, are used for estimating both posterior moments and marginal posterior densities for $\boldsymbol{\theta}$.

To obtain marginal densities for $\boldsymbol{\lambda}$, we write $\boldsymbol{\lambda} = (\boldsymbol{\lambda}^{(k_0)}, \boldsymbol{\lambda}^{(-k_0)})$, where $1 \le k_0 \le k$, $\boldsymbol{\lambda}^{(k_0)}$ is the vector of k_0 components of $\boldsymbol{\lambda}$, and $\boldsymbol{\lambda}^{(-k_0)}$ is the vector of the remaining $k - k_0$ components. The support of the conditional posterior density of $\boldsymbol{\lambda}^{(k_0)}$ given $\boldsymbol{\theta}$ and $\boldsymbol{\lambda}^{(-k_0)}$ is denoted by $\Lambda_{k_0}(\boldsymbol{\theta}, \boldsymbol{\lambda}^{(-k_0)}) = \{\boldsymbol{\lambda}^{(k_0)} : (\boldsymbol{\theta}, \boldsymbol{\lambda}^{(k_0)}, \boldsymbol{\lambda}^{(-k_0)}) \in \Theta \times \Lambda\}$. Let $\boldsymbol{\lambda}^{*(k_0)}$ be a fixed point and denote by $\pi(\boldsymbol{\lambda}^{*(k_0)}|D)$ the joint marginal posterior density for $\boldsymbol{\lambda}^{(k_0)}$. Analogous to (6.2.5), we take

$$\begin{aligned} h(\boldsymbol{\theta}, \boldsymbol{\lambda}) &= \frac{c(\boldsymbol{\lambda}) w^*(\boldsymbol{\lambda}^{(k_0)}|\boldsymbol{\theta}, \boldsymbol{\lambda}^{(-k_0)})}{c(\boldsymbol{\lambda}^{*(k_0)}, \boldsymbol{\lambda}^{(-k_0)})} \\ &\quad \times \frac{L(\boldsymbol{\theta}|D)\pi(\boldsymbol{\theta}|\boldsymbol{\lambda}^{*(k_0)}, \boldsymbol{\lambda}^{(-k_0)})\pi(\boldsymbol{\lambda}^{*(k_0)}, \boldsymbol{\lambda}^{(-k_0)})}{L(\boldsymbol{\theta}|D)\pi(\boldsymbol{\theta}|\boldsymbol{\lambda})\pi(\boldsymbol{\lambda})}, \end{aligned} \tag{6.2.6}$$

where $w^*(\boldsymbol{\lambda}^{(k_0)}|\boldsymbol{\theta}, \boldsymbol{\lambda}^{(-k_0)})$ is a weight conditional density of $\boldsymbol{\lambda}^{(k_0)}$ given $\boldsymbol{\theta}$ and $\boldsymbol{\lambda}^{(-k_0)}$ with support $\Lambda_{k_0}(\boldsymbol{\theta}, \boldsymbol{\lambda}^{(-k_0)})$. Then (6.2.1) and (6.2.2) lead to $\pi(\boldsymbol{\lambda}^{*(k_0)}|D)$ and its estimate $\hat{\pi}(\boldsymbol{\lambda}^{*(k_0)}|D)$, respectively. Note that, if the marginal posterior density $\pi(\boldsymbol{\lambda}^{(k_0)}|D)$ is to be evaluated at L points $\boldsymbol{\lambda}^{*(k_0)l}$, for $l = 1, 2, \ldots, L$, then $\hat{\pi}(\boldsymbol{\lambda}^{*(k_0)}|D)$ requires the evaluation of the normalizing constants $c(\boldsymbol{\lambda}_{(i)})$ and $c(\boldsymbol{\lambda}^{*(k_0)l}, \boldsymbol{\lambda}_i^{(-k_0)})$, where $\boldsymbol{\lambda}_i$ is partitioned as $(\boldsymbol{\lambda}_i^{(k_0)}, \boldsymbol{\lambda}_i^{(-k_0)})$, for $i = 1, 2, \ldots, n$ and $l = 1, 2, \ldots, L$. Therefore, estimation of marginal densities for $\boldsymbol{\lambda}$ is generally much more expensive than for $\boldsymbol{\theta}$.

Finally we note that, to obtain (6.2.4), we assume $\{(\boldsymbol{\theta}_i, \boldsymbol{\lambda}_i), i = 1, 2, \ldots, n\}$ is a random sample from $\pi^*(\boldsymbol{\theta}, \boldsymbol{\lambda}|D)$. However, if one uses an MCMC sample, (6.2.4) is still valid under some regularity conditions, such as ergodicity (see Section 3.2). Also note that $\hat{h}$, $\hat{\pi}(\boldsymbol{\theta}^{*(p_0)}|D)$ and $\hat{\pi}(\boldsymbol{\lambda}^{*(k_0)}|D)$ are not completely determined since the normalizing constants $c(\boldsymbol{\lambda}_i)$ and $c(\boldsymbol{\lambda}^{*(k_0)l}, \boldsymbol{\lambda}_i^{(-k_0)})$ are unknown. In the next section, we consider MC methods to estimate these unknown normalizing constants by an auxiliary MC simulation method.

6.3 Computing Normalizing Constants for Bayesian Estimation

Since marginal posterior densities are special cases of posterior moments, we only consider a general h in the rest of this section. In Chapter 5, we discuss MC based methods for estimating ratios of normalizing constants in detail. Here, however, for a given MC sample $\{(\boldsymbol{\theta}_i, \boldsymbol{\lambda}_i), i = 1, 2, \ldots, n\}$, a total of n or $L \times n$ normalizing constants must be evaluated simultaneously, and it will be inefficient or computationally expensive to estimate these ratios in a pairwise manner. Since $c(\boldsymbol{\lambda})$ is the normalizing constant of the density function $\pi(\boldsymbol{\theta}|\boldsymbol{\lambda})1\{\boldsymbol{\theta} \in \Theta\}$ and not of $\pi^*(\boldsymbol{\theta}, \boldsymbol{\lambda}|D)$, the sample from $\pi^*(\boldsymbol{\theta}, \boldsymbol{\lambda}|D)$ cannot be directly used to estimate $c(\boldsymbol{\lambda})$. Furthermore, there are infinitely many normalizing constants in $\{c(\boldsymbol{\lambda}),\ \boldsymbol{\lambda} \in \Lambda\}$ and the $\boldsymbol{\lambda}_i$ in the MC sample can be any points in Λ. The Bayesian constrained problems with normalizing constants are therefore different from that considered in Geyer (1994, 1995b), although the reweighting mixtures idea of Geyer (1994, 1995b) is still of use.

To develop an MC approach for computing ratios of normalizing constants, we let $\pi_{\mathrm{mix}}(\boldsymbol{\theta})$ be a mixing density with support Θ and known up to a normalizing constant, i.e.,

$$\pi_{\mathrm{mix}}(\boldsymbol{\theta}) = \frac{q_{\mathrm{mix}}(\boldsymbol{\theta})}{c_{\mathrm{mix}}}, \tag{6.3.1}$$

where $q_{\mathrm{mix}}(\boldsymbol{\theta})$ is completely known. Here we use the term "mixing" in the sense that $\pi_{\mathrm{mix}}(\boldsymbol{\theta})$ is a certain mixture of the densities $\pi(\boldsymbol{\theta}|\boldsymbol{\lambda})1\{\boldsymbol{\theta} \in \Theta\}$ such that $\pi_{\mathrm{mix}}(\boldsymbol{\theta})$ will "cover" every $\pi(\boldsymbol{\theta}|\boldsymbol{\lambda})1\{\boldsymbol{\theta} \in \Theta\}$ for $\boldsymbol{\lambda} \in \Lambda$. We will discuss this issue in detail below. In fact, $\pi_{\mathrm{mix}}(\boldsymbol{\theta})$ actually plays the role of an importance sampling density; in Chapter 5, we show how to adapt importance sampling to estimate ratios of normalizing constants. Let $\left\{\boldsymbol{\theta}_l^{\mathrm{mix}},\ l = 1, 2, \ldots, m\right\}$ denote a random sample from $\pi_{\mathrm{mix}}(\boldsymbol{\theta})$. Then $c(\boldsymbol{\lambda}_i)/c_{\mathrm{mix}}$ can be estimated by

$$\hat{c}_m(\boldsymbol{\lambda}_i) = \frac{1}{m} \sum_{l=1}^{m} \frac{\pi(\boldsymbol{\theta}_l^{\mathrm{mix}}|\boldsymbol{\lambda}_i)1\{\boldsymbol{\theta}_l^{\mathrm{mix}} \in \Theta\}}{q_{\mathrm{mix}}(\boldsymbol{\theta}_l^{\mathrm{mix}})}. \tag{6.3.2}$$

Using (6.3.2) and (6.2.2), we can approximate $E_\pi\{h(\boldsymbol{\theta}, \boldsymbol{\lambda})\}$ by

$$\tilde{h}_{n,m} = \sum_{i=1}^{n} \hat{w}_{i,m} h(\boldsymbol{\theta}_i, \boldsymbol{\lambda}_i), \tag{6.3.3}$$

where

$$\hat{w}_{i,m} = \left\{1 + \sum_{j \neq i} \frac{\hat{c}_m(\boldsymbol{\lambda}_i)}{\hat{c}_m(\boldsymbol{\lambda}_j)}\right\}^{-1}. \tag{6.3.4}$$

Note that c_{mix} need not be known because it cancels out in the calculation, as in (6.2.3) or (6.3.4). We define

$$u_j(\boldsymbol{\lambda}) = \int_\Theta \left\{ \frac{\pi(\boldsymbol{\theta}|\boldsymbol{\lambda})}{\pi_{\text{mix}}(\boldsymbol{\theta})} \right\}^j \pi_{\text{mix}}(\boldsymbol{\theta})\, d\boldsymbol{\theta}.$$

Then, the following theorem gives the asymptotic properties of $\tilde{h}_{n,m}$:

Theorem 6.3.1 *Assume that* $\{(\boldsymbol{\theta}_i, \boldsymbol{\lambda}_i),\ i = 1, 2, \ldots, n\}$ *and* $\{\boldsymbol{\theta}_l^{\text{mix}},\ l = 1, 2, \ldots, m\}$ *are two independent random samples from* $\pi^*(\boldsymbol{\theta}, \boldsymbol{\lambda}|D)$ *and* $\pi_{\text{mix}}(\boldsymbol{\theta})$, *respectively, and that*

$$E_{\pi^*}\left\{\frac{u_2(\boldsymbol{\lambda})}{c^2(\boldsymbol{\lambda})}\right\} < \infty,\ E_{\pi*}\left[\frac{\{bh(\boldsymbol{\theta}, \boldsymbol{\lambda}) - a\}^2 u_2(\boldsymbol{\lambda})}{c^4(\boldsymbol{\lambda})}\right] < \infty,\ n/m \to d_0, \tag{6.3.5}$$

for some $0 \le d_0 < \infty$. *Then*

$$\sqrt{n}[\tilde{h}_{n,m} - E_\pi\{h(\boldsymbol{\theta}, \boldsymbol{\lambda})\}] \to N(0, \sigma^2), \tag{6.3.6}$$

in distribution as $n \to \infty$, *where* $a = E_{\pi^*}[h(\boldsymbol{\theta}, \boldsymbol{\lambda})/c(\boldsymbol{\lambda})]$, $b = E_{\pi^*}[1/c(\boldsymbol{\lambda})] = c_w/c^*$,

$$\sigma^2 = b^{-4} E_{\pi*}\left\{\frac{bh(\boldsymbol{\theta}, \boldsymbol{\lambda}) - a}{c(\boldsymbol{\lambda})}\right\}^2 + \sigma^{*2} b^{-4} d_0, \tag{6.3.7}$$

$$\sigma^{*2} = \int_\Theta \left\{ \left[\int_\Omega \frac{bh(\boldsymbol{\theta}, \boldsymbol{\lambda}) - a}{c^2(\boldsymbol{\lambda})} \left\{ \frac{\pi(\boldsymbol{\theta}^{\text{mix}}|\boldsymbol{\lambda}) 1\{\boldsymbol{\theta}^{\text{mix}} \in \Theta\}}{\pi_{\text{mix}}(\boldsymbol{\theta}^{\text{mix}})} - c(\boldsymbol{\lambda}) \right\} \right.\right.$$
$$\left.\left. \times\, \pi^*(\boldsymbol{\theta}, \boldsymbol{\lambda})\, d\boldsymbol{\theta}\, d\boldsymbol{\lambda} \right]^2 \pi_{\text{mix}}(\boldsymbol{\theta}^{\text{mix}}) \right\} d\boldsymbol{\theta}^{\text{mix}}.$$

If, in addition,

$$E_{\pi^*}[\{1 + h(\boldsymbol{\theta}, \boldsymbol{\lambda})\}^2 \{1 + u_4(\boldsymbol{\lambda})/c^4(\boldsymbol{\lambda})\}] < \infty, \tag{6.3.8}$$

then the asymptotic mean-square error of $\tilde{h}_{n,m}$ *is*

$$\lim_{n\to\infty} nE[\tilde{h}_{n,m} - E_\pi\{h(\boldsymbol{\theta}, \boldsymbol{\lambda})\}]^2 = \sigma^2. \tag{6.3.9}$$

The proof is given in the Appendix. Equation (6.3.7) is intuitively appealing. The first term reflects the simulation error due to (6.2.2) for estimating h using the sample $\{(\boldsymbol{\theta}_i, \boldsymbol{\lambda}_i),\ i = 1, 2, \ldots, n\}$, while the second term represents the simulation error due to (6.3.2) for estimating the normalizing constants $c(\boldsymbol{\lambda}_i)$'s using the auxiliary sample $\{\boldsymbol{\theta}_l^{\text{mix}},\ l = 1, 2, \ldots, m\}$.

From (6.3.9), a lower bound of the asymptotic mean-square error of $\tilde{h}_{n,m}$ is

$$\lim_{n\to\infty} nE[\tilde{h}_{n,m} - E_\pi\{h(\boldsymbol{\theta}, \boldsymbol{\lambda})\}]^2 \ge b^{-4} E_{\pi*}\left\{\frac{bh(\boldsymbol{\theta}, \boldsymbol{\lambda}) - a}{c(\boldsymbol{\lambda})}\right\}^2. \tag{6.3.10}$$

It can be observed that, if $n = o(m)$, then $d_0 = 0$ in (6.3.7) and the lower bound in (6.3.10) is achieved. Thus, estimating the normalizing constant $c(\boldsymbol{\lambda}_i)$ does not asymptotically produce any additional simulation errors.

By Theorem 6.3.1, the simulation standard error of $\tilde{h}_{n,m}$ can be estimated by a first-order approximation of the asymptotic mean-square error of $\tilde{h}_{n,m}$:

$$\text{se}(\tilde{h}_{n,m}) = \frac{\hat{\sigma}}{\sqrt{n}}, \tag{6.3.11}$$

where

$$\hat{\sigma}^2 = \hat{\sigma}_1^2 + \hat{\sigma}_2^2, \quad \hat{\sigma}_1^2 = \frac{1}{n}\sum_{i=1}^{n}\left[\frac{h(\boldsymbol{\theta}_i, \boldsymbol{\lambda}_i) - \tilde{h}_{n,m}}{(1/n)\sum_{j=1}^{n}\{\hat{c}_m(\boldsymbol{\lambda}_i)/\hat{c}_m(\boldsymbol{\lambda}_j)\}}\right]^2, \tag{6.3.12}$$

$$\begin{aligned}\hat{\sigma}_2^2 = \frac{n}{m^2}\sum_{l=1}^{m}\Bigg(\frac{1}{n}\sum_{i=1}^{n}\Bigg[&\frac{h(\boldsymbol{\theta}_i, \boldsymbol{\lambda}_i) - \tilde{h}_{n,m}}{(1/n)\sum_{j=1}^{n}\{\hat{c}_m^2(\boldsymbol{\lambda}_i)/\hat{c}_m(\boldsymbol{\lambda}_j)\}} \\ &\times\left\{\frac{\pi(\boldsymbol{\theta}_l^{\text{mix}}|\boldsymbol{\lambda}_i)1\{\boldsymbol{\theta}_l^{\text{mix}} \in \Theta\}}{q_{\text{mix}}(\boldsymbol{\theta}_l^{\text{mix}})} - \hat{c}_m(\boldsymbol{\lambda}_i)\right\}\Bigg]\Bigg)^2.\end{aligned} \tag{6.3.13}$$

The simulation error estimation is important since it provides the magnitude of the simulation accuracy of the estimator $\tilde{h}_{n,m}$.

In order to obtain a good estimator $\tilde{h}_{n,m}$, we need to select a good π_{mix}. It is very difficult to prove which π_{mix} is optimal in the sense of minimizing the asymptotic mean-square error of $\tilde{h}_{n,m}$. However, a good π_{mix} should possess the following properties:

(a) π_{mix} has heavier tails than $\pi(\boldsymbol{\theta}|\boldsymbol{\lambda})$ for all $\boldsymbol{\lambda} \in \Lambda$;

(b) π_{mix} has a shape similar to $\pi(\boldsymbol{\theta}|\boldsymbol{\lambda})$ and a location close to that of $\pi(\boldsymbol{\theta}|\boldsymbol{\lambda})$; and

(c) conditions (6.3.5) and (6.3.8) hold.

Property (c) guarantees (6.3.6) and (6.3.9). In (6.3.2), $\hat{c}_m(\boldsymbol{\lambda}_i)$ is indeed an estimate of the ratio of two normalizing constants $c(\boldsymbol{\lambda}_i)$ and c_{mix} by using the ratio importance sampling method; see Section 5.5. As discussed in Section 5.5, properties (a) and (b) are required in order to obtain an efficient estimator of $c(\boldsymbol{\lambda}_i)/c_{\text{mix}}$. In Section 5.6, we also illustrate how a bad choice of π_{mix} can result in an estimator of $c(\boldsymbol{\lambda}_i)/c_{\text{mix}}$ with a large or possibly infinite asymptotic variance.

Based on the above criteria and using the idea of reweighting mixtures of Geyer (1994, 1995b), a natural choice for π_{mix} is the mixing distribution of $\pi(\boldsymbol{\theta}|\boldsymbol{\lambda})1\{\theta \in \Theta\}$ with mixing parameter $\boldsymbol{\lambda}$. Let $G(\boldsymbol{\lambda})$ be the mixing distribution of $\boldsymbol{\lambda}$. Then π_{mix} is given by

$$\pi_{\text{mix}}(\boldsymbol{\theta}) \propto \int_{\Lambda} \pi(\boldsymbol{\theta}|\boldsymbol{\lambda})1\{\boldsymbol{\theta} \in \Theta\}\, dG(\boldsymbol{\lambda}). \tag{6.3.14}$$

If $\boldsymbol{\lambda}$ is a vector of location parameters, then G may be chosen as a multivariate normal distribution $N_k(\boldsymbol{\mu}, \Sigma)$, where $\boldsymbol{\mu}$ and Σ are specified by the posterior mean and posterior variance–covariance matrix of $\boldsymbol{\lambda}$ with respect to $\pi^*(\boldsymbol{\theta}, \boldsymbol{\lambda})$. If $\boldsymbol{\lambda}$ contains scale parameters, the mixing distribution for each parameter may be chosen as a gamma distribution $\mathcal{G}(\alpha, \tau)$ or an inverse gamma distribution $\mathcal{IG}(\alpha, \tau)$ with shape parameter α and scale parameter τ, where α and τ are specified by the posterior mean and variance of $\boldsymbol{\lambda}$ with respect to $\pi^*(\boldsymbol{\theta}, \boldsymbol{\lambda})$, using method-of-moments estimates. The above choices of G capture the shape of the desired posterior distribution of $\boldsymbol{\lambda}$ with respect to π^*, and the mixing distributions typically have heavier tails than those of $\pi(\boldsymbol{\theta}|\boldsymbol{\lambda})1\{\boldsymbol{\theta} \in \Theta\}$. However, if the parameter space Λ is constrained, the aforementioned approaches may result in intensive computation, and G may instead be simply chosen as a discrete distribution such that the resulting π_{mix} has heavier tails than $\pi(\boldsymbol{\theta}|\boldsymbol{\lambda})1\{\boldsymbol{\theta} \in \Theta\}$ for every $\boldsymbol{\lambda}$. For example, if $\{\pi(\boldsymbol{\theta}|\boldsymbol{\lambda})1\{\boldsymbol{\theta} \in \Theta\},\ \boldsymbol{\lambda} \in \Lambda\}$ is a family of truncated Dirichlet distributions, π_{mix} may be specified as the one from the same Dirichlet family that has heavier tails than any other member in that family. Finally, a good G may be obtained as the mixture of discrete and continuous distributions; see the next section for illustrative examples.

Note that, if $\pi_{\text{mix}}(\boldsymbol{\theta})$ defined by (6.3.14) is not analytically available, a method for estimating a ratio of two normalizing constants with different dimensions described in Section 5.8 can be applied to obtain $\hat{c}_m(\boldsymbol{\lambda}_i)$ by using an MC sample from the distribution $\pi(\boldsymbol{\theta}|\boldsymbol{\lambda})1\{\boldsymbol{\theta} \in \Theta\}\ dG(\boldsymbol{\lambda})$. To illustrate this idea, let $g(\boldsymbol{\lambda})$ be the probability density function of G, and let $\{(\boldsymbol{\theta}_l^{\text{mix}}, \boldsymbol{\lambda}_l^{\text{mix}}),\ l = 1, 2, \ldots, m\}$ be an MC sample from $\pi(\boldsymbol{\theta}|\boldsymbol{\lambda})1\{\boldsymbol{\theta} \in \Theta\}g(\boldsymbol{\lambda})$. Then, instead of (6.3.2), $c(\boldsymbol{\lambda}_i)/c_{\text{mix}}$ is approximated by

$$\hat{c}_m(\boldsymbol{\lambda}_i) = \frac{1}{m} \sum_{l=1}^{m} \frac{\pi(\boldsymbol{\theta}_l^{\text{mix}}|\boldsymbol{\lambda}_i) w_{\text{mix}}(\boldsymbol{\lambda}_l^{\text{mix}}|\boldsymbol{\theta}_l^{\text{mix}})}{\pi(\boldsymbol{\theta}_l^{\text{mix}}|\boldsymbol{\lambda}_l^{\text{mix}}) g(\boldsymbol{\lambda}_l^{\text{mix}})}, \tag{6.3.15}$$

where $w_{\text{mix}}(\boldsymbol{\lambda}_l^{\text{mix}}|\boldsymbol{\theta}_l^{\text{mix}})$ is a completely known density function whose support is contained in or equal to Λ. It directly follows from Theorem 5.8.1 that the optimal choice of $w_{\text{mix}}(\boldsymbol{\lambda}^{\text{mix}}|\boldsymbol{\theta}^{\text{mix}})$ is the conditional density of $\boldsymbol{\lambda}^{\text{mix}}$ given $\boldsymbol{\theta}^{\text{mix}}$ with respect to $\pi(\boldsymbol{\theta}|\boldsymbol{\lambda})1\{\boldsymbol{\theta} \in \Theta\}g(\boldsymbol{\lambda})$.

6.4 Applications

6.4.1 The Meal, Ready-to-Eat (MRE) Model

Consider the MRE data discussed in Example 1.2. For illustrative purposes, we consider here only one entree item, namely, ham–chicken loaf. The primary goal in the study of Chen, Nandram, and Ross (1996) is to investigate the food shelf-life. However, in this example we consider modeling the mean rating scores only. Note that the panelists evaluated only on 23 temperature–time combinations. By design, we have a total of four missing combinations, which are omitted from the analysis.

Let y_{ijl} be the score given by the lth panelist for ham–chicken loaf at temperature c_i and withdrawn at time t_j. The y_{ijl} are independent and identically distributed with $P(y_{ijl} = s|q_{ij}) = q_{ijs}$, where $\boldsymbol{q}_{ij} = (q_{ij1}, q_{ij2}, \ldots, q_{ij9})$ and $\sum_{v=1}^{9} q_{ijv} = 1$, for $i = 1, \ldots, 4$, $j = 1, \ldots, 9$, and $s = 1, \ldots, 9$.

The mean score is $\xi_{ij} = \sum_{s=1}^{9} s q_{ijs}$. For temperature c_i, as the quality of the food deteriorates with time, we have the constraint

$$\xi_{ij} \leq \xi_{i,j-1}, \quad j = 2, 3, \ldots, 9, \tag{6.4.1}$$

and, for withdrawal time t_j, as the quality of food deteriorates with temperature, we have the constraint

$$\xi_{ij} \leq \xi_{i-1,j}, \quad i = 2, 3, 4. \tag{6.4.2}$$

In (6.4.1) and (6.4.2) there is one adjustment, that is, $\xi_{21} \geq \xi_{i2}$ for $i = 2, 3, 4$. For the missing temperature–time combinations there are obvious adjustments to constraints (6.4.1) and (6.4.2).

To facilitate the use of the Bayesian hierarchical model, we introduce latent variables z_{ijl}, where

$$y_{ijl} = s \text{ if } a_{s-1} < z_{ijl} \leq a_s, \quad s = 1, 2, \ldots, 9, \tag{6.4.3}$$

and $z_{ijl}|\theta_{ij} \sim N(\theta_{ij}, \sigma^2)$, independently, for $i = 1, 2, 3, 4$ and $j = 1, 2, \ldots, 9$. In (6.4.3) we take $a_0 = -\infty$, $a_1 = 0$, $a_8 = 1$, $a_9 = \infty$, and $0 \leq a_2 \leq \cdots \leq a_7 \leq 1$. Chen, Nandram, and Ross (1996) use the pastries data obtained from the Natick food experiment as the prior information to specify a_2, a_3, $\ldots$, a_7. The values are $a_2 = 0.0986$, $a_3 = 0.191$, $a_4 = 0.299$, $a_5 = 0.377$, $a_6 = 0.524$, and $a_7 = 0.719$.

It is easy to show that

$$\xi_{ij} = 1 + \sum_{s=1}^{9} \left\{ 1 - \Phi\left(\frac{a_s - \theta_{ij}}{\sigma} \right) \right\},$$

where Φ is the standard normal cumulative distribution function. Since ξ_{ij} is an increasing function of θ_{ij}, it follows that the constraints (6.4.1) and (6.4.2) on the mean scores are equivalent to the constraints

$$\theta_{ij} \leq \theta_{i,j-1}, \quad j = 2, 3, \ldots, 9, \tag{6.4.4}$$
$$\theta_{ij} \leq \theta_{i-1,j}, \quad j = 2, 3, 4. \tag{6.4.5}$$

For the missing temperature–time combinations, constraints (6.4.4) and (6.4.5) require the same adjustment as for constraints (6.4.1) and (6.4.2).

Instead of using a measurement error model $\theta_{ij} = \lambda + \epsilon_{ij}$, as in Chen, Nandram, and Ross (1996), we consider a temperature-effect additive model of the form

$$\theta_{ij} = \lambda_i + \epsilon_{ij}, \tag{6.4.6}$$

subject to constraints (6.4.4) and (6.4.5), where $\epsilon_{ij} \sim N(0, \delta^2)$, independently, and δ^2 is the variance of ϵ_{ij}, for $i = 1, 2, 3, 4$ and $j = 1, 2, \ldots, 9$. In order to incorporate the adjustment in constraints (6.4.4) and (6.4.5) for the room temperature, we set $\theta_{21} = \lambda_1 + \epsilon_{11}$. We also add the constraints

$$\lambda_1 \geq \lambda_2 \geq \lambda_3 \geq \lambda_4 \tag{6.4.7}$$

to ensure consistency with (6.4.5).

We take a diffuse prior for the λ_i over the constrained parameter space defined by (6.4.7) and we choose priors for σ^2 and δ^2 as

$$\frac{\eta}{\sigma^2} \sim \chi^2_\zeta \text{ and } \frac{\tau}{\delta^2} \sim \chi^2_\alpha, \tag{6.4.8}$$

where χ^2_ν denotes a χ^2 distribution with ν degrees of freedom. In (6.4.8) ζ, η, α, and τ are specified. Again, Chen, Nandram, and Ross (1996) use the pastries data as the prior information to obtain $\zeta = 16.88$, $\eta = 0.83$, $\alpha = 4.60$, and $\tau = 0.01$.

Let Θ be the constrained parameter space associated with (6.4.4) and (6.4.5). Also, let $\boldsymbol{\theta} = (\theta_{ij}, \sigma^2)$ and $\boldsymbol{\lambda} = (\lambda_1, \ldots, \lambda_4, \delta^2)$. Therefore, θ is a 24-dimensional vector ($p = 24$), and $\boldsymbol{\lambda}$ is a five-dimensional vector ($k = 5$). Finally, we denote by $\boldsymbol{\theta}^{(-\sigma^2)}$ the vector of all elements of $\boldsymbol{\theta}$ except for σ^2.

As a result of constraints (6.4.4) and (6.4.5) and the temperature-effect additive model (6.4.6), the prior distribution for $\boldsymbol{\theta}$ given $\boldsymbol{\lambda}$ depends on the normalizing constant

$$c(\boldsymbol{\lambda}) = \int_\Theta \left\{ \prod_{i,j} \frac{1}{\delta} \phi\left(\frac{\theta_{ij} - \lambda_i}{\delta} \right) \right\} d\boldsymbol{\theta}^{(-\sigma^2)}, \tag{6.4.9}$$

where ϕ is the standard normal probability density function. Analytical evaluation of $c(\boldsymbol{\lambda})$ does not appear possible. Therefore, we have a constrained parameter problem.

Letting $\boldsymbol{z} = (z_{ijl})$, the posterior distribution is given by

$$\begin{aligned} \pi(\boldsymbol{z}, \boldsymbol{\theta}, \boldsymbol{\lambda}|D) \propto & \prod_{i,j} \prod_{l=1}^{36} \left\{ \sum_{s=1}^{9} 1\{y_{ijl} = s\} 1\{a_{s-1} < z_{ijl} \leq a_s\} \right\} \frac{\pi(\boldsymbol{\theta}^{(-\sigma^2)}|\boldsymbol{\lambda})}{c(\boldsymbol{\lambda})} \\ & \times \frac{1}{\sigma} \phi\left(\frac{z_{ijl} - \theta_{ij}}{\sigma} \right) 1\{\boldsymbol{\theta} \in \Theta\} \pi(\sigma^2|\zeta, \eta) \pi(\boldsymbol{\lambda}), \end{aligned} \tag{6.4.10}$$

where the indicator function $1\{(y_{ijl} = s)\} = 1$ if $y_{ijl} = s$ and 0 otherwise, $\pi(\boldsymbol{\theta}^{(-\sigma^2)}|\boldsymbol{\lambda})$ is determined by (6.4.6),

$$\pi(\boldsymbol{\lambda}) = \pi(\lambda_1, \ldots, \lambda_4) \pi(\delta_2|\alpha, \tau), \quad \pi(\lambda_1, \ldots, \lambda_4) \propto 1,$$

subject to constraint (6.4.7), and $\pi(\sigma^2|\zeta,\eta)$ and $\pi(\delta_2|\alpha,\tau)$ are given in (6.4.8). The pseudo-posterior distribution is

$$\pi^*(\boldsymbol{z},\boldsymbol{\theta},\boldsymbol{\lambda}|D) \propto \prod_{i,j}\prod_{l=1}^{36}\left\{\sum_{s=1}^{9} 1\{y_{ijl}=s\}1\{a_{s-1}<z_{ijl}\leq a_s\}\right\}\pi(\boldsymbol{\theta}^{(-\sigma^2)}|\boldsymbol{\lambda})$$
$$\times\ \frac{1}{\sigma}\phi\left(\frac{z_{ijl}-\theta_{ij}}{\sigma}\right)1\{\boldsymbol{\theta}\in\Theta\}\pi(\sigma^2|\zeta,\eta)\pi(\boldsymbol{\lambda}). \tag{6.4.11}$$

As in Chen, Nandram, and Ross (1996), we use the Gibbs sampler to generate $\boldsymbol{z}$, $\boldsymbol{\theta}$, and $\boldsymbol{\lambda}$ from the pseudo-posterior distribution $\pi^*(\boldsymbol{z},\boldsymbol{\theta},\boldsymbol{\lambda}|D)$. Using several convergence diagnostic procedures discussed in Section 2.9, it is found that the Gibbs sampler converges within 500 iterations. We also find that the autocorrelations are negligible when we take every fifteenth of the Gibbs iterates. Since sampling from the pseudo-posterior distribution $\pi^*(\boldsymbol{z},\boldsymbol{\theta},\boldsymbol{\lambda}|D)$ is much cheaper than computing normalizing constants, every fifteenth Gibbs iterate after convergence is used for estimation, and 30000 Gibbs iterates produce an approximately random sample $\{(\boldsymbol{z}_i,\boldsymbol{\theta}_i,\boldsymbol{\lambda}_i),\ i=1,2,\ldots,n\}$ of size $n=2000$. In this application, $(\lambda_1,\ldots,\lambda_4)$ is a vector of location parameters and δ^2 is a scale parameter. In order to estimate $c(\boldsymbol{\lambda}_i)$ simultaneously for $i=1,2,\ldots,n$, we choose a mixing distribution $G(\boldsymbol{\lambda})=G(\lambda_1,\ldots,\lambda_4)G(\delta^2)$. In view of the constraints (6.4.7), for the sake of computational simplicity $G(\lambda_1,\ldots,\lambda_4)$ is chosen as a degenerate distribution at $(\lambda_1^*,\ldots,\lambda_4^*)$, where λ_j^* is the posterior mean of λ_j with respect to $\pi^*(\boldsymbol{z},\boldsymbol{\theta},\boldsymbol{\lambda}|D)$, $j=1,\ldots,4$. For the scale parameter δ^2, we choose $G(\delta^2)$ to be an inverse gamma distribution with probability density function

$$g(\delta^2)\propto(1/\delta^2)^{(\alpha^*+1)}\exp\{-\tau^*/\delta^2\} \tag{6.4.12}$$

for $\delta^2>0$, where α^* and τ^* are specified by the posterior mean and posterior variance of δ^2 with respect to $\pi^*(\boldsymbol{z},\boldsymbol{\theta},\boldsymbol{\lambda}|D)$ for $j=1,\ldots,4$ using method-of-moments estimates. With the above choice of G and using (6.3.14), we have

$$\pi_{\text{mix}}(\boldsymbol{\theta}^{\text{mix}})\propto\left\{1+\frac{\sum_{i,j}(\theta_{ij}^{\text{mix}}-\lambda_i^*)^2}{2\tau^*}\right\}^{-(23+2\alpha^*)/2}, \tag{6.4.13}$$

where the θ_{ij}^{mix} are subject to constraints (6.4.4) and (6.4.5). For this particular data set, we obtain $\alpha^*=7.65$ and $\tau^*=0.011$. Therefore, $\pi_{\text{mix}}(\boldsymbol{\theta}^{\text{mix}})$ is a truncated multivariate Student t distribution, which has heavier tails than the truncated multivariate normal distribution $\pi(\boldsymbol{\theta}^{(-\sigma^2)}|\boldsymbol{\lambda})$ for every $\boldsymbol{\lambda}$.

We use an algorithm of Geweke (1991) to generate a random sample $\{\boldsymbol{\theta}_l^{\text{mix}},\ l=1,2,\ldots,m\}$, with $m=10000$, from π_{mix}. Then, using (6.3.2),

TABLE 6.1. Estimates of the Mean Rating Scores.

Time	Temperature			
(in months)	4 °C	21 °C	30 °C	38 °C
0	-	5.984	-	-
	-	(0.0046)	-	-
	-	(0.131)	-	-
6	-	-	5.727	5.346
	-	-	(0.0057)	(0.0067)
	-	-	(0.148)	(0.169)
12	5.854	5.739	5.485	5.139
	(0.0040)	(0.0038)	(0.0052)	(0.0065)
	(0.108)	(0.100)	(0.123)	(0.149)
18	-	5.651	5.352	4.992
	-	(0.0037)	(0.0044)	(0.0059)
	-	(0.097)	(0.119)	(0.146)
24	-	5.581	5.204	4.835
	-	(0.0035)	(0.0050)	(0.0076)
	-	(0.095)	(0.129)	(0.172)
30	5.683	5.499	5.082	-
	(0.0037)	(0.0034)	(0.0053)	-
	(0.104)	(0.094)	(0.142)	-
36	5.590	5.428	4.811	-
	(0.0034)	(0.0036)	(0.0082)	-
	(0.099)	(0.099)	(0.206)	-
48	5.485	5.323	-	-
	(0.0038)	(0.0040)	-	-
	(0.105)	(0.111)	-	-
60	5.344	5.137	-	-
	(0.0050)	(0.0051)	-	-
	(0.138)	(0.149)	-	-

(6.3.3), and (6.3.11) and choosing appropriate h's, we obtain the posterior mean rating scores, the simulation standard errors, and their posterior standard deviations, which are reported in Table 6.1.

In Table 6.1, the top entry is the mean, the middle entry is the simulation standard error, and the bottom entry is the posterior standard deviation. As expected, the temperature-effect additive model leads to slightly higher (lower) mean rating scores at low (high) temperatures than does the measurement error model. For example, the estimated mean rating scores for the measurement error model are 5.785, 5.586, 5.487, 5.378, 5.230 for 12, 30, 36, 48, 60 months at temperature 4 °C and 5.470, 5.264, 5.123, 4.965 for 6, 12, 18, 24 months at temperature 38 °C. Note that the simulation standard errors of the posterior means are small and within 5% of the posterior standard deviations.

Finally, we obtain the marginal posterior densities for θ_{21}, θ_{26}, and θ_{45}. We choose $w^*(\theta_{i'j'}|\boldsymbol{\theta}_i^{(-\theta_{i'j'})}, \boldsymbol{z}_i, \boldsymbol{\lambda}_i)$ to be the conditional density of $\theta_{i'j'}$, given the other parameters, where $\boldsymbol{\theta}_i^{(-\theta_{i'j'})}$ is the vector of all elements of $\boldsymbol{\theta}_i$ except $\theta_{i'j'}$. Then, for example, the marginal density of θ_{21} is estimated by

$$\hat{\pi}(\theta_{21}|D) = \sum_{i=1}^{n} \hat{\omega}_{i,m} \left\{ \frac{1}{\varsigma_i} \phi\left(\frac{\theta_{21} - \mu_i}{\varsigma_i} \right) \right\} \left\{ 1 - \Phi\left(\frac{a_i^* - \mu_i}{\varsigma_i} \right) \right\}^{-1},$$

where $\mu_i = \psi_i \bar{z}_{21,i} + (1 - \psi_i)\lambda_{2,i}$, $\varsigma_i^2 = (1 - \psi_i)\delta_i^2$, $\psi_i = \delta_i^2(\delta_i^1 + \sigma_i^2/36)^{-1}$, $\bar{z}_{21,i} = (1/36)\sum_{l=1}^{36} z_{21l,i}$, $a_i^* = \max(\theta_{13,i}, \theta_{23,i}, \theta_{32,i})$, $\boldsymbol{z}_i = (z_{i'jl,i})$, $\boldsymbol{\theta}_i = (\theta_{i'j,i})$, $\boldsymbol{\lambda}_i = (\lambda_{j,i})$, and $\hat{\omega}_{i,m}$ is given in (6.3.4). The results are presented in Figure 6.1. Note that in Figure 6.1 the posterior means (posterior standard deviations) are 0.500 (0.019) for θ_{21}, 0.423 (0.013) for θ_{26}, and 0.346 (0.022) for θ_{45}. Figure 6.1 also shows that the marginal densities are unimodal and approximately symmetric.

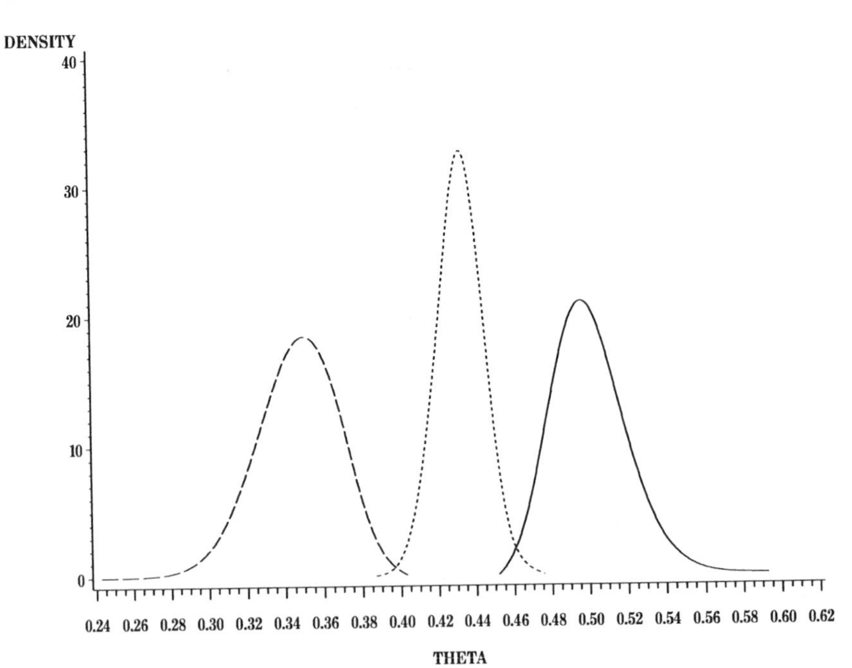

FIGURE 6.1. Marginal posterior densities plots for θ_{21} (solid, right), θ_{26} (dot, middle), and θ_{45} (dash, left).

6.4.2 *Job Satisfaction Example*

We consider the job satisfaction example given in Agresti (1990, pp. 20–21). The data set is reproduced in Table 6.2.

Let $\boldsymbol{n}_i = (n_{i1}, n_{i2}, n_{i3}, n_{i4})$, where n_{ij} is the cell count corresponding to income level i and job satisfaction level j for $i, j = 1, 2, 3, 4$. Then n_i has a multinomial distribution:

$$\boldsymbol{n}_i|\boldsymbol{\theta}_i \sim \text{Multinomial}(\boldsymbol{\theta}_i),$$

where $\boldsymbol{\theta}_i = (\theta_{i1}, \theta_{i2}, \theta_{i3}, \theta_{i4})'$ and $\sum_{j=1}^4 \theta_{ij} = 1$. We write $\boldsymbol{\theta} = (\boldsymbol{\theta}_1', \boldsymbol{\theta}_2', \boldsymbol{\theta}_3', \boldsymbol{\theta}_4')'$. Thus the likelihood function is

$$L(\boldsymbol{\theta}|D) = \prod_{i=1}^4 \left(\sum_{j=1}^4 n_{ij}\right)! \prod_{j=1}^4 \frac{\theta_{ij}^{n_{ij}}}{n_{ij}!}. \tag{6.4.14}$$

As discussed in Agresti (1990), there is a tendency for low job satisfaction to occur with low income and high job satisfaction with high income. Therefore, we naturally have the following constraints: within each income level,

$$\theta_{i1} \le \theta_{i2} \le \theta_{i3} \le \theta_{i4} \ \text{ for } i = 1, 2, 3, 4; \tag{6.4.15}$$

for job dissatisfaction,

$$\begin{aligned} &\theta_{11} \ge \theta_{21} \ge \theta_{31} \ge \theta_{41}, \\ &\theta_{11} + \theta_{12} \ge \theta_{21} + \theta_{22} \ge \theta_{31} + \theta_{32} \ge \theta_{41} + \theta_{42}; \end{aligned} \tag{6.4.16}$$

and, for job satisfaction,

$$\begin{aligned} &\theta_{14} \le \theta_{24} \le \theta_{34} \le \theta_{44}, \\ &\theta_{13} + \theta_{14} \le \theta_{23} + \theta_{24} \le \theta_{33} + \theta_{34} \le \theta_{43} + \theta_{44}. \end{aligned} \tag{6.4.17}$$

Let Θ be the resulting constrained parameter space. We take priors

$$\boldsymbol{\theta}_i|\boldsymbol{\lambda} \sim \text{Dirichlet}(\boldsymbol{\lambda}) \ \text{ for } i = 1, 2, 3, 4,$$

TABLE 6.2. Cross Classification of Job Satisfaction by Income.

		Job Satisfaction j			
		Very Dissatisfied	Little Dissatisfied	Moderately Satisfied	Very Satisfied
Income (US$)	i	1	2	3	4
<6000	1	20	24	80	82
6000–15000	2	22	38	104	125
15000–25000	3	13	28	81	113
>25000	4	7	18	54	92

subject to constraints (6.4.15), (6.4.16), and (6.4.17), where $\boldsymbol{\lambda} = (\lambda_1, \lambda_2, \lambda_3, \lambda_4)$. Therefore, we have

$$\pi(\boldsymbol{\theta}|\boldsymbol{\lambda}) = \prod_{i=1}^{4} \Gamma\left(\sum_{j=1}^{4} \lambda_j\right) \prod_{j=1}^{4} \frac{\theta_{ij}^{\lambda_j - 1}}{\Gamma(\lambda_j)} \tag{6.4.18}$$

and $c(\boldsymbol{\lambda}) = \int_{\Theta} \pi(\boldsymbol{\theta}|\boldsymbol{\lambda})\, d\boldsymbol{\theta}$. We choose a flat prior for $\boldsymbol{\lambda}$:

$$\pi(\boldsymbol{\lambda}) = \left\{\prod_{j=1}^{4} (u_j - 1)\right\}^{-1} \quad \text{for } 1 \le \lambda_j \le u_j < \infty,\ j = 1, 2, 3, 4, \tag{6.4.19}$$

where the u_j are specified. Since we choose a flat prior for $\boldsymbol{\lambda}$, we should not take the u_j too large. For illustrative purposes, we choose $u_1 = 7.5$, $u_2 = 10$, $u_3 = 15$, and $u_4 = 20$ in our calculation. We use the Gibbs sampler to draw $\boldsymbol{\theta}$ and $\boldsymbol{\lambda}$ from the pseudo-posterior $\pi^*(\boldsymbol{\theta}, \boldsymbol{\lambda}|D)$. Note that the conditional distribution of θ_{ij} given the other parameters is a truncated beta distribution, which is easy to sample, while the conditional density of λ_j given the others is log-concave, which can be sampled using the adaptive rejection sampling algorithm of Gilks and Wild (1992). As with the previous example, we check convergence of the Gibbs sampler and autocorrelations of the Gibbs iterates. We find that the autocorrelations are negligible when every fifth Gibbs iterate is taken. Thus, 12500 Gibbs iterates after convergence produce an approximately random sample $\{(\boldsymbol{\theta}_i, \boldsymbol{\lambda}_i),\ i = 1, 2, \ldots, n\}$ of size $n = 2500$. In order to estimate $c(\boldsymbol{\lambda}_i)$ simultaneously, we take

$$\pi_{\text{mix}}(\boldsymbol{\theta}^{\text{mix}}) \propto 1 \quad \text{for } \boldsymbol{\theta}^{\text{mix}} \in \Theta.$$

Note that $\{\pi(\boldsymbol{\theta}|\boldsymbol{\lambda}),\ 1 \le \lambda_j \le u_j, j = 1, \ldots, 4\}$ is indeed a family of truncated Dirichlet distributions and $\pi_{\text{mix}}(\boldsymbol{\theta}^{\text{mix}})$ is a member of this family corresponding to $\lambda_j = 1$ for $j = 1, \ldots, 4$. It can be shown that $\pi_{\text{mix}}(\boldsymbol{\theta}^{\text{mix}})$ has heavier tails than $\pi(\boldsymbol{\theta}|\boldsymbol{\lambda})$ for all $\boldsymbol{\lambda}$ with $1 \le \lambda_j \le u_j$, $j = 1, 2, 3, 4$, and it can also be shown that, with the above $\pi_{\text{mix}}(\boldsymbol{\theta}^{\text{mix}})$, conditions (6.3.5) and (6.3.8) hold as long as the second moment of $h(\boldsymbol{\theta}, \boldsymbol{\lambda})$ with respect to π^* exists. We then generate a random sample $\{\boldsymbol{\theta}_l^{\text{mix}},\ l = 1, 2, \ldots, m\}$ with $m = 50000$ from π_{mix}. Using (6.3.2) and (6.3.3), we obtain the posterior means and standard deviations for $\boldsymbol{\theta}$ and $\boldsymbol{\lambda}$ in Table 6.3. The simulation standard errors of the posterior means are obtained but are not reported here. They are all within 5% of the posterior standard deviations. Note that the Bayesian estimates of θ_{ij} given in Table 6.3 are very close to the maximum likelihood estimates. However, if one ignores the normalizing constant $c(\boldsymbol{\lambda})$ and treats $c(\boldsymbol{\lambda})$ as a constant independent of $\boldsymbol{\lambda}$, the "posterior means" of $\boldsymbol{\theta}$ and $\boldsymbol{\lambda}$ are inaccurate. For example, if we ignore $c(\boldsymbol{\lambda})$, the posterior means (posterior standard deviations) of λ_j, $j = 1, 2, 3, 4$, are 2.983 (0.911), 5.070 (1.343), 12.434 (1.869), and 16.698 (1.495).

TABLE 6.3. Estimates of the Job Satisfaction Cell Probabilities with Posterior Standard Deviations in Parentheses.

i	$\hat{\theta}_{i1}$	$\hat{\theta}_{i2}$	$\hat{\theta}_{i3}$	$\hat{\theta}_{i4}$
1	0.103 (0.012)	0.130 (0.015)	0.362 (0.016)	0.404 (0.016)
2	0.078 (0.010)	0.128 (0.014)	0.357 (0.020)	0.438 (0.018)
3	0.063 (0.010)	0.113 (0.016)	0.346 (0.023)	0.479 (0.021)
4	0.045 (0.012)	0.096 (0.017)	0.326 (0.027)	0.534 (0.028)
	$\hat{\lambda}_1$	$\hat{\lambda}_2$	$\hat{\lambda}_3$	$\hat{\lambda}_4$
	3.465 (1.064)	3.563 (1.389)	12.778 (2.236)	14.045 (3.825)

Next, we conduct a sensitivity study of prior specifications: such a study has not been done before mainly because of the computational difficulty. Let $\pi_1(\boldsymbol{\theta}) \propto 1$ for $\boldsymbol{\theta} \in \Theta$ and $\pi_2(\boldsymbol{\theta}, \boldsymbol{\lambda}) = \pi(\boldsymbol{\theta}|\boldsymbol{\lambda})\pi(\boldsymbol{\lambda})$, where $\pi(\boldsymbol{\theta}|\boldsymbol{\lambda})$ and $\pi(\boldsymbol{\lambda})$ are defined in (6.4.18) and (6.4.19). Denote by $m_1(D)$ and $m_2(D)$ the corresponding marginal likelihoods with respect to π_1 and π_2, and let r be their ratio. Then

$$r = \frac{m_1(D)}{m_2(D)} = \frac{c^{-1}(1,1,1,1) \displaystyle\int_\Theta L(\boldsymbol{\theta}|D)\, d\boldsymbol{\theta}}{\displaystyle\int_\Theta \int_\Lambda L(\boldsymbol{\theta}|D) \frac{\pi(\boldsymbol{\theta}|\boldsymbol{\lambda})}{c(\boldsymbol{\lambda})} \pi(\boldsymbol{\lambda})\, d\boldsymbol{\theta}\, d\boldsymbol{\lambda}}, \tag{6.4.20}$$

where $L(\boldsymbol{\theta}|D)$ is given in (6.4.14) and $\Lambda = \{\boldsymbol{\lambda} : 1 \le \lambda_j \le u_j \text{ for } j = 1,2,3,4\}$. Since the numerator of (6.4.20) contains a 16-dimensional integral and the denominator has a 20-dimensional integral, we need to evaluate a ratio of two normalizing constants for densities of different dimensions. We apply the ratio importance sampling method of Chen and Shao (1997a) (also see Section 5.5) to compute r. In order to use the available random sample $\{(\boldsymbol{\theta}_i, \boldsymbol{\lambda}_i), i = 1, 2, \dots, n\}$, it is natural to choose $\pi^*(\boldsymbol{\theta}, \boldsymbol{\lambda}|D)$ as a ratio importance sampling density. Based on (6.3.2), the estimator of r is

$$\hat{r} = \frac{\displaystyle\sum_{i=1}^n L(\boldsymbol{\theta}_i|D) w^{**}(\boldsymbol{\lambda}_i|\boldsymbol{\theta}_i)\{\hat{c}_m(1,1,1,1)\pi^*(\boldsymbol{\theta}_i, \boldsymbol{\lambda}_i|D)\}^{-1}}{\displaystyle\sum_{i=1}^n L(\boldsymbol{\theta}_i|D)\pi(\boldsymbol{\theta}_i|\boldsymbol{\lambda}_i)\{\hat{c}_m(\boldsymbol{\lambda}_i)\}^{-1}\pi(\boldsymbol{\lambda}_i)\{\pi^*(\boldsymbol{\theta}_i, \boldsymbol{\lambda}_i|D)\}^{-1}}, \tag{6.4.21}$$

where $w^{**}(\boldsymbol{\lambda}|\boldsymbol{\theta})$ is an arbitrary conditional density of $\boldsymbol{\lambda}$ given $\boldsymbol{\theta}$ defined on Λ. Note that $c(1,1,1,1)$ is indeed the normalizing constant of π_{mix}. Simplification of (6.4.21) leads to

$$\hat{r} = \frac{\sum_{i=1}^n w^{**}(\boldsymbol{\lambda}_i|\boldsymbol{\theta}_i)\{\hat{c}_m(1,1,1,1)\pi(\boldsymbol{\theta}_i|\boldsymbol{\lambda}_i)\pi(\boldsymbol{\lambda}_i)\}^{-1}}{\sum_{i=1}^n \{\hat{c}_m(\boldsymbol{\lambda}_i)\}^{-1}}.$$

The simulation standard error based on the first-order approximation of $\mathrm{Var}(\hat{r})$ is thus given by

$$\begin{aligned}\mathrm{se}(\hat{r}) &= \frac{\hat{r}}{\sqrt{n}}\left(\frac{1}{n}\sum_{i=1}^{n}\left[w^{**}(\boldsymbol{\lambda}_i|\boldsymbol{\theta}_i)\{\hat{r}\hat{c}_m(1,1,1,1)\pi(\boldsymbol{\theta}_i|\boldsymbol{\lambda}_i)\pi(\boldsymbol{\lambda}_i)\}^{-1}\right.\right.\\ &\left.\left. \quad - \{\hat{c}_m(\boldsymbol{\lambda}_i)\}^{-1}\right]^2\right)^{1/2} \times \left[\frac{1}{n}\sum_{i=1}^{n}\{\hat{c}_m(\boldsymbol{\lambda}_i)\}^{-1}\right]^{-1}, \qquad (6.4.22)\end{aligned}$$

(see Chen and Shao 1997a and also Section 5.5). For simplicity, we choose $w^{**}(\boldsymbol{\lambda}|\boldsymbol{\theta}) = \pi(\boldsymbol{\lambda})$. Using the same random samples, $\{(\boldsymbol{\theta}_i, \boldsymbol{\lambda}_i),\ i = 1, 2, \ldots, n\}$ and $\{\boldsymbol{\theta}_l^{\mathrm{mix}},\ l = 1, 2, \ldots, m\}$, we obtain $\hat{r} = 0.0153$ and $\mathrm{se}(\hat{r}) = 0.0028$. The small value of $\hat{r}$ indicates that the marginal likelihood is sensitive to the prior specification and π_2 is better than π_1 in the sense of maximizing the marginal likelihood.

6.5 Discussion

In this chapter, we use an MC method to solve problems involving normalizing constants based on constrained parameter spaces that naturally arise in Bayesian hierarchical modeling (Lindley and Smith, 1972). The method discussed in this chapter is essentially an extension of importance sampling. First, we temporarily assume that the importance weights w_i in (6.2.2), which are the functions of $c(\boldsymbol{\lambda})$'s, are known. Then we estimate the w_i's by an auxiliary MC sample from a mixing distribution π_{mix}. Although in this chapter we assume that $\boldsymbol{\lambda}$ has a continuous distribution, the method can easily be extended to the case where $\pi(\boldsymbol{\lambda})$ is a discrete distribution. Moreover, the MC method considered in this chapter can also be used to study prior sensitivity as in Section 6.4.2.

Appendix

Proof of Theorem 6.3.1. Let

$$\tilde{c}_m(\boldsymbol{\lambda}_i) = \hat{c}_m(\boldsymbol{\lambda}_i)c_{\mathrm{mix}} = \frac{1}{m}\sum_{l=1}^{m}\frac{\pi(\boldsymbol{\theta}_l^{\mathrm{mix}}|\boldsymbol{\lambda}_i)1\{\boldsymbol{\theta}_l^{\mathrm{mix}} \in \Theta\}}{\pi_{\mathrm{mix}}(\boldsymbol{\theta}_l^{\mathrm{mix}})},$$

$$\eta(\boldsymbol{\theta}, \boldsymbol{\lambda}) = bh(\boldsymbol{\theta}, \boldsymbol{\lambda}) - a \ \text{ and } \ \eta_i = \eta_i(\boldsymbol{\theta}, \boldsymbol{\lambda}) = bh(\boldsymbol{\theta}_i, \boldsymbol{\lambda}_i) - a,\ i = 1, 2, \ldots.$$

Clearly,

$$\begin{aligned}\tilde{h}_{n,m} - E_\pi h(\boldsymbol{\theta}, \boldsymbol{\lambda}) &= \frac{\sum_{i=1}^n h(\boldsymbol{\theta}_i, \boldsymbol{\lambda}_i)/\tilde{c}_m(\boldsymbol{\lambda}_i)}{\sum_{i=1}^n 1/\tilde{c}_m(\boldsymbol{\lambda}_i)} - \frac{a}{b} \\ &= \frac{\sum_{i=1}^n \eta_i/\tilde{c}_m(\boldsymbol{\lambda}_i)}{b\sum_{i=1}^n 1/\tilde{c}_m(\boldsymbol{\lambda}_i)}\end{aligned}$$

and

$$\begin{aligned}\sum_{i=1}^n \frac{\eta_i}{\tilde{c}_m(\boldsymbol{\lambda}_i)} &= \sum_{i=1}^n \left\{ \frac{\eta_i}{c(\boldsymbol{\lambda}_i)} + \frac{\eta_i}{c^2(\boldsymbol{\lambda}_i)}(c(\boldsymbol{\lambda}_i) - \tilde{c}_m(\boldsymbol{\lambda}_i)) \right\} \\ &\quad + \sum_{i=1}^n \frac{\eta_i}{c^2(\boldsymbol{\lambda}_i)\tilde{c}_m(\boldsymbol{\lambda}_i)}(c(\boldsymbol{\lambda}_i) - \tilde{c}_m(\boldsymbol{\lambda}_i))^2 \\ &= T_{n,1} + T_{n,2}.\end{aligned}$$

One can show that

$$\frac{b}{n}\sum_{i=1}^n 1/\tilde{c}_m(\boldsymbol{\lambda}_i) \to 1 \quad a.s.$$

and

$$T_{n,2}/\sqrt{n} \xrightarrow{\mathcal{P}} 0.$$

Hence, it suffices to show that

$$T_{n,1}/\sqrt{n} \xrightarrow{d} N\left(0, E_{\pi^*}\left\{\frac{bh(\boldsymbol{\theta}, \boldsymbol{\lambda}) - a}{c(\boldsymbol{\lambda})}\right\}^2 + \sigma^{*2} d_0\right). \qquad (6.A.1)$$

Let $g_n(t)$ be the characteristic function of $T_{n,1}/\sqrt{n}$ and put

$$W_n = \sum_{j=1}^n \frac{\eta_j}{c^2(\boldsymbol{\lambda}_j)}(c(\boldsymbol{\lambda}_j) - \tau(\boldsymbol{\theta}^{\text{mix}}, \boldsymbol{\lambda}_j)),$$

where $\tau(\boldsymbol{\theta}^{\text{mix}}, \boldsymbol{\lambda}) = \pi(\boldsymbol{\theta}^{\text{mix}}|\boldsymbol{\lambda})1\{\boldsymbol{\theta}^{\text{mix}} \in \Theta\}/\pi_{\text{mix}}(\boldsymbol{\theta}^{\text{mix}})$. Observe that

$$\begin{aligned}g_n(t) &= E\Bigg\{ \exp\left(\frac{it}{\sqrt{n}}\sum_{j=1}^n \frac{\eta_j}{c(\boldsymbol{\lambda}_j)}\right) \\ &\quad \times \left\{E\left[\exp\left(\frac{it}{m\sqrt{n}}W_n\right)\Big|\boldsymbol{\lambda}_1, \boldsymbol{\lambda}_2, ..., \boldsymbol{\lambda}_n\right]\right\}^m\Bigg\} \\ &= E\Bigg\{ \exp\left(\frac{it}{\sqrt{n}}\sum_{j=1}^n \frac{\eta_j}{c(\boldsymbol{\lambda}_j)}\right) \\ &\quad \times \left\{1 - \frac{t^2}{2m^2 n}E\left(W_n^2|\boldsymbol{\lambda}_1, \boldsymbol{\lambda}_2, ..., \boldsymbol{\lambda}_n\right) + \beta\varepsilon_n\right\}^m\Bigg\},\end{aligned}$$

where $|\beta| \leq 1$ and

$$\begin{aligned} \varepsilon_n &= \frac{t^2}{m^2 n} E(W_n^2 1\{|W_n| > n^{4/3}\} | \boldsymbol{\lambda}_1, \boldsymbol{\lambda}_2, ..., \boldsymbol{\lambda}_n) \\ &+ \frac{t^3}{m^3 n^{3/2}} n^{4/3} E(W_n^2 | \boldsymbol{\lambda}_1, \boldsymbol{\lambda}_2, ..., \boldsymbol{\lambda}_n). \end{aligned}$$

It is easy to see that

$$m\varepsilon_n \xrightarrow{\mathcal{P}} 0 \text{ as } n \to \infty,$$

and that

$$\begin{aligned} &E(W_n^2 | \boldsymbol{\lambda}_1, \boldsymbol{\lambda}_2, ..., \boldsymbol{\lambda}_n) \\ &= \int_\Theta \left(\sum_{j=1}^n \frac{\eta_j}{c^2(\boldsymbol{\lambda}_j)} (\tau(\boldsymbol{\theta}^{\text{mix}}, \boldsymbol{\lambda}_j) - c(\boldsymbol{\lambda}_j)) \right)^2 d\boldsymbol{\theta}^{\text{mix}} \\ &= \int_\Theta \sum_{j=1}^n \frac{\eta_j^2}{c^4(\boldsymbol{\lambda}_j)} (\tau(\boldsymbol{\theta}^{\text{mix}}, \boldsymbol{\lambda}_j) - c(\boldsymbol{\lambda}_j))^2 d\boldsymbol{\theta}^{\text{mix}} \\ &\quad + 2 \int_\Theta \sum_{1 \leq j < l \leq n} \left[\frac{\eta_j \eta_l}{c^2(\boldsymbol{\lambda}_j) c^2(\boldsymbol{\lambda}_l)} (\tau(\boldsymbol{\theta}^{\text{mix}}, \boldsymbol{\lambda}_j) - c(\boldsymbol{\lambda}_j)) \right. \\ &\quad \left. \times \; (\tau(\boldsymbol{\theta}^{\text{mix}}, \boldsymbol{\lambda}_l) - c(\boldsymbol{\lambda}_l)) \right] d\boldsymbol{\theta}^{\text{mix}}. \end{aligned}$$

Hence

$$\begin{aligned} &\frac{1}{mn} E(W_n^2 | \boldsymbol{\lambda}_1, \boldsymbol{\lambda}_2, ..., \boldsymbol{\lambda}_n) \\ &\quad \xrightarrow{\mathcal{P}} d_0 \int_\Theta \left[E\left(\frac{\eta(\boldsymbol{\theta}, \boldsymbol{\lambda})}{c^2(\boldsymbol{\lambda})} (\tau(\boldsymbol{\theta}^{\text{mix}}, \boldsymbol{\lambda}) - c(\boldsymbol{\lambda})) | \boldsymbol{\theta}^{\text{mix}} \right) \right]^2 d\boldsymbol{\theta}^{\text{mix}} \\ &\quad = d_0 \sigma^{*2}. \end{aligned}$$

Thus, we have

$$\begin{aligned} g_n(t) &= E\left\{ \exp\left(\frac{it}{\sqrt{n}} \sum_{j=1}^n \frac{\eta_j}{c(\boldsymbol{\lambda}_j)} \right) \right. \\ &\quad \left. \times \left\{ 1 - \frac{t^2}{2m^2 n} E(W_n^2 | \boldsymbol{\lambda}_1, \boldsymbol{\lambda}_2, ..., \boldsymbol{\lambda}_n) \right\}^m \right\} \\ &= \exp\left(-\frac{t^2 \sigma^{*2} d_0}{2} \right) E\left\{ \exp\left(\frac{it}{\sqrt{n}} \sum_{j=1}^n \frac{\eta_j}{c(\boldsymbol{\lambda}_j)} \right) \right\} + o(1) \\ &= \exp\left(-\frac{t^2}{2} (E(\eta(\boldsymbol{\theta}, \boldsymbol{\lambda})/c(\boldsymbol{\lambda}))^2 + \sigma^{*2} d_0) \right) + o(1), \end{aligned}$$

which yields (6.A.1) immediately. This proves (6.3.6).

Further, it can be shown that $\{n(\tilde{h}_{n,m} - E_\pi[h(\boldsymbol{\theta}, \boldsymbol{\lambda})])^2, n \geq 1\}$ is uniformly integrable. Thus, (6.3.9) follows by (6.3.6). □

Exercises

6.1 Ordered Exponential Family Parameters (Gelfand, Smith, and Lee 1992)

Motivated by graduation problems in actuarial science, Broffitt (1984) considers ordered parameters from a family of models of the form

$$f(y|\theta) = a(y)\theta^{b(y)} \exp\{-\theta c(y)\}, \quad \theta > 0. \tag{6.E.1}$$

(This family includes models such as a gamma distribution with known shape parameter, a normal distribution with known mean, and a Poisson distribution.)

Suppose that conditionally independent observations y_{ji}, $j = 1, 2, \ldots, p$, and $i = 1, 2, \ldots, n_j$ are available from $f(\cdot|\theta_j)$, where it is assumed that

$$\boldsymbol{\theta} \in \Theta = \{\boldsymbol{\theta} = (\theta_1, \theta_2, \ldots, \theta_p)' : 0 < \theta_1 \leq \theta_2 \leq \cdots \leq \theta_p\}.$$

Broffitt (1984) suggests a convenient and flexible prior family for $\boldsymbol{\theta}$ of the form

$$\pi(\boldsymbol{\theta}|\boldsymbol{\lambda}) = \frac{1}{c(\boldsymbol{\lambda})} \prod_{j=1}^{p} \frac{\theta_j^{\delta_j - 1} \gamma_j^{\delta_j}}{\Gamma(\delta_j)} \exp\{-\gamma_j \theta_j\} \text{ for } \boldsymbol{\theta} \in \Theta, \tag{6.E.2}$$

where $\boldsymbol{\lambda} = (\gamma_1, \gamma_2, \ldots, \gamma_p, \delta_1, \delta_2, \ldots, \delta_p)'$, and $c(\boldsymbol{\lambda})$ is the normalizing constant. Using isotonic regression, Broffitt obtains the order-restricted Bayes estimate for θ_j with specified $\boldsymbol{\lambda}$, while Gelfand, Smith, and Lee (1992) provide the Gibbs sampling algorithm to sample $\boldsymbol{\theta}$ from its posterior distribution with fixed $\boldsymbol{\lambda}$.

(i) Consider $\delta_1 = \delta_2 = \cdots = \delta_p = 1$ and assume the γ_j are independent and identically distributed as

$$\pi(\gamma_j) \propto \gamma_j^{a-1} \exp\{-b\gamma_j\}, \tag{6.E.3}$$

where $a > 0$ and $b > 0$ are two specified hyperparameters. Show that $c(\boldsymbol{\lambda})$ does not depend on the γ_j.

(ii) Under the assumptions given in (i), discuss how to implement the Gibbs sampler for sampling $\boldsymbol{\theta}$ and $\boldsymbol{\gamma} = (\gamma_1, \gamma_2, \ldots, \gamma_p)'$ from their joint posterior distribution. Discuss whether the order restriction poses any additional difficulty in the implementation of the Gibbs sampler.

(iii) Discuss the cases where $c(\boldsymbol{\lambda})$ depends on $\boldsymbol{\lambda}$. The methods presented in Sections 6.2 and 6.3 will be useful for computing posterior quantities.

(iv) Assume y given θ follows a Poisson distribution with mean θ in (6.E.1), $\delta_1 = \delta_2 = \cdots = \delta_p = 2$ and $\gamma_j \sim \pi(\gamma_j)$, where $\pi(\gamma_j)$ is given by (6.E.3). Discuss how to choose a good $\pi_{\text{mix}}(\boldsymbol{\theta})$ (see (6.3.1)).

6.2 Show that $\hat{\sigma}$ defined by (6.3.11), (6.3.12), and (6.3.13) is a consistent estimator of σ, where σ is given in (6.3.7).

6.3 Show that $\hat{c}_m(\boldsymbol{\lambda}_i)$ in (6.3.15) is a consistent estimator of $c(\boldsymbol{\lambda}_i)/c_{\text{mix}}$.

6.4 Use the overlapping batch statistics approach given in Section 3.3.2 to obtain an estimate of the standard error of $\tilde{h}_{n,m}$ given by (6.3.3).

6.5 In the MRE data, take $G(\boldsymbol{\lambda}) = G(\lambda_1, \ldots, \lambda_4)G(\delta^2)$, where $G(\lambda_1, \ldots, \lambda_4)$ is chosen as a degenerate distribution at $(\lambda_1^*, \ldots, \lambda_4^*)$, where λ_j^* is the posterior mean of λ_j with respect to $\pi^*(\boldsymbol{z}, \boldsymbol{\theta}, \boldsymbol{\lambda}|D)$, for $j = 1, \ldots, 4$, and $G(\delta^2)$ is chosen to be an inverse gamma distribution with probability density function $g(\delta^2)$ given by (6.4.12). With the above choice of G and using (6.3.14), show that $\pi_{\text{mix}}(\boldsymbol{\theta}^{\text{mix}})$ is given by (6.4.13).

6.6 For the MRE model in Section 6.4.1, compute and plot the marginal posterior distributions for σ^2 and δ^2.

6.7 In the MRE model in Section 6.4.1, discuss the necessity of the constraints given in (6.4.7).

6.8 In the job satisfaction example, choose

$$\pi_{\text{mix}}(\boldsymbol{\theta}^{\text{mix}}) \propto 1 \text{ for } \boldsymbol{\theta}^{\text{mix}} \in \Theta.$$

Show that with the above $\pi_{\text{mix}}(\boldsymbol{\theta}^{\text{mix}})$, conditions (6.3.5) and (6.3.8) hold as long as the second moment of $h(\boldsymbol{\theta}, \boldsymbol{\lambda})$ with respect to π^* exists.

6.9 For the job satisfaction example, compute and plot the marginal posterior distributions for the θ_{ij} using the IWMDE method described in Sections 6.2 and 6.3.

6.10 (a) Similar to (5.7.6), show that the first-order term of $\text{RE}^2(\hat{r}_{\text{RIS}})$ given in (5.5.7) can also be written as

$$\frac{1}{n} E_\pi \left[\frac{\{\pi_1(\boldsymbol{\theta}) - \pi_2(\boldsymbol{\theta})\}^2}{\pi^2(\boldsymbol{\theta})} \right] = \frac{1}{n} \left(\frac{c_\pi}{c_2} \right)^2 E_\pi \left[\left\{ \frac{q_1(\boldsymbol{\theta})/r - q_2(\boldsymbol{\theta})}{q(\boldsymbol{\theta})} \right\}^2 \right]. \tag{6.E.4}$$

(b) Use (6.E.4) to derive (6.4.22).

7

Computing Bayesian Credible and HPD Intervals

One purpose of Bayesian posterior inference is to summarize posterior marginal densities. Graphical presentation of the entire posterior distribution is always desirable if this can be conveniently accomplished. However, summary statistics, which outline important features of the posterior distribution, are sometimes adequate. In particular, when one deals with a high-dimensional problem, graphical display of the entire posterior distribution is generally infeasible, and therefore appropriate summaries of the posterior distribution are most desirable.

Nowadays, it has become a routine practice to summarize marginal posterior distributions by tabulating $100(1-\alpha)\%$ posterior credible intervals for the parameters of interest. The primary reason for this is that credible intervals are easy to obtain. One can obtain such credible intervals analytically or by using a Markov chain Monte Carlo (MCMC) method. However, when the marginal distribution is not symmetric, a $100(1-\alpha)\%$ Highest Probability Density (HPD) interval is more desirable. As discussed in Box and Tiao (1992), an HPD interval has two main properties:

(a) the density for every point inside the interval is greater than that for every point outside the interval; and

(b) for a given probability content, say $1-\alpha$, the interval is of the shortest length.

Unlike Bayesian credible intervals, it is typically computationally intensive to compute HPD intervals unless one is dealing with a simple model such as a standard normal model.

Tanner (1996) provides a Monte Carlo (MC) algorithm to calculate the content and boundary of the HPD region. However, Tanner's algorithm requires evaluating the marginal posterior densities analytically or numerically. The implementation of his algorithm is also quite complicated and computationally intensive. To overcome such difficulties, we present a simple MC method to estimate HPD intervals in this chapter. This new approach requires only an MCMC sample generated from the marginal posterior distribution of the parameter of interest. In particular, we discuss how to compute Bayesian credible intervals in Section 7.2. A detailed treatment of how to compute HPD intervals is given in Section 7.3. In Section 7.4, we extend the MC methods presented in the previous sections to a Bayesian hierarchical model, in which the resulting posterior density contains analytically intractable integrals that depend on the (hyper) parameters under consideration. A simulation study is given in Subsection 7.5.1 and the MC methods considered in the earlier sections are further demonstrated in Subsection 7.5.2.

7.1 Bayesian Credible and HPD Intervals

Consider a Bayesian posterior density having the form

$$\pi(\theta, \varphi|D) = \frac{1}{c(D)} L(\theta, \varphi|D)\pi(\theta, \varphi), \tag{7.1.1}$$

where D denotes *data*, the parameter θ is one-dimensional, and φ may be a multidimensional vector of parameters other than θ in the model. In (7.1.1), $L(\theta, \varphi|D)$ is a likelihood function given D, $\pi(\theta, \varphi)$ is a prior, and $c(D)$ is a normalizing constant. Our objective is to obtain Bayesian credible and HPD intervals for θ.

Let $\pi(\theta|D)$ and $\Pi(\theta|D)$ denote the marginal posterior density function and the marginal posterior cumulative distribution function (cdf) of θ, respectively. Then, one of the widely used $100(1-\alpha)\%$ Bayesian credible intervals for θ takes the form

$$(\theta^{(\alpha/2)}, \theta^{(1-\alpha/2)}),$$

where

$$\Pi(\theta^{(\alpha/2)}|D) = \alpha/2 \text{ and } \Pi(\theta^{(1-\alpha/2)}|D) = 1-\alpha/2. \tag{7.1.2}$$

When $\pi(\theta|D)$ is symmetric and unimodal, the Bayesian credible interval $(\theta^{(\alpha/2)}, \theta^{(1-\alpha/2)})$ is also an HPD interval. However, when $\pi(\theta|D)$ is not symmetric, $(\theta^{(\alpha/2)}, \theta^{(1-\alpha/2)})$ is not an HPD interval in general, and in this case, an HPD interval is more desirable, since it displays more important features of the posterior distribution than a credible interval. A $100(1-\alpha)\%$

HPD interval for θ is given by

$$R(\pi_\alpha) = \{\theta : \pi(\theta|D) \geq \pi_\alpha\}, \tag{7.1.3}$$

where π_α is the largest constant such that $P(\theta \in R(\pi_\alpha)) \geq 1-\alpha$. In (7.1.3), $R(\pi_\alpha)$ can also be viewed as a $100(1-\alpha)\%$ HPD region for θ when $\pi(\theta|D)$ is multimodal.

When closed forms of $\pi(\theta|D)$ and $\Pi(\theta|D)$ are available, a $100(1-\alpha)\%$ credible interval can be obtained by solving the equations given in (7.1.2), while the numerical solution of (7.1.3) gives a $100(1-\alpha)\%$ HPD interval. Further, when $\pi(\theta|D)$ is continuous and unimodal, a $100(1-\alpha)\%$ HPD interval is $(\theta_L, \ \theta_U)$ where θ_L and θ_U are the solution to the following optimization problem

$$\min_{\theta_L < \theta_U} \left(|\pi(\theta_U|D) - \pi(\theta_L|D)| + |\Pi(\theta_U|D) - \Pi(\theta_L|D) - (1-\alpha)| \right). \tag{7.1.4}$$

However, care must be taken when one uses (7.1.4) to obtain the HPD interval (θ_L, θ_U). We present a detailed discussion to address this issue in the following remarks:

Remark 7.1. The solution of (7.1.4) can be obtained using, for example, the Nelder–Mead algorithm implemented by O'Neill (1971).

Remark 7.2. In (7.1.4), if the minimum value is 0, (θ_L, θ_U) is the exact $100(1-\alpha)\%$ HPD interval for θ. However, if the minimum value is greater than 0 and $\pi(\theta|D)$ is a monotone function with support (θ_a, θ_b), then (7.1.4) must be replaced by

$$\min_{\theta_a < \theta_U} |\Pi(\theta_U|D) - \Pi(\theta_a|D) - (1-\alpha)| \tag{7.1.5}$$

if $\pi(\theta|D)$ is decreasing, or

$$\min_{\theta_L < \theta_b} |\Pi(\theta_b|D) - \Pi(\theta_L|D) - (1-\alpha)| \tag{7.1.6}$$

if $\pi(\theta|D)$ is increasing. Therefore, the $100(1-\alpha)\%$ HPD interval for θ is (θ_a, θ_U) or (θ_L, θ_b). Furthermore, if the minimum value is greater than 0 and $\pi(\theta|D)$ is not monotone, then the $100(1-\alpha)\%$ HPD interval for θ is either (θ_a, θ_U) or (θ_L, θ_b) whichever has a smaller interval width.

Remark 7.3. When the solution of the optimization problem given in (7.1.4) is not unique (e.g., $\pi(\theta|D)$ is uniform or $\pi(\theta|D)$ is constant over an interval or several intervals), we take the one with the smallest lower limit of the interval.

We note that the marginal posterior density $\pi(\theta|D)$ is given by

$$\pi(\theta|D) = \int \pi(\theta, \varphi|D)\, d\varphi = \int \frac{1}{c(D)} L(\theta, \varphi|D)\pi(\theta, \varphi)\, d\varphi. \quad (7.1.7)$$

In (7.1.7), the normalizing constant $C(D)$ is often unknown and the analytical evaluation of the integral may not be available. In particular, this is true when φ is high-dimensional. Therefore, when $\pi(\theta|D)$ is analytically intractable, the aforementioned analytical approaches for computing credible and HPD intervals may not be applicable. Due to recent advances in computing technology and the development of MCMC sampling algorithms, it is possible to use an MC approach to approximate Bayesian credible and HPD intervals. In fact, various MC methods have been developed recently; see, for example, Box and Tiao (1992), Wei and Tanner (1990), Tanner (1996), Hyndman (1996), and Chen and Shao (1999b). These methods will be discussed in detail in the subsequent sections.

7.2 Estimating Bayesian Credible Intervals

First, we assume that an MCMC sample, $\{\theta_i,\ i = 1, 2, \ldots, n\}$, is available from the marginal posterior distribution $\pi(\theta|D)$. (Note that if $\{(\theta_i, \varphi_i),\ i = 1, 2, \ldots, n\}$ is an MCMC sample from the joint posterior distribution $\pi(\theta, \varphi|D)$, $\{\theta_i,\ i = 1, 2, \ldots, n\}$ is an MCMC sample from $\pi(\theta|D)$ (see Gelfand and Smith 1990).) Then the order statistics estimator of a $100(1-\alpha)\%$ Bayesian credible interval is given by

$$(\theta_{([(\alpha/2)n])}, \theta_{([(1-\alpha/2)n])}),$$

where $\theta_{([(\alpha/2)n])}$ and $\theta_{([(1-\alpha/2)n])}$ are the $[(\alpha/2)n]^{\text{th}}$ smallest and the $[(1-\alpha/2)n]^{\text{th}}$ smallest of $\{\theta_i\}$, respectively. Here, $[(\alpha/2)n]$ and $[(1-\alpha/2)n]$ are the integer parts of $(\alpha/2)n$ and $(1-\alpha/2)n$. Under certain regularity conditions such as *ergodicity*, it can be shown that $(\theta_{([(\alpha/2)n])}, \theta_{([(1-\alpha/2)n])})$ is a consistent estimator of $(\theta^{(\alpha/2)}, \theta^{(1-\alpha/2)})$. The other properties, such as asymptotic normality, of the sample quantiles can be found in, for example, Sen and Singer (1993).

Second, we assume that an MCMC sample, $\{(\theta_i, \varphi_i),\ i = 1, 2, \ldots n\}$, is readily available from a joint distribution $g(\theta, \varphi)$, which is different than the posterior distribution $\pi(\theta, \varphi|D)$, and we wish to use this MCMC sample to estimate the Bayesian credible interval for θ with respect to the marginal distribution $\pi(\theta|D)$. This is an interesting problem, since, as discussed in Chapter 6, one obtains samples from one distribution but wants to compute posterior quantities with respect to another distribution. The solution to this problem is particularly useful when the direct MCMC generation of θ from its desired marginal posterior distribution is difficult or infeasible. In the context of importance sampling, $g(\theta, \varphi)$ serves as an importance sampling density. It is well known that one can easily approximate posterior expectations using the samples from g. However, it becomes much more difficult to employ the importance sampling approach for estimating non-moment posterior quantities of interest, such as Bayesian credible or HPD intervals. Recently, Chen and Shao (1999b) use the weighted MC method to extend the importance sampling approach for computing Bayesian credible and HPD intervals.

Let $\theta^{(\gamma)}$ denote the γth quantile of θ, that is,

$$\theta^{(\gamma)} = \inf\{\theta : \ \Pi(\theta|D) \geq \gamma\},$$

where $0 < \gamma < 1$ and $\Pi(\theta|D)$ is the marginal posterior cumulative distribution function of θ. It is easy to observe that for a given θ^*

$$\Pi(\theta^*|D) = E\left(1\{\theta \leq \theta^*\}|D\right) = \frac{\int 1\{\theta \leq \theta^*\} \frac{L(\theta, \varphi|D)\pi(\theta, \varphi)}{g(\theta, \varphi)} g(\theta, \varphi) \, d\theta \, d\varphi}{\int \frac{L(\theta, \varphi|D)\pi(\theta, \varphi)}{g(\theta, \varphi)} g(\theta, \varphi) \, d\theta \, d\varphi}, \tag{7.2.1}$$

where $1\{\theta \leq \theta^*\}$ is the indicator function. Then a simulation consistent estimator of $\Pi(\theta^*|D)$ can be obtained by

$$\widehat{\Pi}(\theta^*|D) = \frac{\sum_{i=1}^n 1\{\theta_i \leq \theta^*\} L(\theta_i, \varphi_i|D)\pi(\theta_i, \varphi_i)/g(\theta_i, \varphi_i)}{\sum_{i=1}^n L(\theta_i, \varphi_i|D)\pi(\theta_i, \varphi_i)/g(\theta_i, \varphi_i)}. \tag{7.2.2}$$

Let $\{\theta_{(i)}\}$ denote the ordered values of $\{\theta_i\}$. We rewrite the MCMC sample $\{(\theta_i, \varphi_i), \ i = 1, 2, \ldots, n\}$ as $\{(\theta_{(i)}, \varphi_{(i)}), \ i = 1, 2, \ldots, n\}$. Note that here $\varphi_{(i)}$ is a notation which does not imply an ordered value. Denote

$$w_i = \frac{\dfrac{L(\theta_{(i)}, \varphi_{(i)}|D)\pi(\theta_{(i)}, \varphi_{(i)})}{g(\theta_{(i)}, \varphi_{(i)})}}{\sum_{j=1}^n \dfrac{L(\theta_j, \varphi_j|D)\pi(\theta_j, \varphi_j)}{g(\theta_j, \varphi_j)}} \tag{7.2.3}$$

for $1 \leq i \leq n$. From (7.2.3), it is easy to observe that it is required to know g only up to a normalizing constant, since this normalizing constant cancels out in the calculation of w_i. Thus, a weighted empirical cdf of θ is given by

$$\widehat{\Pi}(\theta^*|D) = \begin{cases} 0 & \text{if } \theta^* < \theta_{(1)}, \\ \sum_{j=1}^i w_j & \text{if } \theta_{(i)} \leq \theta^* < \theta_{(i+1)}, \\ 1 & \text{if } \theta^* \geq \theta_{(n)}. \end{cases} \tag{7.2.4}$$

When the MCMC sample $\{(\theta_i, \varphi_i)\}$ is generated directly from the desired joint posterior distribution $\pi(\theta, \varphi|D)$, $w_i = 1/n$, and thus $\widehat{\Pi}(\theta^*|D)$ reduces to a usual empirical cdf. Therefore, $\widehat{\Pi}(\theta^*|D)$ given in (7.2.4) is a generalization of the usual empirical cdf. Under certain regularity conditions such as *ergodicity*, Chen and Shao (1999b) show that the central limit theorem still holds for $\widehat{\Pi}(\theta^*|D)$. Using (7.2.4), $\theta^{(\gamma)}$ can be estimated by

$$\hat{\theta}^{(\gamma)} = \begin{cases} \theta_{(1)} & \text{if } \gamma = 0, \\ \theta_{(i)} & \text{if } \sum_{j=1}^{i-1} w_j < \gamma \leq \sum_{j=1}^{i} w_j. \end{cases} \tag{7.2.5}$$

In (7.2.5), taking $\gamma = \alpha/2$ and $\gamma = 1 - \alpha/2$, a consistent estimator of the $100(1-\alpha)\%$ Bayesian credible interval is given by

$$(\hat{\theta}^{(\alpha/2)}, \hat{\theta}^{(1-\alpha/2)}).$$

7.3 Estimating Bayesian HPD Intervals

As discussed in Section 7.1, the computation of an HPD interval is more difficult than that of a Bayesian credible interval. An analytical solution of $R(\pi_\alpha)$ defined in (7.1.3) is often not available even when the closed forms of $\pi(\theta|D)$ and $\Pi(\theta|D)$ are known. The computation of $R(\pi_\alpha)$ requires knowing π_α and then calculating the content defined by (7.1.3). Therefore, computing an HPD interval is often quite difficult and challenging. To obtain an approximation of π_α, an MC approach has been developed, see Wei and Tanner (1990), Tanner (1996), or Hyndman (1996) for details. Let $\xi = \pi(\theta|D)$, which is obtained by transforming θ by its own density function. Then, π_α is the αth quantile of ξ so that $P(\xi \geq \pi_\alpha) = 1 - \alpha$. Assume that an MCMC sample $\{\theta_i,\ i = 1, 2, \ldots, n\}$ is available from the marginal posterior distribution $\pi(\theta|D)$. Let $\xi_i = \pi(\theta_i|D)$ for $i = 1, 2, \ldots, n$. Then a consistent estimator of π_α is $\hat{\pi}_\alpha = \xi_{([\alpha n])}$, where $\xi_{([\alpha n])}$ is the $[\alpha n]^{\text{th}}$ smallest of $\{\xi_i\}$. After we obtain $\hat{\pi}_\alpha$, a consistent estimator of $R(\pi_\alpha)$ can be obtained by computing

$$\hat{R}(\hat{\pi}_\alpha) = \{\theta :\ \pi(\theta|D) \geq \hat{\pi}_\alpha\}. \tag{7.3.1}$$

Although the above procedure gives an asymptotically correct approximation of an HPD interval, there are two drawbacks with this procedure. First, it requires a closed-form expression of the marginal posterior distribution $\pi(\theta|D)$. Second, it is difficult to compute $\hat{R}(\hat{\pi}_\alpha)$ in (7.3.1). To overcome these difficulties, Chen and Shao (1999b) propose a much simpler MC method for computing HPD intervals. Chen and Shao's method does not require knowing the closed forms of $\pi(\theta|D)$ and $\Pi(\theta|D)$, and their method can be applied to compute HPD intervals not only for the parameters of interest, but also for functions of the parameters. In addition, their method can also be extended to the case where an MCMC sample is drawn from a different distribution. In the following subsections, we will discuss Chen and Shao's method in detail.

7.3.1 An Order Statistics Approach

For ease of exposition, we assume that $\pi(\theta|D)$ is unimodal. However, possible extensions to multimodal cases will be discussed in Section 7.6. We further assume that $\{(\theta_i, \varphi_i),\ i = 1, 2, \ldots, n\}$ is an MCMC sample from the joint posterior distribution $\pi(\theta, \varphi|D)$.

As discussed earlier, a $100(1-\alpha)\%$ HPD interval must have a probability content of $1-\alpha$ and the density for every point inside the interval must be greater than that for every point outside the interval. Therefore, an HPD interval is a special credible interval and this interval is of the shortest length among all possible credible intervals with the same probability content $1-\alpha$. Based on the main properties of the HPD interval, Chen and Shao (1999b) propose the following procedure for calculating an HPD interval for θ:

Chen–Shao HPD Estimation Algorithm

Step 1. Obtain an MCMC sample $\{\theta_i,\ i = 1, 2, \ldots, n\}$ from $\pi(\theta|D)$.

Step 2. Sort $\{\theta_i,\ i = 1, 2, \ldots, n\}$ to obtain the ordered values:

$$\theta_{(1)} \le \theta_{(2)} \le \cdots \le \theta_{(n)}.$$

Step 3. Compute the $100(1-\alpha)\%$ credible intervals

$$R_j(n) = (\theta_{(j)}, \theta_{(j+[(1-\alpha)n])})$$

for $j = 1, 2, \ldots, n - [(1-\alpha)n]$.

Step 4. The $100(1-\alpha)\%$ HPD interval is the one, denoted by $R_{j^*}(n)$, with *the smallest interval width* among all credible intervals.

Under certain regularity conditions, the above procedure is asymptotically valid. The result is given in the following theorem:

Theorem 7.3.1 *Assume that $\{\theta_i,\ i = 1, 2, \ldots, n\}$ is an ergodic MCMC sample from $\pi(\theta|D)$. If $\pi(\theta|D)$ is unimodal and* (7.1.4) *has a unique solution, then*

$$R_{j^*}(n) \to R(\pi_\alpha) \text{ a.s. as } n \to \infty,$$

where $R(\pi_\alpha)$ is defined in (7.1.3).

The proof is given in the Appendix. Theorem 7.3.1 implies that R_{j^*} is an approximation of the $100(1-\alpha)\%$ HPD interval $R(\pi_\alpha)$. We comment that:

(i) when the derivative of $\pi(\theta|D)$ is not constant over any connected intervals, then (7.1.4) has a unique solution; and

(ii) when the solution of (7.1.4) is not unique, more than one $R_j(n)$ may have the same smallest interval width, and for this case, we recommend taking the one with the smallest lower interval limit to ensure the uniqueness of the choice of $R_{j^*}(n)$.

Theorem 7.3.1 is also useful for computing an HPD interval of a function of θ and φ. To see this, we consider $\eta = h(\theta, \varphi)$ where h is a known function. Unlike a Bayesian credible interval, the HPD interval is not invariant under a nonlinear transformation (see Box and Tiao 1992). Even for a simple case where $\eta = h(\theta)$, the HPD interval of η cannot be obtained by computing $h(\theta_{(j^*)})$ and $h(\theta_{(j^*+[(1-\alpha)n])})$ if h is not a linear function. However, Theorem 7.3.1 can be extended to obtain the HPD interval for $\eta = h(\theta, \varphi)$. The result is given in the following corollary:

Corollary 7.3.1 *Let $\{(\theta_i, \varphi_i),\ i = 1, 2, \ldots, n\}$ be an ergodic MCMC sample from $\pi(\theta, \varphi|D)$. Also let $\eta_i = h(\theta_i, \varphi_i)$ and let $\eta_{(i)}$ be the ordered values of the η_i. Then a $100(1-\alpha)\%$ HPD interval of η can be approximated by*

$$R_{j^*}(n) = (\eta_{(j^*)}, \eta_{(j^*+[(1-\alpha)n])}), \tag{7.3.2}$$

where j^* is chosen so that

$$\eta_{(j^*+[(1-\alpha)n])} - \eta_{(j^*)} = \min_{1 \le j \le n-[(1-\alpha)n]} (\eta_{(j+[(1-\alpha)n])} - \eta_{(j)}). \tag{7.3.3}$$

The proof of Corollary 7.3.1 directly follows from Theorem 7.3.1. This result makes the Chen–Shao algorithm attractive compared to an approach using $\hat{R}(\hat{\pi}_\alpha)$ given in (7.3.1), since in (7.3.1) we need to have a closed-form of the marginal density of $\eta = h(\theta, \varphi)$.

7.3.2 Weighted Monte Carlo Estimation of HPD Intervals

Assume that $\{(\theta_i, \varphi_i),\ i = 1, 2, \ldots n\}$ is an MCMC sample from the joint distribution $g(\theta, \varphi)$. Similar to the construction of Bayesian credible interval estimators, we can obtain a weighted MC estimator of an HPD interval using the sample $\{(\theta_i, \varphi_i)\}$ from g. Let

$$R_j(n) = (\hat{\theta}^{(j/n)}, \hat{\theta}^{(\{j+[(1-\alpha)n]\}/n)}), \tag{7.3.4}$$

for $j = 1, 2, \ldots, n - [(1-\alpha)n]$. In (7.3.4), $\hat{\theta}^{(j/n)}$ is defined by (7.2.5). Then, similar to Theorem 7.3.1, we have the following result:

Theorem 7.3.2 *Let $R_{j^*}(n)$ be the interval that has the smallest width among all $R_j(n)$'s. If $\pi(\theta|D)$ is unimodal and (7.1.4) has a unique solution, then we have*

$$R_{j^*}(n) \to R(\pi_\alpha) \quad as\ n \to \infty,$$

where $R(\pi_\alpha)$ is defined in (7.1.3).

The proof of the theorem is given in the Appendix. Similar to Corollary 7.3.1, we can obtain an HPD interval for $\eta = h(\theta, \varphi)$ as follows:

Corollary 7.3.2 *Let $\eta_i = h(\theta_i, \varphi_i)$ for $i = 1, 2, \ldots, n$. Also let the $\eta_{(i)}$ denote the ordered values of the η_i. Then the γth quantile of the marginal posterior distribution of η can be estimated by*

$$\hat{\eta}^{(\gamma)} = \begin{cases} \eta_{(1)} & \text{if } \gamma = 0, \\ \eta_{(i)} & \text{if } \sum_{j=1}^{i-1} w_{(j)} < \gamma \leq \sum_{j=1}^{i} w_{(j)}, \end{cases} \tag{7.3.5}$$

where $w_{(j)}$ is the weight function associated with the jth ordered value $\eta_{(j)}$. More specifically, we first compute

$$w_j = \frac{\dfrac{L(\theta_j, \varphi_j|D)\pi(\theta_j, \varphi_j)}{g(\theta_j, \varphi_j)}}{\sum_{l=1}^{n} \dfrac{L(\theta_l, \varphi_l|D)\pi(\theta_l, \varphi_l)}{g(\theta_l, \varphi_l)}}.$$

Then we rewrite $\{w_j,\ j = 1, 2, \ldots, n\}$ as $\{w_{(j)},\ j = 1, 2, \ldots, n\}$ so that the jth value $w_{(j)}$ corresponds to the jth ordered value $\eta_{(j)}$. Using (7.3.5), we compute

$$R_j(n) = (\hat{\eta}^{(j/n)}, \hat{\eta}^{(\{j+[(1-\alpha)n]\}/n)}), \tag{7.3.6}$$

and a $100(1-\alpha)\%$ HPD interval of η is $R_{j^*}(n)$ that has the smallest interval width among all $R_j(n)$'s.

We note that the same weight function w_i can be used for computing the HPD interval for θ as well as for any functions of θ and φ. Therefore, the proposed MC methods are advantageous and computationally efficient when one wants to simultaneously compute the HPD intervals for many posterior quantities of interest.

7.4 Extension to the Constrained Parameter Problems

In this section, we apply the weighted MC approach developed in Sections 7.2 and 7.3 to a Bayesian hierarchical model considered in Section 6.1, in which the resulting posterior density contains analytically intractable integrals that depend on hyperparameters.

Suppose that a Bayesian hierarchical model has the following posterior density:

$$\pi(\theta, \varphi, \boldsymbol{\lambda}|D) = \frac{1}{c_w(D)} L(\theta, \varphi|D) \cdot \frac{\pi(\theta, \varphi|\boldsymbol{\lambda})}{c(\boldsymbol{\lambda})} 1\{(\theta, \varphi) \in S\} \cdot \pi(\boldsymbol{\lambda}) 1\{\boldsymbol{\lambda} \in \Lambda\}, \tag{7.4.1}$$

where θ and φ are the parameters of interest, $\boldsymbol{\lambda}$ is a vector of hyperparameters, and $\pi(\theta,\varphi|\boldsymbol{\lambda})$ and $\pi(\boldsymbol{\lambda})$ are proper priors with supports Θ and Λ, i.e., $\int_\Theta \pi(\theta,\varphi|\boldsymbol{\lambda})\, d\theta\, d\varphi = 1$ and $\int_\Lambda \pi(\boldsymbol{\lambda})\, d\boldsymbol{\lambda} = 1$. In (7.4.1), $S \subset \Theta$ is the constrained space that may or may not depend on the data according to the nature of the problem,

$$c(\boldsymbol{\lambda}) = \int_S \pi(\theta,\varphi|\boldsymbol{\lambda})\, d\theta\, d\varphi, \tag{7.4.2}$$

and

$$c_w(D) = \int_\Omega L(\theta,\varphi|D)[\pi(\theta,\varphi|\boldsymbol{\lambda})/c(\boldsymbol{\lambda})]\pi(\boldsymbol{\lambda})\, d\theta\, d\varphi\, d\boldsymbol{\lambda},$$

where Ω is the support of $\pi(\theta,\varphi,\boldsymbol{\lambda}|D)$, defined as

$$\Omega = S \otimes \Lambda = \{(\theta,\varphi,\boldsymbol{\lambda}) : (\theta,\varphi) \in S \text{ and } \boldsymbol{\lambda} \in \Lambda\}.$$

As discussed in Section 6.1, directly sampling from $\pi(\theta,\varphi,\boldsymbol{\lambda}|D)$ is nearly impossible. However, for many Bayesian hierarchical models, it is possible to sample from the so-called pseudo-posterior density $\pi^*(\theta,\varphi,\boldsymbol{\lambda}|D)$ given in (6.1.3) by using an MCMC sampling algorithm. See Section 6.4 for illustrative examples. In order to calculate $100(1-\alpha)\%$ credible and HPD intervals for θ, it is natural to choose g as the pseudo-posterior density $\pi^*(\theta,\varphi,\boldsymbol{\lambda}|D)$. That is,

$$g(\theta,\varphi,\boldsymbol{\lambda}) \propto L(\theta,\varphi|D)\pi(\theta,\varphi|\boldsymbol{\lambda})1\{(\theta,\varphi)\in S\}\pi(\boldsymbol{\lambda})1\{\boldsymbol{\lambda}\in\Lambda\}.$$

For ease of exposition, we assume that $\{(\theta_{(i)},\boldsymbol{\varphi}_{(i)},\boldsymbol{\lambda}_{(i)}),\ i=1,2,\ldots,n\}$ is an MCMC sample from g, where $\theta_{(1)} \le \theta_{(2)} \le \cdots \le \theta_{(n)}$. Similar to (7.2.4), the weighted empirical cdf of θ is given as follows:

$$\widehat{\Pi}(\theta^*|D) = \begin{cases} 0 & \text{if } \theta^* < \theta_{(1)}, \\ \sum_{j=1}^i w_j & \text{if } \theta_{(i)} \le \theta^* < \theta_{(i+1)}, \\ 1 & \text{if } \theta^* \ge \theta_{(n)}, \end{cases} \tag{7.4.3}$$

where

$$w_i = \frac{1/c(\boldsymbol{\lambda}_{(i)})}{\sum_{j=1}^n 1/c(\boldsymbol{\lambda}_{(j)})}. \tag{7.4.4}$$

In (7.4.4), the $c(\boldsymbol{\lambda}_{(i)})$'s are unknown and so is $\widehat{\Pi}_j(\theta^*|D)$. Recall that

$$c(\boldsymbol{\lambda}) = \int_S \pi(\theta,\varphi|\boldsymbol{\lambda})\, d\theta\, d\varphi.$$

Then, using the MC method given in Section 6.3, $c(\boldsymbol{\lambda}_{(i)})$ can be estimated by

$$\hat{c}_m(\boldsymbol{\lambda}_{(i)}) = \frac{1}{m}\sum_{j=1}^m \frac{\pi(\theta_j^{\text{mix}},\boldsymbol{\varphi}_j^{\text{mix}}|\boldsymbol{\lambda}_{(i)})1_S(\theta_j^{\text{mix}},\boldsymbol{\varphi}_j^{\text{mix}})}{\pi_{\text{mix}}(\theta_j^{\text{mix}},\boldsymbol{\varphi}_j^{\text{mix}})}, \tag{7.4.5}$$

where $\pi_{\text{mix}}(\theta, \varphi)$ is a mixing density, which is known up to a normalizing constant and has support S, and $\{(\theta_j^{\text{mix}}, \varphi_j^{\text{mix}}),\ j = 1, 2, \ldots, m\}$ is an MCMC sample from π_{mix}. Using (7.4.3), the weighted MC methods described in Sections 7.2 and 7.3.2 can be directly applied to obtain the estimators of $100(1-\alpha)\%$ credible and HPD intervals. The detailed formulations are omitted here for brevity.

7.5 Numerical Illustration

7.5.1 A Simulation Study

In this subsection, we study the performance of the MC estimator of the HPD interval for θ given in Theorem 7.3.1.

We consider Bayesian inference concerning a variance ratio of two independent normal populations. Suppose that N_j independent observations y_{jl}, $l = 1, 2, \ldots, N_j$, are drawn from the normal population $N(\mu_j, \sigma_j^2)$ for $j = 1, 2$. We take a uniform prior for μ_1, μ_2, $\log \sigma_1^2$, and $\log \sigma_2^2$, that is, $\pi(\mu_1, \mu_2, \sigma_1^2, \sigma_2^2) \propto 1/(\sigma_1^2 \sigma_2^2)$. Let s_j^2 denote the sample variance of the y_{ji}'s and $\nu_j = N_j - 1$ for $j = 1, 2$. We are interested in making inference on the variance ratio $\theta = \sigma_2^2/\sigma_1^2$. In particular, we want to obtain a $100(1-\alpha)\%$ HPD interval for θ since the posterior distribution of θ is skewed. From Box and Tiao (1992), the marginal posterior distribution of θ is given by

$$\pi(\theta|s_1^2, s_2^2) = \frac{\left(\dfrac{s_1^2\nu_1}{s_2^2\nu_2}\right)^{\nu_1/2}}{B(\nu_1/2, \nu_2/2)} \theta^{\nu_1/2-1} \left(1 + \frac{s_1^2\nu_1}{s_2^2\nu_2}\theta\right)^{-(\nu_1+\nu_2)/2}, \ \theta > 0. \tag{7.5.1}$$

For illustrative purposes, we consider $N_1 = 20$, $s_1^2 = 12$, $N_2 = 12$, and $s_2^2 = 50$. Box and Tiao (1992) also use a similar example to illustrate the derivation of an HPD interval for $\ln(\sigma_2^2/\sigma_1^2)$. Since we are interested in an HPD interval of σ_2^2/σ_1^2, we cannot directly use their results because the HPD interval is not invariant under a nonlinear transformation. Therefore, we use (7.1.4) to obtain an exact $100(1-\alpha)\%$ HPD interval, denoted by $(\theta_L(\alpha), \theta_U(\alpha))$, for $\theta = \sigma_2^2/\sigma_1^2$, by the Nelder–Mead algorithm. Because θ is univariate, the Nelder–Mead algorithm is expected to work well. However, this optimization algorithm may become very inefficient in high-dimensional problems; see Nemhauser, Rinnooy Kan, and Todd (1989) for a detailed discussion. Assume that $\{\theta_i,\ i = 1, 2, \ldots, n\}$ is a random sample from $\pi(\theta|s_1^2, s_2^2)$ given by (7.5.1). Then, from the Chen–Shao algorithm, an estimated HPD interval for θ is $(\theta_{(j^*)}, \theta_{(j^*+[(1-\alpha)n])})$. To study convergence of $(\theta_{(j^*)}, \theta_{(j^*+[(1-\alpha)n])})$, we define the following mean relative error (ME):

$$\text{ME}_n = E(|\theta_{(j^*)} - \theta_L(\alpha)| + |\theta_{(j^*+[(1-\alpha)n])} - \theta_U(\alpha)|)/(\theta_U(\alpha) - \theta_L(\alpha)),$$

TABLE 7.1. Mean Relative Errors of the Estimated HPD Intervals of $\theta = \sigma_2^2/\sigma_1^2$ with Simulation Standard Errors in Parentheses.

$1-\alpha$	$(\theta_L(\alpha), \theta_U(\alpha))$		ME_n	
		$n = 500$	$n = 1000$	$n = 5000$
0.75	(1.6435, 6.4546)	0.0891	0.0614	0.0341
		(0.0023)	(0.0016)	(0.0010)
0.90	(1.2407, 8.7862)	0.0636	0.0447	0.0364
		(0.0017)	(0.0012)	(0.0007)
0.95	(1.0263, 10.7439)	0.0650	0.0482	0.0238
		(0.0018)	0.0013)	(0.0006)

where the expectation is taken with respect to the distribution of the θ_i. For a given n, ME_n quantifies the relative difference between the estimated HPD interval $(\theta_{(j^*)}, \theta_{(j^*+[(1-\alpha)n])})$ and the exact HPD interval $(\theta_L(\alpha), \theta_U(\alpha))$ for θ.

Since

$$E(|\theta_{(j^*)} - \theta_L(\alpha)| + |\theta_{(j^*+[(1-\alpha)n])} - \theta_U(\alpha)|))$$

is analytically intractable, we use a standard simulation technique to estimate this expectation. We run K simulations and then calculate

$$\mathrm{ME}_{n,k} = (|\theta_{(j^*),k} - \theta_L(\alpha)| + |\theta_{(j^*+[(1-\alpha)n]),k} - \theta_U(\alpha)|)/(\theta_U(\alpha) - \theta_L(\alpha))$$

for $k = 1, 2, \ldots, K$. Then, ME_n is approximated by $(1/K)\sum_{k=1}^K \mathrm{ME}_{n,k}$ and the simulation standard error is the square root of the sample variance of the $\mathrm{ME}_{n,k}$'s. Table 7.1 gives the ME_n's with the simulation standard errors for various n and $1-\alpha$ using $K = 500$. From Table 7.1, it can be observed that the disagreement between the estimated and exact HPD intervals is within 10% of the length of the exact one for all cases. So, the estimated HPD intervals are quite close to the exact ones even for $n = 500$. Further, based on the 75%, 90%, and 95% HPD intervals, σ_2^2 is significantly greater than σ_1^2 since all three HPD intervals are located on the right-hand side of 1.

7.5.2 Meal, Ready-to-Eat (MRE) Data Example

Consider the MRE data given in Example 1.2 and the associated Bayesian hierarchical model discussed in Section 6.4.1. Following the notation in Section 6.4.1, the resulting posterior distribution in (6.4.10) has the form

$$\pi(\boldsymbol{z}, \boldsymbol{\theta}, \boldsymbol{\lambda}|D) \propto \prod_{i,j}\prod_{l=1}^{36}\left\{\sum_{s=1}^{9} 1\{y_{ijl} = s\}1\{a_{s-1} < z_{ijl} \leq a_s\}\right\}\frac{1}{\sigma}\phi\left(\frac{z_{ijl} - \theta_{ij}}{\sigma}\right)$$
$$\times \frac{\pi(\boldsymbol{\theta}^{(-\sigma^2)}|\boldsymbol{\lambda})}{c(\boldsymbol{\lambda})} 1\{\boldsymbol{\theta} \in \Theta\}\pi(\sigma^2|\zeta, \eta)\pi(\boldsymbol{\lambda}),$$

where

$$c(\boldsymbol{\lambda}) = \int_{\Theta} \left\{ \prod_{i,j} \frac{1}{\delta} \phi \left(\frac{\theta_{ij} - \lambda_i}{\delta} \right) \right\} d\boldsymbol{\theta}^{(-\sigma^2)}.$$

As suggested in Section 7.4, we take $g(\boldsymbol{z}, \boldsymbol{\theta}, \boldsymbol{\lambda})$ to be the pseudo-posterior density in (6.4.11), i.e.,

$$g(\boldsymbol{z}, \boldsymbol{\theta}, \boldsymbol{\lambda}) \propto \prod_{i,j} \prod_{l=1}^{36} \left\{ \sum_{s=1}^{9} 1\{y_{ijl} = s\} 1\{a_{s-1} < z_{ijl} \leq a_s\} \right\} \frac{1}{\sigma} \phi \left(\frac{z_{ijl} - \theta_{ij}}{\sigma} \right)$$
$$\times \pi(\boldsymbol{\theta}^{(-\sigma^2)} | \boldsymbol{\lambda}) 1\{\boldsymbol{\theta} \in \Theta\} \pi(\sigma^2 | \zeta, \eta) \pi(\boldsymbol{\lambda}).$$

We generate an MCMC sample of size 2000 from $g(\boldsymbol{z}, \boldsymbol{\theta}, \boldsymbol{\lambda})$ and another MCMC sample of size 10000 from π_{mix} given in (6.4.12) and (6.4.13). Then, using the MC methods developed in Section 7.4, we compute the 95% HPD intervals for the mean scores ξ_{ij}, which are functions of $\boldsymbol{\theta}$ and σ^2. Table 7.2 gives the results. In Table 7.2, the top entry is the posterior mean and the bottom entry is the 95% HPD interval. From Figure 6.1, it can be observed that the marginal posterior densities of the mean scores are unimodal. Also note that the conventional approaches, such as those described in Box and Tiao (1992) or Hyndman (1996) by using (7.3.1), are difficult to apply for our MRE model. The main reasons are:

(i) the MRE model involves the hyperparameter-dependent normalizing constants $c(\boldsymbol{\lambda})$;

(ii) the mean scores are functions of the model parameters; and

(iii) analytical evaluation of the marginal distributions for the mean scores does not appear possible.

From a data analysis viewpoint, the 95% HPD intervals are informative. For example, the 95% HPD interval for the mean score of the fresh ham–chicken loaf at 21 °C is above all the HPD intervals for the mean scores at 38 °C stored at least 6 months, which implies that the quality of ham–chicken loaf significantly deteriorates with time at high temperatures. Further, it should be mentioned that the HPD intervals are shorter than the frequentist asymptotic t confidence intervals. For instance, after the ham–chicken loaf was stored 6 months at 4 °C, the raw mean score is 5.833, which is comparable to the Bayesian posterior estimate, namely, 5.854. However, the 95% t confidence interval is (5.242, 6.425), which is much wider than the 95% HPD interval (5.606, 6.092). Similar results are obtained for the other temperature–time combinations. The primary reasons that our HPD intervals are shorter than the t confidence intervals are:

(i) we incorporate order restrictions in the hierarchical model; and

(ii) we use the pastries data to fit the hyperparameters.

TABLE 7.2. Bayesian Estimates and 95% HPD Intervals of the Mean Rating Scores.

Time	Temperature			
(in months)	4 °C	21 °C	30 °C	38 °C
0	-	5.984	-	-
	-	(5.700, 6.291)	-	-
6	-	-	5.727	5.346
	-	-	(5.404, 6.027)	(4.953, 5.658)
12	5.854	5.739	5.485	5.139
	(5.606, 6.092)	(5.484, 5.914)	(5.213, 5.710)	(4.797, 5.398)
18	-	5.651	5.352	4.992
	-	(5.421, 5.832)	(5.087, 5.572)	(4.668, 5.264)
24	-	5.581	5.204	4.835
	-	(5.361, 5.751)	(4.899, 5.436)	(4.447, 5.134)
30	5.683	5.499	5.082	-
	(5.424, 5.906)	(5.300, 5.691)	(4.754, 5.325)	-
36	5.590	5.428	4.811	-
	(5.371, 5.805)	(5.192, 5.602)	(4.301, 5.183)	-
48	5.485	5.323	-	-
	(5.256, 5.714)	(5.022, 5.498)	-	-
60	5.344	5.137	-	-
	(5.050, 5.570)	(4.749, 5.384)	-	-

Chen, Nandram, and Ross (1996) find that the Bayesian method based on the hierarchical model which incorporates order restrictions provides improved precision over the non-Bayesian method commonly used in food technology, which does not provide a reliable measure of variability. The HPD intervals in Table 7.2 further support their findings.

7.6 Discussion

In this chapter, we have presented a simple MC method for computing HPD intervals. In particular, it has been shown that this new MC method is useful not only for computing HPD intervals for parameters of interest, but also for functions of the parameters. The small scale simulation study in Section 7.5.1 empirically shows that the Chen–Shao algorithm for estimating HPD intervals performs well even with a moderate simulation sample size, say $n = 1000$. For the MRE data problem, the weighted MC method can easily be implemented to compute HPD intervals for all the mean scores.

Although we state Theorems 7.3.1 and 7.3.2 under the unimodal assumption, these results can be possibly extended to multimodal cases. Here, we state the following conjecture. Assume that $\pi(\theta|D)$ has at most two modes. Let $\{\theta_1, \theta_2, \ldots, \theta_n\}$ be a sample from $\pi(\theta|D)$ and let $\theta_{(j)}$ be the ordered values of the θ_j. For $0 < \alpha < 1$, denote

$$D = \min_{0 \le m \le [(1-\alpha)n]} \min_{0 \le i \le n-[n(1-\alpha)]-2m} \\ \times \min_{i+m \le j \le n-[n(1-\alpha)]-m} \{(\theta_{(i+m)} - \theta_{(i)}) + (\theta_{(j+[n\alpha]-m)} - \theta_{(j)})\}.$$

If $(\theta_{(i^*+m^*)} - \theta_{(i^*)}) + (\theta_{(j^*+[n\alpha]-m^*)} - \theta_{(j^*)}) = D$, then $(\theta_{(i^*)},\ \theta_{(i^*+m^*)}) \cup (\theta_{(j^*)},\ \theta_{(j^*+[n\alpha]-m^*)})$ is an approximate HPD region for θ. We expect that when $\pi(\theta|D)$ is unimodal, $(\theta_{(i^*)},\ \theta_{(i^*+m^*)}) \cup (\theta_{(j^*)},\ \theta_{(j^*+[n\alpha]-m^*)})$ be automatically reduced to one interval. Similarly, we can extend this conjecture to cases where $\pi(\theta|D)$ has more than two modes.

Compared to the other existing methods, the methods presented in Sections 7.2 and 7.3 are nonparametric in the sense that we do not require knowing any parametric forms of the marginal or conditional posterior distributions for θ. Therefore, these methods can be implemented in a routine manner. Note that the methods given in Wei and Tanner (1990) or Tanner (1996) require estimating the marginal posterior density for θ, and therefore, the resulting HPD estimators depend on the quality of the marginal density estimation. In particular, their methods will become computationally expensive when one wants to estimate HPD intervals for many parameters or functions of the parameters of interest.

In contrast to frequentist confidence intervals, HPD intervals do not rely on normality or asymptotic normality assumptions. Therefore, the HPD intervals are advantageous especially when the sample size is small. Thus, we believe that the methodology presented in this chapter is useful to Bayesian practitioners as it is now standard practice to tabulate interval estimates in Bayesian data analysis.

Appendix

Proof of Theorem 7.3.1. Let $Q(t) = \Pi^{-1}(t|D) = \inf\{\theta : \Pi(\theta|D) \ge t\}$ for $0 \le t \le 1$ be the quantile function and let $Q_n(t)$ be the empirical quantile function, i.e.,

$$Q_n(t) = \begin{cases} \theta_{(1)} & \text{if } t = 0, \\ \theta_{(i)} & \text{if } (i-1)/n < t \le i/n. \end{cases}$$

We first show that

$$\min_{1\leq j\leq n-[(1-\alpha)n]}(\theta_{(j+[(1-\alpha)n])}-\theta_{(j)})\to\theta_U-\theta_L \text{ a.s.} \tag{7.A.1}$$

Since $\pi(\theta|D)$ is unimodal, we have

$$\theta_U-\theta_L=\inf_{0\leq t\leq\alpha}(Q(t+1-\alpha)-Q(t)). \tag{7.A.2}$$

By ergodicity (see, e.g., Tierney (1994)), we have

$$\frac{1}{n}\sum_{i=1}^{n}1\{\theta_i\leq\theta\}\to\Pi(\theta|D) \text{ a.s.}$$

for every θ. Hence, we have (see, e.g., Csörgő and Horváth (1993) or Serfling (1980))

$$Q_n(t)\to Q(t) \text{ a.s.} \tag{7.A.3}$$

for every t. Thus, a Glivenko–Cantelli type proof shows that

$$\forall\, A>0,\quad \sup_{|Q(t)|\leq A}|Q_n(t)-Q(t)|\to 0 \text{ a.s.} \tag{7.A.4}$$

(see the proof of Theorem 3 in Mason (1982)). Put

$$a=\inf\{\theta:\pi(\theta|D)>0\}\ \text{ and }\ b=\sup\{\theta:\pi(\theta|D)>0\}.$$

We consider three cases.

Case 1. If $-\infty<a<b<\infty$, then

$$\begin{aligned}\Big|\min_{1\leq j\leq n-[(1-\alpha)n]}&(\theta_{(j+[(1-\alpha)n]}-\theta_{(j)})-\inf_{0\leq t\leq 1-\alpha}(Q(t+1-\alpha)-Q(t))\Big|\\ &\leq 2\sup_{0\leq t\leq 1}|Q_n(t)-Q(t)|+2\sup_{0\leq s\leq t\leq s+2/n}|Q(t)-Q(s)|\\ &\to 0 \text{ a.s.}\end{aligned}$$

by (7.A.4).

Case 2. If $a=-\infty$ and $b=\infty$, then $Q(0)=-\infty$ and $Q(1)=\infty$. It follows from (7.A.2) that there exists a $0<\delta<1-\alpha$ such that

$$\begin{aligned}\inf_{0\leq t\leq 1-\alpha}(Q(t+1-\alpha)-Q(t))=&\inf_{\delta\leq t\leq 1-\alpha-\delta}(Q(t+1-\alpha)-Q(t))\\ =&Q_U-Q_L.\end{aligned} \tag{7.A.5}$$

Choose $0<\varepsilon_0<\delta$ such that

$$Q(\varepsilon_0)<-1-2(\theta_U-\theta_L)-Q(1-\alpha) \tag{7.A.6}$$

and

$$Q(1-\varepsilon_0)>1+2(\theta_U-\theta_L)+Q(\alpha). \tag{7.A.7}$$

Let j^* be an integer satisfying

$$\theta_{(j^*+[(1-\alpha)n])} - \theta_{(j^*)} = \min_{1\le j\le n-[(1-\alpha)n]} (\theta_{(j+[(1-\alpha)n])} - \theta_{(j)}).$$

Observing that

$$\begin{aligned}\{j^*/n < \varepsilon_0\} \subset & \Big\{ \min_{1\le j\le \varepsilon_0 n} (\theta_{(j+[(1-\alpha)n])} - \theta_{(j)}) \\ & \quad \le \min_{\varepsilon_0 n< j\le n+[(1-\alpha)n-\varepsilon_0 n]} (\theta_{(j+[(1-\alpha)n])} - \theta_{(j)}) \Big\} \\ & \subset \Big\{ \min_{1\le j\le \varepsilon_0 n} (\theta_{(j+[(1-\alpha)n])} - \theta_{(j)}) \le 2(\theta_U - \theta_L) \Big\} \\ & \quad \cup \Big\{ \min_{\varepsilon_0 n< j\le n+[(1-\alpha)n-\varepsilon_0 n]} (\theta_{(j+[(1-\alpha)n])} - \theta_{(j)}) > 2(\theta_U - \theta_L) \Big\} \\ & \subset \{ Q_n([(1-\alpha)n]/n) - Q_n([\varepsilon_0 n]/n) \le 2(\theta_U - \theta_L) \} \\ & \quad \cup \Big\{ \min_{\varepsilon_0 n< j\le n+[(1-\alpha)n-\varepsilon_0 n]} (\theta_{(j+[(1-\alpha)n])} - \theta_{(j)}) > 2(\theta_U - \theta_L) \Big\},\end{aligned}$$

$$Q_n([(1-\alpha)n]/n) - Q_n([\varepsilon_0 n]/n) \to Q(1-\alpha) - Q(\varepsilon_0) > 2(\theta_U - \theta_L) \text{ a.s.}$$

and

$$\min_{\varepsilon_0 n< j\le n+[(1-\alpha)n-\varepsilon_0 n]} (Q(j + [(1-\alpha)n]) - Q_{(j)}) \to (\theta_U - \theta_L) \text{ a.s.}$$

we have

$$P(j^*/n < \varepsilon_0 \text{ infinitely often}) = 0. \tag{7.A.8}$$

Similarly,

$$P(j^*/n > 1 - \alpha - \varepsilon_0 \text{ infinitely often}) = 0. \tag{7.A.9}$$

For any $\varepsilon > 0$, let

$$\begin{aligned}Q_n = \Big\{ \Big| & \min_{1\le j\le n-[(1-\alpha)n]} (\theta_{(j+[(1-\alpha)n]} - \theta_{(j)}) \\ & - \inf_{0\le t\le 1-\alpha} (Q(t+1-\alpha) - Q(t)) \Big| > \varepsilon \Big\}.\end{aligned}$$

Then we have

$$\begin{aligned}
Q_n &\le \{j^*/n \le \varepsilon_0\} \cup \{j^*/n \ge 1-\alpha-\varepsilon_0\} \\
&\quad \cup \left\{ \left| \min_{1\le j\le n-[(1-\alpha)n]} (\theta_{(j+[(1-\alpha)n]} - \theta_{(j)}) \right.\right. \\
&\qquad \left.\left. - \inf_{0\le t\le 1-\alpha} (Q(t+1-\alpha) - Q(t)) \right| > \varepsilon, \varepsilon_0 n < j^* < (1-\alpha-\varepsilon_0)n \right\} \\
&\le \{j^*/n \le \varepsilon_0\} \cup \{j^*/n \ge 1-\alpha-\varepsilon_0\} \\
&\quad \cup \left\{ \left| \min_{\varepsilon_0 n\le j\le (1-\alpha-\varepsilon_0)n} (\theta_{(j+[(1-\alpha)n]} - \theta_{(j)}) \right.\right. \\
&\qquad \left.\left. - \inf_{\varepsilon_0\le t\le 1-\alpha-\varepsilon_0} (Q(t+1-\alpha) - Q(t)) \right| > \varepsilon \right\} \\
&\le \{j^*/n \le \varepsilon_0\} \cup \{j^*/n \ge 1-\alpha-\varepsilon_0\} \cup \left\{ 4 \sup_{\varepsilon_0\le t\le 1-\varepsilon_0} |Q_n(t) - Q(t)| > \varepsilon \right\} \\
&\quad \cup \left\{ 2 \sup_{\varepsilon_0\le s\le t\le s+2/n\le 1-\varepsilon_0} |Q(t) - Q(s)| > \varepsilon \right\}.
\end{aligned}$$

Therefore, by (7.A.8), (7.A.9), and (7.A.4)

$$\min_{1\le j\le n-[(1-\alpha)n]} (\theta_{(j+[(1-\alpha)n]} - \theta_{(j)}) - \inf_{0\le t\le 1-\alpha} (Q(t+1-\alpha) - Q(t)) \to 0 \text{ a.s.}$$

Case 3. When $a = -\infty$ and $b < \infty$ or $a > -\infty$ and $b = \infty$, the proof is similar to Case 1 and Case 2.

This proves (7.A.1). Next we show that

$$\theta_{(j^*)} \to \theta_L \text{ a.s.} \tag{7.A.10}$$

Since (7.1.4) has a unique solution, there exists a t^* such that $0 < t^* < 1-\alpha$,

$$\theta_U - \theta_L = \inf_{0\le t\le 1-\alpha} (Q(t+1-\alpha) - Q(t)) = Q(t^*+1-\alpha) - Q(t^*) \tag{7.A.11}$$

and for every $\varepsilon > 0$

$$\inf_{t\in(0,t^*-\varepsilon)\cup(t^*+\varepsilon,1-\alpha)} (Q(t+1-\alpha) - Q(t)) > \theta_U - \theta_L. \tag{7.A.12}$$

So, it suffices to show that

$$\frac{j^*}{n} \to t^* \text{ a.s.} \tag{7.A.13}$$

For any $\varepsilon > 0$ let

$$0 < \eta = \tfrac{1}{2}\left(\inf_{t\in(0,t^*-\varepsilon)\cup(t^*+\varepsilon,1-\alpha)} (Q(t+1-\alpha) - Q(t)) - (\theta_U - \theta_L) \right).$$

It is easy to see that

$$\left\{\frac{j^*}{n} \le t^* - \varepsilon\right\} \subset \left\{\min_{1\le j\le n-[(1-\alpha)n]}\{\theta_{(j+[(1-\alpha)n])} - \theta_{(j)}\}\right.$$

$$\left. = \min_{1\le j\le n(t^*-\varepsilon)}\{\theta_{(j+[(1-\alpha)n])} - \theta_{(j)}\}\right\}$$

$$\subset \left\{\left|\min_{1\le j\le n-[(1-\alpha)n]}\{\theta_{(j+[(1-\alpha)n])} - \theta_{(j)}\} - (\theta_U - \theta_L)\right| > \eta\right\}$$

$$\cup \left\{\left|\min_{1\le j\le n(t^*-\varepsilon)}\{\theta_{(j+[(1-\alpha)n])} - \theta_{(j)}\} - (\theta_U - \theta_L)\right| \le \eta\right\}$$

$$\subset \left\{\left|\min_{1\le j\le n-[(1-\alpha)n]}\{\theta_{(j+[(1-\alpha)n])} - \theta_{(j)}\} - (\theta_U - \theta_L)\right| > \eta\right\}$$

$$\cup \left\{\left|\min_{1\le j\le n(t^*-\varepsilon)}\{\theta_{(j+[(1-\alpha)n])} - \theta_{(j)}\}\right.\right.$$

$$\left.\left. - \inf_{0<t\le t^*-\varepsilon}(Q(t+1-\alpha) - Q(t))\right| \ge \eta\right\}.$$

Following the proof of (7.A.1), we have

$$P\left\{\left|\min_{1\le j\le n(t^*-\varepsilon)}\{\theta_{(j+[(1-\alpha)n])} - \theta_{(j)}\}\right.\right.$$

$$\left.\left. - \inf_{0<t\le t^*-\varepsilon}(Q(t+1-\alpha) - Q(t))\right| \ge \eta \text{ infinitely often}\right\} = 0.$$

Hence,

$$P(j^*/n \le t^* - \varepsilon \text{ infinitely often}) = 0.$$

Similarly,

$$P(j^*/n \ge t^* + \varepsilon \text{ infinitely often}) = 0.$$

This proves (7.A.13). □

Proof of Theorem 7.3.2. It is easy to show that $\hat{\theta}^{(\gamma)}$ is the left continuous inverse of the right continuous function $\widehat{\Pi}(t|D)$. Therefore, for any $0 < t < 1$

$$\hat{\theta}^{(\gamma)} \le t \text{ if and only if } \widehat{\Pi}(t|D) \ge \gamma. \tag{7.A.14}$$

It follows from (7.A.14) that

$$\hat{\theta}^{(\gamma)} - \theta^{(\gamma)} \to 0 \text{ a.s.}$$

for every $0 < \gamma < 1$. Furthermore, we have

$$\forall\, A > 0, \quad \sup_{|\theta^{(\gamma)}|\le A} |\hat{\theta}^{(\gamma)} - \theta^{(\gamma)}| \to 0 \text{ a.s.}$$

The remainder of the proof is similar to that of Theorem 7.3.1. □

Exercises

7.1 Assume θ has an exponential distribution, i.e.,

$$\pi(\theta) \propto \lambda \exp\{-\lambda\theta\}, \quad \theta > 0,$$

where $\lambda > 0$ is a known parameter.

(a) Compute a 95% credible interval for θ.

(b) Use (7.1.4) to obtain an analytical expression of a 95% HPD interval for θ.

(c) Compare the credible interval with the HPD interval and comment on your finding.

7.2 Suppose θ has a gamma distribution with density

$$\pi(\theta) \propto \theta^{\nu-1} \exp\{-\tau\theta\}, \quad \theta > 0, \tag{7.E.1}$$

where $\nu > 0$ and $\tau > 0$ are known parameters.

(a) Use (7.1.4) to obtain 95% HPD intervals for θ for $(\nu, \tau) = (2, 1)$, $(2, 0.5)$, $(10, 0.5)$, and $(20, 0.5)$.

(b) For each $(\nu, \tau) = (2, 1)$, $(2, 0.5)$, $(10, 0.5)$, and $(20, 0.5)$, generate a random sample $\{\theta_i,\ i = 1, 2, \ldots, n\}$ from (7.E.1), and then use the Chen–Shao algorithm to obtain an estimator of the 95% HPD interval for θ, for $n = 100$, 500, and 1000.

7.3 Let $\eta = \text{logit}(\theta) = \ln(\theta/(1-\theta))$, where $0 < \theta < 1$. Assume that $\eta \sim N(0, 1)$.

(a) Compute a 95% HPD interval for η.

(b) Let (η_L, η_U) denote the HPD interval obtained in Part (a). Compute

$$\theta_L = \frac{e^{\eta_L}}{1 + e^{\eta_L}} \quad \text{and} \quad \theta_U = \frac{e^{\eta_U}}{1 + e^{\eta_U}}.$$

Is (θ_L, θ_U) a 95% HPD interval for θ? Why?

(c) Generate a random sample $\{\eta_i,\ i = 1, 2, \ldots, n\}$ from an $N(0, 1)$ using a large sample size n (say, $n = 50000$). Use Corollary 7.3.1 to obtain an estimator of the 95% HPD interval for θ. Is the estimated HPD interval close to (θ_L, θ_U)?

7.4 Classical HPD Intervals

The methods presented in this chapter are also useful for calculating classical HPD intervals. As an illustration, consider frequentist inference concerning a variance ratio of two independent normal populations. Suppose that N_j independent observations y_{jl}, $l = 1, 2, \ldots, N_j$, are drawn from a normal population $N(\mu_j, \sigma_j^2)$ for $j = 1, 2$. Let s_j^2 denote the sample variance of the y_{ji}'s and $\nu_j = N_j - 1$ for $j = 1, 2$. Then, it is well known that $(s_1^2/s_2^2)(\sigma_2^2/\sigma_1^2)$ has an F-distribution with degrees of freedom (ν_1, ν_2).

(a) Let $F_{\nu_1,\nu_2,0.975}$ denote the 0.975^{th} quantile of the F-distribution F_{ν_1,ν_2}. Then, a 95% confidence interval for the variance ratio, σ_2^2/σ_1^2, is given by

$$\left((s_2^2/s_1^2)(1/F_{\nu_1,\nu_2,0.975}), (s_2^2/s_1^2)F_{\nu_1,\nu_2,0.975}\right).$$

Given $N_1 = 20$, $s_1^2 = 12$, $N_2 = 12$, and $s_2^2 = 50$, compute the above confidence interval.

(b) Let $F = (s_1^2/s_2^2)(\sigma_2^2/\sigma_1^2)$ and $F \sim F_{\nu_1,\nu_2}$. Also let $(F_{L,0.95}, F_{U,0.95})$ denote the solution of (7.1.4) with $1 - \alpha = 0.95$. Then a 95% classical HPD interval is defined as

$$\left((s_2^2/s_1^2)F_{L,0.95}, (s_2^2/s_1^2)F_{U,0.95}\right).$$

Use the data given in Part (a) to compute the above classical HPD interval and compare the resulting interval to the one obtained in Part (a).

(c) Generate a random sample $\{F_i,\ i = 1, 2, \ldots, n\}$ from the F-distribution F_{ν_1,ν_2}, and then use the Chen–Shao algorithm to obtain an approximation of $(F_{L,0.95}, F_{U,0.95})$ for $n = 500$, 1000, and 10000.

(d) Compare the intervals obtained from Parts (a) and (b) to a 95% Bayesian HPD interval given in Table 7.1.

7.5 For the job satisfaction example, the posterior means and standard deviations are displayed in Table 6.3. Using the prior distribution specified in Section 6.3, compute the 95% HPD intervals of cell probabilities θ_{ij} and the hyperparameters λ_j, $i, j = 1, 2, 3, 4$.

7.6 Suppose that y_1 and y_2 are independent samples from a Cauchy distribution with unknown location parameter θ and known scale 1. Let $D = (y_1, y_2)$. The likelihood function is given by

$$L(\theta|D) = \prod_{i=1}^{2} \frac{1}{\pi(1 + (y_i - \theta)^2)}.$$

Consider an improper uniform prior for θ, i.e., $\pi(\theta) \propto 1$, and suppose we have the observations $D = (y_1, y_2) = (-2, 2.5)$.

(a) Using the grid approximation, compute and plot the normalized posterior density function

$$\pi(\theta|D) \propto L(\theta|D)$$

as a function of θ. Is this posterior distribution bimodal?

(b) Draw an MCMC sample $\{\theta_i, i = 1, 2, \ldots, n\}$ from $\pi(\theta|D)$ for $n = 10000$, and then use the kernel method or the IWMDE method given in Chapter 4 to obtain an estimator of the posterior distribution $\pi(\theta|D)$.

TABLE 7.3. Number of Subjects with or without the Presence of Positive Colonization with *S. aureus*.

Positive Colonization?	Barcelona	London	Moscow
No	195	168	185
Yes	9	39	15

(c) Using the plot of the posterior distribution obtained from Part (a) or Part (b), compute an approximate 95% HPD region for θ.
(*Hint*: Use the definition of the HPD interval in your derivation.)

(d) Using the MCMC sample from Part (b), obtain an approximate 95% HPD region based on the conjecture given in Section 7.6. Does your approximate HPD interval match the one obtained from Part (c)?

7.7 Comparison of three binomial observations: In 1995, a study on the positive colonization with *S. aureus* was conducted. In this study, 611 women between the ages of 18 and 45 participated. The subjects were randomly sampled from three European cities: Barcelona ($j = 1$), London ($j = 2$), and Moscow ($j = 3$). The results are displayed in Table 7.3. We consider three independent binomial distributions for modeling these data. For $j = 1, 2, 3$, let θ_j denote the proportion of subjects who had positive colonization with *S. aureus* from the jth city. We take the prior distributions for θ_j to be independent uniform on $(0, 1)$.

(a) Write out the joint posterior distribution.

(b) Draw a random sample from the resulting posterior distribution with sample size $n = 10000$, and then use Corollary 7.3.1 to obtain the estimators of 95% HPD intervals for $\theta_1 - \theta_2$, $\theta_1 - \theta_3$, and $\theta_2 - \theta_3$. Do these HPD intervals suggest that there was a higher risk of the positive colonization with *S. aureus* of one city compared to the other two?

7.8 For the New Zealand apple data in Example 1.1, use the Chen–Shao algorithm to compute 90% and 95% HPD intervals for $\boldsymbol{\beta}$ and σ^2 using the constrained multiple linear regression model with the prior specification given in Example 2.2.

7.9 For the 1994 pollen count data in Example 1.3, draw an MCMC sample from the reparameterized posterior $\pi(\boldsymbol{\beta}, \sigma^2, \rho, \boldsymbol{\eta}|D)$ in (2.5.28) with $\delta_0 = 0.01$ and $\gamma_0 = 0.01$. Then use the Chen–Shao algorithm to obtain 95% HPD intervals for all regression coefficients. Based on these HPD intervals, discuss the importance of the pollen count covariates.

7.10 For the rating data in Table 2.1, draw an MCMC sample from the posterior distribution given in (2.6.9), and then compute a 95% HPD interval for $\boldsymbol{\beta}$. Does this HPD interval suggest that gender is an important covariate in predicting the rating score?

7.11 For the lifetime data in Table 2.2, draw an MCMC sample from the posterior distribution specified in Exercise 2.10 and then compute 95% HPD intervals for the regression coefficients for all of the main effects and interactions. Based on these HPD intervals, are there any important main effects or interactions?

8
Bayesian Approaches for Comparing Nonnested Models

Model comparison and model assessment are a crucial part of statistical analysis. Due to recent computational advances, sophisticated techniques for Bayesian model assessment are becoming increasingly popular. We have seen a recent surge in the statistical literature on Bayesian methods for model assessment and model comparison, including articles by George and McCulloch (1993), Madigan and Raftery (1994), Ibrahim and Laud (1994), Laud and Ibrahim (1995), Kass and Raftery (1995), Chib (1995), Chib and Greenberg (1998), Raftery, Madigan, and Volinsky (1995), George, McCulloch, and Tsay (1996), Raftery, Madigan, and Hoeting (1997), Gelfand and Ghosh (1998), Clyde (1999), Sinha, Chen, and Ghosh (1999), Ibrahim, Chen, and Sinha (1998), Ibrahim and Chen (1998), Ibrahim, Chen, and MacEachern (1999), and Chen, Ibrahim, and Yiannoutsos (1999). The scope of Bayesian model comparison and model assessment is quite broad, and can be investigated via Bayes factors, model diagnostics, and goodness of fit measures. In many situations, one may want to compare several models which are not nested. In this particular context, we consider model comparison using marginal likelihood approaches, "super-model" or "sub-model" approaches, and criterion-based methods. The computational techniques involved in these three approaches will be addressed in detail. In addition, several important applications, including scale mixtures of multivariate normal link models and Bayesian discretized semiparametric models for interval-censored data, will be presented.

8.1 Marginal Likelihood Approaches

8.1.1 The Method

Suppose that there are $\mathcal{K}$ models $\mathcal{M}_1, \mathcal{M}_2, \ldots, \mathcal{M}_\mathcal{K}$ under consideration. For model $\mathcal{M}_k$, the posterior distribution takes the form

$$\pi(\boldsymbol{\theta}_k|D, \mathcal{M}_k) \propto L(\boldsymbol{\theta}_k|D, \mathcal{M}_k)\pi(\boldsymbol{\theta}_k|\mathcal{M}_k), \qquad (8.1.1)$$

where $L(\boldsymbol{\theta}_k|D, \mathcal{M}_k)$ is the likelihood function, D denotes the data, and $\pi(\boldsymbol{\theta}_k|\mathcal{M}_k)$ is the prior distribution. Then the marginal likelihood is given by

$$m(D|\mathcal{M}_k) = \int L(\boldsymbol{\theta}_k|D, \mathcal{M}_k)\pi(\boldsymbol{\theta}_k|\mathcal{M}_k)\, d\boldsymbol{\theta}_k. \qquad (8.1.2)$$

To compare different models, we calculate the marginal likelihoods $m(D|\mathcal{M}_k)$ for $k = 1, 2, \ldots, \mathcal{K}$, and choose the model which yields the largest marginal likelihood. We mention that the marginal likelihood approach is essentially the same as the Bayes factor approach, which can be seen through the following identity for comparing models $\mathcal{M}_i$ and $\mathcal{M}_j$:

$$B_{ij} = \exp\{\ln[m(D|\mathcal{M}_i)] - \ln[m(D|\mathcal{M}_j)]\},$$

where B_{ij} is the Bayes factor.

8.1.2 Computation

As discussed in Section 5.10.1, the marginal likelihood $m(D|\mathcal{M}_k)$ in (8.1.2) is essentially the normalizing constant of the posterior distribution $\pi(\boldsymbol{\theta}_k|D, \mathcal{M}_k)$ in (8.1.1). Using (8.1.1) and (8.1.2), Chib (1995) obtains the following identity:

$$m(D|\mathcal{M}_k) = \frac{L(\boldsymbol{\theta}_k|D, \mathcal{M}_k)\pi(\boldsymbol{\theta}_k|\mathcal{M}_k)}{\pi(\boldsymbol{\theta}_k|D, \mathcal{M}_k)}. \qquad (8.1.3)$$

Let $\boldsymbol{\theta}_k^*$ denote the posterior mean or the posterior mode with respect to the posterior distribution $\pi(\boldsymbol{\theta}_k|D, \mathcal{M}_k)$. Then we have

$$m(D|\mathcal{M}_k) = \frac{L(\boldsymbol{\theta}_k^*|D, \mathcal{M}_k)\pi(\boldsymbol{\theta}_k^*|\mathcal{M}_k)}{\pi(\boldsymbol{\theta}_k^*|D, \mathcal{M}_k)}, \qquad (8.1.4)$$

since the identity in (8.1.3) holds for any $\boldsymbol{\theta}_k$. Here we choose $\boldsymbol{\theta}_k^*$ to be either the posterior mean or the posterior mode to ensure numerical stability, since $\boldsymbol{\theta}_k^*$ is a more likely point than the other points. We mention that when $\boldsymbol{\theta}_k^*$ is taken to be a point in the tail of the posterior distribution, it is very difficult to compute $\pi(\boldsymbol{\theta}_k^*|D, \mathcal{M}_k)$. This is particularly true when one uses a Markov chain Monte Carlo (MCMC) method, such as the kernel method or the IWMDE method discussed in Chapter 4, to estimate $\pi(\boldsymbol{\theta}_k^*|D, \mathcal{M}_k)$. The reason behind this is that it is very unlikely to have many MCMC draws falling in the tails of $\pi(\boldsymbol{\theta}_k^*|D, \mathcal{M}_k)$, and in certain extreme cases, $\boldsymbol{\theta}_k^*$ may fall outside the range of the MCMC observations, and this essentially leads to a very unreliable estimate of $\pi(\boldsymbol{\theta}_k^*|D, \mathcal{M}_k)$.

From a computational viewpoint, it may be more efficient to compute $\ln[m(D|\mathcal{M}_k)]$ instead of directly computing $m(D|\mathcal{M}_k)$ using (8.1.4). On the natural logarithmic scale, we can rewrite (8.1.4) as

$$\begin{aligned}\ln[m(D|\mathcal{M}_k)] = & \ln[L(\boldsymbol{\theta}_k^*|D, \mathcal{M}_k)] + \ln[\pi(\boldsymbol{\theta}_k^*|\mathcal{M}_k)] \\ & - \ln[\pi(\boldsymbol{\theta}_k^*|D, \mathcal{M}_k)]. \end{aligned} \tag{8.1.5}$$

For many applications, it may be straightforward to compute $L(\boldsymbol{\theta}_k^*|D, \mathcal{M}_k)$ and $\pi(\boldsymbol{\theta}_k^*|\mathcal{M}_k)$. Therefore, the only difficult computation involved in $\ln[m(D\ |\mathcal{M}_k)]$ is $\ln[\pi(\boldsymbol{\theta}_k^*|D, \mathcal{M}_k)]$. In general, $\pi(\boldsymbol{\theta}_k^*|D, \mathcal{M}_k)$ can be estimated using the kernel method or the IWMDE method via MCMC sampling. However, when data augmentation can be used in the posterior simulation, $\pi(\boldsymbol{\theta}_k^*|D, \mathcal{M}_k)$ can be estimated more efficiently. Chib (1995) examines several situations and illustrates how the data augmentation technique can be used to obtain an efficient Monte Carlo (MC) estimator of $\pi(\boldsymbol{\theta}_k^*|D, \mathcal{M}_k)$.

For illustrative purposes, we assume that $\boldsymbol{\theta}_k = (\boldsymbol{\theta}_{k,1}, \boldsymbol{\theta}_{k,2})$, and the Gibbs sampler is applied to the complete conditional densities

$$\pi(\boldsymbol{\theta}_{k,1}|\boldsymbol{\theta}_{k,2}, \boldsymbol{z}, D, \mathcal{M}_k),\ \pi(\boldsymbol{\theta}_{k,2}|\boldsymbol{\theta}_{k,1}, \boldsymbol{z}, D, \mathcal{M}_k),\ \pi(\boldsymbol{z}|\boldsymbol{\theta}_k, D, \mathcal{M}_k), \tag{8.1.6}$$

where $\boldsymbol{z}$ denotes the vector of latent variables. We further assume that the closed forms of the conditional distributions $\pi(\boldsymbol{\theta}_{k,1}|\boldsymbol{\theta}_{k,2}, \boldsymbol{z}, D, \mathcal{M}_k)$ and $\pi(\boldsymbol{\theta}_{k,2}|\boldsymbol{\theta}_{k,1}, \boldsymbol{z}, D, \mathcal{M}_k)$ are known. Our objective is to estimate $\pi(\boldsymbol{\theta}_k^*|D, \mathcal{M}_k)$, which can be expressed as

$$\pi(\boldsymbol{\theta}_{k,1}^*|D, \mathcal{M}_k)\pi(\boldsymbol{\theta}_{k,2}^*|\boldsymbol{\theta}_{k,1}^*, D, \mathcal{M}_k), \tag{8.1.7}$$

where

$$\pi(\boldsymbol{\theta}_{k,1}^*|D, \mathcal{M}_k) = \int \pi(\boldsymbol{\theta}_{k,1}^*|\boldsymbol{\theta}_{k,2}, \boldsymbol{z}, D, \mathcal{M}_k)\pi(\boldsymbol{\theta}_{k,2}, \boldsymbol{z}|D, \mathcal{M}_k)\ d\boldsymbol{\theta}_{k,2}\ d\boldsymbol{z},$$

and

$$\pi(\boldsymbol{\theta}_{k,2}^*|\boldsymbol{\theta}_{k,1}^*, D, \mathcal{M}_k) = \int \pi(\boldsymbol{\theta}_{k,2}^*|\boldsymbol{\theta}_{k,1}^*, \boldsymbol{z}, D, \mathcal{M}_k)\pi(\boldsymbol{z}|\boldsymbol{\theta}_{k,1}^*, D, \mathcal{M}_k)\ d\boldsymbol{z}$$

is the reduced conditional density ordinate. It should be clear that the normalizing constants of $\pi(\boldsymbol{\theta}_{k,1}|\boldsymbol{\theta}_{k,2}, \boldsymbol{z}, D, \mathcal{M}_k)$ and $\pi(\boldsymbol{\theta}_{k,2}|\boldsymbol{\theta}_{k,1}, \boldsymbol{z}, D, \mathcal{M}_k)$ must be included in the integration for the decomposition in (8.1.7) to be valid. To estimate the first density ordinate $\pi(\boldsymbol{\theta}_{k,1}^*|D, \mathcal{M}_k)$, we let $\{(\boldsymbol{\theta}_{k,1,i}, \boldsymbol{\theta}_{k,2,i}, \boldsymbol{z}_i),\ i = 1, 2, \ldots, n\}$ denote a Gibbs sample from (8.1.6). Then the efficient CMDE method in (4.3.2) gives a consistent estimator of $\pi(\boldsymbol{\theta}_{k,1}|D, \mathcal{M}_k)$ at $\boldsymbol{\theta}_{k,1}^*$ defined by

$$\hat{\pi}(\boldsymbol{\theta}_{k,1}^*|D, \mathcal{M}_k) = \frac{1}{n}\sum_{i=1}^n \pi(\boldsymbol{\theta}_{k,1}^*|\boldsymbol{\theta}_{k,2,i}, \boldsymbol{z}_i, D, \mathcal{M}_k). \tag{8.1.8}$$

We note that the sample $\{z_i,\ i = 1, 2, \ldots, n\}$ from the Gibbs sampler is from the marginal distribution $\pi(z|D, \mathcal{M}_k)$ and not from $\pi(z|\theta^*_{k,1}, D, \mathcal{M}_k)$. Therefore, the second density ordinate $\pi(\theta^*_{k,2}|\theta^*_{k,1}, D, \mathcal{M}_k)$ cannot be estimated directly using the same Gibbs sample. A simple solution to deal with this complication is to continue sampling for an additional n iterations with the complete conditional densities

$$\pi(\theta_{k,2}|\theta^*_{k,1}, z, D, \mathcal{M}_k) \text{ and } \pi(z|\theta^*_{k,1}, D, \mathcal{M}_k),$$

where in each of these densities, $\theta_{k,1}$ is set equal to $\theta^*_{k,1}$. Let $\{\theta_{k,2,i}, z_i,\ i = 1, 2, \ldots, n\}$ denote the resulting Gibbs sample. Then it can be shown that $\{z_i\}$ is a sample from the density $\pi(z|\theta^*_{k,1}, D, \mathcal{M}_k)$. Consequently,

$$\hat{\pi}(\theta^*_{k,2}|\theta^*_{k,1}, D, \mathcal{M}_k) = \frac{1}{n}\sum_{i=1}^{n} \pi(\theta^*_{k,2}|\theta^*_{k,1,i}, z_i, D, \mathcal{M}_k) \tag{8.1.9}$$

is a simulation consistent estimator of $\pi(\theta^*_{k,2}|\theta^*_{k,1}, D, \mathcal{M}_k)$. Although this procedure requires an increase in the number of iterations, it does not require new programming, and thus is straightforward to implement. Finally, substituting these two density estimators into (8.1.7) yields

$$\ln[\hat{\pi}(\theta^*_k|D, \mathcal{M}_k)] = \ln[\hat{\pi}(\theta^*_{k,1}|D, \mathcal{M}_k)] + \ln[\hat{\pi}(\theta^*_{k,2}|\theta^*_{k,1}, D, \mathcal{M}_k)]. \tag{8.1.10}$$

Compared to the other MC methods, such as the bridge sampling or path sampling methods presented in Chapter 5, Chib's method is more efficient when the posterior densities, $\pi(\theta_k|D, \mathcal{M}_k)$, have very little overlap, which is often the case for nonnested models. A partial explanation for this is that Chib's method computes the marginal likelihood for each individual model, and it does require knowing the relationship between the two models. The scale mixtures of multivariate normal link models presented in the next section is a special example, in which the marginal likelihood approaches are particularly useful in determining which link fits the data better. However, in the context of Bayesian variable selection, the computation of the marginal likelihood for each possible subset model becomes time-consuming, since it requires a sample from each subset model, and the number of all possible subset models under consideration can be quite large. Therefore, more feasible approaches are required to compute the posterior model probabilities for all possible subset models. We will discuss this issue in detail in the next chapter.

8.2 Scale Mixtures of Multivariate Normal Link Models

In this section, we consider Bayesian hierarchical generalized linear models using a rich class of scale mixtures of multivariate normal (SMMVN)-link functions for correlated ordinal data. We will illustrate the use of marginal likelihood approaches for comparing different SMMVN-link models. The general approach is an extension of Chib and Greenberg (1998).

8.2.1 The Models

Suppose that we observe an ordinal (1 through L) response y_{ij} on the ith observations and the jth variable and let $\boldsymbol{x}_{ij} = (x_{ij1}, x_{ij2}, \ldots, x_{ijp_j})'$ be the corresponding p_j-dimensional column vector of covariates for $i = 1, 2, \ldots, n$ and $j = 1, 2, \ldots, J$. (Note that x_{ij1} may be 1, which corresponds to an intercept.) Let $\boldsymbol{y}_i = (y_{i1}, y_{i2}, \ldots, y_{iJ})'$ and assume that y_{i1}, y_{i2}, $\ldots$, y_{iJ} are dependent whereas $\boldsymbol{y}_1$, $\boldsymbol{y}_2$, $\ldots$, $\boldsymbol{y}_n$ are independent. Let $D = (n, \boldsymbol{y}, X)$ denote the observed data, where $\boldsymbol{y} = (\boldsymbol{y}_1', \ldots, \boldsymbol{y}_n')'$ and $X = (\boldsymbol{x}_{ij})$. Also let $\boldsymbol{\beta}_j = (\beta_{j1}, \beta_{j2}, \ldots, \beta_{jp_j})'$ be a p_j-dimensional column vector of regression coefficients and let $\boldsymbol{\beta} = (\boldsymbol{\beta}_1', \boldsymbol{\beta}_2', \ldots, \boldsymbol{\beta}_J')'$.

To set up the SMMVN-link models for correlated ordinal response data, we introduce a J-dimensional (latent) random vector $\boldsymbol{w}_i^* = (w_{i1}^*, w_{i2}^*, \ldots, w_{iJ}^*)'$ such that

$$y_{ij} = l, \text{ if } \gamma_{j,l-1}^* \leq w_{ij}^* < \gamma_{jl}^*, \tag{8.2.1}$$

where $-\infty = \gamma_{j0}^* \leq \gamma_{j1}^* \leq \gamma_{j2}^* \leq \gamma_{j,L-1}^* \leq \gamma_{jL}^* = \infty$ are cutpoints for the jth ordinal response that divide the real line into L intervals. As explained by Nandram and Chen (1996) and in Section 2.5.3, we set $\gamma_{j1}^* = 0$ to ensure identifiability of the cutpoint parameters. Here we introduce different sets of cutpoints for different ordinal responses since in many practical problems, each ordinal response may behave quite differently. We further assume that

$$\boldsymbol{w}_i^* \sim N(X_i\boldsymbol{\beta}^*, \kappa(\lambda)\Sigma^*), \tag{8.2.2}$$

and

$$\lambda \sim \pi(\lambda), \ \ \lambda > 0, \tag{8.2.3}$$

where $\kappa(\lambda)$ is a positive function of the one-dimensional scale mixing variable λ, $\pi(\lambda)$ is a mixing distribution which is either discrete or continuous, $X_i = \text{diag}(\boldsymbol{x}_{i1}', \boldsymbol{x}_{i2}', \ldots, \boldsymbol{x}_{iJ}')$, and $\boldsymbol{\beta}^* = (\boldsymbol{\beta}_1^{*\prime}, \boldsymbol{\beta}_2^{*\prime}, \ldots, \boldsymbol{\beta}_J^{*\prime})'$ is a $p = \sum_{j=1}^J p_j$-dimensional column vector of regression coefficients corresponding to the cutpoints $\boldsymbol{\gamma}_j^* = (\gamma_{j2}^*, \gamma_{j3}^*, \ldots, \gamma_{j,L-1}^*)'$ for $j = 1, 2, \ldots, J$. In (8.2.2) we further take $\Sigma^* = \left(\rho_{jj^*}^*\right)_{J \times J}$ to be a correlation matrix with $\rho_{jj}^* = 1$ to ensure identifiability of the parameters. Such a $\boldsymbol{w}_i^*$ is sometimes called a tolerance variable, since in bioassays, for example, $\boldsymbol{w}_i^*$ can denote the lethal dose of a drug.

For the special case $\Sigma^* = I_J$, where I_J is the $J \times J$ identity matrix, Albert and Chib (1993) discuss the independent ordinal probit model using the Gibbs sampler. Even for this model, the Gibbs sampler considered in Albert and Chib (1993) may present challenging problems in achieving convergence. In light of that, Cowles (1996) provides an algorithm which substantially improves convergence for the probit model, the cumulative logit, and complementary log-log link models. Recently, Nandram and Chen (1996) propose an algorithm using a reparameterization technique which improves convergence further. See Subsection 2.5.3 for a detailed discussion. For the above general SMMVN-link models, the computation is even more challenging since we are faced with two difficult sampling problems, i.e.: (i) generating the cutpoints; and (ii) generating the correlation matrix.

To ease the computational burden, we consider the following reparameterization:

$$\delta_j = 1/\gamma^*_{j,L-1}, \quad \gamma_{jl} = \delta_j \gamma^*_{jl}, \quad \boldsymbol{\beta}_j = \delta_j \boldsymbol{\beta}^*_j, \quad \text{and} \quad w_{ij} = \delta_j w^*_{ij} \tag{8.2.4}$$

for $j = 1, 2, \ldots, J$ and $i = 1, 2, \ldots, n$. With the reparameterization in (8.2.4), the SMMVN-link models given by (8.2.1) and (8.2.2) become

$$y_{ij} = l \ \text{ if } \ \gamma_{j,l-1} \le w_{ij} < \gamma_{jl}, \tag{8.2.5}$$

and

$$\boldsymbol{w}_i \sim N(X_i \boldsymbol{\beta}, \kappa(\lambda)\Sigma), \tag{8.2.6}$$

where the reparameterized cutpoints are $-\infty = \gamma_{j0} \le \gamma_{j1} = 0 \le \gamma_{j2} \le \cdots \le \gamma_{j,L-1} = 1 \le \gamma_{jL} = \infty$, $\Sigma = (\sigma_{jj^*})$, $\sigma_{jj} = \delta_j^2$, and $\sigma_{jj^*} = \delta_j \delta_{j^*} \rho^*_{jj^*}$ for $j \ne j^*$. The models given by (8.2.5) and (8.2.6) are thus called the SMMVN-link reparameterized models.

Note that in (8.2.5), for each j, we have only $L-3$ unknown cutpoints, and in (8.2.6), Σ is an unrestricted variance–covariance matrix, which has a great advantage in the implementation of MCMC sampling. We also note that the reparameterization in (8.2.4) does not affect the distribution of the scale mixing variable λ. That is, we still have the same mixing distribution $\pi(\lambda)$ for the mixing variable λ. The SMMVN-link reparameterized models have several attractive features. First, the number of unknown cutpoints is reduced by J. Second, all unknown cutpoints γ_{jl} are between 0 and 1, i.e., $0 \le \gamma_{jl} \le 1$ for $l = 2, 3, \ldots, L-2$ and $j = 1, 2, \ldots, J$. Third, the variance–covariance matrix Σ for w_i is unrestricted. Fourth, when $L = 3$, there are no unknown cutpoints. Because of these nice features, we use the SMMVN-link reparameterized models throughout the rest of this section.

Finally, we note that the distribution of w_i determines the joint distribution of $\boldsymbol{y}_i$ through (8.2.5) and the variance–covariance matrix Σ captures the correlations among the y_{ij}'s. More specifically, we have the joint distribution of the correlated ordinal responses given by

$$f(\boldsymbol{y}_i|\boldsymbol{\beta},\Sigma,\boldsymbol{\gamma},\lambda) = \int_{A_{i1}} \int_{A_{i2}} \cdots \int_{A_{iJ}} \frac{1}{(2\pi\kappa(\lambda))^{J/2} |\Sigma|^{1/2}} \times \exp\left\{ -\frac{[\kappa(\lambda)]^{-1}}{2} (\boldsymbol{w}_i - X_i\boldsymbol{\beta})'\Sigma^{-1}(\boldsymbol{w}_i - X_i\boldsymbol{\beta}) \right\} d\boldsymbol{w}_i, \tag{8.2.7}$$

where $\gamma = (\gamma_1', \gamma_2', \ldots, \gamma_J')'$, $\gamma_j = (\gamma_{j2}, \gamma_{j3}, \ldots, \gamma_{j,L-2})'$, and

$$A_{ij} = (\gamma_{j,l-1}, \gamma_{jl}] \text{ if } y_{ij} = l \text{ for } j = 1, 2, \ldots, J. \tag{8.2.8}$$

The class of SMMVN-link models is very rich and flexible, which includes, for example, multivariate probit (MVP), t-link (MVT), and logit (MVL) models. A brief explanation of these models is given as follows.

Taking $\kappa(\lambda) = 1$ and the mixing distribution $\pi(\{1\}) = 1$, the SMMVN models reduce to the MVP models. Similarly, when we take $\kappa(\lambda) = 1/\lambda$ and $\lambda \sim \mathcal{G}(\nu/2, \nu/2)$, i.e.,

$$\pi(\lambda) = \frac{1}{\Gamma(\nu/2)} \left(\frac{\nu}{2}\right)^{\nu/2} \lambda^{\nu/2-1} \exp\left\{-\frac{\nu}{2}\lambda\right\},$$

the SMMVN-link models give the MVT models. As a special case, the MVT links reduce to the multivariate Cauchy (MVC) link when $\nu = 1$ and the MVP when $\nu \to \infty$.

Logit models are widely used to fit binary data (e.g., see Prentice (1988)). As pointed out by Choy (1995), the SMMVN-link model leads to the MVL model when $\kappa(\lambda) = 4\lambda^2$ and λ follows an asymptotic Kolmogorov distribution with density

$$\pi(\lambda) = \pi_K(\lambda) = 8 \sum_{j=1}^{\infty} (-1)^{j+1} j^2 \lambda \exp\{-2j^2\lambda^2\}. \tag{8.2.9}$$

8.2.2 Prior Distributions and Posterior Computations

First, we choose the same prior distribution for the regression coefficient vector β for all SMMVN-link models presented in Subsection 8.2.1. That is,

$$\pi(\beta|\beta_0, B_0) \propto \exp\{-\tfrac{1}{2}(\beta - \beta_0)' B_0 (\beta - \beta_0)\}, \tag{8.2.10}$$

where B_0 is a precision matrix, β_0 is a location parameter vector, and both β_0 and B_0 are prespecified. Typically, we choose $\beta_0 = 0$ and $B_0 = \text{diag}(B_{11}, B_{12}, \ldots, B_{1p_1}, B_{21}, B_{22}, \ldots, B_{2p_2}, \ldots, B_{J1}, B_{J2}, \ldots, B_{Jp_J})$, where B_{jl} is chosen to be small (e.g., $B_{jl} = 0.01$) so that a vague prior distribution for β is obtained.

Second, we choose

$$\Sigma^{-1} \sim W_J(n_0, Q_0), \tag{8.2.11}$$

where Q_0 is a $J \times J$ symmetric and positive definite matrix, $W_J(n_0, Q_0)$ denotes the Wishart distribution with degrees of freedom n_0 and mean $n_0 Q_0$, and n_0 and Q_0 are prespecified hyperparameters. In the illustrative example given in Subsection 8.2.5, we take $n_0 = 11$ and $Q_0^{-1} = 0.001 I_{10}$, where I_{10} is the 10-dimensional identity matrix, so that the prior is sufficiently diffuse.

Third, we take independent uniform priors on $\boldsymbol{\gamma}_j = (\gamma_{j2}, \gamma_{j3}, \ldots, \gamma_{j,L-2})'$, i.e.,

$$\pi_g(\boldsymbol{\gamma}_j) \propto 1, \quad \text{for } 0 \le \gamma_{j2} \le \gamma_{j3} \le \cdots \le \gamma_{j,L-2} \le 1, \qquad (8.2.12)$$

for $j = 1, 2, \ldots, J$.

We use the Gibbs sampler along with the Metropolis–Hastings algorithm within Gibbs steps to perform the posterior computations. To sample from the posterior distribution, we need to generate $\boldsymbol{\beta}$, Σ, $\boldsymbol{\gamma}_j$, $\boldsymbol{w}_i$, and λ_i from their respective conditional distributions. The technical details of the computational implementation are given as follows.

Let $B = B_0 + \sum_{i=1}^n [\kappa(\lambda_i)]^{-1} X_i' \Sigma^{-1} X_i$ and

$$\hat{\boldsymbol{\beta}} = B^{-1} \left(B_0 \boldsymbol{\beta}_0 + \sum_{i=1}^n [\kappa(\lambda_i)]^{-1} X_i' \Sigma^{-1} \boldsymbol{w}_i \right).$$

Also let $\boldsymbol{w} = (\boldsymbol{w}_1', \boldsymbol{w}_2', \ldots, \boldsymbol{w}_n')'$ and $\boldsymbol{\lambda} = (\lambda_1, \lambda_2, \ldots, \lambda_n)'$. Then, given Σ, $\boldsymbol{w}$, and $\boldsymbol{\lambda}$, we have

$$\boldsymbol{\beta} | \Sigma, \boldsymbol{w}, \boldsymbol{\lambda}, D \sim N\left(\hat{\boldsymbol{\beta}}, B^{-1}\right). \qquad (8.2.13)$$

From (8.2.6) and (8.2.11), it follows that the conditional distribution of Σ^{-1} given $\boldsymbol{\beta}$, $\boldsymbol{w}$, and $\boldsymbol{\lambda}$ is a Wishart distribution,

$$\Sigma^{-1} | \boldsymbol{\beta}, \boldsymbol{w}, \boldsymbol{\lambda}, D \sim W_J \left(n + n_0, \left[Q_0^{-1} + \sum_{i=1}^n [\kappa(\lambda_i)]^{-1} (\boldsymbol{w}_i - X_i \boldsymbol{\beta})(\boldsymbol{w}_i - X_i \boldsymbol{\beta})' \right]^{-1} \right). \qquad (8.2.14)$$

Therefore, generating $\boldsymbol{\beta}$ and Σ from (8.2.13) and (8.2.14) is straightforward.

To generate $\boldsymbol{\gamma}_j$ and $\boldsymbol{w}$ from their conditional distributions, we consider the following MCMC sampling scheme. Let $\boldsymbol{w}^{(j)} = (w_{1j}, w_{2j}, \ldots, w_{nj})'$ and let $\boldsymbol{w}^{(-j)}$ denote $\boldsymbol{w}$ with $\boldsymbol{w}^{(j)}$ deleted for $j = 1, 2, \ldots, J$. Then we use a cycle of J Gibbs steps to generate $\boldsymbol{\gamma}_j$ and $\boldsymbol{w}^{(j)}$ jointly from their conditional distributions for $j = 1, 2, \ldots, J$. To draw $\boldsymbol{\gamma}_j$ and $\boldsymbol{w}^{(j)}$ jointly from the conditional distribution $[\boldsymbol{\gamma}_j, \boldsymbol{w}^{(j)} | \boldsymbol{\beta}, \Sigma, \boldsymbol{w}^{(-j)}, \boldsymbol{\lambda}, D]$, we first draw $\boldsymbol{\gamma}_j$ from $[\boldsymbol{\gamma}_j | \boldsymbol{\beta}, \Sigma, \boldsymbol{w}^{(-j)}, \boldsymbol{\lambda}, D]$, and then draw $\boldsymbol{w}^{(j)}$ from $[\boldsymbol{w}^{(j)} | \boldsymbol{\gamma}_j, \boldsymbol{\beta}, \Sigma, \boldsymbol{w}^{(-j)}, D]$. Given γ_j, β, Σ, $\boldsymbol{w}^{(-j)}$, and Λ, the conditional distribution of w_{ij}, the ith component of $\boldsymbol{w}^{(j)}$, is a truncated normal over interval A_{ij} given in (8.2.8). Therefore, we can use the algorithm of Geweke (1991) to generate w_{ij} from the above truncated normal distribution for $i = 1, 2, \ldots, n$. To sample $\boldsymbol{\gamma}_j$ from the conditional distribution $[\boldsymbol{\gamma}_j | \boldsymbol{\beta}, \Sigma, \boldsymbol{w}^{(-j)}, \Lambda, D]$, we use the Chen–Dey algorithm given in Subsection 2.5.3.

The conditional distribution $[\lambda_i|\boldsymbol{\beta}, \Sigma, \boldsymbol{w}_i, D]$ is

$$\pi(\lambda_i|\boldsymbol{\beta}, \Sigma, \boldsymbol{w}_i, D) \propto \left[\left(\frac{1}{2\pi\kappa(\lambda_i)}\right)^{J/2} |\Sigma|^{-1/2} \right.$$
$$\left. \times \exp\left\{-\frac{[\kappa(\lambda_i)]^{-1}}{2}(\boldsymbol{w}_i - X_i\boldsymbol{\beta})'\Sigma^{-1}(\boldsymbol{w}_i - X_i\boldsymbol{\beta})\right\}\right]\pi(\lambda_i). \quad (8.2.15)$$

To generate λ_i from (8.2.15), we need to know the form of the mixing distribution $\pi(\lambda)$. For an MVP model, we do not need to generate λ_i, since $\pi(\{\lambda_i = 1\}) = 1$. For an MVT model, $\pi(\lambda_i|\boldsymbol{\beta}, \Sigma, \boldsymbol{w}_i, D)$ in (8.2.15) reduces to

$$\mathcal{G}\left(\frac{\nu + J}{2}, \tfrac{1}{2}[\nu + (\boldsymbol{w}_i - X_i\boldsymbol{\beta})'\Sigma^{-1}(\boldsymbol{w}_i - X_i\boldsymbol{\beta})]\right),$$

where $\mathcal{G}(u, v)$ denotes a gamma distribution with density $\pi_{\mathcal{G}}(\lambda|u, v) \propto \lambda^{u-1}e^{-v\xi}$. Therefore, sampling λ_i from its conditional distribution is trivial. For an MVL model, by using an appropriate Student t approximation to the logistic distribution, Chen and Dey (1998) show that a good proposal density for $\pi_K(\lambda)$ given by (8.2.9) is

$$g_L(\lambda|\nu, b) = \frac{(\nu/8b^2)^{\nu/2}}{\Gamma(\nu/2)(\lambda^2)^{\nu/2+1}} \exp\left\{-\left(\frac{\nu}{8b^2}\right)\frac{1}{\lambda^2}\right\} 2\lambda. \quad (8.2.16)$$

They further show that the best choices of ν and b are $\nu = 5$ and $b = 0.712$, and they also provide an efficient way to evaluate $\pi_K(\lambda)$. It is interesting to note that when we take

$$\lambda^2 \sim \mathcal{IG}\left(\frac{\nu}{2}, \frac{\nu}{8b^2}\right),$$

where $\mathcal{IG}(u, v)$ is an inverse gamma distribution with density $\pi_{\mathcal{IG}}(\lambda|u, v) = [v^u/\Gamma(u)\lambda^{u+1}]e^{-v/\lambda}$, $\lambda > 0$, then

$$\lambda \sim g_L(\lambda|\nu, b).$$

Therefore, to draw λ_i from (8.2.15), we can use the Metropolis–Hastings algorithm. Let λ_i be the current value. Generate

$$\lambda_i^{*2} \sim \mathcal{IG}\left(\frac{J+\nu}{2}, \frac{1}{8}\left[(\boldsymbol{w}_i - X_i\boldsymbol{\beta})'\Sigma^{-1}(\boldsymbol{w}_i - X_i\boldsymbol{\beta}) + \frac{\nu}{b^2}\right]\right). \quad (8.2.17)$$

Then a move to the proposal point λ_i^* is made with probability

$$\min\left\{\frac{\pi_K(\lambda_i^*)/g_L(\lambda_i^*|\nu, b)}{\pi_K(\lambda_i)/g_L(\lambda_i|\nu, b)}, 1\right\}, \quad (8.2.18)$$

where $\pi_K(\lambda)$ and $g_L(\lambda_i|\nu, b)$ are given in (8.2.9) and (8.2.16), respectively.

8.2.3 Model Comparison

In this subsection we consider the problem of model uncertainty for the class of SMMVN-link models. We use the marginal likelihood approach discussed in Section 8.1 for model comparison since this approach is particularly suitable for correlated ordinal data models.

Suppose that there are $\mathcal{K}$ models $\mathcal{M}_1$, $\mathcal{M}_2$, $\ldots$, $\mathcal{M}_{\mathcal{K}}$ under consideration. Given model $\mathcal{M}_k$, we let $\pi(\boldsymbol{\beta}, \Sigma^{-1}, \boldsymbol{\gamma}|D, \mathcal{M}_k)$ denote the posterior distribution, given by

$$\pi(\boldsymbol{\beta}, \Sigma^{-1}, \boldsymbol{\gamma}|D, \mathcal{M}_k) = \frac{L(\boldsymbol{\beta}, \Sigma, \boldsymbol{\gamma}|D, \mathcal{M}_k)\pi(\boldsymbol{\beta}, \Sigma^{-1}, \boldsymbol{\gamma})}{m(D|\mathcal{M}_k)}, \tag{8.2.19}$$

where

$$L(\boldsymbol{\beta}, \Sigma, \boldsymbol{\gamma}|D, \mathcal{M}_k) = \prod_{i=1}^{n} L(\boldsymbol{\beta}, \Sigma, \boldsymbol{\gamma}|\boldsymbol{y}_i, \mathcal{M}_k),$$

$$L(\boldsymbol{\beta}, \Sigma, \boldsymbol{\gamma}|\boldsymbol{y}_i, \mathcal{M}_k) = \int_0^\infty \int_{A_{i1}} \int_{A_{i2}} \cdots \int_{A_{iJ}} \frac{1}{(2\pi\kappa_k(\lambda_i))^{J/2} |\Sigma|^{1/2}}$$
$$\times \exp\left\{-\frac{[\kappa_k(\lambda_i)]^{-1}}{2}(\boldsymbol{w}_i - X_i\boldsymbol{\beta})'\Sigma^{-1}(\boldsymbol{w}_i - X_i\boldsymbol{\beta})\right\} \pi_k(\lambda_i)\, d\boldsymbol{w}_i\, d\lambda_i,$$

and $\kappa_k(\lambda_i)$ and $\pi_k(\lambda_i)$ are the scale mixing function and the density function, respectively, of the mixing variable λ_j associated with model $\mathcal{M}_k$. The A_{ij}'s are defined in (8.2.8) based on the observed ordinal responses y_{ij}. Furthermore, the prior distribution, $\pi(\boldsymbol{\beta}, \Sigma^{-1}, \boldsymbol{\gamma})$ in (8.2.19), is given by (8.2.10), (8.2.11), and (8.2.12), which is *the same* across all SMMVN-link models, and $m(D|\mathcal{M}_k)$ is the marginal likelihood.

To compute the marginal likelihood, we use (8.1.5) and let $(\boldsymbol{\beta}^*, \Sigma^*, \boldsymbol{\gamma}^*)$ denote the posterior means of $\boldsymbol{\beta}$, Σ, and $\boldsymbol{\gamma}$. Then the marginal likelihood on the natural logarithmic scale is given by

$$\ln m(D|\mathcal{M}_k) = \sum_{i=1}^{n} \ln L(\boldsymbol{\beta}^*, \Sigma^*, \boldsymbol{\gamma}^*|\boldsymbol{y}_i, \mathcal{M}_k)$$
$$+ \ln \pi(\boldsymbol{\beta}^*, {\Sigma^*}^{-1}, \boldsymbol{\gamma}^*) - \ln \pi(\boldsymbol{\beta}^*, {\Sigma^*}^{-1}, \boldsymbol{\gamma}^*|D, \mathcal{M}_k). \tag{8.2.20}$$

From (8.2.10), (8.2.11), and (8.2.12), it is easy to see that the computation of the second term of (8.2.20) is straightforward. To compute the third term of (8.2.20), we write

$$\ln \pi(\boldsymbol{\beta}^*, {\Sigma^*}^{-1}, \boldsymbol{\gamma}^*|D, \mathcal{M}_k) = \ln \pi(\boldsymbol{\beta}^*|\Sigma^*, \boldsymbol{\gamma}^*, D, \mathcal{M}_k)$$
$$+ \ln \pi({\Sigma^*}^{-1}|\boldsymbol{\gamma}^*, D, \mathcal{M}_k) + \ln \pi(\boldsymbol{\gamma}^*|D, \mathcal{M}_k). \tag{8.2.21}$$

In (8.2.21),

$$\pi(\boldsymbol{\beta}^*|\Sigma^*, \boldsymbol{\gamma}^*, D, \mathcal{M}_k) = \int \pi(\boldsymbol{\beta}^*|\Sigma^*, \boldsymbol{\gamma}^*, \boldsymbol{w}, \boldsymbol{\lambda}, D, \mathcal{M}_k) \times \pi(\boldsymbol{w}, \boldsymbol{\lambda} \mid \Sigma^*, \boldsymbol{\gamma}^*, D, \mathcal{M}_k)\, d\boldsymbol{w}\, d\boldsymbol{\lambda}, \tag{8.2.22}$$

where $\pi(\boldsymbol{w}, \boldsymbol{\lambda}|\Sigma^*, \boldsymbol{\gamma}^*, D, \mathcal{M}_k)$ is the conditional marginal posterior distribution of $[\boldsymbol{w}, \boldsymbol{\lambda}|\Sigma = \Sigma^*, \boldsymbol{\gamma} = \boldsymbol{\gamma}^*]$, $\boldsymbol{w} = (\boldsymbol{w}_1', \boldsymbol{w}_2', \ldots, \boldsymbol{w}_n')'$, and $\boldsymbol{\lambda} = (\lambda_1, \lambda_2, \ldots, \lambda_n)'$. Furthermore,

$$\pi({\Sigma^*}^{-1}|\boldsymbol{\gamma}^*, D, \mathcal{M}_k) = \int \pi({\Sigma^*}^{-1}|\boldsymbol{\beta}, \boldsymbol{w}, \boldsymbol{\lambda}, \boldsymbol{\gamma}^*, D, \mathcal{M}_k) \times \pi(\boldsymbol{\beta}, \boldsymbol{w}, \boldsymbol{\lambda}|\boldsymbol{\gamma}^*, D, \mathcal{M}_k)\, d\boldsymbol{\beta}\, d\boldsymbol{w}\, d\boldsymbol{\lambda}, \tag{8.2.23}$$

where $\pi(\boldsymbol{\beta}, \boldsymbol{w}, \boldsymbol{\lambda}|\boldsymbol{\gamma}^*, D, \mathcal{M}_k)$ is the conditional marginal posterior distribution of $[\boldsymbol{\beta}, \boldsymbol{w}, \boldsymbol{\lambda}|\boldsymbol{\gamma} = \boldsymbol{\gamma}^*]$, and

$$\pi(\boldsymbol{\gamma}^*|D, \mathcal{M}_k) = \int \pi(\boldsymbol{\gamma}^*|\boldsymbol{\beta}, \Sigma, \boldsymbol{w}, \boldsymbol{\lambda}, D, \mathcal{M}_k) \times \pi(\boldsymbol{\beta}, \Sigma^{-1}, \boldsymbol{w}, \boldsymbol{\lambda}|D, \mathcal{M}_k)\, d\boldsymbol{\beta}\, d\Sigma^{-1}\, d\boldsymbol{w}\, d\boldsymbol{\lambda}, \tag{8.2.24}$$

where $\pi(\boldsymbol{\beta}, \Sigma^{-1}, \boldsymbol{w}, \boldsymbol{\lambda}|D, \mathcal{M}_k)$ is the marginal posterior distribution of $\boldsymbol{\beta}$, Σ^{-1}, $\boldsymbol{w}$, and $\boldsymbol{\lambda}$.

To obtain simulation-consistent estimates of (8.2.22), (8.2.23), and (8.2.24), we independently generate $\{(\boldsymbol{w}_{1,r}, \boldsymbol{\lambda}_{1,r}),\ r = 1, 2, \ldots, R\}$ from $\pi(\boldsymbol{w}, \boldsymbol{\lambda}|\Sigma^*, \boldsymbol{\gamma}^*, D, \mathcal{M}_k)$, $\{(\boldsymbol{\beta}_{2,r}, \boldsymbol{w}_{2,r}, \boldsymbol{\lambda}_{2,r}),\ r = 1, 2, \ldots, R\}$ from $\pi(\boldsymbol{\beta}, \boldsymbol{w}, \boldsymbol{\lambda}|\boldsymbol{\gamma}^*, D, \mathcal{M}_k)$, and $\{(\boldsymbol{\beta}_{3,r}, \Sigma_{3,r}, \boldsymbol{w}_{3,r}, \boldsymbol{\lambda}_{3,r}),\ r = 1, 2, \ldots, R\}$ from $\pi(\boldsymbol{\beta}, \Sigma^{-1}, \boldsymbol{w}, \boldsymbol{\lambda}|D, \mathcal{M}_k)$. Note that all three MCMC samples are straightforward to obtain by using the MCMC sampling scheme presented in Subsection 8.2.2. Write $\boldsymbol{w}_{j,r} = (\boldsymbol{w}_{1,jr}', \boldsymbol{w}_{2,jr}', \ldots, \boldsymbol{w}_{n,jr}')'$ and $\boldsymbol{\lambda}_{j,r} = (\lambda_{1,jr}, \lambda_{2,jr}, \ldots, \lambda_{n,jr})'$ for $j = 1, 2, 3$. Then a simulation-consistent estimate of (8.2.22) is

$$\hat{\pi}(\boldsymbol{\beta}^*|\Sigma^*, \boldsymbol{\gamma}^*, D, \mathcal{M}_k) = \frac{1}{R} \sum_{r=1}^{R} \pi(\boldsymbol{\beta}^*|\Sigma^*, \boldsymbol{\gamma}^*, \boldsymbol{w}_{1,r}, \boldsymbol{\lambda}_{1,r}, D, \mathcal{M}_k). \tag{8.2.25}$$

In (8.2.25),

$$\pi(\boldsymbol{\beta}^*|\Sigma^*, \boldsymbol{\gamma}^*, \boldsymbol{w}_{1,r}, \boldsymbol{\lambda}_{1,r}, D, \mathcal{M}_k) = \left(\frac{1}{2\pi}\right)^{p/2} |B_r|^{1/2} \exp\left\{-\frac{(\boldsymbol{\beta}^* - \hat{\boldsymbol{\beta}}_r)' B_r (\boldsymbol{\beta}^* - \hat{\boldsymbol{\beta}}_r)}{2}\right\},$$

where $p = \sum_{j=1}^{J} p_j$,

$$\hat{\boldsymbol{\beta}}_r = (B_r)^{-1} \left(B_0 \boldsymbol{\beta}_0 + \sum_{i=1}^{n} [\kappa_k(\lambda_{i,1r})]^{-1} X_i' (\Sigma^*)^{-1} \boldsymbol{w}_{i,1r} \right),$$

and $B_r = B_0 + \sum_{i=1}^n [\kappa_k(\lambda_{i,1r})]^{-1} X_i'(\Sigma^*)^{-1} X_i$. A simulation-consistent estimate of (8.2.23) is

$$\hat{\pi}(\Sigma^{*-1}|\gamma^*, D, \mathcal{M}_k) = \frac{1}{R}\sum_{r=1}^{R} \pi(\Sigma^{*-1}|\boldsymbol{\beta}_{2,r}, \boldsymbol{w}_{2,r}, \boldsymbol{\lambda}_{2,r}, \boldsymbol{\gamma}^*, D, \mathcal{M}_k). \tag{8.2.26}$$

In (8.2.26),

$$\pi(\Sigma^{*-1}|\boldsymbol{\beta}_{2,r}, \boldsymbol{w}_{2,r}, \boldsymbol{\lambda}_{2,r}, \boldsymbol{\gamma}^*, D, \mathcal{M}_k) = \frac{|V_r|^{-(n+n_0)/2}\exp\{-\frac{1}{2}\mathrm{tr}(V_r^{-1}\Sigma^{*-1})\}|\Sigma^*|^{-(n+n_0-J-1)/2}}{2^{(n+n_0)J/2}\pi^{J(J-1)/4}\prod_{j=1}^{J}\Gamma((n+n_0-j+1)/2)},$$

where $\mathrm{tr}(V_r^{-1}\Sigma^{*-1})$ denotes the trace of matrix $V_r^{-1}\Sigma^{*-1}$, and

$$V_r = \left[Q_0^{-1} + \sum_{i=1}^{n}[\kappa_k(\lambda_{i,2r})]^{-1}(\boldsymbol{w}_{i,2r} - X_i\boldsymbol{\beta}_{2,r})(\boldsymbol{w}_{i,2r} - X_i\boldsymbol{\beta}_{2,r})'\right]^{-1}.$$

Assume that all sets $\{i: \ y_{ij} = l, \ i = 1, 2, \dots, n\}$ for $l = 2, 3, \dots, L-1$ and $j = 1, 2, \dots, J$ are not empty. Under the above assumption, a simulation-consistent estimate of (8.2.24) is given by

$$\hat{\pi}(\boldsymbol{\gamma}^*|D, \mathcal{M}_k) = \frac{1}{R}\sum_{r=1}^{R}\pi(\boldsymbol{\gamma}^*|\boldsymbol{\beta}_{3,r}, \Sigma_{3,r}, \boldsymbol{w}_{3,r}, \boldsymbol{\lambda}_{3,r}, D, \mathcal{M}_k), \tag{8.2.27}$$

where

$$\pi(\boldsymbol{\gamma}^*|\boldsymbol{\beta}_{3,r}, \Sigma_{3,r}, \boldsymbol{w}_{3,r}, \boldsymbol{\lambda}_{3,r}, D, \mathcal{M}_k) = \prod_{j=1}^{J}\prod_{l=2}^{L-2}\frac{1}{\min\{w_{ij,3r}: y_{ij} = l+1\} - \max\{w_{ij,3r}: y_{ij} = l\}} \tag{8.2.28}$$

for $\max\{w_{ij,3r}: y_{ij} = l\} < \gamma_{jl}^* \le \min\{w_{ij,3r}: y_{ij} = l+1\}$, $l = 2, 3, \dots, L-2$, and $j = 1, 2, \dots, J$. The derivation of equation (8.2.28) follows from the fact that if the assumption,

$$\max\{w_{ij,3r}: y_{ij} = l\} < \min\{w_{ij,3r}: y_{ij} = l+1\},$$

for $l = 2, 3, \dots, L-2$ and $j = 1, 2, \dots, J$, holds, then the cutpoints γ_{jl}'s are independent. If the above assumption is violated, which is rare in practice, (8.2.28) still works with an obvious adjustment. However, if L or J are large, the above MC approach may not be efficient because of the high dimensionality of the problem. A more efficient MC method can be obtained by using a sequence of $(J-3)$-dimensional conditional marginal distributions for $\boldsymbol{\gamma}$. To explore this idea, we let $\boldsymbol{\gamma}^{*(+j)} = (\boldsymbol{\gamma}_1^{*\prime}, \boldsymbol{\gamma}_2^{*\prime}, \dots, \boldsymbol{\gamma}_j^{*\prime})'$ for

$j = 1, 2, \ldots, J$. Then we have

$$\pi(\gamma^*|D, \mathcal{M}_k) = \pi(\gamma_1^*|D, \mathcal{M}_k) \times \pi(\gamma_2^*|\gamma^{*(+1)}, D, \mathcal{M}_k) \cdots \pi(\gamma_J^*|\gamma^{*(+(J-1))}, D, \mathcal{M}_k), \qquad (8.2.29)$$

and

$$\pi(\gamma_j^*|\gamma^{*(+(j-1))}, D, \mathcal{M}_k) = \int \pi(\gamma_j^*|\boldsymbol{\beta}, \Sigma, \boldsymbol{w}, \boldsymbol{\lambda}, \gamma^{*(+(j-1))}, D, \mathcal{M}_k) \times \pi(\boldsymbol{\beta}, \Sigma^{-1}, \boldsymbol{w}, \boldsymbol{\lambda}|\gamma^{*(+(j-1))}, D, \mathcal{M}_k)\, d\boldsymbol{\beta}\, d\Sigma^{-1}\, d\boldsymbol{w}\, d\boldsymbol{\lambda}, \qquad (8.2.30)$$

for $j = 1, 2, \ldots, J$. Then, similar to (8.2.27) and (8.2.28), an efficient estimate of $\pi(\gamma_j^*|\gamma^{*(+(j-1))}, D, \mathcal{M}_k)$ can be obtained by using a random sample generated from $\pi(\boldsymbol{\beta}, \Sigma, \boldsymbol{w}, \boldsymbol{\lambda}|\gamma^{*(+(j-1))}, D, \mathcal{M}_k)$.

Next, we discuss an MC method to estimate the probability $L(\boldsymbol{\beta}^*, \Sigma^*, \gamma^*|y_i, \mathcal{M}_k)$. Note that the MC algorithms proposed by Chib and Greenberg (1998) and Chen and Dey (1998) for correlated binary response data problems may not be applicable here because of simulation inefficiency due to the high-dimensional nature of the problem. To overcome this, let $\Sigma_d^* = \text{diag}(\Sigma^*)$, $c_L = L(\boldsymbol{\beta}^*, \Sigma^*, \gamma^*|\boldsymbol{y}_i, \mathcal{M}_k)$, and $c_L^* = L(\boldsymbol{\beta}^*, \Sigma_d^*, \gamma^*|\boldsymbol{y}_i, \mathcal{M}_k)$. Then, c_L^* can be evaluated numerically, since it involves only a one-dimensional integral. Letting

$$\pi^*(\boldsymbol{w}_i, \lambda_i|\boldsymbol{\beta}^*, \Sigma^*, D, \mathcal{M}_k) = \frac{|\Sigma^*|^{-1/2}}{(2\pi\kappa_k(\lambda_i))^{J/2}} \times \exp\left\{-\frac{[\kappa_k(\lambda_i)]^{-1}}{2}(\boldsymbol{w}_i - X_i\boldsymbol{\beta}^*)'(\Sigma^*)^{-1}(\boldsymbol{w}_i - X_i\boldsymbol{\beta}^*)\right\}\pi_k(\lambda_i),$$

we have

$$\text{Ra} = \frac{c_L}{c_L^*} = E\left[\frac{\pi^*(\boldsymbol{w}_i, \lambda_i|\boldsymbol{\beta}^*, \Sigma^*, D, \mathcal{M}_k)}{\pi^*(\boldsymbol{w}_i, \lambda_i|\boldsymbol{\beta}^*, \Sigma_d^*, D, \mathcal{M}_k)}\right], \qquad (8.2.31)$$

where the expectation is taken with respect to $\pi(\boldsymbol{w}_i, \lambda_i|\boldsymbol{\beta}^*, \Sigma_d^*, D, \mathcal{M}_k)$, which is proportional to $\pi^*(\boldsymbol{w}_i, \lambda_i|\boldsymbol{\beta}^*, \Sigma_d^*, D, \mathcal{M}_k)$. Then we use the following steps to obtain an estimate of $L(\boldsymbol{\beta}^*, \Sigma^*, \gamma^*|\boldsymbol{y}_i, \mathcal{M}_k)$:

Step 1. Generate $(\boldsymbol{w}_{i,r}, \lambda_{i,r})$ from $\pi(\boldsymbol{w}_i, \lambda_i|\boldsymbol{\beta}^*, \Sigma_d^*, D, \mathcal{M}_k)$ using the Gibbs sampler for $r = 1, \ldots, R$. The necessary steps required in Gibbs sampling are:

(i) generate $\boldsymbol{w}_{i,r}|\lambda_{i,r-1} \sim N(X_i\boldsymbol{\beta}^*, \kappa_k(\lambda_{i,r-1})\Sigma_d^*)$ over the constrained space $A_{i1}^* \times A_{i2}^* \times \cdots \times A_{iJ}^*$; and

(ii) generate $\lambda_{i,r}$ from $[\lambda_i|\boldsymbol{w}_{i,r}]$ using a procedure presented in Subsection 8.2.2.

Step 2. Calculate the average

$$\widehat{\text{Ra}} = \frac{1}{R}\sum_{r=1}^{R} \frac{\pi(\boldsymbol{w}_{i,r}, \lambda_{i,r}|\boldsymbol{\beta}^*, \Sigma^*, D, \mathcal{M}_k)}{\pi(\boldsymbol{w}_{i,r}, \lambda_{i,r}|\boldsymbol{\beta}^*, \Sigma_d^*, D, \mathcal{M}_k)}, \qquad (8.2.32)$$

and compute $\ln \widehat{L}(\boldsymbol{\beta}^*, \Sigma^*, \boldsymbol{\gamma}^* | \boldsymbol{y}_i, \mathcal{M}_k) = \ln c_L^* + \ln \widehat{\mathrm{Ra}}$.

Chen and Dey (1998) empirically show that the methods, such as bridge sampling and ratio importance sampling, to directly estimate the Bayes factors, are not efficient for the SMMVN-link models. This is partially due to the fact that the posterior distributions in the class of the SMMVN-link models are relatively far apart from each other and the SMMVN-link models are not nested. Therefore, Chib's methods will result in more precision for MC estimation of the marginal likelihoods.

8.2.4 Item Response Data Example

The Department of Mathematical Sciences at Worcester Polytechnic Institute (WPI) recently conducted a survey. The results from the survey were to be used in the renovation of the Master's degree program for secondary teachers. One survey question contained ten items of the Master's degree programs for secondary mathematics teachers, and the teachers were asked to identify which features were important. Each individual responded in one of "not important," "somewhat important," "average importance," "important," and "very important" for each item. The subjects included teachers from two groups: I. Prospective Students; and II. Students who have been part of the WPI program. Prospective Students were defined to be one faculty member (usually the department head) from every high school mathematics department within a 60-mile radius of WPI. The survey was sent to 315 secondary mathematics teachers in Massachusetts in November 1993 and completed surveys were received from 127 teachers. A summary of the data is given in Table 8.1. Note that in Table 8.1, the values of the responses 1, 2, 3, 4, and 5 correspond to "not important," "somewhat important," "average importance," "important," and "very important," respectively, and each entry represents the count. See Rashid, Chen, and Ganter (1999) for a detailed discussion about this survey. We use this example to demonstrate the computational feasibility of the methodology described in Subsections 8.2.2 and 8.2.3.

For illustrative purposes, we consider three SMMVN-link models to fit the WPI survey data. These models are the MVP, MVL, and MVC (i.e., MVT with $\nu = 1$). These models capture different aspects and features of the SMMVN-link models. For example, the MVP and the MVC models correspond to the lightest and heaviest tails, respectively, while the MVL model is roughly "half-way" between the MVP and MVC models. In the implementation of the Gibbs sampler described in Subsection 8.2.2, we use the Chen–Dey algorithm to generate the cutpoints γ_j. We check the convergence of the Gibbs sampler using several diagnostic procedures discussed in Section 2.9. After convergence, we generate a large number of Gibbs iterates for computing the marginal likelihoods under the MVP, MVL, and MVC models. It is worthy to note that after convergence, we calculate the

TABLE 8.1. Summary of the Data.

Group	Response	Items									
		1	2	3	4	5	6	7	8	9	10
I	1	1	2	4	4	1	1	–	1	1	2
	2	–	–	12	10	2	2	8	2	1	5
	3	9	3	36	34	13	7	16	13	9	21
	4	26	25	17	20	31	30	30	33	35	33
	5	40	46	7	8	29	36	22	27	30	15
II	1	–	–	3	12	2	–	5	5	4	4
	2	–	2	6	8	5	–	5	3	7	10
	3	–	9	21	13	7	6	13	10	7	16
	4	12	13	13	16	25	11	18	19	15	15
	5	39	27	8	2	12	34	10	14	18	6

autocorrelations for all model parameters and find that they disappear at lag 10.

To obtain simulation-consistent estimates of the marginal likelihoods, the MC sample sizes in (8.2.25), (8.2.26), (8.2.27), and (8.2.32) are taken to be $R = 10000$. To obtain $\hat{\pi}(\gamma^*|D, \mathcal{M}_k)$, we use (8.2.29) instead of (8.2.28) since $J \times L = 50$ is relatively large. We find that the MC method given in Subsection 8.2.3 works well in this example. Furthermore, we use a procedure provided by Chib (1995) to compute the simulation standard errors for the marginal likelihood estimates. The estimates of $\ln m(D|\mathcal{M}_k)$ with the corresponding simulation standard errors in parentheses are -2055.6 (0.9), -1933.9 (0.6), and -1899.4 (0.6) for the MVC, MVL, and MVP models, respectively. Based on the marginal likelihoods, the MVP model is better than the other two models.

8.3 "Super-Model" or "Sub-Model" Approaches

Suppose we wish to compare two models $\mathcal{M}_1$ and $\mathcal{M}_2$. For model $\mathcal{M}_1$, the posterior distribution has the form

$$\pi(\boldsymbol{\theta}, \boldsymbol{\psi}|D, \mathcal{M}_1) \propto L(\boldsymbol{\theta}, \boldsymbol{\psi}|D, \mathcal{M}_1)\pi(\boldsymbol{\theta}, \boldsymbol{\psi}|\mathcal{M}_1), \tag{8.3.1}$$

and for model $\mathcal{M}_2$, the posterior distribution takes the form

$$\pi(\boldsymbol{\theta}, \boldsymbol{\varphi}|D, \mathcal{M}_2) \propto L(\boldsymbol{\theta}, \boldsymbol{\varphi}|D, \mathcal{M}_2)\pi(\boldsymbol{\theta}, \boldsymbol{\varphi}|\mathcal{M}_2). \tag{8.3.2}$$

In (8.3.1) and (8.3.2), $\pi(\boldsymbol{\theta}, \boldsymbol{\psi}|\mathcal{M}_1)$ and $\pi(\boldsymbol{\theta}, \boldsymbol{\varphi}|\mathcal{M}_2)$ are proper priors. Let $m(D|\mathcal{M}_k)$ denote the marginal likelihood for $k = 1, 2$. Then the Bayes factor for comparing model $\mathcal{M}_1$ to model $\mathcal{M}_2$ is given by

$$B_{12} = \frac{m(D|\mathcal{M}_1)}{m(D|\mathcal{M}_2)}. \tag{8.3.3}$$

Now we give sufficient conditions for applying the "super-model" and "sub-model" approaches. Assume that there exists a reduced model $\mathcal{M}_r$ and a saturated model $\mathcal{M}_s$ so that the posterior distributions are of the form

$$\pi(\boldsymbol{\theta}|D, \mathcal{M}_r) \propto L(\boldsymbol{\theta}|D, \mathcal{M}_r)\pi(\boldsymbol{\theta}|\mathcal{M}_r), \tag{8.3.4}$$

for model $\mathcal{M}_r$, and

$$\pi(\boldsymbol{\theta}, \boldsymbol{\psi}, \boldsymbol{\varphi}|D, \mathcal{M}_s) \propto L(\boldsymbol{\theta}, \boldsymbol{\psi}, \boldsymbol{\varphi}|D, \mathcal{M}_s)\pi(\boldsymbol{\theta}, \boldsymbol{\psi}, \boldsymbol{\varphi}|\mathcal{M}_s) \tag{8.3.5}$$

for model $\mathcal{M}_s$. In (8.3.4) and (8.3.5), we assume that:

(C1) $L(\boldsymbol{\theta}|D, \mathcal{M}_r) = L(\boldsymbol{\theta}, \boldsymbol{\psi} = 0|D, \mathcal{M}_1) = L(\boldsymbol{\theta}, \boldsymbol{\varphi} = 0|D, \mathcal{M}_2)$;

(C2) $\pi(\boldsymbol{\theta}|\mathcal{M}_r) \propto \pi(\boldsymbol{\theta}, \boldsymbol{\psi} = 0|D, \mathcal{M}_1)$ and $\pi(\boldsymbol{\theta}|\mathcal{M}_r) \propto \pi(\boldsymbol{\theta}, \boldsymbol{\varphi} = 0|D, \mathcal{M}_2)$;

(C3) $L(\boldsymbol{\theta}, \boldsymbol{\psi}, \boldsymbol{\varphi} = 0|D, \mathcal{M}_s) = L(\boldsymbol{\theta}, \boldsymbol{\psi}|D, \mathcal{M}_1)$ and $L(\boldsymbol{\theta}, \boldsymbol{\psi} = 0, \boldsymbol{\varphi}|D, \mathcal{M}_s) = L(\boldsymbol{\theta}, \boldsymbol{\varphi}|D, \mathcal{M}_2)$; and

(C4) $\pi(\boldsymbol{\theta}, \boldsymbol{\psi}|\mathcal{M}_1) \propto \pi(\boldsymbol{\theta}, \boldsymbol{\psi}, \boldsymbol{\varphi} = 0|D, \mathcal{M}_s)$ and $\pi(\boldsymbol{\theta}, \boldsymbol{\varphi}|\mathcal{M}_2) \propto \pi(\boldsymbol{\theta}, \boldsymbol{\psi} = 0, \boldsymbol{\varphi}|D, \mathcal{M}_s)$.

The above assumptions essentially imply that $\mathcal{M}_r$ is nested in $\mathcal{M}_1$ and $\mathcal{M}_2$, while $\mathcal{M}_1$ and $\mathcal{M}_2$ are nested in $\mathcal{M}_s$. Let $m(D|\mathcal{M}_r)$ and $m(D|\mathcal{M}_s)$ denote the marginal likelihoods corresponding to models $\mathcal{M}_r$ and $\mathcal{M}_s$, respectively.

We are led to the following theorem:

Theorem 8.3.1 *If conditions* (C1) *and* (C2) *hold, then*

$$\begin{aligned} B_{12} &= \frac{m(D|\mathcal{M}_1)/m(D|\mathcal{M}_r)}{m(D|\mathcal{M}_2)/m(D|\mathcal{M}_r)} \\ &= \frac{\pi(\boldsymbol{\psi} = 0|D, \mathcal{M}_1)/\pi(\boldsymbol{\psi} = 0|\mathcal{M}_1)}{\pi(\boldsymbol{\varphi} = 0|D, \mathcal{M}_2)/\pi(\boldsymbol{\varphi} = 0|\mathcal{M}_2)}. \end{aligned} \tag{8.3.6}$$

Similarly, conditions (C3) *and* (C4) *yield the identity*

$$\begin{aligned} B_{12} &= \frac{m(D|\mathcal{M}_1)/m(D|\mathcal{M}_s)}{m(D|\mathcal{M}_2)/m(D|\mathcal{M}_s)} \\ &= \frac{\pi(\boldsymbol{\varphi} = 0|D, \mathcal{M}_s)/\pi(\boldsymbol{\varphi} = 0|\mathcal{M}_s)}{\pi(\boldsymbol{\psi} = 0|D, \mathcal{M}_s)/\pi(\boldsymbol{\psi} = 0|\mathcal{M}_s)}. \end{aligned} \tag{8.3.7}$$

The proof follows directly from the Savage–Dickey density ratio and, therefore, is left as an exercise. Using Theorem 8.3.1, the "super-model" and "sub-model" approaches for computing the Bayes factor can be stated as follows.

The "Sub-Model" Approach

Step 1. Generate four MCMC samples from the posterior and prior distributions $\pi(\boldsymbol{\theta}, \boldsymbol{\psi}|D, \mathcal{M}_1)$, $\pi(\boldsymbol{\theta}, \boldsymbol{\psi}|\mathcal{M}_1)$ $\pi(\boldsymbol{\theta}, \boldsymbol{\varphi}|D, \mathcal{M}_2)$, and $\pi(\boldsymbol{\theta}, \boldsymbol{\varphi}|\mathcal{M}_2)$, respectively.

Step 2. Use the kernel method or the IWMDE method given in Chapter 4 to obtain the estimates of $\pi(\psi = 0|D, \mathcal{M}_1)$, $\pi(\psi = 0|\mathcal{M}_1)$, $\pi(\varphi = 0|D, \mathcal{M}_2)$, and $\pi(\varphi = 0|\mathcal{M}_2)$.

Step 3. Compute B_{12} using (8.3.6).

The "Super-Model" Approach

Step 1. Generate two MCMC samples from the posterior and prior distributions $\pi(\boldsymbol{\theta}, \psi, \varphi|D, \mathcal{M}_s)$ and $\pi(\boldsymbol{\theta}, \psi, \varphi|\mathcal{M}_s)$, respectively.

Step 2. Use the kernel method or the IWMDE method given in Chapter 4 to obtain the estimates of $\pi(\psi = 0|D, \mathcal{M}_s)$, $\pi(\psi = 0|\mathcal{M}_s)$, $\pi(\varphi = 0|D, \mathcal{M}_s)$, and $\pi(\varphi = 0|\mathcal{M}_s)$.

Step 3. Compute B_{12} using (8.3.7).

We note that the "sub-model" or "super-model" approaches are efficient if the posterior means or modes are not far away from 0. Otherwise, certain adjustments are needed in Step 2 for both procedures. More specifically, more efficient estimates of the posterior densities evaluated at $\psi = 0$ or $\varphi = 0$ can be obtained by using the MC methods for densities with different dimensions as given in Section 5.8. The detailed formulation is omitted here for brevity. From (8.3.1) and (8.3.2), it is easy to see that models $\mathcal{M}_1$ and $\mathcal{M}_2$ are not nested. Therefore, the reduced model $\mathcal{M}_r$ (or the saturated model $\mathcal{M}_s$) serves as a bridge to connect two nonnested models so that the MC methods given in the earlier chapters can be used for computing the Bayes factor. The reduced model and the saturated model can be constructed when one wants to compare two regression models in which both models contain common covariates.

8.4 Criterion-Based Methods

Bayesian methods for model comparison usually rely on posterior model probabilities or Bayes factors, and it is well known that to use these methods, proper prior distributions are needed when the number of parameters in the two competing models are different. In addition, posterior model probabilities are generally sensitive to the choices of prior parameters, and thus one cannot simply select vague proper priors to get around the elicitation issue. We discuss this issue in detail in the next chapter. Alternatively, criterion-based methods can be attractive in the sense that they do not require proper prior distributions in general, and thus have an advantage over posterior model probabilities in this sense. However, posterior model probabilities are intrinsically well calibrated since probabilities are relatively easy to interpret, whereas criterion-based methods are generally not easy to calibrate or interpret. Thus, one potential criticism of criterion-based methods for model comparison is that they generally do not have well-defined calibrations.

Recently, Ibrahim, Chen, and Sinha (1998) propose a Bayesian criterion, called the L *measure*, for model assessment and model comparison, and propose a calibration for it. The L measure can be used as a general model assessment tool for comparing models and assessing goodness of fit for a particular model, and thus in this sense, the criterion is potentially quite versatile. To facilitate the formal comparison of several models, Ibrahim, Chen, and Sinha (1998) also propose a novel calibration for the L measure by deriving the marginal prior predictive density of the difference between the L measures of the candidate model and the true model. This calibrating marginal density is called the *calibration distribution.* Since, in practice, the true model will not be known, we use the criterion minimizing model in place of the true model, and derive the calibration distribution based on the criterion minimizing model. Thus an L measure statistic and its corresponding calibration distribution are computed for each candidate model.

In the remainder of this chapter, we present the general formulation of the L measure criterion and its calibration, discuss MCMC strategies for computing it, and illustrate the method using an example involving right censored or interval censored data.

8.4.1 The L Measure

Consider an experiment that yields the data $\boldsymbol{y} = (y_1, \dots, y_n)'$. Denote the joint sampling density of the y_i's by $f(\boldsymbol{y}|\boldsymbol{\theta})$, where $\boldsymbol{\theta}$ is a vector of indexing parameters. We allow the y_i's to be fully observed, right censored, or interval censored. In the right censored case, y_i may be a failure time or a censored time. In the interval censored case, we only observe the interval $[a_{l_i}, a_{r_i}]$ in which y_i occurred. Let $\boldsymbol{z} = (z_1, \dots, z_n)'$ denote future values of a replicate experiment. That is, $\boldsymbol{z}$ is a future response vector with the same sampling density as $\boldsymbol{y}|\theta$. The idea of using a future response vector $\boldsymbol{z}$ in developing a criterion for assessing a model or comparing several models has been well motivated in the literature by Geisser (1993) and the many references therein, Ibrahim and Laud (1994), Laud and Ibrahim (1995), and Gelfand and Ghosh (1998).

Let $\eta(\cdot)$ be a known function, and let $y_i^* = \eta(y_i)$, $z_i^* = \eta(z_i)$, $\boldsymbol{y}^* = (y_1^*, y_2^*, \dots, y_n^*)'$, and $\boldsymbol{z}^* = (z_1^*, z_2^*, \dots, z_n^*)'$. For example, in survival analysis, it is common to take the logarithms of the survival times, and thus in this case $\eta(y_i) = \ln(y_i) = y_i^*$. Also, $\eta(y_i) = \ln(y_i)$ is a common transformation in Poisson regression. It is also common to take $\eta(\cdot)$ to be the identity function (i.e., $\eta(y_i) = y_i$), as in normal linear regression or logistic regression, so that in this case, $y_i^* = y_i$ and $z_i^* = z_i$.

We modify the general formulation of Gelfand and Ghosh (1998) to develop the L measure. For a given model, we first define the statistic

$$L_1(\boldsymbol{y}^*, \boldsymbol{b}) = E\left[(\boldsymbol{z}^* - \boldsymbol{b})'(\boldsymbol{z}^* - \boldsymbol{b})\right] + \delta(\boldsymbol{y}^* - \boldsymbol{b})'(\boldsymbol{y}^* - \boldsymbol{b}), \quad (8.4.1)$$

where the expectation is taken with respect to the posterior predictive distribution of $\boldsymbol{z}^*|\boldsymbol{y}^*$. The posterior predictive density of $\boldsymbol{z}^*|\boldsymbol{y}^*$ is given by

$$\pi(\boldsymbol{z}^*|\boldsymbol{y}^*) = \int f(\boldsymbol{z}^*|\boldsymbol{\theta})\pi(\boldsymbol{\theta}|\boldsymbol{y}^*)\, d\boldsymbol{\theta}, \quad (8.4.2)$$

where $\boldsymbol{\theta}$ denotes the vector of indexing parameters, $f(\boldsymbol{z}^*|\boldsymbol{\theta})$ is the sampling distribution of the future vector $\boldsymbol{z}^*$, and $\pi(\boldsymbol{\theta}|\boldsymbol{y}^*)$ denotes the posterior distribution of $\boldsymbol{\theta}$. The statistic in (8.4.1) takes the form of a weighted discrepancy measure. The vector $\boldsymbol{b} = (b_1, \ldots, b_n)'$ is an arbitrary location vector to be chosen and δ is a nonnegative scalar that weights the discrepancy based on the future values relative to the observed data. The general criterion in (8.4.1) is a special case of a class considered by Gelfand and Ghosh (1998), which are motivated from a Bayesian decision theoretic viewpoint. We refer the reader to their paper for a more general motivation and discussion. Setting $\boldsymbol{b} = \boldsymbol{y}^*$ in (8.4.1) yields the criterion of Ibrahim and Laud (1994).

In scalar notation, (8.4.1) can be written as

$$L_1(\boldsymbol{y}^*, \boldsymbol{b}) = \sum_{i=1}^{n}\{\mathrm{Var}(z_i^*|\boldsymbol{y}^*) + (\mu_i - b_i)^2 + \delta(y_i^* - b_i)^2\}, \quad (8.4.3)$$

where $\mu_i = E(z_i^*|\boldsymbol{y}^*)$. Thus we see that (8.4.3) has the appealing decomposition as a sum involving the predictive variances plus two squared "bias" terms, $(\mu_i - b_i)^2$ and $\delta(y_i^* - b_i)^2$, where δ is a weight for the second bias component.

We follow Gelfand and Ghosh (1998) by selecting b as the minimizer of (8.4.3). Gelfand and Ghosh (1998) show that the $\boldsymbol{b}$ which minimizes (8.4.3) is

$$\hat{\boldsymbol{b}} = (1 - \nu)\boldsymbol{\mu} + \nu\, \boldsymbol{y}^*, \quad (8.4.4)$$

where $\boldsymbol{\mu} = (\mu_1, \mu_2, \ldots, \mu_n)'$, $\nu = \delta/(\delta + 1)$, which upon substitution in (8.4.3) leads to the criterion

$$L_2(y^*) = \sum_{i=1}^{n} \mathrm{Var}(z_i^*|y_i^*) + \nu \sum_{i=1}^{n}(\mu_i - y_i^*)^2. \quad (8.4.5)$$

Clearly, $0 \leq \nu < 1$, where $\nu = 0$ if $\delta = 0$, and $\nu \to 1$ as $\delta \to \infty$. The quantity ν plays a major role in (8.4.5). It can be interpreted as a weight term in the squared bias component of (8.4.5), and appears to have a lot of potential impact on the ordering of the models, as well as characterizing the properties of the L measure and calibration distribution. Ibrahim and Laud (1994) use $\nu = 1$, and thus give equal weight to the squared bias and variance components. However, there is no theoretical justification for such a weight, and indeed, using $\nu = 1$ may not be desirable in certain situations. Allowing ν to vary between zero and one gives the user a great deal of flexibility in the tradeoff between bias and variance, and therefore results in values of ν that are more desirable than others. This begs the question of whether certain values of ν are "optimal" in some sense for model selection purposes. Ibrahim, Chen, and Sinha (1998) address this optimality issue for the linear model, and theoretically show that certain values of ν yield highly desirable properties of the L measure and the calibration distribution compared to other values of ν. They demonstrate that the choice of ν has much potential influence on the properties of the L measure, calibration distribution, and model choice in general. Based on their theoretical exploration, $\nu = \frac{1}{2}$ is a desirable and justifiable choice for model selection

If $\boldsymbol{y}^*$ is fully observed, then (8.4.5) is straightforward to compute. However, if $\boldsymbol{y}^*$ contains right censored or interval censored observations, then (8.4.5) is computed by taking the expectation of these censored observations with respect to the posterior predictive distribution of the censored observations. Let $\boldsymbol{y}^* = (\boldsymbol{y}^*_{\text{obs}}, \boldsymbol{y}^*_{\text{cens}})$, where $\boldsymbol{y}^*_{\text{obs}}$ denotes the completely observed components of $\boldsymbol{y}^*$, and $\boldsymbol{y}^*_{\text{cens}}$ denotes the censored components. Here, we assume that $\boldsymbol{y}^*_{\text{cens}}$ is a random quantity and $\boldsymbol{a}_l < \boldsymbol{y}^*_{\text{cens}} < \boldsymbol{a}_r$, where $\boldsymbol{a}_l$ and $\boldsymbol{a}_r$ are known. For ease of exposition, we let $D = (n, \boldsymbol{y}^*_{\text{obs}}, \boldsymbol{a}_l, \boldsymbol{a}_r)$ denote the observed data. Then (8.4.5) is modified as

$$L(\boldsymbol{y}^*_{\text{obs}}) = E_{\boldsymbol{y}^*_{\text{cens}}|D}[1\{\boldsymbol{a}_l < \boldsymbol{y}^*_{\text{cens}} < \boldsymbol{a}_r\} L_2(\boldsymbol{y}^*)], \qquad (8.4.6)$$

where $1\{\boldsymbol{a}_l < \boldsymbol{y}^*_{\text{cens}} < \boldsymbol{a}_r\}$ is a generic indicator function taking the value 1 if $\boldsymbol{a}_l < \boldsymbol{y}^*_{\text{cens}} < \boldsymbol{a}_r$ and 0 otherwise, and the expectation $E_{\boldsymbol{y}^*_{\text{cens}}|D}$ is taken with respect to the posterior predictive distribution $f(\boldsymbol{y}^*_{\text{cens}}|\boldsymbol{\theta})\pi(\boldsymbol{\theta}|D)$. Note that $\boldsymbol{a}_l < \boldsymbol{y}^*_{\text{cens}} < \boldsymbol{a}_r$ means that the double inequalities hold for each component of these vectors. If, for example, all n observations are censored, then the above notation means $a_{l_i} < y^*_{\text{cens},i} < a_{r_i}$, $i = 1, \ldots, n$, where $\boldsymbol{a}_l = (a_{l_1}, \ldots, a_{l_n})'$, $\boldsymbol{a}_r = (a_{r_1}, \ldots, a_{r_n})'$, and $\boldsymbol{y}^*_{\text{cens}} = (y^*_{\text{cens},1}, \ldots, y^*_{\text{cens},n})'$. We shall call (8.4.6) the *L measure*. Small values of the L measure imply a good model. Specifically, we can write (8.4.6) as

$$L(\boldsymbol{y}^*_{\text{obs}}) = \int \int_{\boldsymbol{a}_l}^{\boldsymbol{a}_r} L_2(\boldsymbol{y}^*) f(\boldsymbol{y}^*_{\text{cens}}|\boldsymbol{\theta})\pi(\boldsymbol{\theta}|D)\, d\boldsymbol{y}^*_{\text{cens}}\, d\boldsymbol{\theta}, \qquad (8.4.7)$$

where $f(\boldsymbol{y}^*_{\text{cens}}|\boldsymbol{\theta})$ is the sampling density of $\boldsymbol{y}^*_{\text{cens}}$ and $\pi(\boldsymbol{\theta}|D)$ is the posterior density of $\boldsymbol{\theta}$ given the observed data D. If $\boldsymbol{y}^*$ has right censored observations, then $\boldsymbol{a}_r = \infty$, and $\boldsymbol{a}_l$ is a vector of censoring times. If $\boldsymbol{y}^*$ has interval censored observations, then $(\boldsymbol{a}_l, \boldsymbol{a}_r)$ is a sequence of finite interval censoring times. If $\boldsymbol{y}^*$ is fully observed, that is, $\boldsymbol{y}^*_{\text{obs}} = \boldsymbol{y}^*$, then (8.4.6) reduces to (8.4.5), and therefore $L(\boldsymbol{y}^*_{\text{obs}}) \equiv L_2(\boldsymbol{y}^*)$ in this case.

It can be shown that (8.4.5) can be expressed as a posterior expectation, so that

$$L_2(\boldsymbol{y}^*) = \sum_{i=1}^{n}\{E_{\boldsymbol{\theta}|D}(E[(z_i^*)^2|\boldsymbol{\theta}]) - \mu_i^2\} + \nu\sum_{i=1}^{n}(\mu_i - y_i^*)^2, \quad (8.4.8)$$

where $\mu_i = E_{\boldsymbol{\theta}|D}[E(z_i^*|\boldsymbol{\theta})]$, and the expectation $E_{\boldsymbol{\theta}|D}$ is taken with respect to the posterior distribution $\pi(\boldsymbol{\theta}|D)$. Thus (8.4.5) and (8.4.6) can be computed by sampling from the posterior distribution of $\boldsymbol{\theta}$ via MCMC methods. Once the posterior samples of $\boldsymbol{\theta}$ are obtained, (8.4.8) and (8.4.6) can be evaluated. More specifically, suppose that $\{\boldsymbol{\theta}_q,\ q = 1, 2, \ldots, Q\}$ is an MCMC sample from $\pi(\boldsymbol{\theta}|D)$ and $\{\boldsymbol{y}^*_{\text{cens},q},\ q = 1, 2, \ldots, Q\}$ is an MCMC sample from the truncated posterior predictive distribution $1\{\boldsymbol{a}_l < \boldsymbol{y}^*_{\text{cens}} < \boldsymbol{a}_r\}f(\boldsymbol{y}^*_{\text{cens}}|\boldsymbol{\theta})\pi(\boldsymbol{\theta}|D)$. Then an MC estimate of $L(\boldsymbol{y}^*_{\text{obs}})$ is given by

$$\hat{L}(\boldsymbol{y}^*_{\text{obs}}) = \sum_{i=1}^{n}\left\{\frac{1}{Q}\sum_{q=1}^{Q}\left(E\left[(z_i^*)^2|\boldsymbol{\theta}_q\right]\right) - \hat{\mu}_i^2\right\} + \nu\left\{\sum_{\{i:\ y_i^*\ \text{observed}\}}(\hat{\mu}_i - y_i^*)^2 \right.$$
$$\left. + \frac{1}{Q}\sum_{q=1}^{Q}\left[\sum_{\{i:\ y_i^*\ \text{censored}\}}(\hat{\mu}_i - y^*_{\text{cens},iq})^2\right]\right\}, \quad (8.4.9)$$

where $\hat{\mu}_i = (1/Q)\sum_{q=1}^{Q} E(z_i^*|\boldsymbol{\theta}_q)$, and $y^*_{\text{cens},iq}$ is the ith component of $\boldsymbol{y}^*_{\text{cens},q}$. In the cases where $E[(z_i^*)^2|\boldsymbol{\theta}]$ and $E(z_i^*|\boldsymbol{\theta})$ are not analytically available, we need an MCMC sample $\{(\boldsymbol{z}_q^*, \boldsymbol{\theta}_q),\ q = 1, 2, \ldots, Q\}$ from the joint distribution $f(\boldsymbol{z}^*|\boldsymbol{\theta})\pi(\boldsymbol{\theta}|D)$. Then, in (8.4.9), we replace

$$\frac{1}{Q}\sum_{q=1}^{Q}(E[(z_i^*)^2|\boldsymbol{\theta}_q]) \text{ and } \frac{1}{Q}\sum_{q=1}^{Q}E(z_i^*|\boldsymbol{\theta}_q)$$

by

$$\frac{1}{Q}\sum_{r=1}^{Q}\left(z^*_{i,q}\right)^2 \text{ and } \frac{1}{Q}\sum_{q=1}^{Q}z^*_{i,q},$$

where $z^*_{i,q}$ is the ith component of $\boldsymbol{z}^*_q$. Thus, computing $L(\boldsymbol{y}^*_{\text{obs}})$ is relatively straightforward.

8.4.2 The Calibration Distribution

Ibrahim, Chen, and Sinha (1998) propose a calibration for the L measure $L(\boldsymbol{y}^*_{\text{obs}})$. To motivate the calibration distribution, let c denote the candidate model under consideration, and let t denote the true model. Further, let $L_c(\boldsymbol{y}^*_{\text{obs}})$ denote the L measure for the candidate model c, and let $L_t(\boldsymbol{y}^*_{\text{obs}})$ denote the L measure for the true model t. Now consider the difference in

L measures

$$D(\boldsymbol{y}^*_{\text{obs}}, \nu) \equiv L_c(\boldsymbol{y}^*_{\text{obs}}) - L_t(\boldsymbol{y}^*_{\text{obs}}). \tag{8.4.10}$$

The quantity in (8.4.10) is a random variable in $\boldsymbol{y}^*_{\text{obs}}$, and depends on ν. It measures the discrepancy in the L measure values between the candidate model and the true model. To calibrate the L measure, we construct the marginal distribution of $D(\boldsymbol{y}^*_{\text{obs}}, \nu)$, computed with respect to the prior predictive distribution of $\boldsymbol{y}^*_{\text{obs}}$ under the true model t, denoted by

$$p_t(\boldsymbol{y}^*_{\text{obs}}) = \int f_t(\boldsymbol{y}^*_{\text{obs}}|\boldsymbol{\theta})\pi_t(\boldsymbol{\theta})\, d\boldsymbol{\theta}. \tag{8.4.11}$$

Thus, the calibration distribution is defined as

$$p_{L_c} \equiv p(D(\boldsymbol{y}^*_{\text{obs}}, \nu)). \tag{8.4.12}$$

Thus p_{L_c} is the marginal distribution of $D(\boldsymbol{y}^*_{\text{obs}}, \nu)$, computed with respect to $p_t(\boldsymbol{y}^*_{\text{obs}})$. We refer to p_{L_c} as the *calibration distribution* for the candidate model c throughout. We see that p_{L_c} is a univariate distribution, and therefore easily tabulated and plotted. If the candidate model is "close" to the true model, then p_{L_c} should have a mean (or mode) that is close to zero, and much of its mass should be centered around this point. On the other hand, if the candidate model and true model are far apart, then p_{L_c} will have a mean (or mode) that is far from zero. One obvious advantage in having an entire distribution as the calibration is that one is able to make plots of it, and derive various summary statistics from it, such as its mean, mode, and HPD intervals. We see that p_{L_c} is computed for every candidate model c, where $c \neq t$, and therefore changes with every c. We also see from (8.4.12) that for p_{L_c} to be well defined, we need a proper prior distribution for $\boldsymbol{\theta}$. This definition of the calibration distribution in (8.4.12) is appealing since it avoids the potential problem of a double use of the data as discussed by Bayarri and Berger (1999).

The definition of p_{L_c} depends on the data only through $\boldsymbol{y}^*_{\text{obs}}$. When we have right censored data, $\boldsymbol{y}^*_{\text{obs}}$ consists of the observed failure times, and thus p_{L_c} in this case is a function only of the observed failure times. Therefore, its computation does not depend on any of the censoring times. In situations where all of the observations are censored, $\boldsymbol{y}^*_{\text{obs}}$ consists of the empty set. In this case, the definition of p_{L_c} in (8.4.12) must be slightly modified. For interval censored data, we "impute" each interval censored observation by sampling from the truncated prior predictive distribution, where the truncation is taken to be the endpoints of the interval censored observation. Thus, if y_i^* is interval censored in the interval $[a_{l_i}, a_{r_i}]$, then we impute y_i^* by replacing it with a sample of size 1 from

$$p_t(y_i^*) \propto \int f_t(y_i^*|\boldsymbol{\theta})\pi_t(\boldsymbol{\theta})\, d\boldsymbol{\theta}, \quad a_{l_i} < y_i^* < a_{r_i},$$

$i = 1, \ldots, n$. We denote the sampled value by $\tilde{y}_i^*$ for each interval censored observation, thus obtaining $\tilde{\boldsymbol{y}}^* = (\tilde{y}_1^*, \ldots, \tilde{y}_n^*)'$ for the n interval censored observations. We then treat $\tilde{\boldsymbol{y}}^*$ as $\boldsymbol{y}_{\text{obs}}^*$. That is, we set $\tilde{\boldsymbol{y}}^* = \boldsymbol{y}_{\text{obs}}$, and compute p_{L_c} using $\tilde{\boldsymbol{y}}^* = \boldsymbol{y}_{\text{obs}}^*$. Thus, in the interval censored case, $\tilde{\boldsymbol{y}}^*$ can be viewed as *pseudo-observations* needed to form $\boldsymbol{y}_{\text{obs}}^*$ in order to facilitate the computation of p_{L_c}. This is a solid technique for obtaining the calibration distribution p_{L_c} when all of the observations are interval censored, and produces good results as demonstrated in Subsection 8.4.3.

Once p_{L_c} is computed, several statistical summaries can be obtained from it to summarize the calibration. These include various HPD intervals and the mean of $D(\boldsymbol{y}_{\text{obs}}^*, \nu)$. The mean of the calibration distribution is denoted by

$$\mu_c(\nu) = E_t(D(\boldsymbol{y}_{\text{obs}}^*, \nu)), \tag{8.4.13}$$

where $E_t(\cdot)$ denotes the expectation with respect to the prior predictive distribution of the true model. This summary, $\mu_c(\nu)$, is attractive since it measures, on average, how close the centers are of the candidate and true models. If the candidate model is a good model, then $\mu_c(\nu)$ should be close to 0, whereas if the candidate model is far from the true model, then $\mu_c(\nu)$ should be far from 0. We note that $\mu_c(\nu)$ depends on the candidate model and therefore changes with every c. If $c = t$, then $\mu_c(\nu) = 0$ for all ν.

Since the true model t will not be known in practice, we use the criterion minimizing model t_{min} in place of t for computing (8.4.10). Thus, in practice, we compute

$$\hat{D}(\boldsymbol{y}_{\text{obs}}^*, \nu) = L_c(\boldsymbol{y}_{\text{obs}}^*) - L_{t_{\text{min}}}(\boldsymbol{y}_{\text{obs}}^*), \tag{8.4.14}$$

and

$$\hat{p}_{L_c} = p(\hat{D}(\boldsymbol{y}_{\text{obs}}^*, \nu)), \tag{8.4.15}$$

where $\hat{p}_{L_c}$ is computed with respect to the prior predictive distribution of the criterion minimizing model. Also, $\mu_c(\nu)$ is estimated by $\hat{\mu}(\nu)$, where $\hat{\mu}(\nu) = E_{t_{\text{min}}}[\hat{D}(\boldsymbol{y}_{\text{obs}}^*, \nu)]$.

Finally, we briefly describe how to compute the calibration distribution p_{L_c} via MCMC sampling. For illustrative purposes, we consider only the case where $\boldsymbol{y}_{\text{obs}}^*$ is *not empty* as the computation is even much simpler when $\boldsymbol{y}_{\text{obs}}^*$ is empty. From (8.4.12), it can be seen that computing the calibration distribution requires the following two steps: for a candidate model c,

(i) Generate a pseudo-observation $\tilde{\boldsymbol{y}}^*$ from the prior predictive distribution $f_t(\boldsymbol{y}^*|\boldsymbol{\theta})\pi_t(\boldsymbol{\theta})$; and

(ii) Set $\boldsymbol{y}_{\text{obs}}^* = \tilde{\boldsymbol{y}}^*$ and use the method described in Subsection 8.4.1 to obtain an MC estimate of $L(\boldsymbol{y}_{\text{obs}}^*)$.

We repeat (i) and (ii) Q times to obtain an MCMC sample of $L_c(\boldsymbol{y}_{\text{obs}}^*)$. Then we repeat (i) and (ii) Q times using the criterion minimizing model to obtain an MCMC sample of $L_{t_{\min}}(\boldsymbol{y}^*_{\text{obs}})$. Using these MCMC samples, we can compute the entire calibration distribution p_{L_c}, for example, by using the kernel method (see Section 4.2 or Silverman (1986)). We note that step (ii) may be computationally intensive. However, the entire computational procedure is quite straightforward.

8.4.3 Breast Cancer Data Example

We consider the breast cancer data, displayed in Table 8.2, from Finkelstein and Wolf (1985), which consists of a data set of (case-2) interval censored data. In this data set, 46 early breast cancer patients receiving only radiotherapy (covariate value $x = 0$) and 48 patients receiving radio-chemotherapy ($x = 1$) were monitored for cosmetic changes through weekly clinic visits. Some patients missed some of their weekly visits, so the data

TABLE 8.2. The Breast Cancer Data.

Interval	x	Interval	x	Interval	x	Interval	x
(45, −]	0	(6, 10]	0	(0, 7]	0	(46, −]	0
(46, −]	0	(7, 16]	0	(26, 40]	0	(36, 44]	0
(37, −]	0	(46, −]	0	(5, 12]	0	(18, −]	0
(5, 11]	0	(24, −]	0	(19, 26]	0	(36, −]	0
(17, −]	0	(7, 14]	0	(37, 44]	0	(0, 8]	0
(4, 11]	0	(15, −]	0	(46, −]	0	(46, −]	0
(40, −]	0	(11, 18]	0	(37, −]	0	(24, −]	0
(19, 35]	0	(32, −]	0	(37, −]	0	(11, 15]	0
(22, −]	0	(46, −]	0	(46, −]	0	(25, 37]	0
(46, −]	0	(27, 34]	0	(36, 48]	0	(17, 25]	0
(38, −]	0	(0, 5]	0	(36, −]	0	(17, 25]	0
(33, −]	0	(34, −]	0	(17, 26]	1	(35, 39]	1
(22, 32]	1	(8, 12]	1	(35, −]	1	(23, −]	1
(11, 20]	1	(0, 22]	1	(16, 60]	1	(11, 17]	1
(10, 35]	1	(0, 5]	1	(14, 17]	1	(13, −]	1
(12, 20]	1	(17, 27]	1	(8, 21]	1	(33, 40]	1
(24, 30]	1	(11, −]	1	(13, 39]	1	(13, −]	1
(4, 8]	1	(34, −]	1	(16, 20]	1	(30, 36]	1
(16, 24]	1	(32, −]	1	(21, −]	1	(48, −]	1
(30, 34]	1	(5, 8]	1	(24, 31]	1	(10, 17]	1
(11, −]	1	(17, 23]	1	(4, 9]	1	(31, −]	1
(16, 24]	1	(14, 19]	1	(19, 32]	1	(11, 13]	1
(34, −]	1	(13, −]	1	(18, 25]	1	(18, 24]	1
(15, 22]	1	(44, 48]	1				

Source: Finkelstein and Wolf (1985).

TABLE 8.3. The Values of the Prior Parameters.

	η_k	γ_k	β_0	w_k	w_0	v_k	α_0	v_0
$\mathcal{M}_1$	0.2	0.4	0	–	2.0	–	–	–
$\mathcal{M}_2$	0.2	0.4	0	1.0	2.0	–	–	–
$\mathcal{M}_3$	–	–	0	–	2.0	1.0	−0.1	2.0

on the survival time are typically recorded as, for example, $(7, 18]$ (at the seventh week clinic visit patient had shown no change and then in the next clinic visit at the eighteenth week the patient's tissue showed that the change had already occurred). Since the clinic visits of different patients occurred at different times, the censoring intervals in the data set are found to be often overlapping and nondisjoint. We are interested in the effect of the covariate x on the survival time y.

Sinha, Chen, and Ghosh (1999) consider a semiparametric Bayesian analysis of these data using three models based on a discretized version of the Cox model (Cox 1972). Specifically, the hazard, $\lambda(y|x)$, is taken to be a piecewise constant function with $\lambda(y|x) = \lambda_j \theta_j^x$ for $y \in I_j$, where $\theta_j = e^{\beta_j}$, $I_j = (a_{j-1}, a_j]$ for $j = 1, 2, \ldots, g$, $0 = a_0 < a_1 < \cdots < a_g = \infty$, and N is the total number of grid intervals. The length of each grid can be taken to be sufficiently small to approximate any hazard function for all practical purposes.

In this example, we consider the following three models:

$\mathcal{M}_1$: (i) $\lambda_j \overset{\text{i.i.d.}}{\sim} \mathcal{G}(\eta_j, \gamma_j)$ for $j = 1, \ldots, g$; and
(ii) $\beta \sim N(\beta_0, w_0^2)$.

$\mathcal{M}_2$: (i) λ_j's have the same prior as in model $\mathcal{M}_1$; and
(ii) $\beta_{j+1}|\beta_1, \ldots, \beta_{g-1} \sim N(\beta_j, w_j^2)$ for $j = 0, \ldots, g-1$.

$\mathcal{M}_3$: (i) $\alpha_{j+1}|\alpha_1, \ldots, \alpha_j \sim N(\alpha_j, v_j^2)$, where $\alpha_j = \ln(\lambda_j)$; for $j = 0, 1, \ldots, g-1$; and
(ii) same as in $\mathcal{M}_2$.

A detailed description of the motivation for $\mathcal{M}_1$ to $\mathcal{M}_3$ can be found in Sinha, Chen, and Ghosh (1999). Our purpose here is to compute the L measure and the calibration distribution for the three models using noninformative priors. We use the same values of the prior parameters as Sinha, Chen, and Ghosh (1998), which are given in Table 8.3.

Let $D_{\text{obs}} = \{(a_{l_i}, a_{r_i}]; x_i : i = 1, 2, \ldots, n\}$ denote the observed interval-censored data from n patients, where the survival time y_i for the ith patient is known to be within $(a_{l_i}, a_{r_i}]$ and $a_{l_i} < a_{r_i}$ are two of the grid points $(a_1, a_2, \ldots, a_g)$, but are not necessarily consecutive ones, and x_i is the covariate value for the ith patient. Let $D = \{y_i, x_i : i = 1, 2, \ldots, n\}$ denote the complete (augmented) data. Then the complete data likelihood is given by

$$L(\boldsymbol{\lambda}, \boldsymbol{\theta}|D) \propto \prod_{j=1}^{g} \left[\lambda_j^{d_j} \exp\left\{ -\lambda_j \sum_{l \in R_j} \theta_j^{x_l \Delta_{lj}} \right\} \theta_j^{\sum_{l \in R_j^*} x_l} \right], \quad (8.4.16)$$

where $\boldsymbol{\lambda} = (\lambda_1, \lambda_2, \ldots, \lambda_g)'$, $\boldsymbol{\theta} = (\theta_1, \theta_2, \ldots, \theta_g)'$, R_j is the set of patients at risk at a_{j-1}, $\Delta_{lj} = \min(y_l, a_j) - a_{j-1}$, R_j^* is the set of patients failing in $I_j = (a_{j-1}, a_j]$, and d_j is the number of patients in R_j^*. Although the observed data likelihood is difficult to obtain and the joint posterior distribution is very complicated even for $\mathcal{M}_1$, it is quite straightforward to implement the Gibbs sampler to sample from the resulting posterior distributions. The conditional posteriors required for the Gibbs sampler are as follows.

For $\mathcal{M}_2$,

$$\lambda_j | \boldsymbol{\lambda}^{(-j)}, \boldsymbol{\beta}, D \sim \mathcal{G}\left(\eta_j + d_j;\ \gamma_j + \sum_{l \in R_j} \theta_j^{x_l} \Delta_{lj} \right), \quad (8.4.17)$$

where $\mathcal{G}$ denotes a gamma distribution, and

$$\begin{aligned} &\pi(\beta_j | \boldsymbol{\beta}^{(-j)}, \boldsymbol{\lambda}, D) \\ &\quad \propto \phi\left(\beta_j \middle| \frac{(\sum_{l \in R_j^*} x_l) w_j^2 w_{j-1}^2 + \beta_{j-1} w_j^2 + \beta_{j+1} w_{j-1}^2}{w_j^2 + w_{j-1}^2}; \frac{w_j^2 w_{j-1}^2}{w_j^2 + w_{j-1}^2} \right) \\ &\quad \times \exp\left(-\lambda_j \sum_{l \in R_j} \theta_j^{x_l} \Delta_{lj} \right), \end{aligned} \quad (8.4.18)$$

for $j = 1, 2, \ldots, g$, where $\boldsymbol{\lambda}^{(-j)} (\boldsymbol{\beta}^{(-j)})$ is the vector $\boldsymbol{\lambda}$ (vector of $\boldsymbol{\beta}$'s) with $\lambda_j (\beta_j)$ deleted, $\beta_{g+1} = 0$ and $\phi(\cdot|\mu; \sigma^2)$ is the $N(\mu, \sigma^2)$ density function. Finally, for $\mathcal{M}_2$,

$$f(y_i | \boldsymbol{\beta}, \boldsymbol{\lambda}) \propto \frac{\lambda_j \theta_j^{x_i} \exp\left\{ -\sum_{l=l_i+1}^{j-1} \lambda_l \theta_l^{x_i} \tilde{\Delta}_l - \lambda_j \theta_j^{x_i} (y_i - a_{j-1}) \right\}}{1 - \exp\left\{ -\sum_{l=l_i+1}^{r_i} \lambda_l \theta_l^{x_i} \tilde{\Delta}_l \right\}}, \quad (8.4.19)$$

for $y_i \in I_j$, $l_i + 1 \le j \le r_i$, and $\tilde{\Delta}_l = a_l - a_{l-1}$. Note that (8.4.19) can be defined via a product of multinomial and truncated exponential densities.

For $\mathcal{M}_1$, all the θ_k's will be equal to $\theta = e^{\beta}$ in (8.4.17) and

$$\begin{aligned} \pi(\beta | \boldsymbol{\lambda}, D) \propto &\left(\prod_{j=1}^{g} \exp\left\{ -\lambda_j \sum_{l \in R_j} e^{\beta x_l} \Delta_{lj} \right\} \exp\left\{ \beta \sum_{l \in R_j^*} x_l \right\} \right) \\ &\times \phi(\beta | \beta_0; w_0^2). \end{aligned} \quad (8.4.20)$$

The conditional distributions $[\lambda_j|\boldsymbol{\lambda}^{(-j)}, \boldsymbol{\beta}, D]$ and $[y_i|\boldsymbol{\beta}, \boldsymbol{\lambda}]$ for $\mathcal{M}_1$ and $\mathcal{M}_3$ are similar to (8.4.17) and (8.4.19), respectively. For $\mathcal{M}_3$,

$$\pi(\alpha_j|\boldsymbol{\alpha}^{(-j)}, \boldsymbol{\beta}, D)$$
$$\propto \phi\left(\alpha_j \left| \frac{(\sum_{l\in R_j^*} x_l)v_j^2 v_{j-1}^2 + \alpha_{j-1}v_j^2 + \alpha_{j+1}v_{j-1}^2}{v_j^2 + v_{j-1}^2}; \frac{v_j^2 v_{j-1}^2}{v_j^2 + v_{j-1}^2}\right.\right)$$
$$\times \exp\left(- e^{\alpha_j} \sum_{l\in R_j} \theta_j^{x_l} \Delta_{lj}\right), \tag{8.4.21}$$

where $\alpha^{(-j)}$ and $\boldsymbol{\beta}^{(-j)}$ have similar meanings.

Sampling λ_j and y_i from (8.4.17) and (8.4.19) is straightforward. To sample $\boldsymbol{\beta}$ from (8.4.20) for $\mathcal{M}_1$, β_j from (8.4.18) for $\mathcal{M}_2$, and α_j from (8.4.21), we can use the adaptive rejection sampling algorithm of Gilks and Wild (1992), since these conditional distributions are log-concave.

For the breast cancer data, we implement the above Gibbs sampling algorithms, and we use 50000 MCMC iterations for computing the L measures and the calibration distributions. We also choose $y^* = \eta(y) = \ln(y)$ in (8.4.7). Table 8.4 shows the results using $\nu = \frac{1}{2}$, and reveals that model $\mathcal{M}_1$

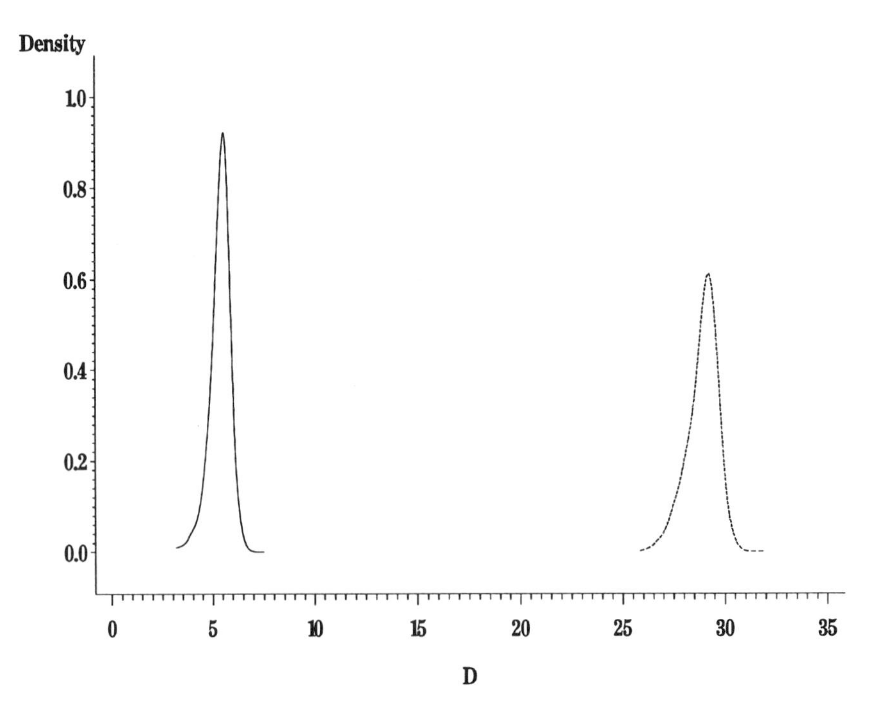

FIGURE 8.1. Calibration distributions for breast cancer data; solid curve: model $\mathcal{M}_2$, and dashed curve: model $\mathcal{M}_3$.

TABLE 8.4. L Measure and Calibration Summaries for Breast Cancer Data.

Model	L Measure	$\mu_c(\frac{1}{2})$	50% HPD	95% HPD
1*	80.45	–	–	–
2	87.24	5.36	(5.23, 5.83)	(4.24, 6.34)
3	113.54	28.91	(28.71, 29.61)	(27.23, 30.23)

* Criterion minimizing model

is the criterion minimizing model with an L measure value of 80.45. Models $\mathcal{M}_2$ and $\mathcal{M}_3$ have $\mu_c(\frac{1}{2})$ values of $\mu_2(\frac{1}{2}) = 5.36$ and $\mu_3(\frac{1}{2}) = 28.91$, respectively, and therefore, model $\mathcal{M}_2$ is much closer to the criterion minimizing model than model $\mathcal{M}_3$. This is also clearly displayed in Figure 8.1, which gives the calibration distributions for models $\mathcal{M}_2$ and $\mathcal{M}_3$. We see from Figure 8.1 that there is a wide separation between p_{L_2} and p_{L_3}, and p_{L_2} has smaller dispersion than p_{L_3}. The HPD intervals for models $\mathcal{M}_2$ and $\mathcal{M}_3$ do not contain 0. We conclude here that both models $\mathcal{M}_2$ and $\mathcal{M}_3$ are sufficiently different from one another as well as being sufficiently different from the criterion minimizing model. We note that other choices of prior parameters yield similar L measure values and calibration distributions, and thus the results are not very sensitive to the choice of the prior distributions.

Exercises

8.1 Using the same MCMC sample $\{(\boldsymbol{\theta}_{k,i,1}, \boldsymbol{\theta}_{k,i,2}, \boldsymbol{z}_i),\ i = 1, 2, \ldots, n\}$, derive the simulation standard error of $\ln[\hat{\pi}(\boldsymbol{\theta}^*_{k,1}|D, \mathcal{M}_k)]$, where $\hat{\pi}(\boldsymbol{\theta}^*_{k,1}| D, \mathcal{M}_k)$ is given in (8.1.8). In addition, use the standard δ method to obtain the simulation standard error of $\ln[\hat{\pi}(\boldsymbol{\theta}^*_k|D, \mathcal{M}_k)]$, where $\hat{\pi}(\boldsymbol{\theta}^*_k|D, \mathcal{M}_k)$ is given by (8.1.10).

8.2 Let t_ν denote a univariate random variable that has a Student t distribution with ν degrees of freedom. Albert and Chib (1993) empirically observe that t_ν is approximately b times a logistic random variable with appropriate choices of positive-valued ν and b. Determine the values of ν and b by matching the first four moments of these two distributions.

8.3 ASYMPTOTIC KOLMOGOROV DISTRIBUTION

(a) Show that the asymptotic Kolmogorov distribution given in (8.2.9) can be written as

$$\pi_L(\lambda) = \text{ch}(\lambda) \sum_{j=0}^{\infty} (-1)^j a_j(\lambda),$$

where

$$\begin{aligned} \mathrm{ch}(\lambda) &= 8\lambda \exp\{-2\lambda^2\}, \quad \lambda > 0, \\ a_j(\lambda) &= (j+1)^2 \exp\{-2\lambda^2((j+1)^2 - 1)\}, \quad j \geq 0 \text{ and } \lambda > 0. \end{aligned}$$

(b) Show that $a_j(\lambda)$ is a decreasing function of j for $\lambda > 0$.
(c) Using (a) and (b), for a given numerical precision $0 < \epsilon < 1$, find the number of terms, $K^*(\lambda)$, required to evaluate $\pi_K(\lambda)$, where

$$K^*(\lambda) = \inf_j \{j : \mathrm{ch}(\lambda) a_j(\lambda) \leq \epsilon\}.$$

8.4 As discussed in Subsection 8.2.2, $[\boldsymbol{w}^{(j)} | \boldsymbol{\gamma}_j, \boldsymbol{\beta}, \Sigma, \boldsymbol{w}^{(-j)}, D]$ is a truncated multivariate normal distribution. Given $\boldsymbol{\gamma}_j$, $\boldsymbol{\beta}$, Σ, $\boldsymbol{w}^{(-j)}$, and $\boldsymbol{\lambda}$, derive closed-form expressions of the mean and variance of the conditional distribution of w_{ij}, the ith component of $\boldsymbol{w}^{(j)}$.

8.5 Consider the item response data given in Table 8.1.

(a) Explain why direct use of the Nandram–Chen algorithm in Subsection 2.5.3 may present a problem in the implementation of the Metropolis algorithm for sampling the cutpoints.
(b) Does the Chen–Dey algorithm in Subsection 2.5.3 have a similar problem? Why?

8.6 Similar to (2.5.18), obtain an expression of the conditional density of $[\boldsymbol{\gamma}_j | \boldsymbol{\beta}, \Sigma, \boldsymbol{w}^{(-j)}, \boldsymbol{\lambda}, D]$ up to a normalizing constant.

8.7 A Skewed Link Model for Binary Response Data
Let $\boldsymbol{y} = (y_1, y_2, \ldots, y_n)'$ denote an $n \times 1$ vector of n independent binary random variables. Also let $\boldsymbol{x}_i = (x_{i1}, \ldots, x_{ip})'$ be a $p \times 1$ vector of covariates, and $\boldsymbol{\beta} = (\beta_1, \ldots, \beta_p)'$ is a $p \times 1$ vector of regression coefficients.
Let $\boldsymbol{w} = (w_1, w_2, \ldots, w_n)'$ be a vector of independent latent variables. Chen, Dey, and Shao (1999) propose a new skewed link model, which is defined as follows:

$$y_i = \begin{cases} 0 & \text{if } w_i < 0, \\ 1 & \text{if } w_i \geq 0, \end{cases} \tag{8.E.1}$$

where

$$w_i = \boldsymbol{x}_i'\boldsymbol{\beta} + \delta z_i + \epsilon_i, \quad z_i \sim G \text{ and } \epsilon_i \sim F, \tag{8.E.2}$$

z_i and ϵ_i are independent, G is the cdf of a skewed distribution, and F is the cdf of a symmetric distribution. In (8.E.2), $-\infty < \delta < \infty$ is a skewness parameter.

(a) Assume that both G and F have finite third moments. Let σ_z^2 and σ_ϵ^2 be the variances of z_i and ϵ_i, and let μ_z^3 denote the standardized third moment of z_i, i.e., $\mu_z^3 = E([z_i - E(z_i)]/\sigma_{z_i})^3$.

(i) Find the standardized third moment μ_w^3 of w_i.

(ii) Provided the distribution G is skewed to the right, discuss the relationship between the skewness of the marginal distribution of w_i and the skewness parameter δ.

(b) Let $D_{\text{obs}} = (n, \boldsymbol{y}, X)$ denote the observed data, where X is the $n \times p$ design matrix with $\boldsymbol{x}_i'$ as its ith row. Derive the likelihood function $L(\boldsymbol{\beta}, \delta | D_{\text{obs}})$ of the parameters $(\boldsymbol{\beta}, \delta)$ based on the observed data.

(c) Assume that F is the standard normal $N(0, 1)$ cdf and G is the cdf of the half-standard normal distribution with density function

$$g(z) = \frac{2}{\sqrt{2\pi}} e^{-z^2/2}, \quad z > 0.$$

Suppose we take an improper uniform prior for $(\boldsymbol{\beta}, \delta)$, i.e., $\pi(\boldsymbol{\beta}, \delta) \propto 1$. Following along the lines given in Subsection 8.1.2, develop an MC procedure for computing the resulting marginal likelihood.

(d) Consider the setting of Part (c), but take F to be the cdf of the univariate logistic distribution. By introducing an additional latent variable that has an asymptotic Kolmogorov distribution π_K in (8.2.9), develop an MC procedure similar to the one obtained in Part (c) for computing the resulting marginal likelihood.

8.8 In Section 8.3:

(i) Show that

$$\pi(\boldsymbol{\theta} | D, \mathcal{M}_r) = \pi(\boldsymbol{\theta} | \boldsymbol{\psi} = 0, D, \mathcal{M}_1) = \pi(\boldsymbol{\theta} | \boldsymbol{\varphi} = 0, D, \mathcal{M}_2),$$

if conditions (C1) and (C2) hold, where $\pi(\boldsymbol{\theta} | D, \mathcal{M}_r)$ is given in (8.3.4) and $\pi(\boldsymbol{\theta} | \boldsymbol{\psi} = 0, D, \mathcal{M}_1)$ and $\pi(\boldsymbol{\theta} | \boldsymbol{\varphi} = 0, D, \mathcal{M}_2)$ are the conditional posterior densities with respect to the posterior distributions given in (8.3.1) and (8.3.2), respectively.

(ii) Show that

$$\begin{aligned} \pi(\boldsymbol{\theta}, \boldsymbol{\psi} | D, \mathcal{M}_1) &= \pi(\boldsymbol{\theta}, \boldsymbol{\psi} | \boldsymbol{\varphi} = 0, D, \mathcal{M}_s), \\ \pi(\boldsymbol{\theta}, \boldsymbol{\varphi} | D, \mathcal{M}_2) &= \pi(\boldsymbol{\theta}, \boldsymbol{\varphi} | \boldsymbol{\psi} = 0, D, \mathcal{M}_s) \end{aligned}$$

if conditions (C3) and (C4) hold, where $\pi(\boldsymbol{\theta}, \boldsymbol{\psi} | \boldsymbol{\varphi} = 0, D, \mathcal{M}_s)$ and $\pi(\boldsymbol{\theta}, \boldsymbol{\varphi} | \boldsymbol{\psi} = 0, D, \mathcal{M}_s)$ are the conditional posterior density with respect to the joint posterior distribution in (8.3.5).

8.9 Prove Theorem 8.3.1.

8.10 Show that the b which minimizes (8.4.3) is

$$\hat{\boldsymbol{b}} = (1 - \nu)\boldsymbol{\mu} + \nu \boldsymbol{y}^*,$$

where $\nu = \delta/(\delta+1)$. Also show that $L_1(\boldsymbol{y}^*, \hat{\boldsymbol{b}})$ in (8.4.3) reduces to $L_2(\boldsymbol{y}^*)$ given by (8.4.5).

8.11 Show that the conditional densities of $[\boldsymbol{\beta}|\boldsymbol{\lambda}, D]$ in (8.4.20) for $\mathcal{M}_1$, $[\beta_j|\boldsymbol{\beta}^{(-j)}, \boldsymbol{\lambda}, D]$ in (8.4.18) for $\mathcal{M}_2$, and $[\alpha_j|\boldsymbol{\alpha}^{(-j)}, \boldsymbol{\beta}, D]$ in (8.4.21) are log-concave.

8.12 A SIMULATION STUDY FOR THE L MEASURE
Generate data y_i from the Weibull model

$$p(y_i|\alpha, \lambda_i) = \alpha^{y_i - 1} \exp\{\lambda_i - y_i^{\alpha} \exp(\lambda_i)\},$$

where $\lambda_i = \beta_0 + \beta_1 x_i$, $i = 1, \ldots, n$, $n = 200$, $\alpha = 2$, $\boldsymbol{\beta} = (\beta_0, \beta_1) = (1, -1)$, and 10% of the observations are randomly right censored with censoring times $t_i = 0.75 * y_i$. Also generate the covariate x_i as i.i.d. $N(0,1)$ variates. Suppose that the prior distribution for $\boldsymbol{\beta}$ is $N_2(0, 4I_2)$, where I_2 is a 2×2 identity matrix, and the prior distribution for α is a gamma density with shape and scale parameters $(1, 0.5)$. Consider three models:

(1) the true Weibull model from which the data are generated;
(2) the Weibull model with a random α parameter; and
(3) the exponential model ($\alpha = 1$).

Take $y_i^* = \eta(y_i) = \ln(y_i)$. Compute the L measures and calibration distributions for these three models.

9

Bayesian Variable Selection

Variable selection is one of the most frequently encountered problems in statistical data analysis. In cancer or AIDS clinical trials, for example, one often wishes to assess the importance of certain prognostic factors such as treatment, age, gender, or race in predicting survival outcome. Most of the existing literature addresses variable selection using criterion-based methods such as the Akaike Information Criterion (AIC) (Akaike 1973) or Bayesian Information Criterion (BIC) (Schwarz 1978). Fully Bayesian approaches to variable selection for these models is now feasible due to recent advances in computing technology and the development of efficient computational algorithms. The Bayesian approach to variable selection is straightforward in principle. One quantifies the prior uncertainties via probabilities for each model under consideration, specifies a prior distribution for each of the parameters in each model, and then uses Bayes' theorem to calculate posterior model probabilities.

In this chapter, we present a comprehensive treatment of Bayesian variable selection. As is well known, Bayesian variable selection is often difficult to carry out because of the challenge in

(i) specifying prior distributions for the regression parameters for all possible models;

(ii) specifying a prior distribution on the model space; and

(iii) computations.

For (i), we discuss classes of informative prior distributions for variable selection that can be elicited in a semiautomatic fashion. Several theoretical and computational properties of the priors will be presented and illustrated with several examples. For (ii), we include methods for specifying an informative prior on the model space, and for (iii) novel methods for computing the marginal distribution and posterior model probabilities will be introduced. In addition, stochastic search variable selection, Bayesian model averaging, and the reversible jump Markov chain Monte Carlo (MCMC) algorithm will also be presented.

9.1 Variable Selection for Logistic Regression Models

There has been a recent surge in the development of Bayesian methods for analyzing logistic regression models. Articles which address informative prior specifications for the logistic regression model include Zellner and Rossi (1984), West (1985), West, Harrison, and Migon (1985), Albert (1988), Zeger and Karim (1991), Albert and Chib (1993), Gelfand, Sahu, and Carlin (1996), Müller and Roeder (1998), and Bedrick, Christensen, and Johnson (1996). These articles mainly address the issue of Bayesian calculations for logistic regression when there is no uncertainty regarding the model itself. In this section, we examine the problem of eliciting informative prior distributions for the regression parameters as well as the elicitation of an informative prior distribution for the model space for Bayesian variable selection in logistic regression. We present a class of informative priors that appears to be quite useful in practice. For computing the analytically intractable prior and posterior model probabilities, we consider the efficient algorithms of Chen, Ibrahim, and Yiannoutsos (1999) that only require Gibbs samples from a single model.

9.1.1 Model and Notation

Let p denote the number of covariates for the full model and let $\mathcal{M}$ denote the model space. We enumerate the models in $\mathcal{M}$ by $k = 1, 2, \ldots, \mathcal{K}$, where $\mathcal{K}$ is the dimension of $\mathcal{M}$ and model $\mathcal{K}$ denotes the full model. Also, let $\boldsymbol{\beta}^{(\mathcal{K})} = (\beta_0, \beta_1, \ldots, \beta_{p-1})'$ denote the regression coefficients for the full model including an intercept, and let $\boldsymbol{\beta}^{(k)}$ denote a $p_k \times 1$ vector of regression coefficients for model k with an intercept, and a specific choice of $p_k - 1$ covariates. We write $\boldsymbol{\beta}^{(\mathcal{K})} = (\boldsymbol{\beta}^{(k)'}, \boldsymbol{\beta}^{(-k)'})'$, where $\boldsymbol{\beta}^{(-k)}$ is $\boldsymbol{\beta}^{(\mathcal{K})}$ with $\boldsymbol{\beta}^{(k)}$ deleted. Under model k, the likelihood function based on n observations for the current study is given by

$$L(\boldsymbol{\beta}^{(k)}|D^{(k)}) = \exp\{y'X^{(k)}\boldsymbol{\beta}^{(k)} - J'Q^{(k)}\}, \tag{9.1.1}$$

where $\boldsymbol{y} = (y_1, \ldots, y_n)'$ denotes the $n \times 1$ vector of binary responses, J is an $n \times 1$ vector of ones, and $X^{(k)}$ is an $n \times p_k$ matrix of fixed covariates of rank

p_k. Also, $Q^{(k)}$ is an $n \times 1$ vector with j^{th} element $\ln(1+\exp((\boldsymbol{x}_j^{(k)})'\boldsymbol{\beta}^{(k)}))$, where $(\boldsymbol{x}_j^{(k)})'$ denotes the jth row of $X^{(k)}$. Finally, $D^{(k)} = (n, \boldsymbol{y}, X^{(k)})$ denotes the data for the current study under model k.

9.1.2 The Prior Distributions

The prior distribution is based on the notion of the existence of a previous study that measures the same response variable and covariates as the current study. For ease of exposition, we assume only one previous study, as the extension to multiple previous studies is straightforward. To this end, let n_0 denote sample size for the previous study, let $\boldsymbol{y}_0$ be an $n_0 \times 1$ response vector for the previous study, let $X_0^{(k)}$ be an $n_0 \times p_k$ matrix of covariates corresponding to $\boldsymbol{y}_0$, and let $D_0^{(k)} \equiv (n_0, \boldsymbol{y}_0, X_0^{(k)})$ denote the historical data for model k. Further, let $\pi(\boldsymbol{\beta}^{(k)}|\cdot)$ denote the prior distribution for $\boldsymbol{\beta}^{(k)}$ from the previous study. Using this information, we wish to construct a prior distribution for $\boldsymbol{\beta}^{(k)}$ for the current study. To this end, we consider a prior of the form

$$\pi(\boldsymbol{\beta}^{(k)}|D_0^{(k)}, a_0) \propto \exp\{a_0[\boldsymbol{y}_0' X_0^{(k)}\boldsymbol{\beta}^{(k)} - J_0' Q_0^{(k)}]\}\ \pi_0(\boldsymbol{\beta}^{(k)}|c_0), \qquad (9.1.2)$$

where J_0 is an $n_0 \times 1$ vector of ones, $Q_0^{(k)}$ is an $n_0 \times 1$ vector with j^{th} component $\ln(1+\exp(\boldsymbol{x}_{j0}^{(k)'}\boldsymbol{\beta}^{(k)}))$, $\boldsymbol{x}_{j0}^{(k)'}$ denotes the jth row of $X_0^{(k)}$, c_0 is a fixed hyperparameter, a_0 is a scalar prior parameter that weights the historical data relative to the likelihood of the current study, and $\pi_0(\boldsymbol{\beta}^{(k)}|c_0)$ is the *initial prior* for $\boldsymbol{\beta}^{(k)}$. That is, $\pi_0(\boldsymbol{\beta}^{(k)}|c_0)$ is the prior for $\boldsymbol{\beta}^{(k)}$ for the previous study. The prior parameter c_0 controls the impact of $\pi_0(\boldsymbol{\beta}^{(k)}|c_0)$ on the entire prior, and the parameter a_0 controls the influence of the historical data on $\pi(\boldsymbol{\beta}^{(k)}|D_0^{(k)}, a_0)$. The parameter a_0 can be interpreted as a dispersion parameter for the prior data. It is reasonable to restrict the range of a_0 to be between 0 and 1, and thus we take $0 \le a_0 \le 1$. One of the main roles of a_0 is that it controls the heaviness of the tails of the prior for $\boldsymbol{\beta}^{(k)}$. As a_0 becomes smaller, the tails of (9.1.2) become heavier.

The most natural specification of $D_0^{(k)}$ is to take $\boldsymbol{y}_0$ to be the raw response vector from the previous study, take $X_0^{(k)}$ to be the raw covariate matrix under model k from the previous study, and take n_0 to be the sample size of the previous study. In this case (9.1.2) has several appealing interpretations. The first term on the right side of (9.1.2) is just the likelihood function of $\boldsymbol{\beta}^{(k)}$ based on the historical data $D_0^{(k)}$ raised to the power a_0. Setting $a_0 = 1$, (9.1.2) corresponds to the update of $\pi_0(\boldsymbol{\beta}^{(k)}|c_0)$ using Bayes' theorem. That is, with $a_0 = 1$, (9.1.2) corresponds to the posterior distribution of $\boldsymbol{\beta}^{(k)}$ from the previous study. When $a_0 = 0$, then the prior does not depend on the historical data, and in this case, $\pi(\boldsymbol{\beta}^{(k)}|D_0^{(k)}, a_0) \equiv \pi_0(\boldsymbol{\beta}^{(k)}|c_0)$. Therefore, the prior (9.1.2) can be viewed as a generalization of the usual

Bayesian update of $\pi_0(\boldsymbol{\beta}^{(k)}|c_0)$. The parameter a_0 allows the investigator to control the influence of the historical data on the current study. Such control is important in cases where there is heterogeneity between the previous and current study, or when the sample sizes of the two studies are quite different.

The prior specification is completed by specifying a prior distribution for a_0. We take a beta prior for a_0, and thus we have a joint prior distribution for $(\boldsymbol{\beta}^{(k)}, a_0)$ of the form

$$\pi(\boldsymbol{\beta}^{(k)}, a_0|D_0^{(k)}) \propto \exp\{a_0[\boldsymbol{y}_0' X_0^{(k)} \boldsymbol{\beta}^{(k)} - J_0' Q_0^{(k)}]\} \times \pi_0(\boldsymbol{\beta}^{(k)}|c_0)\ a_0^{\alpha_0 - 1}(1 - a_0)^{\lambda_0 - 1}, \tag{9.1.3}$$

where (α_0, λ_0) are specified prior parameters. The prior in (9.1.3) does not have a closed form but it has several attractive theoretical and computational properties. First, we note that if $\pi_0(\boldsymbol{\beta}^{(k)}|c_0)$ is proper, then (9.1.3) is guaranteed to be proper. Further, (9.1.3) can be proper even if $\pi_0(\boldsymbol{\beta}^{(k)}|c_0)$ is improper. Chen, Ibrahim, and Yiannoutsos (1999) propose (9.1.3), and give sufficient conditions for the propriety of it in the case that $\pi_0(\boldsymbol{\beta}^{(k)}|c_0)$ is a uniform improper prior and also show that the prior in (9.1.2) converges to a multivariate normal distribution as $n_0 \to \infty$. One attractive feature of (9.1.3) is that it creates heavier tails for the marginal prior of $\boldsymbol{\beta}^{(k)}$ than the prior (9.1.2), which assumes a_0 is a fixed value. This is a desirable feature since it gives the investigator more flexibility in weighting the historical data.

If a previous study does not exist for which to base $D_0^{(k)}$, then $\boldsymbol{y}_0$ can be obtained via a prior prediction, including specifications based on a theoretical prediction model, expert opinion, or case-specific information. For example, a theoretical model of the form $\boldsymbol{y}_0 = g(X^{(k_0)})$ may be available for obtaining the prior predictions, where $X^{(k_0)}$ is the covariate matrix corresponding to some model k_0, and g is a known function. Such prediction models are often used, for example, in respiratory studies measuring forced vital capacity and forced expiratory volume. Also, in these cases, one may take $X_0^{(k)}$ to be the covariate matrix of the current study, i.e., $X_0^{(k)} = X^{(k)}$ and $n_0 = n$. In any case, the existence of a previous study leads to the most natural specification of $D_0^{(k)}$, and serves as the primary motivation for (9.1.3). Taking $D_0^{(k)}$ to be the raw data from a previous study in a more natural, interpretable, and automated specification for (9.1.3).

9.1.3 *A Generalization of the Priors*

When a previous study is available, it sometimes occurs that the set of covariates measured in the previous study is a subset of the covariates measured in the current study. This may occur because the investigators discover "new" and potentially useful covariates to measure in the current study that were not measured in previous studies. In this case, we can modify (9.1.2) as follows. Let $X_1^{(k)}$ denote the $n \times r_k$ matrix of covariates in the current study that are common to the covariates in the previous study, and let $X_2^{(k)}$ be the $n \times s_k$ matrix of new covariates in the current study which are not measured in the previous study. Write

$$\boldsymbol{\beta}^{(k)} = \begin{pmatrix} \boldsymbol{\beta}_1^{(k)} \\ \boldsymbol{\beta}_2^{(k)} \end{pmatrix},$$

and let $X_{01}^{(k)}$ represent the $n_{01} \times r_k$ matrix of covariates from the previous study, $X_{02}^{(k)}$ is an $n_{02} \times s_k$ matrix of covariates representing the new covariates, and $p_k = r_k + s_k$. The most natural choice for $X_{01}^{(k)}$ is the raw covariate matrix from the previous study, and to take $X_{02}^{(k)} = X_2^{(k)}$. In our prior specification, we assume that the new covariates have small or negligible correlation to the common covariates, that is, $\text{Corr}(X_1^{(k)}, X_2^{(k)}) \approx 0$. This seems to be a sensible assumption if in fact the new set of covariates in the current study are being scientifically investigated for the first time. Finally, we assume a priori independence between $\boldsymbol{\beta}_1^{(k)}$ and $\boldsymbol{\beta}_2^{(k)}$, which leads to

$$\begin{aligned} &\pi(\boldsymbol{\beta}^{(k)}|D_0^{(k)}, a_0) \\ &\quad = \pi_1(\boldsymbol{\beta}_1^{(k)}|D_{01}^{(k)}, a_{01})\pi_2(\boldsymbol{\beta}_2^{(k)}|D_{02}^{(k)}, a_{02}) \\ &\quad \propto \exp\{a_{01}[\boldsymbol{y}_{01}' X_{01}^{(k)} \boldsymbol{\beta}_1^{(k)} - J_{01}' Q_{01}^{(k)}]\} \\ &\qquad \times \exp\{a_{02}[\boldsymbol{y}_{02}' X_{02}^{(k)} \boldsymbol{\beta}_2^{(k)} - J_{02}' Q_{02}^{(k)}]\}\pi_0(\boldsymbol{\beta}_1^{(k)}, \boldsymbol{\beta}_2^{(k)}|c_0), \end{aligned} \tag{9.1.4}$$

where $\boldsymbol{y}_{01}$ and $\boldsymbol{y}_{02}$ represent vectors of prior predictions, a_{0j} is a prior parameter, and $D_{0j}^{(k)} = (n_{0j}, \boldsymbol{y}_{0j}, X_{0j}^{(k)})$, $j = 1, 2$. The prior specification is completed by specifying independent beta priors for (a_{01}, a_{02}), leading to the joint prior

$$\begin{aligned} \pi(\boldsymbol{\beta}_1^{(k)}, \boldsymbol{\beta}_2^{(k)}, a_{01}, a_{02}) \propto \prod_{j=1}^{2} &\exp\{a_{0j}[\boldsymbol{y}_{0j}' X_{0j}^{(k)} \boldsymbol{\beta}_j^{(k)} - J_{0j}' Q_{0j}^{(k)}]\} \\ &\times \pi_0(\boldsymbol{\beta}_1^{(k)}, \boldsymbol{\beta}_2^{(k)}|c_0) a_{0j}^{\alpha_{0j}} (1 - a_{0j})^{\lambda_{0j} - 1}. \end{aligned} \tag{9.1.5}$$

A natural choice for $\boldsymbol{y}_{01}$ is the raw response vector from the previous study. The elicitation of $\boldsymbol{y}_{02}$ is less automatic since no a priori information is available for it. One possible choice is to pick $\boldsymbol{y}_{02} = (\frac{1}{2}, \frac{1}{2}, \dots, \frac{1}{2})'$. This choice results in $\pi(\boldsymbol{\beta}_2^{(k)}|D_{02}^{(k)}, a_{02})$ having a mode equal to 0. Also we take $\pi_0(\boldsymbol{\beta}_1^{(k)}, \boldsymbol{\beta}_2^{(k)}|c_0) = \pi_0(\boldsymbol{\beta}_1^{(k)}|c_0)\pi_0(\boldsymbol{\beta}_2^{(k)}|c_0)$. The prior parameters $(\alpha_{02}, \lambda_{02})$ are chosen to reflect vague prior beliefs, and thus values such as $\alpha_{02} = \lambda_{02} = 1$ (i.e., a uniform prior) would be reasonable. We mention that we cannot take $a_{02} = 0$ with probability 1 since this would make the prior improper when a flat initial prior for $\boldsymbol{\beta}_2^{(k)}$ is used, i.e., $\pi_0(\boldsymbol{\beta}_2^{(k)}|c_0) \propto 1$, and thus we would not be able to compute posterior model probabilities when there is no information available to specify the initial prior $\pi_0(\beta_2^{(k)}|c_0)$ for $\beta_2^{(k)}$. The prior in (9.1.5) reduces to (9.1.3) if the sets of covariates from the previous and current studies are identical. If the set of covariates in the current study is a subset of the covariates in the previous study, then we can construct a submatrix by omitting those columns corresponding to covariates not in the current study and take $X_0^{(k)}$ to be that submatrix. For a more detailed discussion on (9.1.5), see Chen, Ibrahim, and Yiannoutsos (1999).

9.1.4 Choices of Prior Parameters

There are several ways one can choose the prior parameters (α_0, λ_0). For the purposes of elicitation, it is often easier to work with $\mu_{a_0} = \alpha_0/(\alpha_0 + \lambda_0)$, and $\sigma_{a_0}^2 = \mu_{a_0}(1-\mu_{a_0})(\alpha_0+\lambda_0+1)^{-1}$. A uniform prior (i.e., $\alpha_0 = \lambda_0 = 1$), which corresponds to $(\mu_{a_0}, \sigma_{a_0}^2) = (\frac{1}{2}, \frac{1}{12})$ may be a suitable noninformative starting point, and facilitates a useful reference analysis for other choices. The investigator may choose μ_{a_0} to be small (say $\mu_{a_0} \leq 0.1$), if he/she wishes to have low prior weight on the historical data. If a large prior weight is desired, then $\mu_{a_0} \geq 0.5$ may be desirable. It is reasonable to choose $\sigma_{a_0}^2$ in the range $\mu_{a_0}/1000 \leq \sigma_{a_0}^2 \leq \mu_{a_0}/10$. For the generalized prior in (9.1.5), the prior parameters can be chosen in a similar manner. Also, it is desirable in this case to take $\mu_{a_{02}} \leq \mu_{a_{01}}$, where $\mu_{a_{0j}} = \alpha_{0j}/(\alpha_{0j} + \lambda_{0j})$. Choices of the form $\mu_{a_{02}} = q_0\mu_{a_{01}}$, where $0 \leq q_0 \leq 1$ are suitable. In any case, in an actual analysis, we recommend that several choices of $(\mu_{a_0}, \sigma_{a_0}^2)$ be used, including ones that give small and large weight to the historical data, and several sensitivity analyses conducted. We do not recommend doing an analysis based on one set of prior parameters. The choices recommended here can be used as starting points from which sensitivity analyses can be based.

It is reasonable to specify a noninformative prior for $\pi_0(\boldsymbol{\beta}^{(k)}|c_0)$ since this is the prior for $\boldsymbol{\beta}^{(k)}$ corresponding to the previous study and contains no information about the historical data $D_0^{(k)}$. To this end, one choice is to take $\pi_0(\boldsymbol{\beta}^{(k)}|c_0)$ to be a normal density with mean 0 and covariance matrix $c_0 W_0^{(k)}$, i.e.,

$$\begin{aligned}\pi_0(\boldsymbol{\beta}^{(k)}|c_0) &= (2\pi)^{-p_k/2} c_0^{-p_k/2} |W_0^{(k)}|^{-1/2} \\ &\quad \times \exp\left\{-\frac{1}{2c_0}(\boldsymbol{\beta}^{(k)\prime}(W_0^{(k)})^{-1}\boldsymbol{\beta}^{(k)})\right\}. \end{aligned} \tag{9.1.6}$$

The quantity $c_0 \geq 0$ is a scalar dispersion parameter which serves to control the impact of $\pi_0(\boldsymbol{\beta}^{(k)}|c_0)$ on $\pi(\boldsymbol{\beta}^{(k)}, a_0|D_0^{(k)})$, and hence influences the marginal distribution of the data. To make $\pi_0(\boldsymbol{\beta}^{(k)}|c_0)$ noninformative, we take large values of c_0 so that $\pi_0(\boldsymbol{\beta}^{(k)}|c_0)$ is flat relative to the other terms in (9.1.3). Small values of c_0 will let $\pi_0(\boldsymbol{\beta}^{(k)}|c_0)$ dominate (9.1.3). Thus, c_0

is an important tuning parameter that allows us to control the impact of the marginal distribution of the data for the calculation of posterior model probabilities.

The actual size of c_0 used will depend on the structure of the data set and the prior parameters for a_0. From the example of Subsection 9.1.7, reasonable choices of c_0 are $c_0 \geq 5$. In any case, we do not recommend an automatic one-time specification for c_0, but rather we emphasize that several sensitivity analyses be conducted with several values of c_0 to examine the impact of $\pi_0(\boldsymbol{\beta}^{(k)}|c_0)$ on the posterior model probabilities.

The matrix $W_0^{(k)}$ has a less crucial role than c_0, and is specified as follows. Let $W_0^{(\mathcal{K})}$ be a diagonal matrix with the ith diagonal element equal to the ith diagonal element of $(X_0^{(\mathcal{K})\prime} V_0^{(\mathcal{K})} X_0^{(\mathcal{K})})^{-1}$, where $V_0^{(\mathcal{K})}$ is the $n_0 \times n_0$ diagonal matrix with i^{th} element

$$v_{0i}^{(\mathcal{K})} = \frac{\exp(\boldsymbol{x}_{0i}^{(\mathcal{K})\prime} \hat{\boldsymbol{\beta}}_0)}{(1 + \exp(\boldsymbol{x}_{0i}^{(\mathcal{K})\prime} \hat{\boldsymbol{\beta}}_0))^2},$$

and $\hat{\boldsymbol{\beta}}_0$ is the MLE of $\boldsymbol{\beta}$ based on the historical data $D_0^{(\mathcal{K})} = (n_0, \boldsymbol{y}_0, X_0^{(\mathcal{K})})$ for the full model. Thus, the diagonal elements of $W_0^{(\mathcal{K})}$ correspond to the asymptotic variances of $\hat{\boldsymbol{\beta}}_0$ based on the full model. Now we take $W_0^{(k)}$ to be the submatrix of the diagonal matrix $W_0^{(\mathcal{K})}$ corresponding to model k. The purpose of picking $W_0^{(k)}$ in this way is to properly adjust for the different scales of the measured covariates. If the covariates are all standardized or are measured on the same scale, then we take $W_0^{(k)} = I$. In any case, $W_0^{(k)}$ plays a minimal role when c_0 is large.

Another choice for $\pi_0(\boldsymbol{\beta}^{(k)}|c_0)$ that we consider is a uniform improper prior, i.e., $\pi_0(\boldsymbol{\beta}^{(k)}|c_0) \propto 1$. This actually corresponds to the case $c_0 \to \infty$ in (9.1.6) and thus can be viewed as a special case of (9.1.6). As shown in Chen, Ibrahim, and Yiannoutsos (1999), under certain minor regularity conditions, $\pi(\boldsymbol{\beta}^{(k)}, a_0|D_0^{(k)})$ is a proper prior when $\pi_0(\boldsymbol{\beta}^{(k)}|c_0) \propto 1$. This is a very important property since it tells us that the prior (9.1.3) remains well defined as $c_0 \to \infty$ which is useful for the purposes of Gibbs sampling from (9.1.3).

9.1.5 *Prior Distribution on the Model Space*

Let

$$\pi_0^*(\boldsymbol{\beta}^{(k)}|D_0^{(k)}) = \exp\{[\boldsymbol{y}_0' X_0^{(k)} \boldsymbol{\beta}^{(k)} - J_0' Q_0^{(k)}]\}\pi_0(\boldsymbol{\beta}^{(k)}|d_0), \quad (9.1.7)$$

where $\pi_0(\boldsymbol{\beta}^{(k)}|d_0)$ is the same density as that described in Subsection 9.1.4 with c_0 replaced by d_0. We take the prior probability of model k as

$$p(k) \equiv p(k|D_0^{(k)}) = \frac{\int \pi_0^*(\boldsymbol{\beta}^{(k)}|D_0^{(k)})\, d\boldsymbol{\beta}^{(k)}}{\sum_{j\in\mathcal{M}} \int \pi_0^*(\boldsymbol{\beta}^{(j)}|D_0^{(j)})\, d\boldsymbol{\beta}^{(j)}} . \tag{9.1.8}$$

The parameter d_0 is a scalar prior parameter that controls the impact of $\pi_0(\boldsymbol{\beta}^{(k)}|d_0)$ on the prior model probability $p(k)$. This choice for $p(k)$ has several nice interpretations. First, $p(k)$ in (9.1.8) corresponds to the posterior probability of model k based on the data $D_0^{(k)}$ using a uniform prior for the previous study, $p_0(k) = 2^{-(p-1)}$ for $k \in \mathcal{M}$. That is, $p(k) \propto p(k|D_0^{(k)})$, and thus $p(k)$ corresponds to the usual Bayesian update of $p_0(k)$ using $D_0^{(k)}$ as the data. Second, as $d_0 \to 0$, $p(k)$ reduces to a uniform prior on the model space. Therefore, as $d_0 \to 0$, the historical data $D_0^{(k)}$ have a minimal impact in determining $p(k)$. On the other hand, with a large value of d_0, $\pi_0(\boldsymbol{\beta}^{(k)}|d_0)$ plays a minimal role in determining $p(k)$, and in this case, the historical data play a larger role in determining $p(k)$. Thus as $d_0 \to \infty$, $p(k)$ will be regulated by the historical data. The parameter d_0 plays the same role as c_0 and thus serves as a tuning parameter to control the impact of $D_0^{(k)}$ on the prior model probability $p(k)$.

It is important to note that we use a scalar parameter c_0 in constructing the prior distribution $\pi(\boldsymbol{\beta}^{(k)}, a_0|D_0^{(k)})$ given by (9.1.3), while we use a *different* scalar parameter d_0 in determining $p(k)$. This development provides us with great flexibility in specifying the prior distribution for $\boldsymbol{\beta}^{(k)}$ as well as the prior model probabilities $p(k)$. In addition, as shown in Chen, Ibrahim, and Yiannoutsos (1999), if $\pi_0(\boldsymbol{\beta}^{(k)}|d_0)$ is a uniform (improper) prior, then under mild conditions,

$$\int \exp\{\boldsymbol{y}_0' X_0^{(k)} \boldsymbol{\beta}^{(k)} - J_0' Q_0^{(k)}\}\, d\boldsymbol{\beta}^{(k)} < \infty,$$

and therefore the formula in (9.1.8) is well defined even if $\pi_0(\boldsymbol{\beta}^{(k)}|d_0)$ is a uniform prior.

We mention here that the prior for $(\boldsymbol{\beta}^{(k)}, a_0)$ in (9.1.3) does not imply a probability structure for $p(k)$ or any specific form for $p(k)$. Thus the prior for a_0 has impact only on the marginal distribution of the data and has no impact whatsoever on $p(k)$. Thus, whether we have large or small weight on the historical data, this does not affect the numerical value of $p(k)$. Therefore $p(k)$ is the same regardless of the choice of prior parameters for a_0. In addition, the prior for $(\boldsymbol{\beta}^{(k)}, a_0)$ is not affected by the choice of $p(k)$, and in particular, the choice of d_0. Finally, we note that if we let $d_0 \to 0$, $a_0 \to 0$, and $c_0 \to \infty$, then the posterior model probability is completely regulated by the likelihood, and in this case, would yield results similar to those of criterion-based likelihood methods such as AIC and BIC.

9.1.6 Computing Prior and Posterior Model Probabilities

In this subsection, we present a novel Monte Carlo method for computing the prior and posterior model probabilities. The method involves computing the marginal distribution of the data via ratios of normalizing constants. The method requires prior and posterior samples *only* from the *full model* for computing prior and posterior probabilities for all possible models. The method is thus very efficient for variable selection. For our discussion, it suffices to consider (9.1.3), since the extension to (9.1.4) is clear.

Computing Prior Model Probabilities

To compute $p(k)$ in (9.1.8), we adopt a Monte Carlo approach similar to Ibrahim, Chen, and MacEachern (1999) to estimate all of the prior model probabilities using a single Gibbs sample from the full model. The technical details of this procedure are given as follows.

Suppose that under the full model, we have a sample $\{\boldsymbol{\beta}_{0,l}^{(\mathcal{K})}, l = 1, \ldots, L\}$ from $\pi_0(\boldsymbol{\beta}^{(\mathcal{K})}|D_0^{(\mathcal{K})})$, where

$$\pi_0(\boldsymbol{\beta}^{(\mathcal{K})}|D_0^{(\mathcal{K})}) \propto \pi_0^*(\boldsymbol{\beta}^{(\mathcal{K})}|D_0^{(\mathcal{K})}), \tag{9.1.9}$$

and $\pi_0^*(\boldsymbol{\beta}^{(\mathcal{K})}|D_0^{(\mathcal{K})})$ is given by (9.1.7). Also, let

$$p(D_0^{(k)}|k) = \int \pi_0^*(\boldsymbol{\beta}^{(k)}|D_0^{(k)})\, d\boldsymbol{\beta}^{(k)}. \tag{9.1.10}$$

Then, using the result given in Section 5.8, we have the key identity

$$\frac{p(D_0^{(k)}|k)}{p(D_0^{(\mathcal{K})}|\mathcal{K})} = E\left(\frac{\pi_0^*(\boldsymbol{\beta}^{(k)}|D_0^{(k)})\, w(\boldsymbol{\beta}^{(-k)}|\boldsymbol{\beta}^{(k)})}{\pi_0^*(\boldsymbol{\beta}^{(\mathcal{K})}|D_0^{(\mathcal{K})})}\right), \tag{9.1.11}$$

where the expectation is taken with respect to the density $\pi_0(\boldsymbol{\beta}^{(\mathcal{K})}|D_0^{(\mathcal{K})})$, and $w(\boldsymbol{\beta}^{(-k)}|\boldsymbol{\beta}^{(k)})$ is a *completely* known conditional density whose support is contained in, or equal to, the support of the conditional density of $\boldsymbol{\beta}^{(-k)}$ given $\boldsymbol{\beta}^{(k)}$ with respect to the full model joint prior distribution (9.1.9). Note that the choice of the weight function $w(\boldsymbol{\beta}^{(-k)}|\boldsymbol{\beta}^{(k)})$ is somewhat arbitrary. However, in Subsection 5.8.4, it has been shown that the best choice of $w(\boldsymbol{\beta}^{(-k)}|\boldsymbol{\beta}^{(k)})$ is the conditional density of $\boldsymbol{\beta}^{(-k)}$ given $\boldsymbol{\beta}^{(k)}$ with respect to the density $\pi_0(\boldsymbol{\beta}^{(\mathcal{K})}|D_0^{(\mathcal{K})})$. Since a closed-form expression of this conditional density is not available, we follow an empirical procedure given in Section 4.3 to select $w(\boldsymbol{\beta}^{(-k)}|\boldsymbol{\beta}^{(k)})$. Specifically, using the sample $\{\boldsymbol{\beta}_{0,l}^{(\mathcal{K})},\ l = 1, \ldots, L\}$, we construct the mean and covariance matrix, denoted by $(\tilde{\boldsymbol{\beta}}_0, \tilde{\Sigma}_0)$, and then we choose $w(\boldsymbol{\beta}^{(-k)}|\boldsymbol{\beta}^{(k)})$ to be the conditional density of the p-dimensional normal distribution, $N_p(\tilde{\boldsymbol{\beta}}_0, \tilde{\Sigma}_0)$, for $\boldsymbol{\beta}^{(-k)}$

given $\boldsymbol{\beta}^{(k)}$. Thus, $w(\boldsymbol{\beta}^{(-k)}|\boldsymbol{\beta}^{(k)})$ is given by

$$w(\boldsymbol{\beta}^{(-k)}|\boldsymbol{\beta}^{(k)}) = (2\pi)^{-(p-p_k)/2}|\tilde{\Sigma}_{11.2k}|^{-1/2} \times \exp\{-\tfrac{1}{2}(\boldsymbol{\beta}^{(-k)} - \tilde{\boldsymbol{\mu}}_{11.2k})'\tilde{\Sigma}_{11.2k}^{-1}(\boldsymbol{\beta}^{(-k)} - \tilde{\boldsymbol{\mu}}_{11.2k})\}, \quad (9.1.12)$$

where

$$\tilde{\Sigma}_{11.2k} = \tilde{\Sigma}_{11k} - \tilde{\Sigma}_{12k}\tilde{\Sigma}_{22k}^{-1}\tilde{\Sigma}_{12k}',$$

$\tilde{\Sigma}_{11k}$ is the covariance matrix from the marginal distribution of $\boldsymbol{\beta}^{(-k)}$, $\tilde{\Sigma}_{12k}$ consists of the covariances between $\boldsymbol{\beta}^{(-k)}$ and $\boldsymbol{\beta}^{(k)}$, and $\tilde{\Sigma}_{22k}$ is the covariance matrix of the marginal distribution of $\boldsymbol{\beta}^{(k)}$ with respect to the joint normal distribution $N_p(\tilde{\boldsymbol{\beta}}_0, \tilde{\Sigma}_0)$ for $\boldsymbol{\beta}^{(\mathcal{K})}$. Also in (9.1.12),

$$\tilde{\boldsymbol{\mu}}_{11.2k} = \tilde{\boldsymbol{\mu}}^{(-k)} + \tilde{\Sigma}_{12k}\tilde{\Sigma}_{22k}^{-1}(\boldsymbol{\beta}^{(k)} - \tilde{\boldsymbol{\mu}}^{(k)}),$$

where $\tilde{\boldsymbol{\mu}}^{(-k)}$ is the mean of the normal marginal distribution of $\boldsymbol{\beta}^{(-k)}$ and $\tilde{\boldsymbol{\mu}}^{(k)}$ is the mean of the normal marginal distribution of $\boldsymbol{\beta}^{(k)}$. A nice feature of this procedure is that $w(\boldsymbol{\beta}^{(-k)}|\boldsymbol{\beta}^{(k)})$ is calculated in an automatic fashion.

It can be seen that using (9.1.11), $p(k)$ can be rewritten as

$$p(k) = \frac{E\left(\dfrac{\pi_0^*(\boldsymbol{\beta}^{(k)}|D_0^{(k)})w(\boldsymbol{\beta}^{(-k)}|\boldsymbol{\beta}^{(k)})}{\pi_0^*(\boldsymbol{\beta}^{(\mathcal{K})}|D_0^{(\mathcal{K})})}\right)}{\sum_{j=1}^{\mathcal{K}} E\left(\dfrac{\pi_0^*(\boldsymbol{\beta}^{(j)}|D_0^{(j)})w(\boldsymbol{\beta}^{(-j)}|\boldsymbol{\beta}^{(j)})}{\pi_0^*(\boldsymbol{\beta}^{(\mathcal{K})}|D_0^{(\mathcal{K})})}\right)}. \quad (9.1.13)$$

Thus, the prior probability of model k can be estimated by

$$\hat{p}(k) \equiv \hat{p}(k|D_0^{(k)}) = \frac{\dfrac{1}{L}\sum_{l=1}^{L}\dfrac{\pi_0^*(\boldsymbol{\beta}_{0,l}^{(k)}|D_0^{(k)})w(\boldsymbol{\beta}_{0,l}^{(-k)}|\boldsymbol{\beta}_{0,l}^{(k)})}{\pi_0^*(\boldsymbol{\beta}_{0,l}^{(\mathcal{K})}|D_0^{(\mathcal{K})})}}{\dfrac{1}{L}\sum_{j=1}^{\mathcal{K}}\sum_{l=1}^{L}\dfrac{\pi_0^*(\boldsymbol{\beta}_{0,l}^{(j)}|D_0^{(j)})w(\boldsymbol{\beta}_{0,l}^{(-j)}|\boldsymbol{\beta}_{0,l}^{(j)})}{\pi_0^*(\boldsymbol{\beta}_{0,l}^{(\mathcal{K})}|D_0^{(\mathcal{K})})}}. \quad (9.1.14)$$

There are several advantages of the above Monte Carlo procedure:

(i) we need only one random draw from $\pi_0(\boldsymbol{\beta}^{(\mathcal{K})}|D_0^{(\mathcal{K})})$, which greatly eases the computational burden;

(ii) it is more numerically stable since we calculate ratios of the densities in (9.1.14); and

(iii) in (9.1.14), $\pi_0(\boldsymbol{\beta}^{(\mathcal{K})}|D_0^{(\mathcal{K})})$ plays the role of a ratio importance sampling density (see Section 5.5) which needs to be known only up to a normalizing constant since this common constant cancels out in the calculation.

Computing Posterior Model Probabilities

Using Bayes' theorem, the posterior probability of model k can be written as

$$p(k|D^{(k)}) = \frac{p(D^{(k)}|k)p(k)}{\sum_{j\in\mathcal{M}} p(D^{(j)}|j)p(j)}, \tag{9.1.15}$$

where

$$p(D^{(k)}|k) = \int L(\boldsymbol{\beta}^{(k)}|D^{(k)})\ \pi(\boldsymbol{\beta}^{(k)}, a_0|D_0^{(k)})\ d\boldsymbol{\beta}^{(k)}\ da_0 \tag{9.1.16}$$

denotes the marginal distribution of the data $D^{(k)}$ for the current study under model k, and $p(k)$ is estimated by (9.1.14). The marginal density $p(D^{(k)}|k)$ is precisely the normalizing constant of the joint posterior density of $(\boldsymbol{\beta}^{(k)}, a_0)$.

Computing the posterior model probability $p(k|D^{(k)})$ given by (9.1.15) requires a different Monte Carlo method other than the one for computing the prior model probability $p(k)$ given by (9.1.8). We give a brief explanation as follows. From (9.1.16), it can be seen that the calculation of posterior probabilities requires evaluating

$$\begin{aligned} p(D^{(k)}|k) &= \int L(\boldsymbol{\beta}^{(k)}|D^{(k)})\pi(\boldsymbol{\beta}^{(k)}, a_0|D_0^{(k)})\ d\boldsymbol{\beta}^{(k)}\ da_0 \\ &= \int L(\boldsymbol{\beta}^{(k)}|D^{(k)})\frac{\pi^*(\boldsymbol{\beta}^{(k)}, a_0|D_0^{(k)})}{c_k}\ d\boldsymbol{\beta}^{(k)}\ da_0, \end{aligned} \tag{9.1.17}$$

where the unnormalized joint prior density

$$\begin{aligned} \pi^*(\boldsymbol{\beta}^{(k)}, a_0|D_0^{(k)}) &= \exp\{a_0[\boldsymbol{y}_0' X_0^{(k)}\boldsymbol{\beta}^{(k)} - J_0' Q_0^{(k)}]\} \\ &\quad \times \pi_0(\boldsymbol{\beta}^{(k)}|c_0)a_0^{\alpha_0-1}(1-a_0)^{\lambda_0-1}, \end{aligned} \tag{9.1.18}$$

and the normalizing constant for the joint prior density is given by

$$c_k = \int \pi^*(\boldsymbol{\beta}^{(k)}, a_0|D_0^{(k)})\ d\boldsymbol{\beta}^{(k)}\ da_0. \tag{9.1.19}$$

Due to the complexity of (9.1.18), a closed form of c_k is not available. Therefore, computing $p(D^{(k)}|k)$ requires evaluating the ratio of two analytically intractable integrals, which is essentially a ratio of two normalizing constants. However, to compute similar quantities for the prior model probability $p(k)$ given by (9.1.8), we only need to evaluate

$$\int \exp\{[\boldsymbol{y}_0' X_0^{(k)}\boldsymbol{\beta}^{(k)} - J_0' Q_0^{(k)}]\}\ \pi_0(\boldsymbol{\beta}^{(k)}|d_0)\ d\boldsymbol{\beta}^{(k)},$$

since a closed-form of $\pi_0(\boldsymbol{\beta}^{(k)}|d_0)$ is available.

To develop a more efficient Monte Carlo method to calculate posterior model probabilities, we first present several theoretical results.

Under model k, let

$$\pi(\boldsymbol{\beta}^{(k)}|D_0^{(k)}) = \int \pi(\boldsymbol{\beta}^{(k)}, a_0|D_0^{(k)})\, da_0$$

denote the marginal prior distribution of $\boldsymbol{\beta}^{(k)}$ and let

$$\pi(\boldsymbol{\beta}^{(k)}|D^{(k)}) = \int \pi(\boldsymbol{\beta}^{(k)}, a_0|D^{(k)})\, da_0$$

denote the marginal posterior distribution of $\boldsymbol{\beta}^{(k)}$, where

$$\pi(\boldsymbol{\beta}^{(k)}, a_0|D^{(k)}) \propto L(\boldsymbol{\beta}^{(k)}|D^{(k)})\pi(\boldsymbol{\beta}^{(k)}, a_0|D_0^{(k)}).$$

Using (8.1.3), we can rewrite the marginal distribution of the data, $p(D^{(k)}|k)$, as

$$p(D^{(k)}|k) = \frac{L(\boldsymbol{\beta}^{(k)}|D^{(k)})\pi(\boldsymbol{\beta}^{(k)}|D_0^{(k)})}{\pi(\boldsymbol{\beta}^{(k)}|D^{(k)})}, \tag{9.1.20}$$

for all $\boldsymbol{\beta}^{(k)}$ and $k \in \mathcal{M}$. Using standard distribution theory, we are led to the following lemma:

Lemma 9.1.1 *From* (9.1.1), (9.1.3), *and the construction of* $\pi_0(\boldsymbol{\beta}^{(k)}|c_0)$, *we have*

(i) $L(\boldsymbol{\beta}^{(k)}|D^{(k)}) = L(\boldsymbol{\beta}^{(k)}, \boldsymbol{\beta}^{(-k)} = 0|D^{(\mathcal{K})})$ *where* $L(\boldsymbol{\beta}^{(k)}, \boldsymbol{\beta}^{(-k)} = 0|D^{(\mathcal{K})})$ *is the likelihood function for the full model evaluated at* $\boldsymbol{\beta}^{(\mathcal{K})} = (\boldsymbol{\beta}^{(k)}, \boldsymbol{\beta}^{(-k)} = 0)$.

(ii) $\pi(\boldsymbol{\beta}^{(k)}|D^{(m)}) = \pi(\boldsymbol{\beta}^{(k)}|\boldsymbol{\beta}^{(-k)} = 0, D^{(\mathcal{K})})$ *where* $\pi(\boldsymbol{\beta}^{(k)}|\boldsymbol{\beta}^{(-k)} = 0, D^{(\mathcal{K})})$ *is the conditional posterior density of* $\boldsymbol{\beta}^{(k)}$ *given* $\boldsymbol{\beta}^{(-k)} = 0$ *obtained from the marginal posterior density based on the full model,* $\pi(\boldsymbol{\beta}^{(\mathcal{K})}|D^{(\mathcal{K})})$.

(iii) $\pi(\boldsymbol{\beta}^{(k)}|D_0^{(k)}) = \pi(\boldsymbol{\beta}^{(k)}|\boldsymbol{\beta}^{(-k)} = 0, D_0^{(\mathcal{K})})$ *where* $\pi(\boldsymbol{\beta}^{(k)}|\boldsymbol{\beta}^{(-k)} = 0, D_0^{(\mathcal{K})})$ *is the conditional prior distribution of* $\boldsymbol{\beta}^{(k)}$ *given* $\boldsymbol{\beta}^{(-k)} = 0$ *obtained from the marginal prior density based on the full model,* $\pi(\boldsymbol{\beta}^{(\mathcal{K})}|D_0^{(\mathcal{K})})$.

The proof of this lemma is relatively straightforward, and thus is left as an exercise. Identity (9.1.20) and Lemma 9.1.1 yield the following theorem:

Theorem 9.1.1 *Let* $\pi(\boldsymbol{\beta}^{(-k)}|D_0^{(\mathcal{K})})$ *and* $\pi(\boldsymbol{\beta}^{(-k)}|D^{(\mathcal{K})})$ *denote the respective marginal prior and posterior distributions of* $\boldsymbol{\beta}^{(-k)}$ *obtained from the full model. Then*

$$\frac{p(D^{(k)}|k)}{p(D^{(\mathcal{K})}|\mathcal{K})} = \frac{\pi(\boldsymbol{\beta}^{(-k)} = 0|D^{(\mathcal{K})})}{\pi(\boldsymbol{\beta}^{(-k)} = 0|D_0^{(\mathcal{K})})}, \quad m = 1, \ldots, \mathcal{K}. \tag{9.1.21}$$

The proof follows directly from Lemma 9.1.1 and the Savage–Dickey density ratio given in Subsection 5.10.3. Using (9.1.15), we have

$$p(k|D^{(k)}) = \frac{p(D^{(k)}|k)p(k)}{\sum_{j\in\mathcal{M}} p(D^{(j)}|j)p(j)} = \frac{\dfrac{p(D^{(k)}|k)}{p(D^{(k)}|\mathcal{K})}p(k)}{\displaystyle\sum_{j=1}^{\mathcal{K}} \frac{p(D^{(j)}|j)}{p(D^{(j)}|\mathcal{K})}p(j)}.$$

This equation, along with (9.1.21), yields

$$p(k|D^{(k)}) = \frac{\dfrac{\pi(\boldsymbol{\beta}^{(-k)} = 0|D^{(\mathcal{K})})}{\pi(\boldsymbol{\beta}^{(-k)} = 0|D_0^{(\mathcal{K})})}p(k)}{\displaystyle\sum_{j=1}^{\mathcal{K}} \frac{\pi(\boldsymbol{\beta}^{(-j)} = 0|D^{(\mathcal{K})})}{\pi(\boldsymbol{\beta}^{(-j)} = 0|D_0^{(\mathcal{K})})}p(j)}, \tag{9.1.22}$$

for $k = 1, 2, \ldots, \mathcal{K}$. In (9.1.22), we define $\pi(\boldsymbol{\beta}^{(-\mathcal{K})} = 0|D^{(\mathcal{K})}) = 1$. Furthermore, it can be shown that the posterior model probabilities given by (9.1.22) are invariant to scale changes in the covariates.

The results given in Theorem 9.1.1 and (9.1.22) are very attractive since they show that the posterior probability $p(k|D^{(k)})$ is simply a function of the prior model probabilities $p(k)$ and the marginal prior and posterior density functions of $\boldsymbol{\beta}^{(-k)}$ for the full model evaluated at $\boldsymbol{\beta}^{(-k)} = 0$. Therefore, to estimate the posterior model probabilities for all $k \in \mathcal{M}$, we use (9.1.14) to estimate the prior model probabilities and compute the marginal prior and posterior density functions only for the full model via the marginal posterior density method given in Chapter 4. These results also demonstrate the importance and usefulness of marginal posterior density estimation, which is discussed in detail in Chapter 4.

Due to the complexity of the prior and posterior distributions, the analytical forms of $\pi(\boldsymbol{\beta}^{(-k)}|D_0^{(\mathcal{K})})$ and $\pi(\boldsymbol{\beta}^{(-k)}|D^{(\mathcal{K})})$ are not available. However, we can use, for example, the IWMDE method given in Section 4.3 to estimate these marginal prior and posterior densities. The IWMDE method requires using only two respective MCMC samples from the prior and posterior distributions for the full model, making the computation of complicated posterior model probabilities feasible. It directly follows from the IWMDE method that a simulation consistent estimator of $\pi(\boldsymbol{\beta}^{(-k)} = 0|D^{(\mathcal{K})})$ is given by

$$\begin{aligned} &\hat{\pi}(\boldsymbol{\beta}^{(-k)} = 0|D^{(\mathcal{K})}) \\ &\quad = \frac{1}{L}\sum_{l=1}^{L} w(\boldsymbol{\beta}_l^{(-k)}|\boldsymbol{\beta}_l^{(k)}, a_{0,l})\frac{\pi(\boldsymbol{\beta}_l^{(k)}, \boldsymbol{\beta}^{(-k)} = 0, a_{0,l}|D^{(\mathcal{K})})}{\pi(\boldsymbol{\beta}_l^{(\mathcal{K})}, a_{0,l}|D^{(\mathcal{K})})}, \end{aligned}$$

where $w(\boldsymbol{\beta}^{(-k)}|\boldsymbol{\beta}^{(k)}, a_0)$ is a completely known conditional density of $\boldsymbol{\beta}^{(-k)}$ given $\boldsymbol{\beta}^{(k)}$ and a_0, whose support is contained in, or equal to, the support of the conditional density of $\boldsymbol{\beta}^{(-k)}$ given $\boldsymbol{\beta}^{(k)}$ and a_0 with respect to the full model joint posterior distribution, $\{(\boldsymbol{\beta}_l^{(\mathcal{K})}, a_{0,l}), l = 1, 2, \ldots, L\}$ is a sample from the joint posterior distribution $\pi(\boldsymbol{\beta}^{(\mathcal{K})}, a_0 | D^{(\mathcal{K})})$ of $(\boldsymbol{\beta}^{(\mathcal{K})}, a_0)$. To construct a good $w(\boldsymbol{\beta}^{(-k)}|\boldsymbol{\beta}^{(k)}, a_0)$, we can use a similar procedure that is used to construct $w(\boldsymbol{\beta}^{(-k)}|\boldsymbol{\beta}^{(k)})$ in (9.1.14) for calculating the prior model probabilities. Similarly, we can obtain $\hat{\pi}(\boldsymbol{\beta}^{(-k)} = 0|D_0^{(\mathcal{K})})$, an estimate of $\pi(\boldsymbol{\beta}^{(-k)} = 0|D_0^{(\mathcal{K})})$, using a sample from the joint prior distribution $\pi(\boldsymbol{\beta}^{(\mathcal{K})}, a_0|D_0^{(\mathcal{K})})$. We use an example given in Chen, Ibrahim, and Yiannoutsos (1999) to illustrate the above Bayesian variable selection method.

Example 9.1. AIDS ACTG019 and ACTG036 data. We consider an analysis of the AIDS study ACTG036 using the data from ACTG019 as prior information. The purpose of this example is to demonstrate the Bayesian variable selection procedure, and show that, by incorporating prior information from ACTG019, different results can be obtained than those of criterion-based procedures such as AIC and BIC. A detailed description of the data from the ACTG036 and ACTG019 studies can be found in Example 1.4.

The sample size for the ACTG019 study was $n_0 = 823$. The response variable (y_0) for these data is binary with a 1 indicating death, development of AIDS, or an AIDS related complex (ARC), and a 0 indicates otherwise. The covariates used in our analysis are CD4 count (x_{01}) (cell count per mm^3 of serum), age (x_{02}), treatment (x_{03}), and race (x_{04}). The sample size in the ACTG019 study was $n = 183$. The response variable (y) for these data is binary with a 1 indicating death, development of AIDS, or an AIDS related complex (ARC), and a 0 indicates otherwise. Several covariates were measured for these data. The covariates from this study include CD4 count (x_1), age (x_2), treatment (x_3), race (x_4), hemophilia factor type (x_5), and monoclonal factor concentrate use (x_6).

The SAS stepwise logistic procedure identifies the (x_1) model as the best model for the ACTG036 data using an entry and exit p-value criterion of 0.2. Table 9.1 gives the top two models based on the AIC and BIC criteria, which also identify (x_1) as the best model. For model k, AIC and BIC are given by

$$\text{AIC}_k = -2 \ln L(\hat{\boldsymbol{\beta}}^{(k)}|D^{(k)}) + 2p_k,$$

and

$$\text{BIC}_k = -2 \ln L(\hat{\boldsymbol{\beta}}^{(k)}|D^{(k)}) + \ln(n)p_k,$$

where $\hat{\boldsymbol{\beta}}^{(k)}$ is the maximum likelihood estimate of $\boldsymbol{\beta}^{(k)}$. Since the covariates in the previous study (ACTG019) are a subset of the covariates in the current study (ACTG036), we use the priors developed in (9.1.5) to carry

TABLE 9.1. Top Two Models Based on AIC and BIC.

Model	AIC	BIC
(x_1)	65.8	72.3
(x_1, x_2)	67.6	77.2

out the variable subset selection. An intercept is included in every model and 50000 Gibbs iterations were used to get convergence.

Table 9.2 shows the results of a Bayesian variable selection for several values of c_0 using $d_0 = 0.5$, $(\mu_{a_{01}}, \sigma^2_{a_{01}}) = (0.5, 0.005)$ (i.e., $\alpha_{01} = \lambda_{01} = 25$), $(\mu_{a_{02}}, \sigma^2_{a_{02}}) = (0.5, 0.083)$ (i.e., $\alpha_{02} = \lambda_{02} = 1$). We see that for this choice, the top model is (x_1, x_2, x_3), which is quite different from the one selected by AIC and BIC. The second best model is (x_1, x_2) with a posterior model probability of 0.08. Thus, we see that with a moderate incorporation of the historical data and a nearly uniform prior on the model space (i.e., $d_0 = 0.5$), a different top model is obtained than the one given by AIC and BIC. We note that for $c_0 = 3$, the x_1 model has posterior model probability of 0.023 and the (x_1, x_3) model has a posterior probability of 0.04. For $c_0 \geq 3$ and $d_0 \geq 0.5$, the top model remains (x_1, x_2, x_3) and its prior and posterior probabilities increase monotonically as (d_0, c_0) increase. For example, when $c_0 = 3$ and $d_0 = 5$, the prior probability of (x_1, x_2, x_3) is 0.17 and its posterior probability is 0.28. When $c_0 = 50$ and $d_0 = 10$, the prior model probability is 0.20 and the posterior probability is 0.31. When $d_0 \geq 5$, the (x_1, x_2, x_3) model also obtains the largest prior model probability. We see that model choice is not sensitive when $c_0 \geq 3$ and $d_0 \geq 0.5$, for which (x_1, x_2, x_3) is consistently the top model. To obtain a result similar to AIC and BIC, we let $d_0 \to 0$. With $d_0 = .001$, and $c_0 = 50$, the top model is x_1 with posterior model probability of 0.22. In general, we see that our prior elicitation scheme is quite flexible, and is able to obtain criterion-based results with appropriate choices of prior parameters.

Table 9.3 shows the results of a sensitivity analysis on a_{02}. In each case, the (x_1, x_2, x_3) model obtains the largest posterior probability and the results are not sensitive to the choice of prior parameters. We observe a monotonic decrease in the posterior probability of (x_1, x_2, x_3) as more prior

TABLE 9.2. The Posterior Model Probabilities for $d_0 = 0.5$, $(\mu_{a_{01}}, \sigma^2_{a_{01}}) = (0.5, 0.008)$, $(\mu_{a_{02}}, \sigma^2_{a_{02}}) = (0.5, 0.083)$ for Various Choices of c_0.

c_0	Model k	$p(k)$	$p(D \mid k)$	$p(k\|D)$
3	(x_1, x_2, x_3)	0.057	0.053	0.12
5	(x_1, x_2, x_3)	0.057	0.059	0.12
10	(x_1, x_2, x_3)	0.057	0.061	0.12

TABLE 9.3. The Posterior Model Probabilities for $d_0 = 3$, $c_0 = 10$, $(\mu_{a_{01}}, \sigma^2_{a_{01}}) = (0.5, 0.008)$, and Various Choices of $(\mu_{a_{02}}, \sigma^2_{a_{02}})$.

$(\mu_{a_{02}}, \sigma^2_{a_{02}})$	Model k	$p(k)$	$p(D \mid k)$	$p(k\|D)$
$(0.5, 0.083)$	(x_1, x_2, x_3)	0.14	0.06	0.24
$(0.5, 0.023)$	(x_1, x_2, x_3)	0.14	0.06	0.23
$(0.98, 3.7 \times 10^{-4})$	(x_1, x_2, x_3)	0.14	0.05	0.20

weight is given to the part of the prior that incorporates the new covariates. This is expected since the new covariates in the current study do not involve age (x_2) or treatment (x_3). Tables 9.2 and 9.3 demonstrate that the incorporation of the ACTG019 data into the current analysis reveals the importance of age (x_2) and treatment (x_3) as well as CD4 count (x_1) in predicting the response. By incorporating the prior information from the ACTG019 study, the model with the largest posterior probability includes two covariates, treatment and age, which are not included in the best model based on the AIC and BIC procedures. Moreover, after incorporation of the prior information from ACTG019, model (x_1) gets very small posterior probability for several choices of c_0 and d_0. With an analysis of the ACTG019 data alone, the BIC criterion and the stepwise procedure yield the model containing age, treatment, and CD4 count as the best model. Thus the prior distributions incorporate the importance of these two additional covariates (age and treatment) into the ACTG036 analysis, and as a result, have an impact on the final results. The result obtained here is important since it shows the importance of the treatment and age covariates when the prior information from a previous study is incorporated. Such results play a crucial role in decision making and public policy regarding the treatment of AIDS. Such a result would not have been obtained using criterion-based methods such as AIC and BIC. In fact, for the ACTG036 data, the (x_1, x_2, x_3) model obtained the ninth smallest AIC and BIC criterion values. We see in this analysis how the incorporation of data from a previous study can affect the model choice and yield results different from an analysis using criterion-based methods.

9.2 Variable Selection for Time Series Count Data Models

Correlated count data arise often in practice, especially in repeated measures situations or instances in which observations are collected over time. In this section, we consider a parametric model for a time series of counts by constructing a likelihood-based generalization of a model considered by Zeger (1988). We consider a Bayesian approach and propose a class of informative prior distributions for the model parameters that are useful for variable subset selection. Similar to the logistic regression model, we discuss the prior specification based on historical data. We present the computational methods of Ibrahim, Chen, and Ryan (1999) for sampling from the posterior distribution of the parameters and computing posterior model probabilities using the idea of hierarchical centering discussed in Subsection 2.5.2. These computational methods are slightly different than those given in the previous section and are particularly suitable for time series count data models.

9.2.1 The Likelihood Function

Following the notation given in Subsection 9.1.1, let $\boldsymbol{\beta}^{(\mathcal{K})} = (\beta_0, \beta_1, \ldots, \beta_{p-1})'$ denote the regression coefficients for the full model including an intercept, and let $\boldsymbol{\beta}^{(k)}$ denote a $p_k \times 1$ vector of regression coefficients for model k with an intercept, and a specific choice of $p_k - 1$ covariates. We write $\boldsymbol{\beta}^{(\mathcal{K})} = (\boldsymbol{\beta}^{(k)'}, \boldsymbol{\beta}^{(-k)'})'$, where $\boldsymbol{\beta}^{(-k)}$ is $\boldsymbol{\beta}^{(\mathcal{K})}$ with $\boldsymbol{\beta}^{(k)}$ deleted.

Consider a time series of counts y_t, $t = 1, \ldots, n$, where each y_t has corresponding $p_k \times 1$ covariate vector $x_t^{(k)}$ under model k. Under model k, conditional on $\boldsymbol{\beta}^{(k)}$ and a stationary unobserved process ϵ_t, the y_t's are assumed to be independent discrete random variables from a distribution in the exponential family, leading to the conditional likelihood function

$$\begin{aligned} L(\boldsymbol{\beta}^{(k)}|\boldsymbol{\epsilon}, D^{(k)}) &= \prod_{t=1}^{n} f(y_t|\boldsymbol{\beta}^{(k)}, \epsilon_t) \\ &= \prod_{t=1}^{n} \exp\{\tau_t[y_t\theta(\boldsymbol{x}_t^{(k)}, \boldsymbol{\beta}^{(k)}, \epsilon_t) - q(\theta(\boldsymbol{x}_t^{(k)}, \boldsymbol{\beta}^{(k)}, \epsilon_t))] - c(y_t, \tau_t)\}, \end{aligned} \tag{9.2.1}$$

indexed by the canonical parameter $\theta(\boldsymbol{x}_t^{(k)}, \boldsymbol{\beta}^{(k)}, \epsilon_t)$ and the scale parameter τ_t. In (9.2.1), $\boldsymbol{\epsilon} = (\epsilon_1, \ldots, \epsilon_n)'$, $D^{(k)} = (n, \boldsymbol{y}, X^{(k)})$ denotes the observed data, $\boldsymbol{y} = (y_1, \ldots, y_n)'$, and $X^{(k)}$ is the $n \times p_k$ matrix of covariates with t^{th} row equal to $(\boldsymbol{x}_t^{(k)})'$, Further, suppose $\theta(\boldsymbol{x}_t^{(k)}, \boldsymbol{\beta}^{(k)}, \epsilon_t)$ satisfies the equation

$$\theta(\boldsymbol{x}_t^{(k)}, \boldsymbol{\beta}^{(k)}, \epsilon_t) = h((\boldsymbol{x}_t^{(k)})'\boldsymbol{\beta}^{(k)} + \epsilon_t), \;\; t = 1, \ldots, n, \tag{9.2.2}$$

where h is a monotonic differentiable function, often referred to as the link function. In (9.2.1), the functions q and c determine a particular family in the class, such as the binomial and Poisson distributions. For example, if we take y_t to have a Poisson distribution with conditional mean $\lambda_t = \exp((\boldsymbol{x}_t^{(k)'}\boldsymbol{\beta}^{(k)} + \epsilon_t)$, then $\tau_t = 1$, $h((\boldsymbol{x}_t^{(k)})'\boldsymbol{\beta}^{(k)} + \epsilon_t) = (\boldsymbol{x}_t^{(k)})'\boldsymbol{\beta}^{(k)} + \epsilon_t$, $q(\theta(\boldsymbol{x}_t^{(k)}, \boldsymbol{\beta}^{(k)}, \epsilon_t)) = \exp\{(\boldsymbol{x}_t^{(k)})'\boldsymbol{\beta}^{(k)} + \epsilon_t\}$, and $c(y_t, \tau_t) = \ln(y_t!)$. We emphasize here that the likelihood in (9.2.1) is a general exponential family model for discrete outcomes, with the Poisson model being a special case. Throughout this section, we assume a general exponential family model with discrete outcomes. For ease of exposition, we also assume $\tau_t = 1$ and denote $c(y_t) = c(y_t, \tau_t)$ throughout, since this is in fact the case for many models in the exponential family, including the binomial and Poisson models. In addition, it will be convenient to write (9.2.1) in vector notation as

$$L(\boldsymbol{\beta}^{(k)}|\boldsymbol{\epsilon}, D^{(k)}) \\ = \exp\{y'\theta(X^{(k)}, \boldsymbol{\beta}^{(k)}, \boldsymbol{\epsilon}) - J_n' Q(X^{(k)}, \boldsymbol{\beta}^{(k)}, \boldsymbol{\epsilon}) - J_n' C(\boldsymbol{y})\}, \quad (9.2.3)$$

where J_n is an $n \times 1$ vector of ones, $\theta(X^{(k)}, \boldsymbol{\beta}^{(k)}, \boldsymbol{\epsilon})$, $Q(X^{(k)}, \boldsymbol{\beta}^{(k)}, \boldsymbol{\epsilon})$, and $C(\boldsymbol{y})$ are $n \times 1$ vectors with the tth components equal to $\theta_t = h((\boldsymbol{x}_t^{(k)})'\boldsymbol{\beta}^{(k)} + \epsilon_t)$, $q_t = q(\theta_t)$, and $c_t = c(y_t)$, respectively.

The latent process ϵ_t is assumed to have normal distribution with mean 0. We assume an AR(1) structure for the covariance matrix of $\boldsymbol{\epsilon}$. Thus, $\boldsymbol{\epsilon}$ has a multivariate normal distribution with mean 0 and covariance matrix $\sigma^2\Sigma$, where the $(i, j)^{\text{th}}$ element of Σ has the form $\sigma_{ij} = \rho^{|i-j|}$, where $\rho^{|i-j|}$ is the correlation between (ϵ_i, ϵ_j), and $-1 < \rho < 1$. The unobserved process ϵ_t is analogous to a "random effect" in a random effects model, with the exception that the latent process is correlated.

Let $\phi_n(\boldsymbol{\epsilon}|\boldsymbol{\mu}, \sigma^2\Sigma)$ denote the n-dimensional normal density of the latent process $\boldsymbol{\epsilon}$ with mean $\boldsymbol{\mu}$ and covariance matrix $\sigma^2\Sigma$, i.e.,

$$\phi_n(\boldsymbol{\epsilon}|\boldsymbol{\mu}, \sigma^2\Sigma) = (2\pi\sigma^2)^{-n/2}|\Sigma|^{-1/2} \exp\left\{-\frac{1}{2\sigma^2}(\boldsymbol{\epsilon} - \boldsymbol{\mu})'\Sigma^{-1}(\boldsymbol{\epsilon} - \boldsymbol{\mu})\right\}. \quad (9.2.4)$$

We note that in (9.2.4), $|\Sigma| = (1 - \rho^2)^{n-1}$. Then the complete data likelihood function can be written as

$$L(\boldsymbol{\beta}^{(k)}, \sigma^2, \rho, \boldsymbol{\epsilon}|D^{(k)}) \\ = \exp\{\boldsymbol{y}'\theta(X^{(k)}, \boldsymbol{\beta}^{(k)}, \boldsymbol{\epsilon}) - J_n' Q(X^{(k)}, \boldsymbol{\beta}^{(k)}, \boldsymbol{\epsilon}) - J_n' C(\boldsymbol{y})\} \\ \times \phi_n(\boldsymbol{\epsilon}|0, \sigma^2\Sigma). \quad (9.2.5)$$

To induce the correlation structure on $\boldsymbol{y}$, we integrate out $\boldsymbol{\epsilon}$ from (9.2.5) leading to the "marginal" likelihood of $\boldsymbol{\beta}^{(k)}$, σ^2, and ρ given by

$$L(\boldsymbol{\beta}^{(k)}, \sigma^2, \rho|D^{(k)}) = \int L(\boldsymbol{\beta}^{(k)}, \sigma^2, \rho, \boldsymbol{\epsilon}|D^{(k)})\, d\boldsymbol{\epsilon}. \quad (9.2.6)$$

9.2.2 *Prior Distributions for $\boldsymbol{\beta}^{(m)}$*

We consider a class of informative priors for the regression coefficients $\boldsymbol{\beta}^{(k)}$ similar to those for the logistic regression models. Suppose there are N historical data sets and the sample size of the ith historical study is n_{0i}. Let $\boldsymbol{y}_{0i}$ denote the $n_{0i} \times 1$ vector of time series counts for the ith historical study and let $X_{0i}^{(k)}$ denote the $n_{0i} \times p_k$ matrix of covariates corresponding to the ith historical study. In addition, let $\boldsymbol{\epsilon}_{0i}$ denote the latent process for the ith historical study, where $\boldsymbol{\epsilon}_{0i}$ is an $n_{0i} \times 1$ vector, $i = 1, \ldots, N$, and $\boldsymbol{\epsilon}_{0i}$ has an n_{0i}-dimensional multivariate normal distribution with mean 0 and covariance matrix $\sigma^2 \Sigma_{0i}$, where Σ_{0i} is an $n_{0i} \times n_{0i}$ matrix with the $(j, j^*)^{\text{th}}$ element equal to $\rho^{|j-j^*|}$. Finally, let $D_{0i}^{(k)} = (n_{0i}, \boldsymbol{y}_{0i}, X_{0i}^{(k)})$ denote the data from the ith historical study, and let $D_0^{(k)} = (D_{01}^{(k)}, D_{02}^{(k)}, \ldots, D_{0N}^{(k)})$ denote the data from all of the historical studies.

We take the prior distribution for $\boldsymbol{\beta}^{(k)}$ based on the ith historical study to be

$$\pi(\boldsymbol{\beta}^{(k)} | \sigma^2, \rho, a_{0i}, D_{0i}^{(k)}) \propto \int L(\boldsymbol{\beta}^{(k)} | \boldsymbol{\epsilon}_{0i}, D_{0i}^{(k)})^{a_{0i}} \phi_{n_{0i}}(\boldsymbol{\epsilon}_{0i} | 0, \sigma^2 \Sigma_{0i}) \, d\boldsymbol{\epsilon}_{0i}, \tag{9.2.7}$$

where

$$\begin{aligned} L(\boldsymbol{\beta}^{(k)} | \boldsymbol{\epsilon}_{0i}, D_{0i}^{(k)}) = \exp\{ & \boldsymbol{y}_{0i}' \theta(X_{0i}^{(k)}, \boldsymbol{\beta}^{(k)}, \boldsymbol{\epsilon}_{0i}) \\ & - J_{n_{0i}}' Q(X_{0i}^{(k)}, \boldsymbol{\beta}^{(k)}, \boldsymbol{\epsilon}_{0i}) - J_{n_{0i}}' C(\boldsymbol{y}_{0i})\}, \end{aligned} \tag{9.2.8}$$

is the conditional likelihood function for the ith study, and a_{0i} is a scalar prior parameter that controls the weight of the ith historical study relative to the likelihood of the current study. The parameter a_{0i} can be interpreted as a precision parameter which takes into account the between and within study variability in the historical data sets. The prior distribution of $\boldsymbol{\beta}^{(k)}$ based on all of the historical studies is thus given by

$$\pi(\boldsymbol{\beta}^{(k)} | \sigma^2, \rho, \boldsymbol{a}_0 | D_0^{(k)}) \propto \prod_{i=1}^{N} \int L(\boldsymbol{\beta}^{(k)} | \boldsymbol{\epsilon}_{0i}, D_{0i}^{(k)})^{a_{0i}} \phi_{n_{0i}}(\boldsymbol{\epsilon}_{0i} | 0, \sigma^2 \Sigma_{0i}) \, d\boldsymbol{\epsilon}_{0i}, \tag{9.2.9}$$

where $\boldsymbol{a}_0 = (a_{01}, \ldots, a_{0N})'$.

The prior specification is completed by specifying priors for $(\sigma^2, \rho, \boldsymbol{a}_0)$. We take these parameters to be independent a priori. We specify an inverse gamma prior for σ^2, denoted $\mathcal{IG}(\delta_0, \gamma_0)$, a scaled beta prior for ρ, denoted scbeta(ν_0, ψ_0), and independent identically distributed beta priors for each a_{0i}, denoted beta(α_0, λ_0). Here $(\delta_0, \gamma_0, \nu_0, \psi_0, \alpha_0, \lambda_0)$ are specified prior hyperparameters. Thus, the joint prior distribution is of the form

$$\begin{aligned} \pi(\boldsymbol{\beta}^{(k)}, \sigma^2, \rho, \boldsymbol{a}_0 | D_0^{(k)}) & \propto \pi_0^*(\boldsymbol{\beta}^{(k)}, \sigma^2, \rho, \boldsymbol{a}_0 | D_0^{(k)}) \\ = & \prod_{i=1}^{N} \left(\int L(\boldsymbol{\beta}^{(k)} | \boldsymbol{\epsilon}_{0i}, D_{0i}^{(k)})^{a_{0i}} \phi_{n_{0i}}(\boldsymbol{\epsilon}_{0i} | 0, \sigma^2 \Sigma_{0i}) \, d\boldsymbol{\epsilon}_{0i} \right) (1 + \rho)^{\nu_0 - 1} \\ & \times (1 - \rho)^{\psi_0 - 1} (\sigma^2)^{-(\delta_0 + 1)} \exp(-\sigma^{-2} \gamma_0) \prod_{i=1}^{N} a_{0i}^{\alpha_0 - 1} (1 - a_{0i})^{\lambda_0 - 1}, \end{aligned} \tag{9.2.10}$$

where $\pi_0^*(\boldsymbol{\beta}^{(k)}, \sigma^2, \rho, \boldsymbol{a}_0 | D_0^{(k)})$ is the unnormalized prior density. The prior in (9.2.10) does not have a closed form, in general, but it has several attractive theoretical and computational properties. Ibrahim, Chen, and Ryan (1999) propose the prior in (9.2.10), and show that it is proper under certain mild regularity conditions. The propriety of (9.2.10) is important since it is required for carrying out Bayesian variable selection. In addition, the propriety of the prior distribution automatically guarantees the propriety of the resulting posterior distribution, which assures the stability of the Gibbs sampler in posterior computations.

In the context of model selection, (ρ, σ^2) are viewed as nuisance parameters, and therefore we take vague choices for their prior hyperparameters. In particular, it is reasonable to take $\nu_0 = \psi_0 = 1$ which yields a uniform prior for ρ on $[-1, 1]$. Also, we take $\delta_0 \to 0$ and $\gamma_0 \to 0$, which yields a noninformative prior for σ^2. For a_{0i}, we recommend that several values of the hyperparameters be chosen and sensitivity analyses conducted. For elicitation purposes, it is easier to work with the prior mean and variance of a_{0i}, given by $\mu_{a_0} = \alpha_0/(\alpha_0 + \lambda_0)$, and $\sigma^2_{a_0} = \mu_{a_0}(1 - \mu_{a_0})(\alpha_0 + \lambda_0 + 1)^{-1}$. From Ibrahim, Chen, and Ryan (1999), a sufficient condition for the propriety of the prior distribution is $\alpha_0 > p/N$ for the full model (see Exercise 9.6). Therefore, a reasonable starting point for the analysis is to choose $\alpha_0 = \lambda_0 = (p+1)/N$, which gives $\mu_{a_0} = \frac{1}{2}$. Then we conduct several sensitivity analyses within a suitable range of the uniform prior, using various values of $(\mu_{a_0}, \sigma^2_{a_0})$. Small and large values of $(\mu_{a_0}, \sigma^2_{a_0})$ should be considered.

9.2.3 Prior Distribution on the Model Space

Let

$$\pi_0^*(\boldsymbol{\beta}^{(k)} | D_0^{(k)}) = \int \pi_0^*(\boldsymbol{\beta}^{(k)}, \sigma^2, \rho, \boldsymbol{a}_0 | D_0^{(k)}) \, d\sigma^2 \, d\rho \, d\boldsymbol{a}_0, \quad (9.2.11)$$

where $\pi_0^*(\boldsymbol{\beta}^{(k)}, \sigma^2, \rho, \boldsymbol{a}_0 | D_0^{(k)})$ is given by (9.2.10). We see that $\pi_0^*(\boldsymbol{\beta}^{(k)} | D_0^{(k)})$ is proportional to the marginal prior of $\boldsymbol{\beta}^{(k)}$. We take the prior probability of model k, denoted $p(k)$, as

$$p(k) = \frac{\int \pi_0^*(\boldsymbol{\beta}^{(k)} | D_0^{(k)}) \, d\boldsymbol{\beta}^{(k)}}{\sum_{j=1}^{\mathcal{K}} \int \pi_0^*(\boldsymbol{\beta}^{(j)} | D_0^{(j)}) \, d\boldsymbol{\beta}^{(j)}} . \quad (9.2.12)$$

This choice for $p(k)$ in (9.2.12) is a natural one since the numerator is just the normalizing constant of the joint prior of $(\boldsymbol{\beta}^{(k)}, \sigma^2, \rho, \boldsymbol{a}_0)$ under model k. The prior model probabilities in (9.2.12) are based on coherent Bayesian updating and this results in several attractive interpretations. First, $p(k)$ in (9.2.12) corresponds to the posterior probability of model k based on the data $D_0^{(k)}$ under model k, using a uniform prior for the previous study, $p_0(k) = 2^{-p-1}$ for $k \in \mathcal{M}$ as $\alpha_0 \to \infty$. That is, $p(k) \equiv p(k | D_0^{(k)})$, and thus

$p(k)$ corresponds to the usual Bayesian update of $p_0(k)$ using $D_0^{(k)}$ as the data. Second, as $\lambda_0 \to \infty$, $p(k)$ reduces to a uniform prior on the model space. Therefore, as $\lambda_0 \to \infty$, the historical data $D_0^{(k)}$ have a minimal impact in determining $p(k)$. On the other hand, $p(k)$ in (9.2.12) has a nice theoretical property, which greatly eases the computational burden for calculating posterior model probabilities using an MCMC sample. These properties are discussed in more detail in the subsequent subsections.

9.2.4 Sampling from the Posterior Distribution

Let $\boldsymbol{\epsilon}_0 = (\boldsymbol{\epsilon}_{01}', \boldsymbol{\epsilon}_{02}', \ldots, \boldsymbol{\epsilon}_{0N}')'$. Using (9.2.10), the joint posterior distribution of $(\boldsymbol{\beta}^{(k)}, \sigma^2, \rho, \boldsymbol{a}_0, \boldsymbol{\epsilon}, \boldsymbol{\epsilon}_0)$ under model k is given by

$$\begin{aligned}
\pi(\boldsymbol{\beta}^{(k)}, \sigma^2, \rho, \boldsymbol{a}_0, \boldsymbol{\epsilon}, \boldsymbol{\epsilon}_0 | D^{(k)}) &\propto L(\boldsymbol{\beta}^{(k)}, \sigma^2, \rho, \boldsymbol{\epsilon} | D^{(k)}) \\
&\times \prod_{i=1}^{N} (L(\boldsymbol{\beta}^{(k)} |\, \boldsymbol{\epsilon}_{0i}, D_{0i}^{(k)})^{a_{0i}} \phi_{n_{0i}}(\boldsymbol{\epsilon}_{0i} | 0, \sigma^2 \Sigma_{0i}))(1+\rho)^{\nu_0 - 1} \\
&\times (1-\rho)^{\psi_0 - 1} (\sigma^2)^{-(\delta_0 + 1)} \exp(-\sigma^{-2}\gamma_0) \prod_{i=1}^{N} a_{0i}^{\alpha_0 - 1}(1 - a_{0i})^{\lambda_0 - 1},
\end{aligned} \tag{9.2.13}$$

where $L(\boldsymbol{\beta}^{(k)}, \sigma^2, \rho, \boldsymbol{\epsilon} | D^{(k)})$ is given by (9.2.5). To sample from the posterior distribution, we use the hierarchical centering reparameterization technique of Gelfand, Sahu, and Carlin (1995, 1996). Similar to the Poisson random effects model given in Subsection 2.5.4, we consider the following reparameterization:

$$\boldsymbol{\eta} = \boldsymbol{\epsilon} + X^{(k)} \boldsymbol{\beta}^{(k)} \tag{9.2.14}$$

and

$$\boldsymbol{\eta}_{0i} = \boldsymbol{\epsilon}_{0i} + X_{0i}^{(k)} \boldsymbol{\beta}^{(k)}, \tag{9.2.15}$$

for $i = 1, 2, \ldots, N$. Let $\boldsymbol{\eta}_0 = (\boldsymbol{\eta}_{01}', \cdots, \boldsymbol{\eta}_{0N}')'$. Now the reparameterized posterior under model k is given by

$$\begin{aligned}
&\pi(\boldsymbol{\beta}^{(k)}, \sigma^2, \rho, \boldsymbol{a}_0, \boldsymbol{\eta}, \boldsymbol{\eta}_0 | D^{(k)}) \\
&\quad \propto \exp\{\boldsymbol{y}'\boldsymbol{\theta}(\boldsymbol{\eta}) - J_n' Q(\boldsymbol{\eta})\} \, \phi_n(\boldsymbol{\eta} | X^{(k)} \boldsymbol{\beta}^{(k)}, \sigma^2 \Sigma) \\
&\quad \times \left(\prod_{i=1}^{N} \exp\{a_{0i}[\boldsymbol{y}_{0i}' \boldsymbol{\theta}_0(\boldsymbol{\eta}_{0i}) - J_{n_{0i}}' Q_0(\boldsymbol{\eta}_{0i}) - J_{n_{0i}}' C(y_{0i})]\} \right. \\
&\quad \left. \times \, \phi_{n_{0i}}(\boldsymbol{\eta}_{0i} | X_{0i}^{(k)} \boldsymbol{\beta}^{(k)}, \sigma^2 \Sigma_{0i}) \right) (1+\rho)^{\nu_0 - 1}(1-\rho)^{\psi_0 - 1} \\
&\quad \times (\sigma^2)^{-(\delta_0 + 1)} \exp\left(-\frac{\gamma_0}{\sigma^2}\right) \prod_{i=1}^{N} a_{0i}^{\alpha_0 - 1}(1 - a_{0i})^{\lambda_0 - 1}.
\end{aligned} \tag{9.2.16}$$

To run the Gibbs sampler for sampling from the reparameterized posterior, we need the following five steps:

Step 1. We sample $(\boldsymbol{\eta}, \boldsymbol{\eta}_0)$ from their conditional posterior distributions. After the hierarchical centering reparameterization, it is straightforward to show that the conditional posterior density of $\boldsymbol{\eta}, \boldsymbol{\eta}_0$, denoted $\pi(\boldsymbol{\eta}, \boldsymbol{\eta}_0 | \boldsymbol{\beta}^{(k)}, \sigma^2, \rho, \boldsymbol{a}_0, D^{(k)})$, is log-concave in each component of $\boldsymbol{\eta}$ or $\boldsymbol{\eta}_0$ as long as $f(y_t | \boldsymbol{\beta}^{(k)}, \epsilon_t)$ and $f(y_{0it} | \boldsymbol{\beta}^{(k)}, \epsilon_{0it})$ are log-concave, which is the case for the binomial and Poisson models. Thus, we use the adaptive rejection sampling algorithm of Gilks and Wild (1992) to sample $(\boldsymbol{\eta}, \boldsymbol{\eta}_0)$.

Step 2. We sample $\boldsymbol{\beta}^{(k)}$ from its conditional posterior distribution. Here, the hierarchical centering technique makes the generation of $\boldsymbol{\beta}^{(k)}$ quite easy. As a result of hierarchical centering, it can be shown that

$$(\boldsymbol{\beta}^{(k)} | \boldsymbol{\eta}, \boldsymbol{\eta}_0, \sigma^2, \rho, D^{(k)}) \sim N_{p_k}(\hat{\boldsymbol{\beta}}^{(k)}, B_k^{-1}), \tag{9.2.17}$$

where

$$B_k = \frac{1}{\sigma^2} \left((X^{(k)})' \Sigma^{-1} X^{(k)} + \sum_{i=1}^{N} (X_{0i}^{(k)})' \Sigma_{0i}^{-1} X_{0i}^{(k)} \right),$$

and

$$\hat{\boldsymbol{\beta}}^{(k)} = \frac{1}{\sigma^2} B_k^{-1} \left((X^{(k)})' \Sigma^{-1} \boldsymbol{\eta} + \sum_{i=1}^{N} (X_{0i}^{(k)})' \Sigma_{0i}^{-1} \boldsymbol{\eta}_{0i} \right).$$

Thus, it is straightforward to generate $\boldsymbol{\beta}^{(k)}$ from the normal distribution in (9.2.17).

Step 3. We sample σ^2 from

$$(\sigma^2 | \boldsymbol{\beta}^{(k)}, \rho, \boldsymbol{\eta}, \boldsymbol{\eta}_0, \boldsymbol{a}_0, D^{(k)}) \sim \mathcal{IG}(\delta^*, \gamma^*)$$

where

$$\delta^* = \delta_0 + \frac{n + \sum_{i=1}^{N} n_{0i}}{2},$$

$$\gamma^* = \gamma_0 + \frac{(\boldsymbol{\eta} - X^{(k)} \boldsymbol{\beta}^{(k)})' \Sigma^{-1} (\boldsymbol{\eta} - X^{(k)} \boldsymbol{\beta}^{(k)})}{2} + \frac{\sum_{i=1}^{N} (\boldsymbol{\eta}_{0i} - X_{0i}^{(k)} \boldsymbol{\beta}^{(k)})' \Sigma_{0i}^{-1} (\boldsymbol{\eta}_{0i} - X_{0i}^{(k)} \boldsymbol{\beta}^{(k)})}{2},$$

and $\mathcal{IG}(\delta^*, \gamma^*)$ is an inverse gamma distribution.

Step 4. We use a Metropolis–Hastings algorithm given in Example 2.3 to sample ρ. The conditional posterior distribution of ρ is given by

$$\begin{aligned}\pi(\rho|\boldsymbol{\beta}^{(k)},&\sigma^2,\boldsymbol{\eta},\boldsymbol{\eta}_0,D^{(k)})\\ &\propto \exp\left\{-\frac{1}{2\sigma^2}(\boldsymbol{\eta}-X^{(k)}\boldsymbol{\beta}^{(k)})'\Sigma^{-1}(\boldsymbol{\eta}-X^{(k)}\boldsymbol{\beta}^{(k)})\right.\\ &\quad\left.-\frac{1}{2\sigma^2}\sum_{i=1}^{N}(\boldsymbol{\eta}_{0i}-X_{0i}^{(k)}\boldsymbol{\beta}^{(k)})'\Sigma_{0i}^{-1}(\boldsymbol{\eta}_{0i}-X_{0i}^{(k)}\boldsymbol{\beta}^{(k)})\right\}\\ &\quad\times(1+\rho)^{\nu_0-1}(1-\rho)^{\psi_0-1}. \end{aligned} \tag{9.2.18}$$

Step 5. To sample each a_{0i} from its conditional posterior distribution, we use a very similar Metropolis–Hastings algorithm as given in Example 2.3. In this case

$$a_{0k}=\frac{\exp(\zeta_i)}{1+\exp(\zeta_i)},$$

and the conditional posterior distribution of $(\zeta_i|\boldsymbol{\beta}^{(k)},\sigma^2,\rho,D^{(k)})$ is given by

$$\pi(\zeta_i|\boldsymbol{\beta}^{(k)},\sigma^2,\rho,D^{(k)}) \;\propto\; \pi^*(a_{0i}|\boldsymbol{\beta}^{(k)},\sigma^2,\rho,D^{(k)})\frac{\exp(\zeta_i)}{(1+\exp(\zeta_i))^2},$$

where $\pi(a_{0i}|\boldsymbol{\beta}^{(k)},\sigma^2,\rho,\boldsymbol{\eta},\boldsymbol{\eta}_0,D^{(k)})$ is given by

$$\begin{aligned}\pi^*(a_{0i}|\boldsymbol{\beta}^{(k)},&\sigma^2,\rho,D^{(k)})\\ &\propto\exp\{a_{0i}[\boldsymbol{y}_{0i}'\theta_0(\boldsymbol{\eta}_{0i})-J_{n_{0i}}'Q_0(\boldsymbol{\eta}_{0i})-J_{n_{0i}}'C(\boldsymbol{y}_{0i})]\}\\ &\quad\times a_{0i}^{\alpha_0-1}(1-a_{0i})^{\lambda_0-1},\end{aligned}$$

and a_{0i} is evaluated at $a_{0i}=\exp(\zeta_i)/(1+\exp(\zeta_i))$.

Other implementational details for this Metropolis–Hastings algorithm can be found in Example 2.3.

9.2.5 Computation of Posterior Model Probabilities

The posterior probability of model k is given by

$$p(k|D^{(k)})=\frac{p(D^{(k)}|k)p(k)}{\sum_{j=1}^{\mathcal{K}}p(D^{(j)}|j)p(j)}, \tag{9.2.19}$$

where $p(D^{(k)}|k)$ denotes the marginal distribution of the data under model k for the current study, and $p(k)$ is given by (9.2.12).

From (9.2.10), the joint prior distribution for $(\boldsymbol{\beta}^{(k)},\sigma^2,\rho)$ is given by

$$\begin{aligned}\pi(\boldsymbol{\beta}^{(k)},\sigma^2,\rho|D_0^{(k)}) &\propto \pi_0^*(\boldsymbol{\beta}^{(k)},\sigma^2,\rho|D_0^{(k)})\\ &= \int\pi_0^*(\boldsymbol{\beta}^{(k)},\sigma^2,\rho,\boldsymbol{a}_0|D_0^{(k)})\,d\boldsymbol{a}_0,\end{aligned} \tag{9.2.20}$$

where $\pi_0^*(\boldsymbol{\beta}^{(k)}, \sigma^2, \rho, \boldsymbol{a}_0 | D_0^{(k)})$ is given by (9.2.10). Then, using (9.2.20), the joint posterior distribution of $(\boldsymbol{\beta}^{(k)}, \sigma^2, \rho)$ under model k is given by

$$\begin{aligned}\pi(\boldsymbol{\beta}^{(k)}, \sigma^2, \rho | D^{(k)}) &\propto \pi^*(\boldsymbol{\beta}^{(k)}, \sigma^2, \rho | D^{(k)}) \\ &= L(\boldsymbol{\beta}^{(k)}, \sigma^2, \rho | D^{(k)}) \pi(\boldsymbol{\beta}^{(k)}, \sigma^2, \rho | D_0^{(k)}),\end{aligned} \tag{9.2.21}$$

where $L(\boldsymbol{\beta}^{(k)}, \sigma^2, \rho | D^{(k)})$ and $\pi(\boldsymbol{\beta}^{(k)}, \sigma^2, \rho | D_0^{(k)})$ are given by (9.2.6) and (9.2.20), respectively, and $\pi^*(\boldsymbol{\beta}^{(k)}, \sigma^2, \rho | D^{(k)})$ is an unnormalized joint posterior density function.

We are now led to the following lemma:

Lemma 9.2.1 *Under model k, let*

$$\pi(\beta^{(k)} | D_0^{(k)}) = \int \pi(\boldsymbol{\beta}^{(k)}, \sigma^2, \rho | D_0^{(k)}) \, d\sigma^2 \, d\rho$$

denote the marginal prior distribution of $\boldsymbol{\beta}^{(k)}$, and let

$$\pi(\boldsymbol{\beta}^{(k)} | D^{(k)}) = \int \pi(\boldsymbol{\beta}^{(k)}, \sigma^2, \rho | D^{(k)}) \, d\sigma^2 \, d\rho$$

denote the marginal posterior distribution of $\boldsymbol{\beta}^{(k)}$, where $\pi(\boldsymbol{\beta}^{(k)}, \sigma^2, \rho | D_0^{(k)})$ and $\pi(\boldsymbol{\beta}^{(k)}, \sigma^2, \rho | D^{(k)})$ are given by (9.2.20) and (9.2.21). Then, from (9.2.6) and (9.2.20), we have:

(i) $L(\boldsymbol{\beta}^{(k)}, \sigma^2, \rho | D^{(k)}) = L(\boldsymbol{\beta}^{(k)}, \boldsymbol{\beta}^{(-k)} = 0, \sigma^2, \rho | D^{(\mathcal{K})})$ *where* $L(\boldsymbol{\beta}^{(k)}, \boldsymbol{\beta}^{(-k)} = 0, \sigma^2, \rho | D^{(\mathcal{K})})$ *is the marginal likelihood function for the full model evaluated at* $\boldsymbol{\beta}^{(\mathcal{K})} = (\boldsymbol{\beta}^{(k)}, \boldsymbol{\beta}^{(-k)} = 0)$.

(ii) $\pi(\boldsymbol{\beta}^{(k)}, \sigma^2, \rho | D^{(k)}) = \pi(\boldsymbol{\beta}^{(k)}, \sigma^2, \rho | \boldsymbol{\beta}^{(-k)} = 0, D^{(\mathcal{K})})$, *where* $\pi(\boldsymbol{\beta}^{(k)}, \sigma^2, \rho | \boldsymbol{\beta}^{(-k)} = 0, D^{(\mathcal{K})})$ *is the conditional posterior density of* $\boldsymbol{\beta}^{(k)}$, σ^2, *and* ρ *given* $\boldsymbol{\beta}^{(-k)} = 0$ *obtained from the full model joint posterior density* $\pi(\boldsymbol{\beta}^{(\mathcal{K})}, \sigma^2, \rho | D^{(\mathcal{K})})$.

(iii) $\pi(\boldsymbol{\beta}^{(k)}, \sigma^2, \rho | D_0^{(k)}) = \pi(\boldsymbol{\beta}^{(k)}, \sigma^2, \rho | \boldsymbol{\beta}^{(-k)} = 0, D^{(\mathcal{K})})$ *where* $\pi(\boldsymbol{\beta}^{(k)}, \sigma^2, \rho | \boldsymbol{\beta}^{(-k)} = 0, D^{(\mathcal{K})})$ *is the conditional prior distribution of* $\boldsymbol{\beta}^{(k)}$, σ^2, *and* ρ *given* $\boldsymbol{\beta}^{(-k)} = 0$ *obtained from the full model joint prior density* $\pi(\boldsymbol{\beta}^{(\mathcal{K})}, \sigma^2, \rho | D_0^{(\mathcal{K})})$.

The proof of Lemma 9.2.1 is similar to that of Lemma 9.1.1, and thus is left as an exercise. From Lemma 9.2.1, we have the following key identity:

$$\frac{p(D^{(k)} | k)}{p(D^{(k)} | \mathcal{K})} = \frac{\pi(\boldsymbol{\beta}^{(-k)} = 0 | D^{(\mathcal{K})})}{\pi(\boldsymbol{\beta}^{(-k)} = 0 | D_0^{(\mathcal{K})})}, \quad k = 1, \ldots, \mathcal{K}, \tag{9.2.22}$$

where $\pi(\boldsymbol{\beta}^{(-k)} | D_0^{(\mathcal{K})})$ and $\pi(\boldsymbol{\beta}^{(-k)} | D^{(\mathcal{K})})$ denote the respective marginal prior and posterior distributions of $\boldsymbol{\beta}^{(-k)}$ obtained from the full model.

Finally, we are led to the following key result for computing the posterior model probability $p(k | D^{(k)})$:

Theorem 9.2.1 (i) *We can rewrite* $p(k)$ *given by* (9.2.12) *as*

$$p(k) = c_0^* \; \pi(\boldsymbol{\beta}^{(-k)} = 0|D^{(\mathcal{K})}), \tag{9.2.23}$$

where c_0^* *is a constant that does not depend on the model index* k.

(ii) *Equations* (9.2.23), (9.2.22), *and* (9.2.19) *yield*

$$p(k|D^{(k)}) = \frac{\pi(\boldsymbol{\beta}^{(-k)} = 0|D^{(\mathcal{K})})}{\sum_{j=1}^{\mathcal{K}} \pi(\boldsymbol{\beta}^{(-j)} = 0|D^{(\mathcal{K})})}, \tag{9.2.24}$$

$k = 1, \ldots, \mathcal{K}$, *where* $\pi(\boldsymbol{\beta}^{(-\mathcal{K})} = 0|D^{(\mathcal{K})}) = 1$.

The proof of the theorem is given in the Appendix.

The result in (9.2.24) is very attractive since it shows that the posterior model probability $p(k|D^{(k)})$ is simply a function of the marginal posterior density function of $\boldsymbol{\beta}^{(-k)}$ for the full model evaluated at $\boldsymbol{\beta}^{(-k)} = 0$. Thus, this result is very different from the one given in Theorem 9.1.1. The posterior model probability $p(k|D^{(k)})$ does not algebraically depend on the prior model probability $p(k)$ since it cancels out in the derivation due to the structure of $p(k)$. This is an important feature since it allows us to compute the posterior model probabilities directly *without* numerically computing the prior model probabilities. This has a clear computational advantage and as a result, allows us to compute posterior model probabilities very efficiently. We note that this computational device works best if all of the covariates are standardized to have mean 0 and variance 1. This is not restrictive since this is a typical transformation used quite often in practice to numerically stabilize the Gibbs sampler and the adaptive rejection sampling algorithm of Gilks and Wild (1992). If the covariates are not standardized, the posterior model probability $p(k|D^{(k)})$ is not invariant to scale changes in the covariates. Although $p(k|D^{(k)})$ given by (9.2.24) does not have the scale invariance property, the simulation study conducted by Ibrahim, Chen, and Ryan (1999) demonstrates that the above Bayesian variable selection procedure performs quite well in general, in which the true model obtains the largest posterior probability. In addition, the above procedure can be modified so that the posterior model probability is scale invariant. This modification can be achieved by specifying a prior distribution on model space similar to the one given in Subsection 9.1.5. However, the computation of the resulting posterior model probabilities will become much more expensive. We mention that $\pi(\boldsymbol{\beta}^{(-k)} = 0|D^{(\mathcal{K})})$ in (9.2.24) can be estimated by the efficient CMDE method given in Section 4.3, based on an MCMC sample from the reparameterized posterior $\pi(\boldsymbol{\beta}^{(k)}, \sigma^2, \rho, \boldsymbol{a}_0, \boldsymbol{\eta}, \boldsymbol{\eta}_0|D^{(k)})$ given in (9.2.16). The derivation of a Monte Carlo estimate of $p(k|D^{(k)})$ is left as an exercise. Finally, we note that the method discussed in this section can be used for variable selection in generalized linear mixed models (GLMMs). The time series model in (9.2.1) is essentially a generalization of a GLMM, and therefore, the methodology discussed here is applicable to the class of GLMMs. Next, we use the pollen count data example given in Ibrahim, Chen, and Ryan (1999) to illustrate the methodology.

Example 9.2. Pollen count data example. In Example 1.3, we present a detailed description of the pollen count data, which were collected daily in Kalamazoo, Michigan, from 1991 to 1994. The response variable y, is the pollen count for a particular day in the season for a given year. We take the 1991, 1992, and 1993 data as the historical data and the 1994 data as the current data. The full model contains an intercept and seven covariates. These are x_1 = rain, x_2 = day in the pollen season, x_3 = log(day), x_4 and x_5, which are the lowess smoothed function of temperature and the deviation from the daily average temperature to the lowess line, respectively, x_6 = windspeed, and x_7 = cold. Tables 1.3 and 1.4 summarize the response variable and covariate data for the four years.

We model the pollen counts as a Poisson distribution as in (9.2.3) with covariates $(x_1, \ldots, x_7)$. The model space $\mathcal{M}$ contains 2^7 models. We specify noninformative priors for ρ and σ^2. Specifically, we take a uniform prior for ρ on $[-1, 1]$ (i.e., $\nu_0 = \psi_0 = 1$) and take $\sigma^2 \sim \mathcal{IG}(0.005, 0.005)$. Table 9.4 give results for the model with the largest posterior probability based on several values of $(\mu_{a_0}, \sigma^2_{a_0})$. From Table 9.4, we see that the top model in each case is $(x_1, x_2, x_3, x_4, x_5)$. In addition, we see that the posterior model probabilities increase monotonically as more weight is given to the historical data. When we put very small weight on the historical data, such as $(\mu_{a_0}, \sigma^2_{a_0}) = (0.01, 9.7 \times 10^{-6})$ the $(x_1, x_2, x_3, x_4, x_5)$ model still obtains the largest posterior probability, with value 0.117. When we put extremely small weight on the historical data such as $(\mu_{a_0}, \sigma^2_{a_0}) = (0.001, 1.0 \times 10^{-7})$, the $(x_2, x_3, x_4, x_5, x_7)$ model obtains the largest posterior probability, with value 0.122 and the $(x_1, x_2, x_3, x_4, x_5)$ model obtains the fourth largest posterior probability with value 0.101. Thus, we see that model choice is reasonably robust to the choice of $(\mu_{a_0}, \sigma^2_{a_0})$, consistently yielding the $(x_1, x_2, x_3, x_4, x_5)$ model as the top model for a suitable range of $(\mu_{a_0}, \sigma^2_{a_0})$. Based on these analyses, it does not appear that the variables x_6 (windspeed) and x_7 (coldness of temperature) are important predictors of pollen count.

TABLE 9.4. Posterior Model Probabilities for Pollen Data.

Model	$(\mu_{a_0}, \sigma^2_{a_0})$	$p(k \mid D^{(k)})$
$(x_1, x_2, x_3, x_4, x_5)$	(0.50, 0.0119)	0.142
$(x_1, x_2, x_3, x_4, x_5)$	(0.50, 0.0061)	0.290
$(x_1, x_2, x_3, x_4, x_5)$	(0.50, 0.0041)	0.385
$(x_1, x_2, x_3, x_4, x_5)$	(0.50, 0.0025)	0.420
$(x_1, x_2, x_3, x_4, x_5)$	(0.98, 0.0004)	0.421

9.3 Stochastic Search Variable Selection

George and McCulloch (1993) develop a novel procedure called Stochastic Search Variable Selection (SSVS) for variable subset selection in linear regression. The basic idea is based on embedding the entire regression problem in a hierarchical Bayes normal mixture model, where latent variables are used to identify subset choices. In this framework, good models can be identified as those with higher posterior probability. SSVS then proceeds by using the Gibbs sampler to indirectly sampling from the resulting multinomial posterior distribution defined on the set of possible subset choices. Those subsets with higher probability can then be identified by their more frequent appearance in the Gibbs sample. In this way, SSVS avoids the problem of calculating posterior probabilities for all 2^p possible subset models. SSVS is controlled by various tuning parameters that can be prespecified by the user. With different specifications, the user can address the particular goals of variable selection that are appropriate for the problem under consideration. A distinguishing feature of SSVS is that it allows the user to let the practical importance of a variable influence its selection, rather than just its statistical significance.

The SSVS method can be described as follows. Consider the linear regression model

$$\boldsymbol{y} = X\boldsymbol{\beta} + \boldsymbol{\epsilon}, \tag{9.3.1}$$

where $\boldsymbol{y}$ is an $n \times 1$ vector of response variables, $X = (X_1, X_2, \ldots, X_p)$ is an $n \times p$ matrix of fixed covariates, $\boldsymbol{\beta} = (\beta_1, \ldots, \beta_p)'$, $\boldsymbol{\epsilon} \sim N_n(0, \sigma^2 I)$, and $(\boldsymbol{\beta}, \sigma^2)$ are considered unknown. For the model in (9.3.1), selecting a subset of covariates is equivalent to setting to zero those β_j's corresponding to the nonselected covariates. Let $D = (n, \boldsymbol{y}, X)$ denote the observed data.

To extract information relevant to variable selection, (9.3.1) is embedded in a larger hierarchical model. The key feature of the hierarchical model is that each component of $\boldsymbol{\beta}$ is modeled as having come from a mixture of two normal distributions with different variances. A similar setup in this context is also considered by Mitchell and Beauchamp (1988), who instead use "spike and slab" mixtures. An important distinction in the SSVS approach is that it does not put a probability mass on $\beta_j = 0$. By introducing the latent variable $\gamma_j = 0$ or 1, the normal mixture is represented by

$$\beta_j | \gamma_j \sim (1 - \gamma_j) N(0, \tau_j^2) + \gamma_j N(0, c_j^2 \tau_j^2) \tag{9.3.2}$$

and

$$P(\gamma_j = 1) = 1 - P(\gamma_j = 0) = p_j. \tag{9.3.3}$$

When $\gamma_j = 0$, $\beta_j \sim N(0, \tau_j^2)$, and when $\gamma_j = 1$, $\beta_j \sim N(0, c_j^2 \tau_j^2)$. Thus, setting τ_j (> 0) small so that if $\gamma_j = 0$, then β_j would probably be so small that it could "safely" be estimated by 0. Second, c_j is set large ($c_j > 1$ always) so that if $\gamma_j = 1$, then a nonzero estimate of β_j should probably be included in the final model. Based on this interpretation, p_j can be viewed as the prior probability that β_j will require a nonzero estimate, or equivalently that X_j should be included in the model.

Writing (9.3.2) in matrix notation, we get

$$\boldsymbol{\beta}|\boldsymbol{\gamma} \sim N_p(0, D_{\boldsymbol{\gamma}} R D_{\boldsymbol{\gamma}}), \tag{9.3.4}$$

where $\boldsymbol{\gamma} = (\gamma_1, \ldots, \gamma_p)'$, R is the prior correlation matrix, and

$$D_{\boldsymbol{\gamma}} = \text{diag}(d_1\tau_1, \ldots, d_p\tau_p),$$

with $d_j = 1$ if $\gamma_j = 0$ and $d_j = c_j$ if $\gamma_j = 1$. The matrix $D_{\boldsymbol{\gamma}}$ determines the scaling of the prior covariance matrix in such a way that (9.3.2) is satisfied. Common choices of R include $R = I$ or $R \propto (X'X)^{-1}$. Specific choices of τ_j and c_j are discussed below. To complete the hierarchical model, an inverse gamma conjugate prior is specified for $\sigma^2|\boldsymbol{\gamma}$, denoted $\sigma^2|\boldsymbol{\gamma} \sim \mathcal{IG}(\nu_{\boldsymbol{\gamma}}/2, \nu_{\boldsymbol{\gamma}}\lambda_{\boldsymbol{\gamma}}/2)$.

To identify the best subset models, the marginal posterior distribution of $\boldsymbol{\gamma}$ is obtained, which is given by

$$\pi(\boldsymbol{\gamma}|D) \propto \pi(\boldsymbol{y}|\boldsymbol{\gamma})\pi(\boldsymbol{\gamma}), \tag{9.3.5}$$

where $\pi(\boldsymbol{\gamma})$ is the prior distribution of $\boldsymbol{\gamma}$ implied by (9.3.3). Therefore, $\pi(\boldsymbol{\gamma})$ is the prior distribution for all of the possible subset models, and $\pi(\boldsymbol{\gamma}|D)$ is the posterior distribution for all of the subset models. SSVS specifies the hierarchical normal mixture model so that $\pi(\boldsymbol{\gamma}|D)$ puts most weight on the more "promising" subset models. Possible choices of $\pi(\boldsymbol{\gamma})$ include

$$\pi(\boldsymbol{\gamma}) = \prod_{j=1}^{p} p_j^{\gamma_j}(1-p_j)^{1-\gamma_j}, \tag{9.3.6}$$

which implies that the γ_j's are independent Bernoulli distributions a priori. Note that the uniform prior $\pi(\boldsymbol{\gamma}) = 2^{-p}$ is a special case of (9.3.6), which is obtained by setting $p_j = \frac{1}{2}$.

Rather than calculate all 2^p posterior probabilities in $\pi(\boldsymbol{\gamma}|D)$, SSVS uses the Gibbs sampler to generate an MCMC sample $\{\boldsymbol{\gamma}_l,\ l = 1, 2, \ldots, L\}$, which in many cases, converges rapidly to the posterior distribution of $\boldsymbol{\gamma}$. The Gibbs sampling scheme can be described as follows:

Step 1. Sample

$$\boldsymbol{\beta}_l \sim \pi(\boldsymbol{\beta}_l|\sigma_{l-1}, \boldsymbol{\gamma}_{l-1}, D) = N_p(A_{\boldsymbol{\gamma}_{l-1}}\sigma_{l-1}^{-2}X'X\hat{\boldsymbol{\beta}}, A_{\boldsymbol{\gamma}_{l-1}}), \tag{9.3.7}$$

where

$$A_{\boldsymbol{\gamma}_{l-1}} = [\sigma_{l-1}^{-2}X'X + D_{\boldsymbol{\gamma}_{l-1}}^{-1}R^{-1}D_{\boldsymbol{\gamma}_{l-1}}^{-1}]^{-1}.$$

Step 2. Sample

$$\begin{aligned}\sigma_l &\sim \pi(\sigma_l|\boldsymbol{\beta}_l, \gamma_{l-1}, D) \\ &= \mathcal{IG}\left(\frac{n+\nu_{\gamma_{l-1}}}{2}, \frac{(\boldsymbol{y}-X\boldsymbol{\beta}_l)'(\boldsymbol{y}-X\boldsymbol{\beta}_l)+\nu_{\gamma_{l-1}}\lambda_{\gamma_{l-1}}}{2}\right). \quad (9.3.8)\end{aligned}$$

Step 3. The vector $\boldsymbol{\gamma}_l$ is obtained componentwise by sampling from

$$\begin{aligned}\gamma_{j,l} &\sim \pi(\gamma_{j,l}|\boldsymbol{\beta}_l, \sigma_l, \gamma_{1,l}, \ldots, \gamma_{j-1,l}, \gamma_{j+1,l-1}, \ldots, \gamma_{p,l-1}, D) \\ &= \pi(\gamma_{j,l}|\boldsymbol{\beta}_l, \sigma_l, \gamma_{1,l}, \ldots, \gamma_{j-1,l}, \gamma_{j+1,l-1}, \ldots, \gamma_{p,l-1}), \quad (9.3.9)\end{aligned}$$

for $j = 1, 2, \ldots, p$.

Note that (9.3.9) does not depend on D, which results from the hierarchical structure of the model whereby $\boldsymbol{\gamma}$ affects D only through $\boldsymbol{\beta}$. Each distribution in (9.3.9) is Bernoulli with success probability

$$P(\gamma_{j,l} = 1|\boldsymbol{\beta}_l, \sigma_l, \gamma_{1,l}, \ldots, \gamma_{j-1,l}, \gamma_{j+1,l-1}, \ldots, \gamma_{p,l-1}) = \frac{a}{a+b}, \quad (9.3.10)$$

where

$$\begin{aligned}a &= \pi(\boldsymbol{\beta}_l|\gamma_{j,l} = 1, \gamma_{1,l}, \ldots, \gamma_{j-1,l}, \gamma_{j+1,l-1}, \ldots, \gamma_{p,l-1}) \\ &\times\ \pi(\sigma_l|\gamma_{j,l} = 1, \gamma_{1,l}, \ldots, \gamma_{j-1,l}, \gamma_{j+1,l-1}, \ldots, \gamma_{p,l-1}) \\ &\times\ \pi(\gamma_{j,l} = 1, \gamma_{1,l}, \ldots, \gamma_{j-1,l}, \gamma_{j+1,l-1}, \ldots, \gamma_{p,l-1})\end{aligned}$$

and

$$\begin{aligned}b &= \pi(\boldsymbol{\beta}_l|\gamma_{j,l} = 0, \gamma_{1,l}, \ldots, \gamma_{j-1,l}, \gamma_{j+1,l-1}, \ldots, \gamma_{p,l-1}) \\ &\times\ \pi(\sigma_l|\gamma_{j,l} = 0, \gamma_{1,l}, \ldots, \gamma_{j-1,l}, \gamma_{j+1,l-1}, \ldots, \gamma_{p,l-1}) \\ &\times\ \pi(\gamma_i^{(j)} = 0, \gamma_{1,l}, \ldots, \gamma_{j-1,l}, \gamma_{j+1,l-1}, \ldots, \gamma_{p,l-1}).\end{aligned}$$

When the prior parameters for σ are constant ($\nu_\gamma = \nu$ and $\lambda_\gamma = \lambda$), (9.3.10) can be obtained more simply by

$$a = \pi(\boldsymbol{\beta}_l|\gamma_{j,l} = 1, \gamma_{1,l}, \ldots, \gamma_{j-1,l}, \gamma_{j+1,l-1}, \ldots, \gamma_{p,l-1})p_j$$

and

$$b = \pi(\boldsymbol{\beta}_l|\gamma_{j,l} = 0, \gamma_{1,l}, \ldots, \gamma_{j-1,l}, \gamma_{j+1,l-1}, \ldots, \gamma_{p,l-1})(1 - p_j).$$

Further simplifications result when $R = I$.

Peng (1998) proposes several efficient weighted Monte Carlo methods for computing the normalizing constant of the posterior distribution, $\pi(\boldsymbol{\gamma}|D)$, given by (9.3.5). She obtains the fixed weight and data-dependent weight estimators of the normalizing constant. She also shows that the weighted estimators are better than the ones proposed by George and McCulloch (1997). Her methods are particularly useful for computing the normalizing constant of a discrete posterior distribution.

The choice of τ_j in (9.3.2) should be such that if $\beta_j \sim N(0, \tau_j^2)$, then β_j can be safely replaced by 0. Because $|\beta_j| \leq 3\tau_j$ with high probability, as a rough guide, one may want to select $3\tau_j$ equal to the maximum size at which β_j would, for practical purposes, be equivalent to zero. Unfortunately, this may not be easy or even possible, because ascertaining this maximum requires understanding the potential effect of β_j in the final model. The choice of c_j in (9.3.2) should be such that if $\beta_j \sim N(0, c_j^2\tau_j^2)$, then a nonzero estimate of β_j should be included in the final model. To help guide the choice of c_j, it may be useful to observe that the densities of $N(0, \tau_j^2)$ and $N(0, c_j^2\tau_j^2)$ intersect at $\xi(c_j)\tau_j$ when $\xi(c_j) = (2\ln(c_j)c_j^2/(c_j^2 - 1))^{1/2}$. This implies that the density of $N(0, c_j^2\tau_j^2)$ will be larger than the density of $N(0, \tau_j^2)$ if and only if $|\beta_j| > \xi(c_j)\tau_j$. This intersection point increases very slowly; for example, the choices $c_j = 10, 100, 1000, 10000$ correspond to $\xi(c_j) \approx 2.1, 3.1, 3.7, 4.3, 4.8$. It is useful to also observe that c_j is the ratio of the heights of $N(0, \tau_j^2)$ and $N(0, c_j^2\tau_j^2)$ at zero. Thus c_j can be interpreted as the prior odds that X_j should be excluded when β_j is very close to zero.

A semiautomatic approach to selecting τ_j and c_j may be obtained by considering the intersection point and relative heights at zero of the marginal densities $(\hat{\beta}_j|\sigma_{\beta_j}, \gamma_j = 0) \sim N(0, \sigma_{\beta_j}^2 + \tau_j^2)$ and $(\hat{\beta}_j|\sigma_{\beta_j}, \gamma_j = 1) \sim N(0, \sigma_{\beta_j}^2 + c_j^2\tau_j^2)$. Let $t_j\sigma_{\beta_j}$ denote the intersection point, where $\sigma_{\beta_j}^2$ is the variance of the least squares estimator $\hat{\beta}_j$. Because

$$P(\gamma_j = 1|\hat{\beta}_j, \sigma_{\beta_j}) > p_j \tag{9.3.11}$$

if and only if $\hat{\beta}_j/\sigma_{\beta_j} > t_j$, the point t_j may be thought of as the threshold at which the t statistic corresponds to an increased marginal probability that X_i should be included in the model. Small t_j would tend to favor more saturated models, whereas large t_j would yield more parsimonious models. The relative heights of the marginal densities of $\hat{\beta}_j$ at zero is given by

$$r_j = \left(\frac{\sigma_{\beta_j}^2/\tau_j^2 + c_j^2}{\sigma_{\beta_j}^2/\tau_j^2 + 1} \right). \tag{9.3.12}$$

The value of r_j is the marginal posterior probability of including X_j when $\hat{\beta}_j = 0$. The values of t_j and r_j in (9.3.11) and (9.3.12) are functions only of $\sigma\beta_j/\tau_j$ and c_j. Thus one might consider fixing $\hat{\sigma}\beta_j/\tau_j$ and c_j to obtain the desired values of t_j and r_j. George and McCulloch (1993) discuss the choices of c_j and τ_j and their implications in detail.

A strong feature of the SVSS algorithm is that it is computationally efficient and tailored to very large regression problems. However, it does require a lot of prior elicitation since the c_j's, τ_j's, and R have to be specified. In addition, the method does not allow for informative prior elicitation, and therefore one cannot incorporate real prior information. The SVSS methodology is quite general and can be adapted to other models including generalized linear models, time series models (see George, McCulloch, and Tsay, 1996), models for survival data, and models for longitudinal data.

The SVSS algorithm has been used in various contexts by several authors including Clyde, Desimone, and Parmigiani (1996), Chipman, Kolaczyk, and McCulloch (1997), and Chipman, George, and McCulloch (1998).

9.4 Bayesian Model Averaging

A popular approach to model selection is Bayesian Model Averaging (BMA). In this approach, one bases inference on an average of all possible models in the model space $\mathcal{M}$, instead of a single "best" model. Suppose $\mathcal{M} = \{\mathcal{M}_1, \ldots, \mathcal{M}_\mathcal{K}\}$, and let $\boldsymbol{\theta}$ denote the quantity of interest such as a future observation, a set of regression coefficients, or the utility of a course of action. The posterior distribution of $\boldsymbol{\theta}$ is then given by

$$\pi(\boldsymbol{\theta}|D) = \sum_{k=1}^{K} \pi(\boldsymbol{\theta}|D, \mathcal{M}_k) p(\mathcal{M}_k|D), \tag{9.4.1}$$

where D denotes the data, $\pi(\boldsymbol{\theta}|D, \mathcal{M}_k)$ is the posterior distribution of $\boldsymbol{\theta}$ under model $\mathcal{M}_k$, and $p(\mathcal{M}_k|D)$ is the posterior model probability. Equation (9.4.1), called BMA, consists of an average of the posterior distributions under each model weighted by the corresponding posterior model probabilities. The motivation behind BMA is based on the notion that a single "best" model ignores uncertainty about the model itself, which can result in underestimated uncertainties about quantities of interest, whereas BMA in (9.4.1) incorporates model uncertainty.

Averaging over all possible models as in (9.4.1) provides better predictive ability, as measured by a logarithmic scoring rule, than using any single model $\mathcal{M}_k$:

$$-E\left[\ln\left\{\sum_{j=1}^{\mathcal{K}} \pi(\boldsymbol{\theta}|D, \mathcal{M}_j) p(\mathcal{M}_j|D)\right\}\right] \le -E[\ln\{\pi(\boldsymbol{\theta}|D, \mathcal{M}_k)\}] \tag{9.4.2}$$

for $k = 1, \ldots, \mathcal{K}$, where $\boldsymbol{\theta}$ is the observable to be predicted and the expectation is taken with respect to $\sum_{j=1}^{\mathcal{K}} \pi(\boldsymbol{\theta}|D, \mathcal{M}_j) p(\mathcal{M}_j|D)$. This result follows from the nonnegativity of the Kullback–Leibler information divergence.

The implementation of BMA is difficult for two reasons. First, $p(\mathcal{M}_k|D)$ can be difficult to compute. Second, the number of terms in (9.4.1) can be enormous. One solution to reduce the number of possible models in (9.4.1) involves applying the Occam's window algorithm of Madigan and Raftery (1994). Two basic principles underlie this ad hoc approach. First, if a model predicts the data far less well than the model that provides the best predictions, then it has effectively been discredited and should no longer be considered. Thus models not belonging to

$$\mathcal{A}' = \left\{\mathcal{M}_k : \frac{\max_l\{p(\mathcal{M}_l|D)\}}{p(\mathcal{M}_k|D)} \le C\right\} \tag{9.4.3}$$

are excluded from (9.4.1), where C is chosen by the data analyst and $\max_l\{p(\mathcal{M}_l|D)\}$ denotes the model with the highest posterior probability. A common choice of C is $C = 20$. The number of models in Occam's window increases as C decreases. Second, appealing to Occam's razor, models that receive less support from the data than any other simpler models are excluded. That is, models from (9.4.1) are excluded if they belong to

$$\mathcal{B} = \left\{\mathcal{M}_k : \exists\, \mathcal{M}_l \in \mathcal{M}, \mathcal{M}_l \subset \mathcal{M}_k, \frac{p(\mathcal{M}_l|D)}{p(\mathcal{M}_k|D)} > 1\right\}. \qquad (9.4.4)$$

Thus (9.4.1) is replaced by

$$\pi(\boldsymbol{\theta}|D) = \frac{\sum_{\mathcal{M}_k\in\mathcal{A}} \pi(\boldsymbol{\theta}|D,\mathcal{M}_k)p(D|\mathcal{M}_k)p(\mathcal{M}_k)}{\sum_{\mathcal{M}_k\in\mathcal{A}} p(D|\mathcal{M}_k)p(\mathcal{M}_k)} \qquad (9.4.5)$$

where $\mathcal{A} = \mathcal{A}'\backslash\mathcal{B} \in \mathcal{M}$, $p(D|\mathcal{M}_k)$ is the marginal likelihood of the data D under model $\mathcal{M}_k$, and $p(\mathcal{M}_k)$ denotes the prior model probability.

This strategy greatly reduces the number of possible models in (9.4.1), and now all that is required is a search strategy to identify the models in $\mathcal{A}$. Two further principles underlie the search strategy. The first principle–Occam's window–concerns interpreting the ratio of posterior model probabilities $p(\mathcal{M}_1|D)/p(\mathcal{M}_0|D)$, where $\mathcal{M}_0$ is a model with one less predictor than $\mathcal{M}_1$. If there is evidence for $\mathcal{M}_0$, then $\mathcal{M}_1$ is rejected, but to reject $\mathcal{M}_0$, stronger evidence for the larger model $\mathcal{M}_1$ is required. These principles fully define the strategy. Madigan and Raftery (1994) provide a detailed description of the algorithm and mention that the number of terms in (9.4.1) is often reduced to fewer than 25.

The second approach for reducing the number of terms in (9.4.1) is to approximate (9.4.1) using an MCMC approach. Madigan and York (1995) propose the MCMC model composition (MC^3) methodology, which generates a stochastic process that moves through the model space. A Markov chain $\{\mathcal{M}(l), l = 1, 2, \ldots\}$ is constructed with state space $\mathcal{M}$ and equilibrium distribution $p(\mathcal{M}_k|D)$. If this Markov chain is simulated for $l = 1, \ldots, L$, then under certain regularity conditions, for any function $g(\mathcal{M}_k)$ defined on $\mathcal{M}$, the average

$$\hat{G} = \frac{1}{L}\sum_{l=1}^{L} g(\mathcal{M}(l))$$

converges almost surely to $E(g(\mathcal{M}_k))$ as $L \to \infty$. To compute (9.4.1) in this fashion, set $g(\mathcal{M}_k) = \pi(\boldsymbol{\theta}|D,\mathcal{M}_k)$. To construct the Markov chain, define a neighborhood $\text{nbd}(\mathcal{M}_*)$ for each $\mathcal{M}_* \in \mathcal{M}$ that consists of the model $\mathcal{M}_*$ itself and the set of models with either one variable more or one variable fewer than $\mathcal{M}_*$. Define a transition matrix q by setting $q(\mathcal{M}_* \to \mathcal{M}'_*) = 0$ for all $\mathcal{M}'_* \notin \text{nbd}(\mathcal{M}_*)$ and $q(\mathcal{M}_* \to \mathcal{M}'_*)$ constant for all $\mathcal{M}'_* \in \text{nbd}(\mathcal{M}_*)$. If the chain is currently in state $\mathcal{M}_*$, then we proceed by drawing $\mathcal{M}'_*$ from

$q(\mathcal{M}_* \to \mathcal{M}'_*)$. It is then accepted with probability

$$\min\left\{1, \frac{p(\mathcal{M}'_*|D)}{p(\mathcal{M}_*|D)}\right\}.$$

Otherwise, the chain stays in state $\mathcal{M}_*$.

To compute $p(D|\mathcal{M}_k)$, Raftery (1996) suggests the use of the Laplace approximation, leading to

$$\ln(p(D|\mathcal{M}_k)) = \ln(L(\hat{\boldsymbol{\theta}}_k|D, \mathcal{M}_k)) - p_k/2\ln(n) + O(1),$$

where n is the sample size, $L(\hat{\boldsymbol{\theta}}_k|D, \mathcal{M}_k))$ is the likelihood function, $\hat{\boldsymbol{\theta}}_k$ is the MLE of $\boldsymbol{\theta}$ under model $\mathcal{M}_k$, and p_k is the number of parameters in model $\mathcal{M}_k$.

We now describe BMA for the linear regression model as in Raftery, Madigan, and Hoeting (1997). For the linear model with conjugate priors, $p(D|\mathcal{M}_k)$ has a closed form, and therefore the Laplace approximation is not needed. Consider the priors $\boldsymbol{\beta} \sim N_p(\boldsymbol{\mu}, \sigma^2 V)$ and $\nu\lambda/\sigma^2 \sim \chi^2_\nu$, where ν, λ, the $p \times p$ matrix V, and the $p \times 1$ vector $\boldsymbol{\mu}$ are hyperparameters to be chosen. For this model, it can be shown that

$$\begin{aligned} p(D|\mathcal{M}_k) &= \frac{\Gamma([\nu+n]/2)(\nu\lambda)^{\nu/2}}{\pi^{n/2}\Gamma(\nu/2)|I + X_k V_k X'_k|^{1/2}} \\ &\quad \times [\lambda\nu + (\boldsymbol{y} - X_k\boldsymbol{\mu}_k)'((I|X_k V_k X'_k)^{-1}(\boldsymbol{y} - X_k\boldsymbol{\mu}_k)]^{-(\nu+n)/2}, \end{aligned} \tag{9.4.6}$$

where $\boldsymbol{y}$ is the vector of the observed values of the response variable, X_k is the covariate matrix, and $\boldsymbol{\mu}_k$ and V_k are the prior mean and covariance matrix of $\boldsymbol{\beta}$ under model $\mathcal{M}_k$. The Bayes factor for M_0 versus M_1 (i.e., the ratio of (9.4.6) for $k=0$ and $k=1$) is then given by

$$B_{01} = \left(\frac{|I + X_1V_1X'_1|}{|I + X_0V_0X'_0|}\right)^{1/2} (d_0/d_1)^{-(\nu+n)/2},$$

where $d_l = \lambda\nu + (\boldsymbol{y} - X_l\boldsymbol{\mu}_l)'(I + X_lV_lX'_l)^{-1}(\boldsymbol{y} - X_l\boldsymbol{\mu}_l)$, $l = 0, 1$.

To select the prior distributions, Raftery, Madigan, and Hoeting (1997) recommend the following. For noncategorical covariates, the individual $\boldsymbol{\beta}$'s are assumed independent a priori. The prior mean vector is taken to be $\boldsymbol{\mu} = (\hat{\boldsymbol{\beta}}_0, 0, \ldots, 0)'$, where $\hat{\boldsymbol{\beta}}_0$ is the ordinary least squares estimate of the intercept $\boldsymbol{\beta}_0$. The covariance matrix V is equal to σ^2 multiplied by a diagonal matrix with entries $(s^2_{\boldsymbol{y}}, \phi^2 s_1^{-2}, \phi^2 s_2^{-2}, \ldots, \phi^2 s_p^{-2})$, where $s^2_{\boldsymbol{y}}$ denotes the sample variance of $\boldsymbol{y}$, s^2_k denotes the sample variance of X_k for $k = 1, \ldots, p$, and ϕ is a hyperparameter to be chosen. The prior variance of $\boldsymbol{\beta}$ is chosen conservatively and represents an upper bound on the reasonable variance for this parameter. The variances of the remaining $\boldsymbol{\beta}$ parameters are chosen to reflect increasing precision about each $\boldsymbol{\beta}_k$ as the variance of the corresponding X_k increases. They are also chosen so that they are invariant to scale changes in both the predictor variables and the response variable.

For a categorical covariate X_k with $(c+1)$ possible outcomes $(c \geq 2)$, the Bayes factor should be invariant to the selection of the corresponding dummy variables $(X_{k1}, \ldots, X_{kc})$. Thus, the prior variance of $(\beta_{k1}, \ldots, \beta_{kc})$ is set equal to $\sigma^2\phi^2(1/nX^{k'}X^k)^{-1}$, where X^k is the $n \times c$ design matrix for the dummy variables, where each dummy variable has been centered by subtracting its sample mean. The complete prior covariance matrix for $\boldsymbol{\beta}$ is now given by

$$V(\boldsymbol{\beta}) = \sigma^2 \text{diag}(s_{\boldsymbol{y}}^2, \phi^2 s_1^{-2}, \ldots, \phi^2 s_{k-1}^{-2}, \phi^2(1/nX^{k'}X^k)^{-1}, \\ \phi^2 s_{k+1}^{-2}, \ldots, \phi^2 s_p^{-2}).$$

Assuming that all variables have been standardized to have mean 0 and variance 1, the remaining hyperparameters ν, λ, and ϕ, are chosen to satisfy the following conditions:

(i) the prior density $\pi(\beta_1, \ldots, \beta_p)$ is reasonably flat over the unit hypercube $[-1, 1]^p$;

(ii) $\pi(\sigma^2)$ is reasonably flat over $(d, 1)$ for some small d; and

(iii) $P(\sigma^2 \leq 1)$ is large.

For (iii), $P(\sigma^2 \leq 1)$ is maximized subject to the following conditions:

(a) $P(\beta_1 = 0, \ldots, \beta_p = 0)/P(\beta_2 = 1, \ldots, \beta_p = 1) \leq K_1$, where $K_1 = \sqrt{10}$ according to Jeffreys (1961);

(b) $\max_{d<\sigma^2<1} \left\{P(\sigma^2 = d)/\pi(\sigma^2)\right\} \leq K_2$; and

(c) $\max_{d<\sigma^2<1} \left\{P(\sigma^2 = 1)/\pi(\sigma^2)\right\} \leq K_2$.

A suitable choice of K_2 is $K_2 = 10$. For $d = 0.05$, this procedure yields $\nu = 2.58$, $\lambda = 0.28$ and $\phi = 2.85$, yielding $P(\sigma^2 \leq 1) = 0.81$.

BMA has also been extensively discussed for various other contexts. Madigan and Raftery (1994) and Kass and Raftery (1995) give a general development and motivation of BMA. Raftery, Madigan, and Volinsky (1995) and Volinsky, Madigan, Raftery, and Kronmal (1997) discuss BMA for proportional hazards models, and Raftery (1996) examines BMA for generalized linear models.

9.5 Reversible Jump MCMC Algorithm for Variable Selection

The Monte Carlo methods given in Sections 9.1 and 9.2 may not be feasible for problems involving more than 20 covariates. The main reason is that it is impossible to enumerate all possible models when the number of covariates is large. To overcome such computational limitations, Green (1995) proposes a novel reversible jump MCMC algorithm, which is attractive for Bayesian variable selection with a large number of covariates.

Suppose that we have a countable collection of candidate models $\{\mathcal{M}_k, k \in \mathcal{M}\}$, where model $\mathcal{M}_k$ has a vector $\boldsymbol{\theta}^{(k)}$ of unknown parameters, with dimension p_k, which may vary from model to model. Under model $\mathcal{M}_k$, the posterior distribution of $\boldsymbol{\theta}^{(k)}$ takes the form

$$\pi(\boldsymbol{\theta}^{(k)}|D, \mathcal{M}_k) \propto \pi^*(\boldsymbol{\theta}^{(k)}|D, \mathcal{M}_k) = L(\boldsymbol{\theta}^{(k)}|D, \mathcal{M}_k)\pi(\boldsymbol{\theta}_k|\mathcal{M}_k), \quad (9.5.1)$$

where $L(\boldsymbol{\theta}^{(k)}|D, \mathcal{M}_k)$ is the likelihood function, D denotes the data, $\pi(\boldsymbol{\theta}^{(k)}|\mathcal{M}_k)$ is the prior distribution, and $\pi^*(\boldsymbol{\theta}^{(k)}|D, \mathcal{M}_k)$ is the unnormalized posterior density. Then the joint distribution of $(k, \boldsymbol{\theta}^{(k)})$ given the data D takes the form

$$\pi(k, \boldsymbol{\theta}^{(k)}|D) \propto p(k)\pi^*(\boldsymbol{\theta}^{(k)}|D, \mathcal{M}_k). \quad (9.5.2)$$

Reversible jump MCMC is a flexible MCMC sampling strategy for generating samples from the joint distribution $\pi(k, \boldsymbol{\theta}^{(k)}|D)$ given in (9.5.2). The algorithm is based on constructing a Markov chain which can "jump" between models with parameter spaces of different dimension, while retaining a detailed balance that ensures the correct limiting distribution, provided the chain is irreducible and aperiodic.

The reversible jump MCMC algorithm has been discussed by several authors including Green (1995), Dellaportas, Forster, and Ntzoufras (1997), and Clyde (1999). It involves sampling from $\pi(k, \boldsymbol{\theta}_k|D)$, which can be described as follows:

Reversible Jump MCMC Algorithm

If the current state of the chain is $(k, \boldsymbol{\theta}^{(k)})$, then:

Step 1. Propose a new model $\mathcal{M}_{k^*}$ with probability $j(k^*|k)$.

Step 2. Generate $\boldsymbol{u}$ from a specified proposal density $q(\boldsymbol{u}|\boldsymbol{\theta}^{(k)}, k, k^*)$.

Step 3. Set $(\boldsymbol{\theta}^{*(k^*)}, \boldsymbol{u}^*) = g_{k,k^*}(\boldsymbol{\theta}^{(k)}, \boldsymbol{u})$, where g_{k,k^*} is a bijection between $(\boldsymbol{\theta}^{(k)}, \boldsymbol{u})$ and $(\boldsymbol{\theta}^{*(k^*)}, \boldsymbol{u}^*)$, and the lengths of $\boldsymbol{u}$ and $\boldsymbol{u}'$ must satisfy $p_k + \dim(\boldsymbol{u}) = p_{k^*} + \dim(\boldsymbol{u}^*)$.

Step 4. Accept the proposed move to $(k^*, \boldsymbol{\theta}^{*(k^*)})$ with probability

$$\alpha = \min\left\{1, \frac{p(k^*)\pi^*(\boldsymbol{\theta}^{*(k^*)}|D, \mathcal{M}_{k^*})j(k|k^*)q(\boldsymbol{u}^*|\boldsymbol{\theta}^{*(k^*)}, k^*, k)}{p(k)\pi^*(\boldsymbol{\theta}^{(k)}|D, \mathcal{M}_k)j(k^*|k)q(\boldsymbol{u}|\boldsymbol{\theta}^{(k)}, k, k^*)} \right.$$
$$\left. \times \left| \frac{\partial g_{k,k^*}(\boldsymbol{\theta}^{(k)}, \boldsymbol{u})}{\partial(\boldsymbol{\theta}^{(k)}, \boldsymbol{u})} \right| \right\}, \quad (9.5.3)$$

where $\pi^*(\boldsymbol{\theta}^{(k)}|D, \mathcal{M}_k)$ is given by (9.5.1).

Once an MCMC sample $\{k_l,\ l = 1, 2, \ldots, L\}$ is generated by the reversible jump MCMC algorithm, the posterior model probability $p(k|D)$ can be estimated by

$$\hat{p}(k|D) = \frac{1}{L} \sum_{l=1}^{L} 1_k(k_l), \tag{9.5.4}$$

where the indicator function $1_k(k_l) = 1$ if $k_l = k$ and $1_k(k_l) = 0$ if $k_l \neq k$. The simulation standard error is also easy to compute, and can be estimated by the usual standard error of the sample mean of $\{1_k(k_l),\ l = 1, 2, \ldots, L\}$, or more accurately by the overlapping batch means method given in Subsection 3.3.2.

Dellaportas, Forster, and Ntzoufras (1997) point out that when $q(\cdot)$ is the posterior distribution of $\boldsymbol{\theta}^{*(k^*)}$, then the acceptance probability simplifies to

$$\alpha = \min \left\{ 1, \frac{p(k^*)p(D|\mathcal{M}_{k^*})j(k|k^*)}{p(k)p(D|\mathcal{M}_k)j(k^*|k)} \right\}, \tag{9.5.5}$$

where $p(D|\mathcal{M}_k)$ the marginal distribution of the data D under model $\mathcal{M}_k$. In this case, there is no need to actually generate $\boldsymbol{u} = \boldsymbol{\theta}^{*(k^*)}$. The acceptance probability α given by (9.5.5) is useful only if the marginal distribution of the data is available in closed form, or can be computed using certain Monte Carlo methods such as those given in Subsections 9.1.6 and 9.2.5. In addition, Clyde (1999) points out that in linear models with conjugate prior distributions, both the SSVS (George and McCulloh 1997) and MC^3 (Raftery, Madigan, and Hoeting 1997) algorithms given in Sections 9.3 and 9.4 can be viewed as special cases of the reversible jump MCMC algorithm. Clyde (1999) also provides a detailed explanation for this, which we omit here for brevity.

Finally, we note that a more general version of the reversible jump MCMC algorithm is also available. This algorithm, called the Metropolized Carlin–Chib algorithm, was proposed by Godsill (1998), which is a generalization of Carlin and Chib's method (Carlin and Chib 1995). We describe this algorithm as follows. Let $\boldsymbol{\theta}^{(-k)}$ denote the vector of parameters that are not included in model $\mathcal{M}_k$, and also let $\boldsymbol{\theta} = (\boldsymbol{\theta}^{(k)}, \boldsymbol{\theta}^{(-k)})$. Consider a joint posterior distribution of $(k, \boldsymbol{\theta})$ that has the form

$$\begin{aligned} \pi(k, \boldsymbol{\theta}|D) &\propto \pi^*(k, \boldsymbol{\theta}|D) \\ &= p(k)L(\boldsymbol{\theta}^{(k)}|D, \mathcal{M}_k)\pi(\boldsymbol{\theta}^{(k)}|\mathcal{M}_k)\pi(\boldsymbol{\theta}^{(-k)}|\boldsymbol{\theta}^{(k)}, \mathcal{M}_k), \end{aligned} \tag{9.5.6}$$

where $\pi^*(k, \boldsymbol{\theta}|D)$ is the unnormalized posterior density, and $\pi(\boldsymbol{\theta}^{(-k)}|\boldsymbol{\theta}^{(k)}, \mathcal{M}_k)$ is called a pseudo-prior, also called a link prior density as in Carlin and Chib (1995). To sample from the joint distribution $\pi(k, \boldsymbol{\theta}|D)$ given by (9.5.6), Godsill (1998) proposes the following generalized reversible jump MCMC algorithm:

Metropolized Carlin–Chib Algorithm

If the current state of the chain is $(k, \boldsymbol{\theta})$, then:

Step 1. Generate $(k^*, \boldsymbol{\theta}^*)$ from a proposal transition kernel $q(k^*, \boldsymbol{\theta}^*|k, \boldsymbol{\theta})$.

Step 2. Accept the proposed move to $(k^*, \boldsymbol{\theta}^*)$ with probability

$$\alpha = \min\left\{1, \frac{\pi^*(k^*, \boldsymbol{\theta}^*|D)q(k, \boldsymbol{\theta}|k^*, \boldsymbol{\theta}^*)}{\pi^*(k, \boldsymbol{\theta}|D)q(k^*, \boldsymbol{\theta}^*|k, \boldsymbol{\theta})}\right\}, \tag{9.5.7}$$

where $\pi^*(k, \boldsymbol{\theta}|D)$ is given by (9.5.6).

The Metropolized Carlin–Chib algorithm is very simple and general, which includes the reversible jump MCMC algorithm as a special case. For instance, when we choose

$$q(k^*, \boldsymbol{\theta}^*|k, \boldsymbol{\theta}) = j(k^*|k)\pi(\boldsymbol{\theta}^{*(k^*)}|D, \mathcal{M}_{k^*})\pi(\boldsymbol{\theta}^{*(-k^*)}|\boldsymbol{\theta}^{*(k^*)}, \mathcal{M}_{k^*}), \tag{9.5.8}$$

where $\pi(\boldsymbol{\theta}^{*(k^*)}|D, \mathcal{M}_{k^*})$ is the posterior distribution of $\boldsymbol{\theta}^{*(k^*)}$ under model $\mathcal{M}_{k^*}$, then it can be shown that the acceptance probability α given by (9.5.7) reduces to (9.5.5). Unlike the reversible jump MCMC algorithm, a Markov chain induced by the Metropolized Carlin–Chib algorithm always moves in the parameter space of the same dimension. In addition, if $q(k, \boldsymbol{\theta}|k^*, \boldsymbol{\theta}^*)$ is chosen to have the form similar to (9.5.8), then: (i) no random generation is needed from the pseudo-prior; and (ii) no calculation of the pseudo-prior is required, since $\pi(\boldsymbol{\theta}^{(-k^*)}|\boldsymbol{\theta}^{(k^*)}, \mathcal{M}_{k^*})$ cancels out in the ratio of α.

Appendix

Proof of Theorem 9.2.1. From (9.2.20) and (9.2.11), it can be observed that

$$\int \pi_0^*(\boldsymbol{\beta}^{(\mathcal{K})}, \sigma^2, \rho|D_0^{(\mathcal{K})})\, d\boldsymbol{\beta}^{(\mathcal{K})}\, d\sigma^2\, d\rho = \frac{\pi_0^*(\boldsymbol{\beta}^{(k)}, \boldsymbol{\beta}^{(-k)} = 0, \sigma^2, \rho|D_0^{(\mathcal{K})})}{\pi(\boldsymbol{\beta}^{(k)}, \boldsymbol{\beta}^{(-k)} = 0, \sigma^2, \rho|D_0^{(\mathcal{K})})}, \tag{9.A.1}$$

and

$$\int \pi_0^*(\boldsymbol{\beta}^{(k)}|D_0^{(k)})\, d\boldsymbol{\beta}^{(k)} = \frac{\pi_0^*(\boldsymbol{\beta}^{(k)}, \sigma^2, \rho|D_0^{(k)})}{\pi(\boldsymbol{\beta}^{(k)}, \sigma^2, \rho|D_0^{(k)})}. \tag{9.A.2}$$

Then, (9.2.20) and Lemma 9.2.1 lead to

$$\pi_0^*(\boldsymbol{\beta}^{(k)}, \boldsymbol{\beta}^{(-k)} = 0, \sigma^2, \rho|D_0^{(\mathcal{K})}) = \pi_0^*(\boldsymbol{\beta}^{(k)}, \sigma^2, \rho|D_0^{(k)}),$$

and

$$\pi(\boldsymbol{\beta}^{(k)}, \boldsymbol{\beta}^{(-k)} = 0, \sigma^2, \rho | D_0^{(\mathcal{K})})$$
$$= \pi(\boldsymbol{\beta}^{(-k)} = 0 | D_0^{(\mathcal{K})}) \pi(\boldsymbol{\beta}^{(k)}, \sigma^2, \rho | D_0^{(k)}). \tag{9.A.3}$$

The above two identities yield

$$\int \pi_0^*(\boldsymbol{\beta}^{(\mathcal{K})}, \sigma^2, \rho | D_0^{(\mathcal{K})}) \, d\boldsymbol{\beta}^{(\mathcal{K})} \, d\sigma^2 \, d\rho = \frac{\int \pi_0^*(\boldsymbol{\beta}^{(k)} | D_0^{(k)}) \, d\boldsymbol{\beta}^{(k)}}{\pi(\boldsymbol{\beta}^{(-k)} = 0 | D_0^{(\mathcal{K})})}. \tag{9.A.4}$$

Thus, the result given in (9.2.23) directly follows from (9.A.4) and (9.2.12). Note that in (9.2.23),

$$c_0^* = \frac{\int \pi_0^*(\boldsymbol{\beta}^{(\mathcal{K})}, \sigma^2, \rho | D_0^{(\mathcal{K})}) \, d\boldsymbol{\beta}^{(\mathcal{K})} \, d\sigma^2 \, d\rho}{\sum_{j=1}^{\mathcal{K}} \int \pi_0^*(\boldsymbol{\beta}^{(j)} | D_0^{(j)}) \, d\boldsymbol{\beta}^{(j)}},$$

which is independent of the model index k. Therefore, (9.2.24) immediately follows from (9.2.23), (9.2.22), and (9.2.19).

Finally, we note that unlike Theorem 9.1.1, the Savage–Dickey density ratio cannot be used to prove Theorem 9.2.1. We give a brief explanation as follows. If we treat $\pi_0(\boldsymbol{\beta}^{(\mathcal{K})} | D_0^{(\mathcal{K})})$ as a "posterior" distribution based on data $D_0^{(\mathcal{K})}$, then, from (9.2.11), the "prior" distribution corresponding to this "posterior" distribution is uniform, and therefore is improper. Thus, the condition for the Savage–Dickey density ratio is not satisfied. Therefore, we cannot use the Savage–Dickey density ratio to simplify the ratio, $p(k)/p(\mathcal{K})$, to compute the prior model probabilities. □

Exercises

9.1 Use standard distribution theory to prove Lemma 9.1.1.

9.2 Use Lemma 9.1.1 and the Savage–Dickey density ratio to prove Theorem 9.1.1.

9.3 Similar to (9.1.14), derive an estimator, denoted by $\hat{p}(k|D^{(k)})$, of the posterior model probability $p(k|D^{(k)})$ using (9.1.22) along with the IWMDE method.

9.4 Derive the simulation standard error (s.e.) of $\hat{p}(k|D^{(k)})$ obtained in Exercise 9.3, based on a first-order approximation of the asymptotic mean square error of $\hat{p}(k|D^{(k)})$ as discussed in Section 5.7.

9.5 Let $\alpha_0 > 0$, $\lambda_0 > 0$. Show that there exists a constant $K = K(\alpha_0, \lambda_0) > 0$, such that $\forall\, 0 \le \xi \le 1$,

$$\int_0^1 \xi^{a_0} a_0^{\alpha_0 - 1} (1 - a_0)^{\lambda_0 - 1} \, da_0 \le K(1 + \ln(1/\xi))^{-\alpha_0}. \tag{9.E.1}$$

9.6 For the general exponential family model with discrete outcomes given in Subsections 9.2.1 and 9.2.2, assume that

$$\exp\{(y_{0it}\theta_{0it} - q(\theta_{0it})) - c(y_{0it})\} \le M, \qquad (9.E.2)$$

for $t = 1, 2, \ldots, n_{0i}$, $i = 1, 2, \ldots, N$, where M is some finite constant. Suppose there exist $y_{0it_{i1}}$, $y_{0it_{i2}}$, $\ldots$, $y_{0it_{ip_k}}$ $(1 \le t_{i1} \le t_{i2} \le \cdots \le t_{ip_k})$ such that

$$\int_{-\infty}^{\infty} e^{d_0|\eta|} \exp\{(y_{0it_j} h(\eta) - q(h(\eta))\} \, d\eta < \infty \qquad (9.E.3)$$

for some $d_0 > 0$ and $j = 1, 2, \ldots, p_k$, and the corresponding design matrix $(x_{0it_1}^{(k)}, x_{0it_2}^{(k)}, \ldots, x_{0it_{p_k}}^{(k)})'$ has full rank p_k. Show that if $\alpha_0 > p_k/N$, $\lambda_0 > 0$, and (9.E.3) holds, then the joint prior distribution $\pi(\boldsymbol{\beta}^{(k)}, \sigma^2, \rho, \boldsymbol{a}_0 | D_0^{(k)})$ given by (9.2.10) is proper.
(*Hint*: Use Exercise 9.5.)

9.7 Prove Lemma 9.2.1.

9.8 Prove the identity given by (9.2.22).

9.9 Assume that $\{(\boldsymbol{\beta}_l^{(\mathcal{K})}, \sigma_l^2, \rho_l, \boldsymbol{a}_{0,l}, \boldsymbol{\eta}_l, \boldsymbol{\eta}_{0,l}),\ l = 1, 2, \ldots, L\}$ is an MCMC sample from the reparameterized posterior $\pi(\boldsymbol{\beta}^{(k)}, \sigma^2, \rho, \boldsymbol{a}_0, \boldsymbol{\eta}, \boldsymbol{\eta}_0 | D^{(k)})$ given by (9.2.16). Use the CMDE method given in Section 4.3 to derive a consistent estimate of the posterior model probability $p(k|D^{(k)})$ given by (9.2.24).

9.10 Derive formulas (9.3.7) and (9.3.8)

9.11 Consider the following simulation: generate $n = 200$ independent observations from the linear model

$$y_i = -1.0 - 0.5x_{i1} - 2.0x_{i3} + \epsilon_i, \quad i = 1, \ldots, n, \qquad (9.E.4)$$

where x_{i1} and x_{i3} are i.i.d. normal random variables with means 1.0 and 0.8, and variances 1.0, and 0.8, respectively, and $\epsilon \sim N(0, 0.25)$. Generate two additional covariates (x_{i2}, x_{i4}) such that the joint distribution of $x_i = (x_{i1}, \ldots, x_{i4})'$ is $N_4(\mu, \Sigma)$, where $\mu = (1.0, 0.5, 0.8, 1.4)$ and

$$\Sigma = \begin{pmatrix} 1.0 & 0.353 & 0 & 0 \\ 0.353 & 0.5 & 0 & 0 \\ 0 & 0 & 0.8 & 0.588 \\ 0 & 0 & 0.588 & 1.2 \end{pmatrix}.$$

Thus the full model consists of the four covariates $(x_1, \ldots, x_4)$ and the true model contains (x_1, x_3).

(a) Use the semiautomatic method described in Section 9.3 to compute c_j and τ_j for $j = 1, \ldots, 4$.

(b) Using the c_j and τ_j values in Part (a), $p_j = \frac{1}{2}$, and $R = I$, carry out the SVSS algorithm and summarize the posterior distribution of γ.

(c) Do a sensitivity analysis on the posterior distribution of γ in Part (b) by varying c_j, τ_j, and R.

(d) Logistic Regression: Suppose instead of model (9.E.4) we generate $n = 200$ independent Bernoulli observations with success probability

$$p_i = \frac{\exp\{-1.0 - 0.5x_{i1} - 2.0x_{i3}\}}{1 + \exp\{-1.0 - 0.5x_{i1} - 2.0x_{i3}\}}, \quad i = 1, \ldots, n,$$

where $(x_{i1}, \ldots, x_{i4})$ are the same covariate values as those generated above. Using $c_j = 5$, $\tau_j = 0.5$, $p_j = 0.5$, $j = 1, \ldots, 4$, and $R = I$, carry out the SVSS procedure and summarize the posterior distribution of γ.

9.12 Prove (9.4.2).

9.13 Derive formula (9.4.6).

9.14 Consider the simulation described in Exercise 9.11 for the linear regression model.

(a) Compute $\pi(D|\mathcal{M}_j)$ for $j = 1, \ldots, 16$, using the priors described in Section 9.4 with $\phi = 5$, $\nu = \lambda = 0.01$.

(b) Use Part (a) to compute the Bayes factor of model $\mathcal{M}_0 = \{(x_1, x_3)\}$ against the full model $\mathcal{M}_1 = \{(x_1, \ldots, x_4)\}$. What is your conclusion?

9.15 For the reversible jump MCMC algorithm, show that when $q(\cdot)$ is the posterior distribution of $\boldsymbol{\theta}^{(k^*)}$, then the acceptance probability α given by (9.5.3) simplifies to (9.5.5).

9.16 Show that Chib's Metropolized algorithm with the proposal transition kernel $q(k^*, \boldsymbol{\theta}^* | k, \boldsymbol{\theta})$ given by (9.5.8) reduces to the reversible jump MCMC algorithm with the acceptance probability given by (9.5.5).

10

Other Topics

In this last chapter of the book, we discuss several other related Monte Carlo methods commonly used in Bayesian computation. More specifically, we present various Bayesian methods for model adequacy and related computational techniques, including Monte Carlo estimation of Conditional Predictive Ordinates (CPO) and various Bayesian residuals. This chapter also provides a detailed treatment of the computation of posterior modes, and sampling from posterior distributions for proportional hazards models and mixture of Dirichlet process models.

10.1 Bayesian Model Adequacy

10.1.1 Predictive Approach

Assessing model adequacy is very important and fundamental in Bayesian data analysis, since the analysis can be misleading when the model is not adequate. The literature on Bayesian model adequacy is very extensive; for example, see Box (1980), Geisser (1987, 1993), Gelfand, Dey, and Chang (1992), Gelman, Meng, and Stern (1996), Dey, Kuo and Sahu (1995), Dey, Chen, and Chang (1997), and many others. Regarding the complementary roles of the predictive and posterior distributions in Bayesian data analysis, Box (1980) notes that the posterior distribution provides a basis for "estimation of parameters conditional on the adequacy of the entertained model" while the predictive distribution enables "criticism of the entertained model in light of current data." In this spirit, Gelfand, Dey, and

Chang (1992) consider a cross-validation approach, in which the predictive distribution is used in various ways to assess model adequacy. The main idea of this cross-validation approach is to validate conditional predictive distributions arising from single observation deletion against observed responses. A detailed formulation and related computations of this method will be discussed in this subsection. Other related methods are also available, which can be found in Gelman, Carlin, Stern, and Rubin (1995) and the references therein.

Let $\boldsymbol{y} = (y_1, y_2, \ldots, y_n)'$ denote the $n \times 1$ vector of the observed responses. Let X denote the $n \times p$ matrix of covariates whose i^{th} row $\boldsymbol{x}_i'$ is associated with y_i. Then, the observed data can be written as $D = (n, \boldsymbol{y}, X)$. Also let $\boldsymbol{y}^{(-i)}$ denote the $(n-1) \times 1$ response vector with y_i deleted, let $X^{(-i)}$ denote the $(n-1) \times p$ matrix that is X with the ith row $\boldsymbol{x}_i'$ deleted, and the resulting observed data are written as $D^{(-i)} = ((n-1), \boldsymbol{y}^{(-i)}, X^{(-i)})$. In addition, let $\boldsymbol{\theta}$ be the vector of model parameters. We assume that $y_i \sim f(y_i|\boldsymbol{\theta}, \boldsymbol{x}_i)$ and we let $\pi(\theta)$ denote the prior distribution of θ. Then, the posterior distribution of $\boldsymbol{\theta}$ based on the data D is given by

$$\pi(\boldsymbol{\theta}|D) \propto \left[\prod_{i=1}^{n} f(y_i|\boldsymbol{\theta}, \boldsymbol{x}_i)\right] \pi(\theta), \tag{10.1.1}$$

and the posterior distribution of $\boldsymbol{\theta}$ based on the data $D^{(-i)}$ is given by

$$\pi(\boldsymbol{\theta}|D^{(-i)}) \propto \left[\prod_{j \neq i} f(y_j|\boldsymbol{\theta}, \boldsymbol{x}_j)\right] \pi(\theta). \tag{10.1.2}$$

Let $\boldsymbol{z} = (z_1, z_2, \ldots, z_n)'$ denote future values of a replicate experiment. The usual prior predictive density is given by

$$\pi(z_i) = \int f(z_i|\boldsymbol{\theta}, \boldsymbol{x}_i)\pi(\boldsymbol{\theta})\, d\boldsymbol{\theta}.$$

Gelfand, Dey, and Chang (1992) note that $\pi(z_i)$ is improper if $\pi(\boldsymbol{\theta})$ is improper, making it difficult to use in model checking. Let $\pi(z_i|\boldsymbol{x}_i, D^{(-i)})$ denote the conditional density of z_i given $\boldsymbol{x}_i$ and $D^{(-i)}$ defined as

$$\pi(z_i|\boldsymbol{x}_i, D^{(-i)}) = \int f(z_i|\boldsymbol{\theta}, \boldsymbol{x}_i)\pi(\theta|D^{(-i)})\, d\boldsymbol{\theta}, \tag{10.1.3}$$

for $i = 1, 2, \ldots, n$. Then, $\pi(z_i|\boldsymbol{x}_i, D^{(-i)})$ is proper, since $\pi(\boldsymbol{\theta}|D^{(-i)})$ is proper. We note that when $\pi(\boldsymbol{\theta})$ is improper, $\pi(\boldsymbol{\theta}|D^{(-i)})$ is still proper under some very mild regularity conditions.

The conditional predictive density $\pi(z_i|\boldsymbol{x}_i, D^{(-i)})$ is also called the cross-validated predictive density. This density is to be checked against y_i, for $i = 1, 2, \ldots, n$ in the sense that, if the model holds, y_i may be viewed as a random observation from $\pi(z_i|\boldsymbol{x}_i, D^{(-i)})$. To do this, we consider a checking function $g(z_i, y_i)$ (Box 1980), whose expectation under $\pi(z_i|\boldsymbol{x}_i, D^{(-i)})$ is calculated and is denoted by g_i. One possible choice of $g(z_i, y_i)$ is

$$g_\epsilon(z_i, y_i) = \frac{1}{2\epsilon} 1\{z_i \in I_i(\epsilon)\},$$

where $\epsilon > 0$, $1\{z_i \in I_i(\epsilon)\}$ denotes the indicator function of the interval $I_i(\epsilon)$, with $I_i(\epsilon) = \{z_i : |z_i - y_i| \leq \epsilon\}$, yielding

$$g_i(\epsilon) = \frac{1}{2\epsilon} \int_{I_i(\epsilon)} \pi(z_i|\boldsymbol{x}_i, D^{(-i)})\, dz_i.$$

The Conditional Predictive Ordinate (CPO), which was first proposed by Geisser (1980) and further discussed in Gelfand, Dey, and Chang (1992), is obtained by letting $\epsilon \to 0$, i.e.,

$$\text{CPO}_i = \lim_{\epsilon \to 0} g_i(\epsilon) = \pi(y_i|\boldsymbol{x}_i, D^{(-i)}). \tag{10.1.4}$$

CPO_i is a very useful quantity for model checking, since it describes how much the ith observation supports the model. Large CPO values indicate a good fit. Another possible choice of $g(z_i, y_i)$ is

$$g(z_i, y_i) = \frac{y_i - z_i}{\sqrt{\text{Var}(z_i|\boldsymbol{x}_i, D^{(-i)})}},$$

which yields the Bayesian standardized residual

$$d_i = E[g(z_i, y_i)|\boldsymbol{x}_i, D^{(-i)}] = \frac{y_i - E(z_i|\boldsymbol{x}_i, D^{(-i)})}{\sqrt{\text{Var}(z_i|\boldsymbol{x}_i, D^{(-i)})}}, \tag{10.1.5}$$

where $\text{Var}(z_i|\boldsymbol{x}_i, D^{(-i)})$ is the variance of z_i with respect to the predictive distribution $\pi(z_i|\boldsymbol{x}_i, D^{(-i)})$ given by (10.1.3). The Bayesian standardized residuals, d_i, play a similar role as the Studentized residuals with the current observation deleted. Large $|d_i|$'s cast doubt upon the model but retaining the sign of d_i allows patterns of under or over fitting to be revealed. Gelfand, Dey, and Chang (1992) also consider several other choices of $g(z_i, y_i)$.

In general, given the checking function $g(z_i, y_i)$, we want to compute

$$\begin{aligned} g_i &= E(g(z_i, y_i)|\boldsymbol{x}_i, D^{(-i)}) \\ &= \int\int g(z_i, y_i) f(z_i|\boldsymbol{\theta}, \boldsymbol{x}_i)\pi(\boldsymbol{\theta}|D^{(-i)}))\, dz_i\, d\boldsymbol{\theta}. \end{aligned} \tag{10.1.6}$$

Since the right-hand side of (10.1.6) contains a multidimensional integral, it is very difficult or even impossible to find an analytical expression for g_i. To circumvent this problem, we use Monte Carlo integration. One possible approach is: (i) to generate a Markov chain Monte Carlo (MCMC) sample $\{(z_{i,l}, \boldsymbol{\theta}_l),\ l = 1, 2, \ldots, L\}$ from the joint distribution $f(z_i|\boldsymbol{\theta}, \boldsymbol{x}_i)\pi(\boldsymbol{\theta}|D^{(-i)}))$; and (ii) to approximate g_i by $\hat{g}_i = \sum_{l=1}^L g(z_{i,l})$. Although this approach is straightforward, sampling from the joint distribution of $(z_i, \boldsymbol{\theta})$ is expensive, since $f(z_i|\boldsymbol{\theta}, \boldsymbol{x}_i)\pi(\boldsymbol{\theta}|D^{(-i)}))$ depends on i. To overcome this difficulty, using (10.1.1) and (10.1.2), we can rewrite (10.1.6) as

$$g_i = \int\int g(z_i, y_i) f(z_i|\boldsymbol{\theta}, \boldsymbol{x}_i)\pi(\boldsymbol{\theta}|D^{(-i)})) \, d\boldsymbol{\theta} \, dz_i$$
$$= \frac{\int\int [g(z_i, y_i)/f(y_i|\boldsymbol{\theta}, \boldsymbol{x}_i)] f(z_i|\boldsymbol{\theta}, \boldsymbol{x}_i)\pi(\boldsymbol{\theta}|D) \, dz_i \, d\boldsymbol{\theta}}{\int [1/f(y_i|\boldsymbol{\theta}, \boldsymbol{x}_i)]\pi(\boldsymbol{\theta}|D) \, d\boldsymbol{\theta}}. \tag{10.1.7}$$

Assume $\{(\boldsymbol{z}_l = (z_{1,l}, z_{2,l}, \ldots, z_{n,l})', \boldsymbol{\theta}_l), \; l = 1, 2, \ldots, L\}$ is an MCMC sample from the joint distribution $\prod_{i=1}^n f(z_i|\boldsymbol{\theta}, \boldsymbol{x}_i)\pi(\boldsymbol{\theta}|D)$. Then, g_i can be estimated simultaneously by

$$\hat{g}_i = \frac{(1/L)\sum_{l=1}^L [g(z_{i,l}, y_i)/f(y_i|\boldsymbol{\theta}_l, \boldsymbol{x}_i)]}{(1/L)\sum_{l=1}^L [1/f(y_i|\boldsymbol{\theta}_l, \boldsymbol{x}_i)]}, \tag{10.1.8}$$

for $i = 1, 2, \ldots, n$. When a closed form of

$$E[(g_i(z_i, y_i)|\boldsymbol{\theta}, \boldsymbol{x}_i)] = \int g(z_i, y_i) f(z_i|\boldsymbol{\theta}, \boldsymbol{x}_i) \, dz_i$$

is available, (10.1.8) can be simplified as

$$\hat{g}_i = \frac{(1/L)\sum_{l=1}^L E[g(z_i, y_i|\boldsymbol{\theta}_l, \boldsymbol{x}_i)]/f(y_i|\boldsymbol{\theta}_l, \boldsymbol{x}_i)}{(1/L)\sum_{l=1}^L 1/f(y_i|\boldsymbol{\theta}_l, \boldsymbol{x}_i)},$$

and in this case, the sample $\{\boldsymbol{z}_l\}$ is no longer needed. Interestingly, the reciprocal of the denominator of (10.1.8) is indeed a Monte Carlo estimator of CPO_i. To see this, we can rewrite CPO_i given by (10.1.4) as

$$\text{CPO}_i = f(y_i|\boldsymbol{x}_i, D^{(-i)}) = \left(\int \frac{1}{f(y_i|\boldsymbol{\theta}_l, \boldsymbol{x}_i)} \pi(\boldsymbol{\theta}|D) \, d\boldsymbol{\theta}\right)^{-1}.$$

Thus, a Monte Carlo approximation of CPO_i is given by

$$\widehat{\text{CPO}}_i = \left(\frac{1}{L}\sum_{l=1}^L \frac{1}{f(y_i|\boldsymbol{\theta}_l, \boldsymbol{x}_i)}\right)^{-1}. \tag{10.1.9}$$

Next, we use the constrained multiple linear regression model and the bivariate normal model for human twin data to illustrate the derivation of the CPO_i's, univariate and bivariate Bayesian standardized residuals.

Example 10.1. Constrained multiple linear regression model (Example 2.2 continued). For the constrained multiple linear regression model defined in (1.3.1), the joint posterior distribution $\pi(\boldsymbol{\beta}, \sigma^2|D)$ is given by (2.1.7). Using (4.1.7), we have

$$f(z_i|\boldsymbol{\beta}, \sigma^2, \boldsymbol{x}_i) = \frac{1}{\sqrt{2\pi}\sigma} \exp\left\{-\frac{(z_i - \boldsymbol{x}_i'\boldsymbol{\beta})^2}{2\sigma^2}\right\},$$

where $\boldsymbol{x}_i = (x_{i1}, x_{i2}, \ldots, x_{i,10})'$. Thus,

$$E(z_i|\boldsymbol{x}_i, D^{(-i)}) = \int (\boldsymbol{x}_i'\boldsymbol{\beta})\pi(\boldsymbol{\beta}, \sigma^2|D^{(-i)})\, d\boldsymbol{\beta}\, d\sigma^2.$$

Let $\{(\boldsymbol{\beta}_l, \sigma_l^2),\ l = 1, 2, \ldots, L\}$ denote an MCMC sample from $\pi(\boldsymbol{\beta}, \sigma^2|D)$ using the Gibbs sampler given in Section 2.1. Then, the Monte Carlo estimate of CPO_i is given by

$$\widehat{\text{CPO}}_i = L\left[\sum_{l=1}^{L} \left(f(y_i|\boldsymbol{\beta}_l, \sigma_l^2, \boldsymbol{x}_i)\right)^{-1}\right]^{-1}, \tag{10.1.10}$$

and the Monte Carlo estimates of $E(z_i|\boldsymbol{x}_i, D^{(-i)})$ and $\text{Var}(z_i|\boldsymbol{x}_i, D^{(-i)})$ are given by

$$\hat{E}(z_i|\boldsymbol{x}_i, D^{(-i)})) = \widehat{\text{CPO}}_i L^{-1} \sum_{l=1}^{L} \frac{\boldsymbol{x}_i'\boldsymbol{\beta}_l}{f(y_i|\boldsymbol{\beta}_l, \sigma_l^2, \boldsymbol{x}_i)}, \tag{10.1.11}$$

and

$$\begin{aligned}
&\widehat{\text{Var}}(z_i|\boldsymbol{x}_i, D^{(-i)})) \\
&\quad = \hat{E}(z_i^2|\boldsymbol{x}_i, D^{(-i)}) - [\hat{E}(z_i|\boldsymbol{x}_i, D^{(-i)})]^2 \\
&\quad = \widehat{\text{CPO}}_i L^{-1} \sum_{l=1}^{L} \frac{\sigma_l^2 + (\boldsymbol{x}_i'\boldsymbol{\beta}_l)^2}{f(y_i|\boldsymbol{\beta}_l, \sigma_l^2, \boldsymbol{x}_i)} - [\hat{E}(z_i|\boldsymbol{x}_i, D^{(-i)})]^2,
\end{aligned} \tag{10.1.12}$$

respectively. Using (10.1.11) and (10.1.12), the Monte Carlo estimate of the Bayesian standardized residual d_i is

$$\hat{d}_i = \frac{y_i - \hat{E}(z_i|\boldsymbol{x}_i, D^{(-i)})}{\sqrt{\widehat{\text{Var}}(z_i|\boldsymbol{x}_i, D^{(-i)})}}. \tag{10.1.13}$$

For the New Zealand apple data, Chen and Deely (1996) use 50,000 Gibbs iterations to obtain the $\hat{d}_i$'s, and the results are displayed in Figure 10.1.

From Figure 10.1, it can be seen that: (i) the $\hat{d}_i$'s are small when the $\hat{E}(z_i|\boldsymbol{x}_i,\ D^{(-i)})$'s are small; and (ii) the $\hat{d}_i$'s are roughly symmetric about zero, which implies that the model is neither over-fitted nor under-fitted. Chen and Deely (1996) also check the distribution of $\hat{d}_i$ and find that the $\hat{d}_i$'s roughly follow a Student t distribution. Noting that $f(y_i|\boldsymbol{\beta}, \sigma^2, \boldsymbol{x}_i)$ is a normal distribution and $\hat{f}(y_i|\boldsymbol{x}_i, D^{(-i)})$ in (10.1.10) is a finite mixture of normal distributions, it follows from a result of Johnson and Geisser (1983) that $f(y_i|\boldsymbol{x}_i, D^{(-i)})$ is approximately a Student t distribution. Hence the results obtained by Chen and Deely (1996) are consistent with the theoretical result of Johnson and Geisser (1983), and give further support that the normal assumption of the error terms in the constrained multiple linear regression model is appropriate.

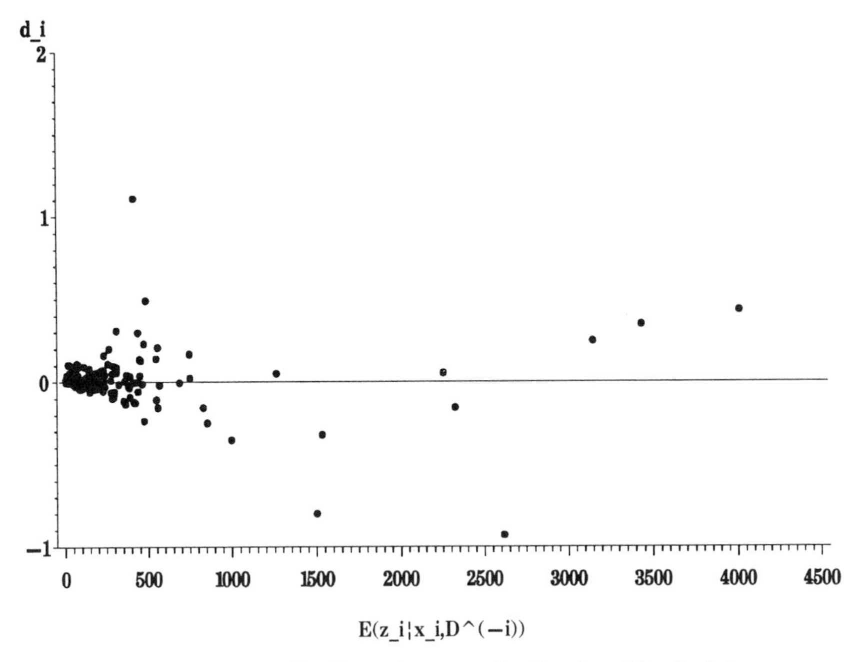

FIGURE 10.1. The Bayesian standardized residual plot.

Example 10.2. The bivariate normal model for human twin data. Chen, Manatunga, and Williams (1998) consider a bivariate normal model for human twin data. Suppose that the data from a twin sample consist of n_1 monozygotic (MZ) pairs $\boldsymbol{y}_{1j} = (y_{1j1}, y_{1j2})'$, $j = 1, \ldots, n_1$, and n_2 dizygotic (DZ) pairs $\boldsymbol{y}_{2j} = (y_{2j1}, y_{2j2})'$, $j = 1, \ldots, n_2$. Typical analyses of twin data assume a bivariate normal distribution of the variable of interest, and focus on estimation of variance components or correlations. One model for these data is

$$\boldsymbol{y}_{ij} \sim N_2(x_{ij}\beta, \Sigma_i), \tag{10.1.14}$$

where N_2 is a bivariate normal distribution, and

$$\Sigma_i = \begin{pmatrix} \sigma_{i11} & \sigma_{i12} \\ \sigma_{i21} & \sigma_{i22} \end{pmatrix},$$

which is specific to zygosity i with $\sigma_{i11} = \sigma_{i22} = \sigma^2$ and $\sigma_{i12} = \sigma_{i21} = \sigma^2 \rho_i$, and the covariates $x_{ij} = (\boldsymbol{x}_{ij1}, \boldsymbol{x}_{ij2})'$, $\boldsymbol{x}_{ijk} = (x_{ijk1}, x_{ijk2}, \ldots, x_{ijkp})'$, $k = 1, 2$, for $j = 1, 2, \ldots, n_i$ and $i = 1, 2$. Note that x_{ijk1} may be 1, which corresponds to an intercept, for $k = 1, 2$ and that $\rho_1 = \rho_{\text{MZ}}$ and $\rho_2 = \rho_{\text{DZ}}$ denote the intraclass correlation coefficients of MZ and DZ twins. Also in (10.1.14), we let $\boldsymbol{\beta} = (\beta_1, \beta_2, \ldots, \beta_p)'$ be a p-dimensional column vector of regression coefficients. Let $D = (\boldsymbol{y}, X, n)$ denote the observed data, where $n = (n_1, n_2)$, $\boldsymbol{y} = (\boldsymbol{y}_{ij},\ j = 1, 2, \ldots, n_i,\ i = 1, 2)$ and $X = (x_{ij},\ j = 1, 2, \ldots, n_i,\ i = 1, 2)$. Then the likelihood function for the unknown parameters $\boldsymbol{\beta}$, σ^2, ρ_1 and ρ_2 is

$$L(\boldsymbol{\beta},\sigma^2,\rho_1,\rho_2|D)$$
$$= \prod_{i=1}^{2}\prod_{j=1}^{n_i} \frac{|\Sigma_i|^{-1/2}}{2\pi} \exp\{-\tfrac{1}{2}(\boldsymbol{y}_{ij} - x_{ij}\boldsymbol{\beta})'\Sigma_i^{-1}(\boldsymbol{y}_{ij} - x_{ij}\boldsymbol{\beta})\}.$$

Suppose we specify a noninformative prior on the parameters $\boldsymbol{\beta}$, σ^2, ρ_1, and ρ_2, i.e.,

$$\pi(\boldsymbol{\beta},\sigma^2,\rho_1,\rho_2) \propto \frac{1}{\sigma^2}.$$

Then the posterior distribution for $\boldsymbol{\beta}$, σ^2, ρ_1, and ρ_2 given the data D can be written as

$$\begin{aligned}\pi(\boldsymbol{\beta},\sigma^2,\rho_1,\rho_2|D) &\propto L(\boldsymbol{\beta},\sigma^2,\rho_1,\rho_2|D)\pi(\boldsymbol{\beta},\sigma^2,\rho_1,\rho_2)\\ &= L(\boldsymbol{\beta},\sigma^2,\rho_1,\rho_2|D) \times \frac{1}{\sigma^2}. \qquad (10.1.15)\end{aligned}$$

Let $D^{(-ij)}$ denote the data D with the jth twin pair of zygosity i deleted for $j = 1,2,\ldots,n_i$ and $i = 1,2$. Let $f(\boldsymbol{z}_{ij}|x_{ij}, D^{(-ij)})$ be the conditional predictive density of the trait $\boldsymbol{z}_{ij} = (z_{ij1}, z_{ij2})'$ for the jth pair of zygosity i twin given x_{ij} and $D^{(-ij)}$. This density evaluated at $\boldsymbol{z}_{ij} = \boldsymbol{y}_{ij}$ is known as the CPO since it describes how much the observation from the jth pair of zygosity i twin supports the model. Therefore,

$$\begin{aligned}\text{CPO}_{ij} &= f(\boldsymbol{y}_{ij}|x_{ij}, D_{(ij)})\\ &= \int f(\boldsymbol{y}_{ij}|\boldsymbol{\beta},\sigma^2,\rho_i,x_{ij})\pi(\boldsymbol{\beta},\sigma^2,\rho_1,\rho_2|D^{(-ij)})\, d\boldsymbol{\beta}\, d\sigma^2\, d\rho_1\, d\rho_2,\end{aligned}$$

where $\pi(\boldsymbol{\beta},\sigma^2,\rho_1,\rho_2|D^{(-ij)})$ is the posterior distribution given the data $D^{(-ij)}$, and

$$f(\boldsymbol{y}_{ij}|\boldsymbol{\beta},\sigma^2,\rho_i,x_{ij})$$
$$= \frac{|\Sigma_i|^{-1/2}}{2\pi} \exp\{-\tfrac{1}{2}(\boldsymbol{y}_{ij} - x_{ij}\boldsymbol{\beta})'\Sigma_i^{-1}(\boldsymbol{y}_{ij} - x_{ij}\boldsymbol{\beta})\}. \qquad (10.1.16)$$

Based on CPO_{ij}, the bivariate Bayesian standardized residual for the jth twin pair of zygosity i is defined as

$$\begin{aligned}\boldsymbol{d}_{ij} &= (d_{ij1}, d_{ij2})'\\ &= V^{-1/2}(\boldsymbol{z}_{ij}|x_{ij}, D^{(-ij)})(\boldsymbol{y}_{ij} - E(\boldsymbol{z}_{ij}|x_{ij}, D^{(-ij)})), \qquad (10.1.17)\end{aligned}$$

where $E(\boldsymbol{z}_{ij}|x_{ij}, D^{(-ij)})$ is the two-dimensional expected value of $\boldsymbol{z}_{ij}$ and $V(\boldsymbol{z}_{ij}|x_{ij}, D^{(-ij)})$ is the 2×2 variance–covariance matrix of $\boldsymbol{z}_{ij}$ under the predictive distribution $f(\boldsymbol{z}_{ij}|x_{ij}, D^{(-ij)})$ for $j = 1,2,\ldots,n_i$ and $i = 1,2$.

Since the quantities defined in (10.1.17) are not available in closed form, we now describe how to approximate them using a simulation-based approach. Assume that $\{(\boldsymbol{\beta}_l, \sigma_l^2, \rho_{1,l}, \rho_{2,l}),\ l = 1,2,\ldots,L\}$ is a Gibbs sample from the posterior distribution $\pi(\boldsymbol{\beta}, \sigma^2, \rho_1, \rho_2 | D)$. Then the Monte Carlo estimate of CPO_{ij} is given by

$$\begin{aligned}\widehat{\text{CPO}}_{ij} &= \hat{f}(\boldsymbol{y}_{ij} | x_{ij}, D^{(-ij)}) \\ &= L\left[\sum_{l=1}^{L} (f(\boldsymbol{y}_{ij} | \boldsymbol{\beta}_l, \sigma^2{}_l, \rho_{i,l}, x_{ij}))^{-1}\right]^{-1},\end{aligned} \tag{10.1.18}$$

where $f(\boldsymbol{y}_{ij} | \beta, \sigma^2, \rho_i, x_{ij})$ is given by (10.1.16). To compute d_{ij}, we need to estimate $E(\boldsymbol{z}_{ij} | x_{ij}, D^{(-ij)})$, $\text{Var}(z_{ijk} | x_{ij}, D^{(-ij)})$ $(k = 1, 2)$, and $\text{Cov}(z_{ij1}, z_{ij2} | x_{ij}, D^{(-ij)})$. Using the Gibbs sample $\{(\boldsymbol{\beta}_l, \sigma_l^2, \rho_{1,l}, \rho_{2,l}),\ l = 1, \ldots, L\}$, the conditional means, variances, and covariance can be approximated by

$$\hat{E}(\boldsymbol{z}_{ij} | x_{ij}, D^{(-ij)}) = \widehat{\text{CPO}}_{ij} L^{-1} \sum_{l=1}^{L} \frac{x_{ij}\boldsymbol{\beta}_l}{f(\boldsymbol{y}_{ij} | \boldsymbol{\beta}_l, \sigma_l^2, \rho_{i,l}, x_{ij})}, \tag{10.1.19}$$

$$\begin{aligned}\widehat{\text{Var}}(z_{ijl} | x_{ij}, D^{(-ij)}) &= \widehat{\text{CPO}}_{ij} L^{-1} \sum_{l=1}^{L} \frac{\sigma_l^2 + (\boldsymbol{x}'_{ijl}\boldsymbol{\beta}_l)^2}{f(\boldsymbol{y}_{ij} | \boldsymbol{\beta}_l, \sigma_l^2, \rho_{i,l}, x_{ij})} \\ &\quad - (\hat{E}(z_{ijl} | x_{ij}, D^{(-ij)}))^2,\end{aligned} \tag{10.1.20}$$

and

$$\begin{aligned}&\widehat{\text{Cov}}(z_{ij1}, z_{ij2} | x_{ij}, D^{(-ij)}) \\ &\quad = \widehat{\text{CPO}}_{ij} L^{-1} \sum_{l=1}^{L} \frac{\sigma_l^2 \rho_{i,l} + (\boldsymbol{x}'_{ij1}\boldsymbol{\beta}_l)(\boldsymbol{x}'_{ij2}\boldsymbol{\beta}_l)}{f(\boldsymbol{y}_{ij} | \boldsymbol{\beta}_l, \sigma_l^2, \rho_{i,l}, x_{ij})} \\ &\quad - \hat{E}(z_{ij1} | x_{ij}, D^{(-ij)}) \hat{E}(z_{ij2} | x_{ij}, D^{(-ij)}),\end{aligned} \tag{10.1.21}$$

where $\hat{E}(z_{ijk} | x_{ij}, D^{(-ij)})$ is given by (10.1.19) for $k = 1, 2$. Therefore, the Monte Carlo estimate of $\boldsymbol{d}_{ij}$ is

$$\hat{\boldsymbol{d}}_{ij} = \hat{V}^{-1/2}(\boldsymbol{z}_{ij} | x_{ij}, D^{(-ij)})(\boldsymbol{y}_{ij} - \hat{E}(\boldsymbol{z}_{ij} | x_{ij}, D^{(-ij)})), \tag{10.1.22}$$

where $\hat{V}(\boldsymbol{z}_{ij} | x_{ij}, D^{(-ij)})$ can be easily obtained by using (10.1.20) and (10.1.21). Under some mild regularity conditions, it can be shown that $\hat{\boldsymbol{d}}_{ij}$ is a consistent estimator of $\boldsymbol{d}_{ij}$ as $L \to \infty$.

Chen, Manatunga, and Williams (1998) implement the Bayesian standardized residuals using data from the NHLBI Veteran Twin Study (Feinleib et al. 1977) to address the problem of model adequacy and model diagnostics. The NHLBI Twin Study is a longitudinal study of white male twins who were veterans of World War II and were born between 1917 and 1927. Here we are interested in estimating the heritability of high density lipoprotein cholesterol (HDL) as measured during the first of several examinations that were conducted on these twins. These data have been previously analyzed in Christian et al. (1990). The data set used in this example contains $n_1 = 123$ pairs of MZ twins and $n_2 = 102$ pairs of DZ

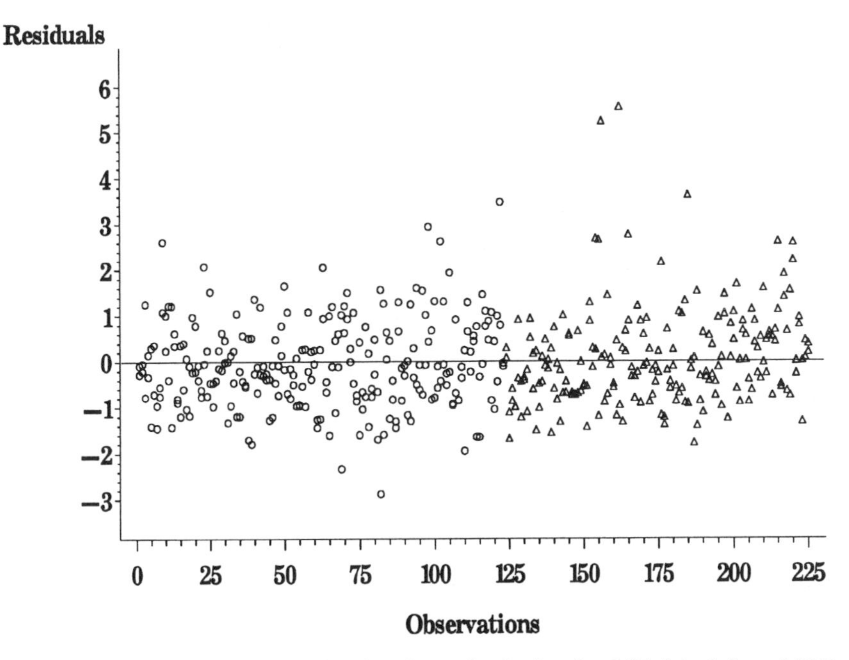

FIGURE 10.2. Bayesian standardized residual plot for MZ (circle) and DZ (triangle) twins with noninformative prior.

twins. In the HDL data, the response (y_{ijl}) is HDL, and Alcohol and Body mass index (BMI) are covariates.

Chen, Manatunga, and Williams (1998) use 50,000 Gibbs iterations to compute $\hat{\boldsymbol{d}}_{ij}$ given by (10.1.22), and the plot of the $(\hat{\boldsymbol{d}}_{ij})$'s is given in Figure 10.2. From Figure 10.2, it can be seen that all of the points are fairly symmetric about zero and no specific patterns are evident. Therefore, we can conclude that the model fits the data fairly well. Furthermore, there are four points whose values are greater than 3 and, therefore, these four points can be viewed as the aberrant points based on this plot. Indeed, after we further inspect the data, we find that these four points have certain aberrant features. The HDL values for these twin pairs are $(65, 85)$, $(54, 108)$, $(43, 106)$, and $(42, 85)$, respectively, whereas the mean value for the entire data set is approximately 46. Note that the HDL values for these four pairs of twins are much larger than the others in the data set.

10.1.2 Latent Residual Approach

Albert and Chib (1995) propose Bayesian latent residuals for binary response regression models. Due to the discrete nature of the binary response variable, classical residuals are difficult to define and interpret. In contrast, Bayesian residuals are attractive, since they have continuous-valued posterior distributions which can be graphed and used to examine outlying observations.

Let $\boldsymbol{y} = (y_1, y_2, \dots, y_n)'$ denote the vector of binary $(0, 1)$ responses, and let $\boldsymbol{x}_i = (x_{i1}, x_{i2}, \dots, x_{ip})'$ be the p-dimensional column vector of covariates for the ith observation. Also let $\boldsymbol{\beta} = (\beta_1, \beta_2, \dots, \beta_p)'$ denote the p-dimensional column vector of regression coefficients, and let $D = (n, \boldsymbol{y}, X)$ denote the data, where X is a $n \times p$ design matrix with $\boldsymbol{x}_i'$ as its ith row. Assume that $y_i = 1$ with probability p_i and $y_i = 0$ with probability $1 - p_i$. In the binary response regression models, it is usually assumed that

$$p_i = F(\boldsymbol{x}_i'\boldsymbol{\beta}), \tag{10.1.23}$$

where $F(\cdot)$ denotes a cumulative distribution function, and F^{-1} is called a link function.

From a frequentist viewpoint, outlier detection in these models is based on the difference $y_i - \hat{p}_i$, where $\hat{p}_i = F(\boldsymbol{x}_i\hat{\boldsymbol{\beta}})$ is the fitted probability for the ith observation, and $\hat{\boldsymbol{\beta}}$ is the maximum likelihood estimate of $\boldsymbol{\beta}$. One approach to detecting outliers is based on the set of Pearson residuals

$$\frac{y_i - \hat{p}_i}{[\hat{p}_i(1-\hat{p}_i)]^{1/2}},$$

and another on the deviance residuals

$$\text{sign}(y_i - \hat{p}_i)\left[2y_i \ln\left(\frac{y_i}{\hat{p}_i}\right) + 2(1-y_i)\ln\left(\frac{1-y_i}{1-\hat{p}_i}\right)\right]^{1/2}.$$

As pointed out by Albert and Chib (1995), the Pearson and deviance residuals can be useful in outlier detection for binomial data. However, in the context of binary data, they have unknown sampling distributions, and so the residual plots can be difficult to interpret.

As an alternative to the frequentist approach, Albert and Chib (1995) define a Bayesian latent residual, which is based on the concept of a tolerance random variable, also called a latent variable. Corresponding to each binary observation y_i, we define an unknown real-valued latent variable z_i that follows the linear model

$$z_i = \boldsymbol{x}_i\boldsymbol{\beta} + \epsilon_i \tag{10.1.24}$$

such that $z_i \sim F$, and

$$y_i = \begin{cases} 1 & \text{if } z_i > 0, \\ 0 & \text{if } z_i \le 0. \end{cases} \tag{10.1.25}$$

Then it is easy to check that $p_i = P(y_i = 1) = F(\boldsymbol{x}_i'\boldsymbol{\beta})$. In the bioassay setting, z_i can be interpreted as an insect's tolerance to a pesticide, and the insect survives ($y_i = 1$) if the tolerance exceeds some constant value.

Using (10.1.24), Albert and Chib (1995) propose the following latent residual:

$$\epsilon_i = \epsilon_i(z_i, \boldsymbol{\beta}) = z_i - \boldsymbol{x}_i\boldsymbol{\beta} \tag{10.1.26}$$

for $i = 1, 2, \ldots, n$. For ease of exposition, we consider F^{-1} to be the probit link. However, the method can be easily extended to other links, such as the scale mixtures of normal links discussed in Section 8.2.1. For the probit link, it follows from (10.1.24), $\{\epsilon_i,\ i = 1, 2, \ldots, n\}$ is, a priori, a random sample from $N(0,1)$, which provides a convenient base with which to compare the posterior distribution. To understand how the observation y_i changes the distribution of these residuals, consider the posterior distribution of $\{\epsilon_i\}$ conditional on β and D. Using (10.1.25), straightforward algebra yields

$$\pi(\epsilon_i|\boldsymbol{\beta}, y_i) = \begin{cases} \dfrac{\phi(\epsilon_i)}{\Phi(\boldsymbol{x}_i'\boldsymbol{\beta})} 1\{\epsilon_i > -\boldsymbol{x}_i\boldsymbol{\beta}\} & \text{if } y_i = 1, \\ \dfrac{\phi(\epsilon_i)}{\Phi(-\boldsymbol{x}_i'\boldsymbol{\beta})} 1\{\epsilon_i \le -\boldsymbol{x}_i\boldsymbol{\beta}\} & \text{if } y_i = 0, \end{cases} \tag{10.1.27}$$

where ϕ and Φ are the $N(0,1)$ probability density and cumulative distribution functions, respectively. When $y_i = 1$, the posterior mean and variance of ϵ_i, conditional on $\boldsymbol{\beta}$, are given by

$$E(\epsilon_i|\boldsymbol{\beta}, y_i = 1) = q_i, \quad \mathrm{Var}(\epsilon_i|\boldsymbol{\beta}, y_i = 1) = 1 - q_i(\boldsymbol{x}_i'\boldsymbol{\beta} + q_i), \tag{10.1.28}$$

where $q_i = \phi(\boldsymbol{x}_i'\boldsymbol{\beta})/\Phi(\boldsymbol{x}_i'\boldsymbol{\beta})$. These moments are significantly different from the prior moments, $E(\epsilon_i) = 0$ and $\mathrm{Var}(\epsilon_i) = 1$, when q_i is large, or equivalently, when the linear predictor $\boldsymbol{x}_i'\boldsymbol{\beta}$ is smaller than some negative constant C. Also, for a prespecified value $K > -\boldsymbol{x}_i\boldsymbol{\beta}$,

$$P(|\epsilon_i| > K|\boldsymbol{\beta}, y_i = 1) = \Phi(-K)/\Phi(\boldsymbol{x}_i'\boldsymbol{\beta}). \tag{10.1.29}$$

These latent residuals are very attractive, since they can be easily simulated by the Gibbs sampler. For ease of exposition, we assume that $\boldsymbol{\beta}$ has an improper uniform prior, i.e., $\pi(\boldsymbol{\beta}) \propto 1$. Then the joint posterior distribution of $(\boldsymbol{\beta}, \boldsymbol{z})$ is given by

$$\pi(\boldsymbol{\beta}, \boldsymbol{z}|D) \propto \prod_{i=1}^{n} \exp\{-\tfrac{1}{2}(z_i - \boldsymbol{x}_i'\boldsymbol{\beta})^2\} 1\{z_i \in A_i\}, \tag{10.1.30}$$

where $\boldsymbol{z} = (z_1, z_2, \ldots, z_n)'$, $A_i = (-\infty, 0]$ if $y_i = 0$, and $A_i = (0, \infty)$ if $y_i = 1$. Thus, similar to the Albert–Chib algorithm given in Subsection 2.5.3, the Gibbs sampler requires the following steps:

Step 1. Generate $\boldsymbol{\beta}|\boldsymbol{z}, D \sim N_p((X'X)^{-1}X'\boldsymbol{z}, (X'X)^{-1})$.

Step 2. Sample z_i from $z_i|\boldsymbol{\beta}, D \sim N(\boldsymbol{x}_i'\boldsymbol{\beta}, 1)$, $z_i \in A_i$.

Let $\{(\boldsymbol{\beta}_t, \boldsymbol{z}_t),\ t = 1, 2, \ldots, T\}$ denote a Gibbs sample from the posterior distribution given by (10.1.30). Also, let $\epsilon_{i,t} = z_{i,t} - \boldsymbol{x}_i'\boldsymbol{\beta}_t$, where $z_{i,t}$ is the ith component of $\boldsymbol{z}_t$, and $\boldsymbol{\epsilon}_t = (\epsilon_{1,t}, \epsilon_{2,t}, \ldots, \epsilon_{n,t})'$. Then

$\{\epsilon_t,\ t = 1, 2, \ldots, T\}$ is a Gibbs sample from the posterior distribution of the latent residuals ϵ_i. For a particular observation, the posterior distribution of the residual can be summarized by sample quantiles of the simulated values $\{\epsilon_{i,t}\}$. For example, we can use graphical tools, such as boxplots of $\{\epsilon_{i,t}\}$ to identify outlying observations. If the boxplots cross the parallel lines K^* and $-K^*$, the corresponding observations are viewed as outliers. Alternatively, we can estimate the posterior expectation of $E[P(|\epsilon_i| > K|\boldsymbol{\beta}, y_i = 1)|D]$ by

$$\hat{E}[P(|\epsilon_i| > K|\boldsymbol{\beta}, y_i = 1)|D] = \frac{1}{T}\sum_{t=1}^{T} 1\{|\epsilon_{i,t}| > K\},$$

or it can be estimated by

$$\hat{E}[P(|\epsilon_i| > K|\boldsymbol{\beta}, y_i = 1)|D] = \frac{1}{T}\sum_{t=1}^{T} \Phi(-K)/\Phi(\boldsymbol{x}_i'\boldsymbol{\beta}_t).$$

The observations associated with large values of $\hat{E}[P(|\epsilon_i| > K|\boldsymbol{\beta}, y_i = 1)|D]$ are viewed as outliers. In practice, several values of K and K^* should be chosen. Albert and Chib (1995) use $K = 2$, $K^* = 0.75$, and $K^* = 2$ in their illustrative examples.

Chen and Dey (1996) generalize the univariate Bayesian residuals of Albert and Chib (1995) for correlated ordinal data. From Subsection 8.2.1, the SMMVN-link reparameterized models for correlated ordinal response data can be defined as

$$y_{ij} = l \text{ if } \gamma_{j,l-1} \le w_{ij} < \gamma_{jl}, \tag{10.1.31}$$

where $\boldsymbol{w}_i = (w_{i1}, w_{i2}, \ldots, w_{iJ})'$ is a J-dimensional (latent) random vector, and $-\infty = \gamma_{j0} \le \gamma_{j1} = 0 \le \gamma_{j2} \le \gamma_{j,L-1} = 1 \le \gamma_{jL} = \infty$ are cutpoints for the jth ordinal response that divide the real line into L intervals. We further assume that

$$\boldsymbol{w}_i \sim N(X_i\boldsymbol{\beta}, \kappa(\lambda)\Sigma), \tag{10.1.32}$$

and

$$\lambda \sim \pi(\lambda),\ \lambda > 0, \tag{10.1.33}$$

where $\kappa(\lambda)$, $\pi(\lambda)$, X_i, and Σ are defined in Subsection 8.2.1. Then, Chen and Dey (1996) define the Bayesian latent residuals as

$$\epsilon_{ij} = \frac{w_{ij} - \mu_{ij}}{\sigma_{ij}}, \tag{10.1.34}$$

where $\mu_{ij} = E(w_{ij}|D)$ and $\sigma_{ij}^2 = \text{Var}(w_{ij}|D)$, that is, μ_{ij} and σ_{ij}^2 are the posterior mean and variance of w_{ij}, for $j = 1, 2, \ldots, J$, $i = 1, 2, \ldots, n$. Note that μ_{ij} and σ_{ij} can simply be calculated by using the readily available

MCMC samples of w_{ij}'s generated by the Gibbs sampler given in Subsection 8.2.2. Therefore, no additional MCMC samples are needed in order to obtain the latent residuals ϵ_{ij}'s.

Based on the Bayesian latent residuals ϵ_{ij}'s, we can use similar tools such as boxplots of the posterior distributions of the ϵ_{ij}'s to detect outlying observations. Alternatively, we can calculate $P(|\epsilon_{ij}| \geq K^*|D)$ and plot $P(|\epsilon_{ij}| \geq K^*|D)$ versus $E(y_{\text{new},ij}|D)$, where the expectation is taken with respect to the posterior predictive distribution $\pi(\boldsymbol{y}_{\text{new},ij}|D)$, where $y_{\text{new},ij}$ denotes the future ordinal response value of a replicate experiment. Note that to obtain an efficient Monte Carlo estimate of $E(y_{\text{new},ij}|D)$, we can use the following identity:

$$E(y_{\text{new},ij}|D) = E[E(y_{\text{new},ij}|\boldsymbol{x}_{ij}, \boldsymbol{\beta}_j, \Sigma, \boldsymbol{\gamma}_j, D)],$$

where the first expectation is taken with respect to the posterior distribution $\pi(\boldsymbol{\beta}_j, \Sigma, \boldsymbol{\gamma}_j|D)$ and the second expectation is

$$\begin{aligned} &E(y_{\text{new},ij}|\boldsymbol{x}_{ij}, \boldsymbol{\beta}_j, \Sigma, \boldsymbol{\gamma}_j, D) \\ &\quad = \int_0^\infty \sum_{l=1}^L l \left[\Phi\left(\frac{\gamma_{jl} - \boldsymbol{x}_{ij}'\boldsymbol{\beta}_j}{\sqrt{\kappa(\lambda)\sigma_{jj}}}\right) - \Phi\left(\frac{\gamma_{j,l-1} - \boldsymbol{x}_{ij}'\boldsymbol{\beta}_j}{\sqrt{\kappa(\lambda)\sigma_{jj}}}\right)\right] \pi(\lambda)\, d\lambda, \end{aligned} \tag{10.1.35}$$

where $\boldsymbol{x}_{ij}$ and $\boldsymbol{\beta}_j$ are the covariates and regression coefficients corresponding to the ordinal response y_{ij}. In (10.1.35), we have $\Phi([\gamma_{jl} - \boldsymbol{x}_{ij}'\boldsymbol{\beta}_j]/\sqrt{\kappa(\lambda)\sigma_{jj}})$ equal to 1 when $l = L$ and 0 when $l = 0$. We use the item response data given in Subsection 8.2.4 to illustrate the methodology.

Example 10.3. Item response data. In Subsection 8.2.4, we consider three SMMVN-link models, i.e., the multivariate probit (MVP), multivariate logit (MVL), and multivariate Cauchy (MVC) link models to fit the item response data collected at WPI in November 1993. Based on the marginal likelihoods, we find that the MVP model is better than the other two models.

For the model diagnostics, we use 50,000 Gibbs iterations after convergence to compute $P(|\epsilon_{ij}| \geq K^*|D)$, and then plot posterior probabilities, $P(|\epsilon_{ij}| \geq K^*|D)$, of the absolute values of the standardized Bayesian residuals greater than or equal to K^* versus $E(y_{\text{new},ij}|D)$ for the MVP model. Figure 10.3 gives the plot for $K^* = 2$. In Figure 10.3, the symbols • (dot), ⋆ (star), ∘ (circle), △ (triangle), and □ (square) correspond to ordinal responses $y_{ij} = 1$ to $y_{ij} = 5$. Several other values of K^* are also considered, and resulted in similar plots. From Figure 10.3, it can been seen that the MVP fits the data fairly well and no aberrant features are found.

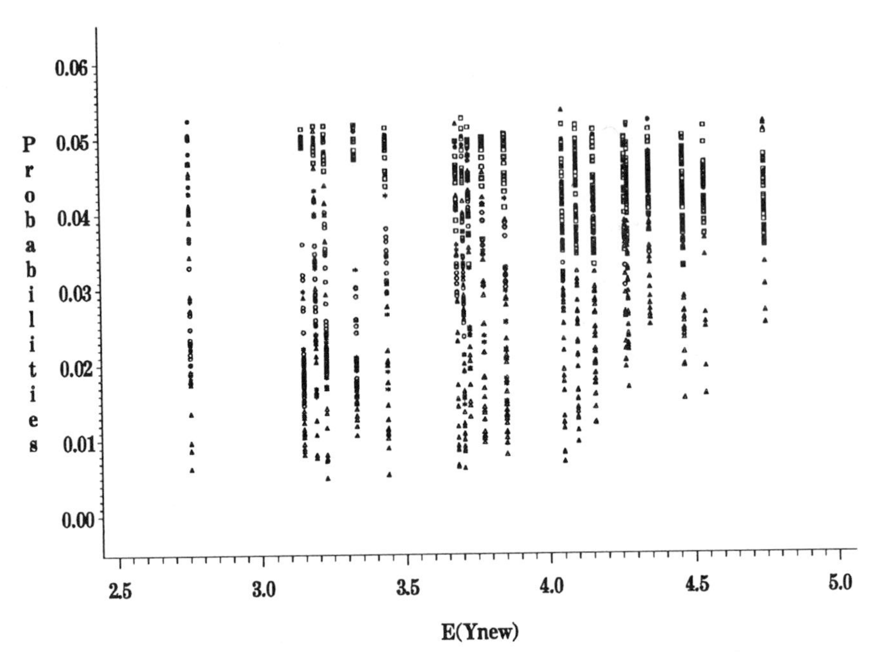

FIGURE 10.3. Plot of posterior probabilities $P(|\epsilon_{ij}| \geq 2|D)$ versus $E(y_{\text{new},ij}|D)$ for the MVP model.

10.2 Computing Posterior Modes

10.2.1 Lindley–Smith Optimization

Lindley and Smith (1972) propose a deterministic optimization algorithm to find joint posterior modes. Let

$$\pi(\boldsymbol{\theta}|D) \propto \pi^*(\boldsymbol{\theta}|D) = L(\boldsymbol{\theta}|D)\pi(\boldsymbol{\theta}) \tag{10.2.1}$$

denote the posterior distribution, where $\boldsymbol{\theta}$ is the vector of model parameters, D denotes the data, $L(\boldsymbol{\theta}|D)$ is the likelihood function, $\pi(\boldsymbol{\theta})$ is the prior, and $\pi^*(\boldsymbol{\theta}|D)$ is the unnormalized posterior density.

First, we consider $\boldsymbol{\theta} = (\theta_1, \theta_2)$ to be a two-dimensional vector. Let $\tilde{\boldsymbol{\theta}} = (\tilde{\theta}_1, \tilde{\theta}_2)'$ denote the joint posterior mode. Then the modal values satisfy the equations

$$\left.\frac{\partial}{\partial\theta_1}\pi(\theta_1, \theta_2|D)\right|_{\boldsymbol{\theta}=\tilde{\boldsymbol{\theta}}} = \left.\frac{\partial}{\partial\theta_2}\pi(\theta_1, \theta_2|D)\right|_{\boldsymbol{\theta}=\tilde{\boldsymbol{\theta}}} = 0. \tag{10.2.2}$$

These equations may be rewritten in terms of conditional and marginal distributions. More specifically, (10.2.2) can be expressed as

$$\frac{\partial}{\partial \theta_1} \pi(\theta_1|\theta_2, D)\pi(\theta_2|D)\bigg|_{\boldsymbol{\theta}=\tilde{\boldsymbol{\theta}}} = \frac{\partial}{\partial \theta_2} \pi(\theta_2|\theta_1, D)\pi(\theta_1|D)\bigg|_{\boldsymbol{\theta}=\tilde{\boldsymbol{\theta}}} = 0, \quad (10.2.3)$$

or

$$\frac{\partial}{\partial \theta_1} \pi(\theta_1|\theta_2, D)\bigg|_{\boldsymbol{\theta}=\tilde{\boldsymbol{\theta}}} = \frac{\partial}{\partial \theta_2} \pi(\theta_2|\theta_1, D)\bigg|_{\boldsymbol{\theta}=\tilde{\boldsymbol{\theta}}} = 0, \quad (10.2.4)$$

provided that $\pi(\tilde{\theta}_1|D) \neq 0$ and $\pi(\tilde{\theta}_2|D) \neq 0$. In (10.2.3) and (10.2.4), $\pi(\theta_1|\,\theta_2, D)$ and $\pi(\theta_2|\,\theta_1, D)$ denote the conditional densities, while $\pi(\theta_1|D)$ and $\pi(\theta_2|D)$ denote the marginal densities.

Equations (10.2.3) and (10.2.4) indicate that the joint posterior mode $\tilde{\boldsymbol{\theta}}$ can be obtained via iterative conditional maximizations. Since both conditional densities are proportional to $\pi^*(\boldsymbol{\theta}|D) = L(\boldsymbol{\theta}|D)\pi(\theta)$, and each of them is a function of a one-dimensional parameter, the conditional maximization can be effectively achieved by using the Newton–Raphson algorithm or the Nelder–Mead algorithm implemented by O'Neill (1971). The detailed steps of the Lindley–Smith optimization algorithm are given as follows:

Lindley–Smith Optimization

Step 0. Choose a starting point $\tilde{\boldsymbol{\theta}}_0 = (\tilde{\theta}_{1,0}, \tilde{\theta}_{2,0})'$, and set $i = 0$.

Step 1. Compute the modal values $\tilde{\boldsymbol{\theta}}_{i+1} = (\tilde{\theta}_{1,i+1}, \tilde{\theta}_{2,i+1})'$ as follows:

- Compute the model value of $\pi(\theta_1|\tilde{\theta}_{2,i}, D)$, denoted by $\theta_{1,i+1}$.
- Compute the modal value of $\pi(\theta_2|\tilde{\theta}_{1,i+1}, D)$, denoted by $\theta_{2,i+1}$.

Step 2. Set $i = i + 1$, and go to Step 1.

Thus each component of $\boldsymbol{\theta}$ is visited in a natural order, and a cycle in this algorithm requires two conditional maximizations. The Lindley–Smith optimization algorithm stops if convergence is reached.

The Lindley–Smith optimization algorithm is very similar to the Gibbs sampler given in Section 2.1, and it can easily be extended to more than two parameters. Suppose $\boldsymbol{\theta}$ is partitioned into J groups of parameters, $\boldsymbol{\theta} = (\boldsymbol{\theta}_1', \boldsymbol{\theta}_2', \ldots, \boldsymbol{\theta}_J')'$. Let $\pi(\boldsymbol{\theta}_j|\boldsymbol{\theta}_1, \ldots, \boldsymbol{\theta}_{j-1}, \boldsymbol{\theta}_{j+1}, \ldots, \boldsymbol{\theta}_J, D)$ denote the conditional distribution of $\boldsymbol{\theta}_j$ given the other parameters. The Lindley–Smith optimization algorithm can be modified as follows:

Step 0. Choose a starting point $\tilde{\boldsymbol{\theta}}_0 = (\tilde{\boldsymbol{\theta}}_{1,0}, \ldots, \tilde{\boldsymbol{\theta}}_{J,0})'$, and set $i = 0$.

Step 1. Compute the modal values $\tilde{\boldsymbol{\theta}}_{i+1} = (\tilde{\boldsymbol{\theta}}_{1,i+1}, \ldots, \tilde{\boldsymbol{\theta}}_{J,i+1})'$ as follows:

- Compute the model value of $\pi(\boldsymbol{\theta}_1|\tilde{\boldsymbol{\theta}}_{2,i},\ldots,\tilde{\boldsymbol{\theta}}_{J,i},D)$, denoted by $\theta_{1,i+1}$.
- Compute the modal value of $\pi(\boldsymbol{\theta}_2|\tilde{\boldsymbol{\theta}}_{1,i+1},\tilde{\boldsymbol{\theta}}_{3,i},\ldots,\tilde{\boldsymbol{\theta}}_{J,i},D)$, denoted by $\boldsymbol{\theta}_{2,i+1}$.

  ... ...
- Compute the modal value of $\pi(\boldsymbol{\theta}_J|\tilde{\boldsymbol{\theta}}_{1,i+1},\tilde{\boldsymbol{\theta}}_{2,i+1},\ldots,\tilde{\boldsymbol{\theta}}_{J-1,i+1},D)$, denoted by $\boldsymbol{\theta}_{J,i+1}$.

Step 2. Set $i=i+1$, and go to Step 1.

The Lindley–Smith optimization algorithm always converges to a mode. If the conditional posterior distributions are not unimodal, then $\{\tilde{\boldsymbol{\theta}}_i\}$ may converge to a local mode. However, if the posterior conditional distributions are unimodal, $\{\tilde{\boldsymbol{\theta}}_i\}$ will converge to the global mode. We consider a simple bivariate normal model to illustrate this method.

Example 10.4. Bivariate normal model. In this example, we apply the Lindley–Smith optimization algorithm for computing the joint mode of a bivariate normal distribution $N_2(\boldsymbol{\mu},\Sigma)$, where $\boldsymbol{\mu}=(\mu_1,\mu_2)'$, and

$$\Sigma=\begin{pmatrix}\sigma_1^2 & \rho\sigma_1\sigma_2\\ \rho\sigma_1\sigma_2 & \sigma_2^2\end{pmatrix},$$

with $\sigma_1>0$, $\sigma_2>0$, and $-1<\rho<1$. Let $\boldsymbol{\theta}=(\theta_1,\theta_2)'\sim N_2(\boldsymbol{\mu},\Sigma)$. We use the Lindley–Smith optimization algorithm to obtain a sequence $\{\tilde{\boldsymbol{\theta}}_i=(\tilde{\theta}_{1,i},\tilde{\theta}_{2,i})',\ i=0,1,2,\ldots\}$, where $\tilde{\boldsymbol{\theta}}_0$ is an arbitrary starting point. For this bivariate normal distribution, the conditional distributions, $\pi(\theta_1|\theta_2)$ and $\pi(\theta_2|\theta_1)$, are

$$N\left(\mu_1+\rho\frac{\sigma_1}{\sigma_2}(\theta_2-\mu_2),\sigma_1^2(1-\rho^2)\right),$$

and

$$N\left(\mu_2+\rho\frac{\sigma_2}{\sigma_1}(\theta_1-\mu_1),\sigma_2^2(1-\rho^2)\right),$$

respectively. Then it is easy to show that

$$\tilde{\theta}_{1,i+1}=\mu_1+\rho^i(\tilde{\theta}_{1,i}-\mu_1),$$

and

$$\tilde{\theta}_{2,i+1}=\mu_2+\rho^i(\tilde{\theta}_{2,i}-\mu_2).$$

Since, $|\rho|<1$, $\lim_{i\to\infty}\tilde{\theta}_{1,i+1}=\mu_1$, and $\lim_{i\to\infty}\tilde{\theta}_{2,i+1}=\mu_2$. That is, $\lim_{i\to\infty}\tilde{\boldsymbol{\theta}}_{i+1}=\boldsymbol{\mu}$, which is the global mode of the bivariate normal distribution $N_2(\boldsymbol{\mu},\Sigma)$.

10.2.2 Stochastic Approximation

Robbins and Monro (1951) introduce a stochastic approximation approach to solve the univariate fixed point problem

$$g(\varphi) = \int h(\boldsymbol{z}, \varphi) f(\boldsymbol{z}|\varphi)\, d\boldsymbol{z} = \alpha, \tag{10.2.5}$$

where φ is a scalar, $\boldsymbol{z}$ is a vector, and $f(\boldsymbol{z}|\varphi)$ is a conditional density function. The fixed point, denoted by $\tilde{\varphi}$, is assumed to be unique so that g must be monotonic, at least in the vicinity of $\tilde{\varphi}$. This can be expressed as

$$(\varphi - \tilde{\varphi})(g(\varphi) - \alpha) > 0$$

in a neighborhood of $\tilde{\varphi}$. Then the stochastic approximation approach for finding $\tilde{\varphi}$ can be described as follows:

Stochastic Approximation Algorithm

Step 0. Choose a starting point $\tilde{\varphi}_0$, and set $i = 0$.

Step 1. Generate $\boldsymbol{z}_i \sim f(\boldsymbol{z}|\tilde{\varphi}_i)$.

Step 2. Set $\tilde{\varphi}_{i+1} = \tilde{\varphi}_i + a_i(h(\boldsymbol{z}_i, \tilde{\varphi}_i) - \alpha)$.

Step 3. Set $i = i + 1$, and go to Step 1.

Let $\{\tilde{\varphi}_i,\ i = 0, 1, \dots\}$ denote the sequence induced by the stochastic approximation algorithm. A nice feature of the stochastic approximation algorithm is that it produces a nonstationary Markov chain $\{\tilde{\varphi}_i,\ i = 0, 1, \dots\}$ without requiring the integration in (10.2.5). A sufficient condition for convergence of the chain to $\tilde{\varphi}$ is that the companion sequence $\{a_i,\ i = 0, 1, 2, \dots\}$ satisfies the conditions

$$\sum a_i = \infty \text{ and } \sum a_i^2 = \infty.$$

Gelfand and Banerjee (1998) point out that Step 2 in the stochastic approximation algorithm is closely related to the damped Newton–Raphson algorithm. We give a brief explanation as follows. Assume that $g(\varphi)$ is differentiable. A damped Newton–Raphson algorithm, as in Thisted (1988, Chap. 4), sets

$$\tilde{\varphi}_{i+1} = \tilde{\varphi}_i - (1/(i+1))(g(\tilde{\varphi}_i) - \alpha)/g'(\tilde{\varphi}_i)$$

for $i \geq 0$. Hence, the stochastic approximation replaces $g(\tilde{\varphi}_i) - \alpha$ by $h(\boldsymbol{z}_i, \tilde{\varphi}_i) - \alpha$, whose expectation given $\tilde{\varphi}_i$ is $g(\tilde{\varphi}_i) - \alpha$, and uses $a_i = -1/((i+1)g'(\tilde{\varphi}_i))$. To improve convergence of the chain $\{\tilde{\varphi}_i,\ i = 0, 1, \dots\}$, the stochastic approximation algorithm can be modified as follows. Instead of generating a single $\boldsymbol{z}_i$ given $\tilde{\varphi}_i$ in Step 1, we generate an MCMC sample, $\{\boldsymbol{z}_{i,t},\ t = 1, 2, \dots, T_i\}$, from $f(\boldsymbol{z}|\tilde{\varphi}_i)$, and then modify the updating step (i.e., Step 2) to

$$\tilde{\varphi}_{i+1} = \tilde{\varphi}_i + \frac{a_i}{T_i} \sum_{t=1}^{T_i} (h(\boldsymbol{z}_{i,t}, \tilde{\varphi}_i) - \alpha).$$

Gelfand and Banerjee (1998) present a novel application of the stochastic approximation approach for the marginal posterior mode problem. From (10.2.1), the marginal posterior distribution of θ_1 has the form

$$\pi(\theta_1|D) = \int \pi(\theta_1, \boldsymbol{\theta}_2|D) \, d\boldsymbol{\theta}_2 = \frac{1}{m(D)} \int \pi^*(\theta_1, \boldsymbol{\theta}_2|D) \, d\boldsymbol{\theta}_2,$$

where θ_1 is one-dimensional, $\boldsymbol{\theta}_2$ may be a vector of the remaining parameters, $m(D)$ is the normalizing constant, and $\pi^*(\theta_1, \boldsymbol{\theta}_2|D)$ is the unnormalized posterior density. Assume that $\pi(\theta_1|D)$ is unimodal and twice differentiable. Under the usual regularity conditions, the marginal posterior mode $\tilde{\theta}_1$ satisfies

$$\begin{aligned} 0 = \frac{\partial \ln \pi(\theta_1|D)}{\partial \theta_1} &= \frac{(\partial/\partial\theta_1) \int \pi^*(\theta_1, \boldsymbol{\theta}_2|D) \, d\boldsymbol{\theta}_2}{\int \pi^*(\theta_1, \boldsymbol{\theta}_2|D) \, d\boldsymbol{\theta}_2} \\ &= \frac{\int [\partial \pi^*(\theta_1, \boldsymbol{\theta}_2|D)/\partial\theta_1] \, d\boldsymbol{\theta}_2}{\int \pi^*(\theta_1, \boldsymbol{\theta}_2|D) \, d\boldsymbol{\theta}_2} \\ &= \int \frac{\partial \ln \pi^*(\theta_1, \boldsymbol{\theta}_2|D)}{\partial \theta_1} \pi(\boldsymbol{\theta}_2|\theta_1, D) \, d\boldsymbol{\theta}_2, \end{aligned} \tag{10.2.6}$$

where $\pi(\boldsymbol{\theta}_2|\theta_1, D)$ is the conditional posterior density of $\boldsymbol{\theta}_2$ given θ_1. Thus, (10.2.6) becomes the fixed point problem given in (10.2.5) with $h(\theta_1, \boldsymbol{\theta}_2) = \partial\pi^*(\theta_1, \boldsymbol{\theta}_2|D)/\partial\theta_1$ and $f(\boldsymbol{\theta}_2|\theta_1) = \pi(\boldsymbol{\theta}_2|\theta_1, D)$. The assumption of unimodality ensures that

$$(\theta_1 - \tilde{\theta}_1) \left(-\frac{\partial \ln \pi(\theta_1|D)}{\partial \theta_1} \right) > 0,$$

which implies that the fixed-point problem has a unique solution. Taking the second derivative, we have

$$\begin{aligned} \frac{\partial^2 \ln \pi(\theta_1|D)}{\partial \theta_1^2} &= \frac{\int [\partial^2 \pi^*(\theta_1, \boldsymbol{\theta}_2|D)/\partial\theta_1^2] \, d\boldsymbol{\theta}_2}{\int \pi^*(\theta_1, \boldsymbol{\theta}_2|D) \, d\boldsymbol{\theta}_2} \\ &\quad - \left(\frac{\int [\partial \pi^*(\theta_1, \boldsymbol{\theta}_2|D)/\partial\theta_1] \, d\boldsymbol{\theta}_2}{\int \pi^*(\theta_1, \boldsymbol{\theta}_2|D) \, d\boldsymbol{\theta}_2} \right)^2. \end{aligned} \tag{10.2.7}$$

Since

$$\frac{\partial^2 \ln \pi^*(\theta_1, \boldsymbol{\theta}_2|D)}{\partial \theta_1^2} = \frac{1}{\pi^*(\theta_1, \boldsymbol{\theta}_2|D)} \frac{\partial^2 \pi^*(\theta_1, \boldsymbol{\theta}_2|D)}{\partial \theta_1^2} - \left(\frac{\partial \pi^*(\theta_1, \boldsymbol{\theta}_2|D)}{\partial \theta_1} \right)^2,$$

after some algebra, (10.2.7) reduces to

$$\frac{\partial^2 \ln \pi(\theta_1|D)}{\partial \theta_1^2} = \text{Var}\left(\frac{\partial \pi^*(\theta_1, \boldsymbol{\theta}_2|D)}{\partial \theta_1} \middle| \theta_1, D \right) + E\left(\frac{\partial^2 \ln \pi^*(\theta_1, \boldsymbol{\theta}_2|D)}{\partial \theta_1^2} \middle| \theta_1, D \right), \tag{10.2.8}$$

where the variance and expectation are taken with respect to the conditional posterior distribution $\pi(\boldsymbol{\theta}_2|\theta_1, D)$. Thus, the stochastic approximation algorithm takes the form

$$\tilde{\theta}_{1,i+1} = \tilde{\theta}_{1,i} + \frac{a_i}{T_i} \sum_{t=1}^{T_i} \left. \frac{\partial \pi^*(\theta_1, \boldsymbol{\theta}_2|D)}{\partial \theta_1} \right|_{\boldsymbol{\theta}=(\tilde{\theta}_{1,i}, \boldsymbol{\theta}_{2,it})'}, \tag{10.2.9}$$

where $\{\boldsymbol{\theta}_{2,it},\ t = 1, 2, \ldots, T_i\}$ is an MCMC sample from $\pi(\boldsymbol{\theta}_2|\tilde{\theta}_{1,i}, D)$. As discussed earlier, a theoretical choice of a_i is

$$-\left((i+1) \left. \frac{\partial^2 \ln \pi(\theta_1|D)}{\partial \theta_1^2} \right|_{\theta_1=\tilde{\theta}_{1,i}} \right)^{-1},$$

which requires (10.2.8) to be evaluated at $\theta_1 = \tilde{\theta}_{1,i}$. A convenient Monte Carlo approximation for (10.2.8) at the ith iteration, $i \geq 1$, is the ergodic average

$$d_i = \frac{1}{i} \sum_{j=0}^{i} (v_j - \bar{v}_i)^2 + \frac{1}{i+1} \sum_{j=0}^{i} w_j,$$

where

$$v_j = \frac{1}{T_j} \sum_{t=1}^{T_j} \left. \frac{\partial \pi^*(\theta_1, \boldsymbol{\theta}_2|D)}{\partial \theta_1} \right|_{\boldsymbol{\theta}=(\tilde{\theta}_{1,i}, \boldsymbol{\theta}_{2,it})'}, \quad \bar{v}_i = (i+1)^{-1} \sum_{j=1}^{i} v_j,$$

and

$$w_j = \frac{1}{T_j} \sum_{t=1}^{T_j} \left. \frac{\partial^2 \pi^*(\theta_1, \boldsymbol{\theta}_2|D)}{\partial \theta_1^2} \right|_{\boldsymbol{\theta}=(\tilde{\theta}_{1,i}, \boldsymbol{\theta}_{2,it})'}.$$

Then we take $a_i = -[(i+1)d_i]^{-1}$. Gelfand and Banerjee (1998) also consider the multiple-dimensional extension of the stochastic approximation algorithm for both the fixed-point problem and the marginal posterior mode problem. The details can be found in their paper, and thus are omitted here for brevity.

10.3 Bayesian Computation for Proportional Hazards Models

Semiparametric Bayesian analyses of proportional hazards models are becoming computationally feasible due to modern technology and recent advances in computing techniques such as the MCMC methods given in Chapter 2. Sinha and Dey (1997) give a nice overview of Bayesian semiparametric methods for the Cox model. The potential advantage of using Bayesian methods to jointly model the baseline hazard and the regression coefficients is that one can accurately compute posterior quantities of interest using MCMC simulation techniques. In this section, we provide only a brief introduction to this subject, and discuss the related computational issues. A comprehensive treatment of Bayesian analysis of survival models can be found in the forthcoming book of Ibrahim, Sinha, and Chen (2000).

10.3.1 Model

A proportional hazards model is defined by a hazard function of the form

$$h(t_i, \boldsymbol{x}) = h_b(t_i)\exp(\boldsymbol{x}_i'\boldsymbol{\beta}), \tag{10.3.1}$$

where $h_b(t_i)$ denotes the baseline hazard function at time t_i, $\boldsymbol{x}_i$ denotes the p-dimensional vector of covariates for the ith individual, and $\boldsymbol{\beta} = (\beta_1, \beta_2, \dots, \beta_p)'$ denotes a vector of regression coefficients. The likelihood function for a set of right censored data on n individuals in a proportional hazards model based on (10.3.1) is given by

$$L(\boldsymbol{\beta}, h_b(\boldsymbol{t})|D) = \prod_{i=1}^{n} [h_b(t_i)\exp(\eta_i)]^{\nu_i} \left(S_b(t_i)^{\exp(\eta_i)}\right), \tag{10.3.2}$$

where $\eta_i = \boldsymbol{x}_i'\boldsymbol{\beta}$, t_i is an observed failure time or censoring time for the ith individual and ν_i is the indicator variable taking on the value 1 if t_i is a failure time, and 0 if it is a censoring time, and $\boldsymbol{t} = (t_1, t_2, \dots, t_n)'$. Moreover, $D = (n, \boldsymbol{t}, \boldsymbol{\nu}, X)$, where X denotes the $n \times p$ covariate matrix of rank p with $\boldsymbol{x}_i$ as its ith row, and $\boldsymbol{\nu} = (\nu_1, \nu_2, \dots, \nu_n)'$ denotes the corresponding n-dimensional vector of censoring indicators. Further, $F_b(\cdot)$ denotes the baseline cumulative distribution function, and $S_b(\cdot) = 1 - F_b(\cdot)$ is the baseline survivor function, which, since we consider continuous survival distributions, is related to $h_b(\cdot)$ by $S_b(t_i) = \exp(-\int_0^{t_i} h_b(u)\,du)$.

10.3.2 Prior Distribution for $h_b(\cdot)$

We consider a discrete gamma process prior for the baseline hazard function. The gamma process can be described as follows. Let $\mathcal{G}(\alpha(t), \lambda)$ denote the gamma distribution with shape parameter $\alpha(t) > 0$ and scale parameter $\lambda > 0$, where the density is given by

$$f(z|\alpha(t), \lambda) = \begin{cases} \dfrac{\lambda^{\alpha(t)}}{\Gamma(\alpha(t))} z^{\alpha(t)-1} e^{-\lambda z} & \text{if } z > 0, \\ 0 & \text{otherwise.} \end{cases}$$

Let $\alpha(t), t \geq 0$, be an increasing left continuous function such that $\alpha(0) = 0$, and let $z(t), t \geq 0$, be a stochastic process with the properties, $z(0) = 0, z(t)$ has independent increments, and for $t > s$, $z(t) - z(s)$ is $\mathcal{G}(\alpha(t) - \alpha(s), \lambda)$. Then the process $\{z(t) : t \geq 0\}$ is called a gamma process. The sample paths of the gamma process are almost surely increasing functions. Therefore, by definition, the gamma process prior on the hazard rate implies that the underlying hazard rate is increasing.

There has been some previous work on modeling the cumulative baseline hazard rate. Kalbfleisch (1978) considers gamma process priors for the cumulative baseline hazard and Clayton (1991) illustrates Gibbs sampling techniques for frailty models using gamma process priors on the cumulative baseline hazard rate. The prior specifications of Kalbfleisch (1978) and Clayton (1991) are quite different from the ones considered here. As Kalbfleisch (1978) points out, the assumption of independent increments for the prior on the baseline cumulative hazard may not be a very satisfactory representation of the prior distribution for the baseline hazard. Alternatively, we directly specify a prior distribution on the baseline hazard rate. Hjort (1990) and Laud, Damien, and Smith (1998) consider a beta process prior on the cumulative baseline hazard function. We refer the reader to these papers for this type of approach. Here we focus on a gamma process prior for the baseline hazard function.

There are many situations in which an increasing hazard rate is appropriate as demonstrated in Example 10.5. However, there are also situations in which the increasing hazard rate assumption is inappropriate, for example, when a significant proportion of the patients are "cured". We note that such studies require sufficient follow-up. Ibrahim and Chen (1998) and Ibrahim, Chen, and MacEachern (1999) empirically demonstrate that the posterior model probabilities and model choice in general are not sensitive to the increasing hazard rate assumption, and this assumption appears to have little impact on the analysis for the data sets we consider in Example 10.5.

To define the discrete gamma process, we first construct a finite partition of the time axis. Let $0 \leq s_0 < s_1 < \cdots < s_M$ denote this finite partition, with $s_M > t_j$, for all $j = 1, \ldots, n$. Let

$$\delta_i = h_b(s_i) - h_b(s_{i-1})$$

denote the increment in the baseline hazard in the interval $(s_{i-1}, s_i], i = 1, \ldots, M$. The δ_i's are random variables since the baseline hazard is assumed random. The δ_i's are independent a priori, and have gamma distributions, which are induced by the underlying gamma process. Thus, the δ_i's have independent gamma distributions with shape parameters $\alpha(s_i) - \alpha(s_{i-1})$ and scale parameter λ. The variance of the gamma process is controlled by choosing λ large (small) to reflect sharp (vague) prior beliefs at various time intervals. Letting $\boldsymbol{\delta} = (\delta_1, \ldots, \delta_M)'$, the prior density of $\boldsymbol{\delta}$ is given by

$$\pi(\boldsymbol{\delta}) = \prod_{i=1}^{M} f(\delta_i), \tag{10.3.3}$$

where $f(\delta_i)$ is a $\mathcal{G}(\alpha(s_i) - \alpha(s_{i-1}), \lambda)$ density.

10.3.3 *The Likelihood Function*

To construct the likelihood function, we use a piecewise-constant baseline hazard model and use only information about which interval the failure times fall into. The cumulative distribution function for the proportional hazards model at time s is given by

$$\begin{aligned} F(s) &= 1 - \exp\left\{-\exp(\eta) \int_0^s h_b(t)\, dt\right\} \\ &\simeq 1 - \exp\left[-\exp(\eta)\left\{(s - s_0)^+ h_b(s_0) + \sum_{i=1}^{M} \delta_i (s - s_{i-1})^+\right\}\right], \end{aligned} \tag{10.3.4}$$

where $(t)^+ = t$ if $t > 0$, 0 otherwise, $\eta = \boldsymbol{x}'\boldsymbol{\beta}$, and $\boldsymbol{x}$ is a p-dimensional vector of covariates. We assume here that $h_b(s_0) = 0$, and $F(s) = 1$ for $s > s_M$, so that (10.3.4) is slightly simplified. We take the increment in the hazard rate, δ_i, to occur immediately after s_{i-1}. Let p_i denote the probability of a failure in the interval $(s_{i-1}, s_i], i = 1, \ldots, M$. Using the fact that $h_b(s_0) = 0$, we have

$$\begin{aligned} p_i &= F(s_i) - F(s_{i-1}) \\ &\simeq \exp\left\{-\exp(\eta) \sum_{j=1}^{i-1} \delta_j (s_{i-1} - s_{j-1})\right\} \\ &\quad \times \left[1 - \exp\left\{-\exp(\eta)(s_i - s_{i-1}) \sum_{j=1}^{i} \delta_j\right\}\right]. \end{aligned}$$

Thus, in the ith interval $(s_{i-1}, s_i]$, the contribution to the likelihood function for an exact observation (i.e., a failure) is p_i and $1 - F(s_i)$ for a right censored observation. Let d_i be the number of failures and let c_i be the number of right censored observations in the ith interval, respectively, $i = 1, \ldots, M$. For ease of exposition, we order the observations so that in the ith interval, the first d_i are failures and the remaining c_i are censored. Define

$$u_{il}(\boldsymbol{\beta}) = \exp\{\boldsymbol{x}'_{i_l}\boldsymbol{\beta}\}, \quad a_i = \sum_{j=i+1}^{M}\sum_{l=1}^{d_j} u_{jl}(\boldsymbol{\beta})(s_{j-1} - s_{i-1}),$$

$$b_i = \sum_{j=i}^{M}\sum_{l=d_j+1}^{d_j+c_j} u_{jl}(\boldsymbol{\beta})(s_j - s_{i-1}), \quad T_i(\boldsymbol{\delta}) = (s_i - s_{i-1})\sum_{j=1}^{i}\delta_j.$$

The likelihood function over all M intervals is given by

$$L(\boldsymbol{\beta}, \boldsymbol{\delta}|D) = \left[\prod_{i=1}^{M} \exp\{-\delta_i(a_i + b_i)\}\right] \times \left(\prod_{i=1}^{M}\prod_{l=1}^{d_i}[1 - \exp\{-u_{il}(\boldsymbol{\beta})T_i(\boldsymbol{\delta})\}]\right). \tag{10.3.5}$$

10.3.4 Prior Distribution for the Regression Coefficients

We assume a priori independence between the baseline hazard rate and the regression coefficients, and thus the joint prior density of $(\boldsymbol{\beta}, \boldsymbol{\delta})$ is given by

$$\pi(\boldsymbol{\beta}, \boldsymbol{\delta}) = \pi(\boldsymbol{\beta})\pi(\boldsymbol{\delta}). \tag{10.3.6}$$

We consider a fully parametric multivariate normal prior for $\boldsymbol{\beta}$, since the normal prior has proved to be a flexible and useful class of priors for many regression problems (see Geisser 1993). Let $N_p(\boldsymbol{\mu}, \tau_0 T^{-1})$ denote the p-dimensional multivariate normal distribution with mean $\boldsymbol{\mu}$ and covariance matrix $\tau_0 T^{-1}$. Thus, we take

$$\boldsymbol{\beta} \sim N_p(\boldsymbol{\mu}, \tau_0 T^{-1}), \tag{10.3.7}$$

where τ_0 is a scalar quantifying the degree of prior belief one wishes to attach to $\boldsymbol{\mu}$. Assume we have the historical data $D_0 = (n_0, \boldsymbol{t}_0, X_0, \nu_0)$ and τ_0, where X_0 is an $n_0 \times p$ design matrix, $\boldsymbol{t}_0$ is an $n_0 \times 1$ vector of prior predictions, and ν_0 is the corresponding $n_0 \times 1$ vector of censoring indicators. We take the prior mean of $\boldsymbol{\beta}$ to be the solution to Cox's partial likelihood equations for $\boldsymbol{\beta}$ using D_0 as data. Suppose there are r failures and $n_0 - r$ right censored values in $\boldsymbol{t}_0$. Cox's partial likelihood for $\boldsymbol{\beta}$ based on D_0 is given by

$$L^*(\boldsymbol{\beta}|D_0) = \prod_{i=1}^{r}\left[\frac{\exp\{\boldsymbol{x}'_{0i}\boldsymbol{\beta}\}}{\sum_{\ell\in\mathcal{R}(t_{0i})}\exp\{\boldsymbol{x}'_{0\ell}\boldsymbol{\beta}\}}\right], \tag{10.3.8}$$

where $\boldsymbol{x}'_{0i}$ is the ith row of X_0, $(t_{01}, \ldots, t_{0r})$ are the ordered failures, and $\mathcal{R}(t_{0i})$ is the set of labels attached to the individuals at risk just prior to

t_{0i}. Now we take $\boldsymbol{\mu}$ to be the solution to

$$\frac{\partial \ln L^*(\boldsymbol{\beta}|D_0)}{\partial \beta_j} = 0, \tag{10.3.9}$$

$j = 1, \ldots, p$. The matrix T is taken to be the Fisher information matrix of $\boldsymbol{\beta}$ based on the partial likelihood in (10.3.8). Thus

$$T = \left[\frac{-\partial^2}{\partial \beta_j \partial \beta_j^*} \ln\{L^*(\boldsymbol{\beta}|D_0)\} \right] \Bigg|_{\boldsymbol{\beta}=\boldsymbol{\mu}}. \tag{10.3.10}$$

An attractive feature of the priors for $\boldsymbol{\beta}$ is that they are semiautomatic in the sense that one only needs a one time input of (D_0, τ_0) to generate the prior distribution. Our proposed priors represent a summary of the historical data D_0 through $(\boldsymbol{\mu}, T)$ which are obtained via Cox's partial likelihood. This is a practical and useful summary of the data D_0 as indicated by many authors including Cox (1972, 1975) and Tsiatis (1981).

10.3.5 Sampling from the Posterior Distribution

To obtain samples from $[\boldsymbol{\beta}, \boldsymbol{\delta}|D]$, we describe a Gibbs sampling strategy for sampling from $[\boldsymbol{\delta}|\boldsymbol{\beta}, D]$ and $[\boldsymbol{\beta}|\boldsymbol{\delta}, D]$. The conditional posterior density of $[\boldsymbol{\delta}|\boldsymbol{\beta}, D]$ is given by

$$\begin{aligned}\pi(\boldsymbol{\delta}|\boldsymbol{\beta}, D) \propto & \prod_{i=1}^{M} \exp(-\delta_i(a_i + b_i)) \\ & \times \prod_{i=1}^{M} \prod_{l=1}^{d_i} (1 - \exp\{-u_{il}(\beta) T_i(\boldsymbol{\delta})\}) \times \prod_{i=1}^{M} \pi(\delta_i),\end{aligned} \tag{10.3.11}$$

where $u_{il}(\boldsymbol{\beta})$,$a_i$, b_i, and $T_i(\boldsymbol{\delta})$ are defined in Subsection 10.3.3.

Following, Laud, Smith, and Damien (1996), an efficient method of sampling from (10.3.11) is to define latent variables in order to make the components of $\boldsymbol{\delta}$ independent a posteriori. We do this by first defining

$$e_i = (e_{i1}, \ldots, e_{id_i})', \;\; l = 1, 2, \ldots, M,$$

to be independent exponential random variables truncated at 1 with mean equal to $(T_i(\boldsymbol{\delta}) u_{il}(\beta))^{-1}$. Thus each e_{il} has density

$$f(e_{il}) = \begin{cases} \left(\dfrac{T_i(\boldsymbol{\delta}) u_{il}(\boldsymbol{\beta})}{1 - \exp\{-T_i(\boldsymbol{\delta}) u_{il}(\boldsymbol{\beta})\}} \right) \exp\{-e_{il} T_i(\boldsymbol{\delta}) u_{il}(\boldsymbol{\beta})\} & \text{if } e_{il} \le 1, \\ 0 & \text{otherwise.} \end{cases}$$

Letting $\boldsymbol{e} = (e_1, \dots, e_M)'$, we can write the posterior distribution of $[\boldsymbol{\delta}|\boldsymbol{\beta}, \boldsymbol{e}, D]$ as

$$\pi(\boldsymbol{\delta}|\boldsymbol{\beta}, \boldsymbol{e}, D) \propto \left\{\prod_{i=1}^{M} (T_i(\boldsymbol{\delta}))^{d_i}\right\} \left\{\exp\left\{-\sum_{i=1}^{M}\sum_{l=1}^{d_i} e_{il} T_i(\boldsymbol{\delta}) u_{il}(\boldsymbol{\beta})\right\}\right\} \times \left\{\prod_{i=1}^{M} \exp\{-\delta_i(a_i + b_i)\}\right\} \left\{\prod_{i=1}^{M} \pi(\delta_i)\right\}.$$

Next we consider additional latent variables $\boldsymbol{q}_i = (q_{i1}, \dots, q_{ii})'$, $i = 1, \dots, M$, where q_i are independent multinomial variates. Each q_i is an i-cell multinomial of d_i independent trials with probability of the lth cell defined to be $p_l = \delta_l / \sum_{j=1}^{i} \delta_j$. Letting $\boldsymbol{q} = (\boldsymbol{q}_1', \dots, \boldsymbol{q}_M')'$, we are led to

$$\pi(\boldsymbol{\delta}|\boldsymbol{\beta}, \boldsymbol{e}, \boldsymbol{q}, D) \propto \prod_{i=1}^{M}\prod_{l=1}^{i} \left\{\frac{\delta_l^{q_{il}}}{\sum_{j=1}^{i} \delta_j^{q_{il}}}\right\} \left\{\prod_{i=1}^{M} \left[(s_i - s_{i-1}) \sum_{j=1}^{i} \delta_j\right]^{d_i}\right\} \times \exp\left\{-\sum_{i=1}^{M}\sum_{l=1}^{d_i} e_{il} T_i(\boldsymbol{\delta}) u_{il}(\boldsymbol{\beta})\right\} \times \left\{\prod_{i=1}^{M} \exp\{-\delta_i(a_i + b_i)\}\right\} \left\{\prod_{i=1}^{M} \pi(\delta_i)\right\}. \quad (10.3.12)$$

Equation (10.3.12) can be simplified further. Define $w_{il}(\boldsymbol{\beta}) = u_{il}(\boldsymbol{\beta}) e_{il}$ and let $w_{i+}(\boldsymbol{\beta}) = \sum_{l=1}^{d_i} w_{il}(\boldsymbol{\beta})$. Since

$$\exp\left\{-\sum_{i=1}^{M}\sum_{j=1}^{i} \delta_j w_{i+}(\boldsymbol{\beta})(s_i - s_{i-1})\right\} = \prod_{i=1}^{M} \exp\left\{-\delta_i \sum_{k=i}^{M} w_{k+}(\boldsymbol{\beta})(s_k - s_{k-1})\right\},$$

we can write (10.3.12) as

$$\pi(\boldsymbol{\delta}|\boldsymbol{\beta}, \boldsymbol{e}, \boldsymbol{q}, D) \propto \left\{\prod_{i=1}^{M} \delta_i^{\sum_{l=i}^{M} q_{li}}\right\} \times \prod_{i=1}^{M} \exp\left\{-\delta_i \left(a_i + b_i + \sum_{k=i}^{M} w_{k+}(\boldsymbol{\beta})(s_k - s_{k-1})\right)\right\} \times \prod_{i=1}^{M} \pi(\delta_i). \quad (10.3.13)$$

We see that from (10.3.13) that given the latent variables $(\boldsymbol{e}, \boldsymbol{q})$, the posterior density of $\boldsymbol{\delta}$ consists of a product of the marginal posterior densities of the δ_i's, thus implying independence. We use (10.3.13) in the Gibbs sampler to sample $\boldsymbol{\delta}$.

The posterior density of $[\boldsymbol{\beta}|\boldsymbol{\delta}, D]$ is given by

$$\pi(\boldsymbol{\beta}|\boldsymbol{\delta}, D) \propto \prod_{i=1}^{M} \exp\{-\delta_i(a_i + b_i)\}$$
$$\times \prod_{i=1}^{M}\prod_{l=1}^{d_i}(1 - \exp\{-u_{il}(\boldsymbol{\beta})T_i(\boldsymbol{\delta})\})\pi(\boldsymbol{\beta}). \tag{10.3.14}$$

To obtain samples from the posterior distribution of $(\boldsymbol{\beta}, \boldsymbol{\delta})$, we use the Gibbs sampler to sample from the following four distributions: (a) $[\boldsymbol{\delta}|\boldsymbol{\beta}, \boldsymbol{e}, \boldsymbol{q}, D]$; (b) $[\boldsymbol{e}|\boldsymbol{\beta}, \boldsymbol{\delta}, \boldsymbol{q}, D]$; (c) $[\boldsymbol{q}|\boldsymbol{\beta}, \boldsymbol{\delta}, \boldsymbol{e}, D]$; and (d) $[\boldsymbol{\beta}|\boldsymbol{\delta}, D]$. As pointed out by Laud, Smith, and Damien (1996), the prior density of $\boldsymbol{\delta}$ is infinitely divisible, and thus the distribution in (a) has the form of a gamma density times an infinitely divisible density. Bondesson (1982) and Damien, Laud, and Smith (1995) propose an algorithm for sampling from infinitely divisible distributions. Here, we use Bondesson's algorithm to sample from the prior density of $\boldsymbol{\delta}$, and follow the same basic steps as Laud, Smith, and Damien (1996) to obtain samples from (a). Thus, sampling each δ_i requires the following steps:

Step 1. Independently generate ξ_j from an exponential distribution with parameter $\lambda^* = \alpha(s_i) - \alpha(s_{i-1})$, $j = 1, 2, \ldots, N$, and define an N-dimensional vector $\boldsymbol{\zeta} = (\zeta_1, \zeta_2, \ldots, \zeta_N)'$, where $\zeta_j = \sum_{l=1}^{j} \xi_l$ for $j = 1, 2, \ldots, N$.

Step 2. Generate N independent random variables $v_1, \ldots, v_N$ with distribution proportional to $\alpha(s)$ restricted to $(s_{i-1}, s_i]$. Thus the v_j's have density of the form

$$f_{v_j}(s) = \begin{cases} \dfrac{\alpha(s)}{\int_{s_{i-1}}^{s_i} \alpha(u)\, du} & \text{if } s_{i-1} < s \leq s_i, \\ 0 & \text{otherwise.} \end{cases}$$

Step 3. Independently generate z_j from an exponential distribution with parameter $\lambda(v_j)\exp\{\zeta_j\}$, $j = 1, \ldots, N$. Note that $\lambda(v_j)$ is the scale parameter of the discrete gamma process prior. Define $z = \sum_{l=1}^{N} z_l$. Then $z \sim \mathcal{G}(\alpha(s_i), \lambda(s_i))$.

Step 4. Given z, we use a rejection algorithm with the gamma density as the envelope to obtain a sample from the distribution in (a). The gamma density used in the rejection algorithm proportional to

$$\left\{\prod_{i=1}^{M} \delta_i^{\sum_{l=i}^{M} q_{li}}\right\} \prod_{i=1}^{M} \exp\left\{-\delta_i\left(a_i + b_i + \sum_{l=i}^{M} w_{l+}(\boldsymbol{\beta})(s_l - s_{l-1})\right)\right\}, \tag{10.3.15}$$

which has mode equal to

$$\tilde{m} = \frac{\sum_{l=i}^{M} q_{li}}{a_i + b_i + \sum_{l=i}^{M} w_{l+}(\boldsymbol{\beta})(s_l - s_{l-1})} .$$

Now we use the gamma envelope in (10.3.15) along with the mode $\tilde{m}$ in a standard rejection algorithm to decide upon acceptance or rejection of z from the conditional density of δ_i.

Cycling through (a), (b), and (c) via the Gibbs sampler yields samples from the posterior distribution of $[\boldsymbol{\delta}|\boldsymbol{\beta}, D]$. Once a sample of $\boldsymbol{\delta}$ is obtained from $[\boldsymbol{\delta}|\boldsymbol{\beta}, D]$, we complete the Gibbs cycle by sampling from $[\boldsymbol{\beta}|\boldsymbol{\delta}, D]$. To obtain a sample $\boldsymbol{\beta}$ from this distribution, we can show that $[\boldsymbol{\beta}|\boldsymbol{\delta}, D]$ is log-concave in each component of $\boldsymbol{\beta}$. Therefore, we may directly use the adaptive rejection sampling algorithm of Gilks and Wild (1992) to sample from this posterior distribution. Next, we use the myeloma data to illustrate these posterior computations.

Example 10.5. Myeloma data. In this example, we consider two studies in multiple myeloma. Krall, Uthoff, and Harley (1975) analyze data from a study (Study 1) on multiple myeloma in which researchers treated $n_0 = 65$ patients with alkylating agents. Of those patients, 48 died during the study and 17 survived. A few years later, another multiple myeloma study (Study 2) using similar alkylating agents was undertaken by the Eastern Cooperative Oncology Group (ECOG). This study, labeled E2479, had $n = 479$ patients with the same set of covariates being measured as Study 1. The results of E2479 are available in Kalish (1992). The two studies have similar patient populations, and thus serve as good examples in which to apply the methodology discussed in this section.

The response variable for these data was survival time in months from diagnosis. Several covariates were measured for these data at diagnosis. These are blood urea nitrogen (x_1), hemoglobin (x_2), platelet count (x_3) (1 if normal, 0 if abnormal), age (x_4), white blood cell count (x_5), bone fractures (x_6), percentage of the plasma cells in bone marrow (x_7), and serum calcium (x_8). These are typical covariates measured in multiple myeloma studies. In this example, we use the historical data (D_0) from Study 1 to construct a prior distribution for the regression parameters in Study 2. The prior parameters are chosen as follows. For the prior distribution of $\boldsymbol{\beta}$, the prior mean was chosen to be the solution to Cox's partial likelihood using Study 1 as data, and the prior precision matrix was computed using formula (10.3.10) with data D_0. The prior for $\pi(\boldsymbol{\delta})$ was $\mathcal{G}(s_i - s_{i-1}, 0.1)$ for $i = 1, \ldots, M-1$, and $\mathcal{G}(s_i - s_{i-1}, 10)$ for $i = M$. We implement the Gibbs sampler described in this section. In this example, 100,000 Gibbs iterations are used in all of the computations after a burn-in of 1000 iterations. Also, all covariates are standardized to numerically stabilize the

TABLE 10.1. Posterior Estimates for Myeloma Data.

	Posterior Mean			Posterior Std. Error		
Variable	$\tau_0 = 0.19$	$\tau_0 = 2$	$\tau_0 = 10$	$\tau_0 = 0.19$	$\tau_0 = 2$	$\tau_0 = 10$
x_1	0.101	0.145	0.253	0.051	0.047	0.036
x_2	−0.157	−0.157	−0.143	0.050	0.045	0.036
x_3	0.016	−0.013	−0.066	0.057	0.049	0.036
x_4	0.310	0.293	0.247	0.054	0.050	0.040
x_5	0.070	0.099	0.135	0.062	0.054	0.038
x_6	0.014	0.006	−0.012	0.055	0.050	0.039
x_7	0.359	0.341	0.314	0.062	0.055	0.042
x_8	0.192	0.182	0.164	0.065	0.056	0.040

Gibbs sampler. Convergence is checked using the methods discussed in Section 2.9. Specifically, trace plots, autocorrelations, and PSRs are computed, and convergence is observed to occur before 500 iterations. The posterior estimates of the regression coefficients for three choices of τ_0's are given in Table 10.1. From Table 10.1, it can be seen that the posterior estimates are fairly robust, especially when $\tau_0 \leq 2$. Other values of τ_0 are also tried, but the results are not reported in the table. We note that the posterior estimates are almost identical when $\tau_0 \leq 1$. Overall, the posterior standard errors get smaller when τ_0 becomes large. That is, the posterior estimates become more accurate when more prior information is incorporated into the analysis. A detailed analysis of these data, including variable selection, can be found in Ibrahim and Chen (1998) and Ibrahim, Chen, and MacEachern (1999).

10.4 Posterior Sampling for Mixture of Dirichlet Process Models

The Mixture of Dirichlet Process (MDP) model arises in cases of the following general situation. Suppose an $n_i \times 1$ random vector $\boldsymbol{y}_i$ has a parametric distribution indexed by the $w \times 1$ vector $\boldsymbol{\theta}_i$, $i = 1, \ldots, N$. Then suppose the $\boldsymbol{\theta}_i$ themselves have a prior distribution with known hyperparameters $\boldsymbol{\psi}_0$. Thus

$$\begin{aligned} &\text{Stage 1:} \quad [\boldsymbol{y}_i|\boldsymbol{\theta}_i] \sim D_{n_i}(h_1(\boldsymbol{\theta}_i)), \\ &\text{Stage 2:} \quad [\boldsymbol{\theta}_i|\boldsymbol{\psi}_0] \sim D_w(h_2(\boldsymbol{\psi}_0)), \end{aligned} \tag{10.4.1}$$

where $D_w(\cdot)$ is a generic label for a w-dimensional parametric multivariate distribution and $h_1(\cdot)$ and $h_2(\cdot)$ are functions. The MDP model (Escobar 1994 and MacEachern 1994) removes the assumption of a parametric prior at the second stage, and replaces it with a general distribution G. The distribution G then in turn has a Dirichlet process prior (Ferguson 1973), leading to

$$\begin{aligned} &\text{Stage 1:} \quad [\boldsymbol{y}_i|\theta_i] \sim D_{n_i}(h_1(\boldsymbol{\theta}_i)),\\ &\text{Stage 2:} \quad \boldsymbol{\theta}_i|G \overset{\text{i.i.d.}}{\sim} G,\\ &\text{Stage 3:} \quad [G|M,\boldsymbol{\psi}_0] \sim DP(M \cdot G_0(h_2(\boldsymbol{\psi}_0))), \end{aligned} \tag{10.4.2}$$

where G_0 is a w-dimensional parametric distribution, often called the base measure, and M is a positive scalar. The parameters of a Dirichlet process are $G_0(\cdot)$, a probability measure, and M, a positive scalar. The parameter $MG_0(\cdot)$ contains a distribution, $G_0(\cdot)$, which approximates the true nonparametric shape of G, and the scalar M, which reflects our prior belief about how similar the nonparametric distribution G is to the base measure $G_0(\cdot)$.

There are two special cases in which the MDP model leads to the fully parametric case. As $M \to \infty$, $G \to G_0(\cdot)$, so that the base measure is the prior distribution for $\boldsymbol{\theta}_i$. Also, if $\boldsymbol{\theta}_i \equiv \boldsymbol{\theta}$ for all i, the same is true. For a more hierarchical modeling approach, it is possible to place prior distributions on $(M, \boldsymbol{\psi}_0)$. In Subsection 10.4.4, we place a prior on $\boldsymbol{\psi}_0$, but we do not do so for M. The specification in (10.4.2) results in a semiparametric specification in that a fully parametric distribution is given in Stage 1 and a nonparametric distribution is given in Stages 2 and 3.

The Polya urn representation of the Dirichlet Process is developed by Blackwell and MacQueen (1973) and is useful for sampling purposes. We describe it as follows. The draw of $\boldsymbol{\theta}_1$ is always from the base measure, $G_0(\cdot)$. The draw of $\boldsymbol{\theta}_2$ is equal to θ_1 with probability p_1 and is from the base measure with probability $p_0 = 1 - p_1$. The draw of $\boldsymbol{\theta}_3$ is equal to θ_1 with probability p_1, equal to θ_2 with probability p_2; and is a draw from the base measure with probability $p_0 = 1 - (p_1 + p_2)$. The values of the p_i's change with each new draw. This process continues until $\boldsymbol{\theta}_N$ is equal to each of the preceding $\boldsymbol{\theta}$'s with probability p_i, $i \in \{1, \ldots, N-1\}$ and is a draw from the base measure with probability $p_0 = 1 - \sum_{i=1}^{N-1} p_i$. We determine the values of p_i, $i = 0, \ldots, N-1$, from the Dirichlet Process parameters. In other words, the $\boldsymbol{\theta}$'s are actually drawn from a mixture distribution, where the mixing probabilities are determined by the Dirichlet Process of Stage 3, thus giving rise to the MDP label. From this representation, it is clear that if all of the $\boldsymbol{\theta}_i \equiv \boldsymbol{\theta}$ for all i, then we draw $\boldsymbol{\theta}$ from the base measure with probability 1 and thus the base measure is the prior.

The MDP model is simplified in practice by the Polya urn representation, using the fact that, marginally, the $\boldsymbol{\theta}_i$ are distributed as the base measure along with the added property that $P(\boldsymbol{\theta}_i = \boldsymbol{\theta}_j, i \neq j) > 0$. The Dirichlet process prior results in what MacEachern (1994) calls a "cluster structure" among the $\boldsymbol{\theta}_i$'s. This cluster structure partitions the N $\boldsymbol{\theta}_i$'s into k sets or clusters, $0 < k \leq N$. All of the observations in a cluster share an identical value of $\boldsymbol{\theta}$ and subjects in different clusters have differing values of $\boldsymbol{\theta}$.

As described by Escobar (1994), conditional on the other $\boldsymbol{\theta}$'s, $\boldsymbol{\theta}_i$ has the following mixture distribution:

$$\pi(\boldsymbol{\theta}_i|\boldsymbol{y}, \boldsymbol{\theta}^{(-i)}) \propto \sum_{j \neq i} q_j \delta_{\boldsymbol{\theta}_j} + M q_0 g_0(\boldsymbol{\theta}_i) f(\boldsymbol{y}_i|\boldsymbol{\theta}_i), \tag{10.4.3}$$

where $\boldsymbol{y} = (\boldsymbol{y}_1', \boldsymbol{y}_2', \ldots, \boldsymbol{y}_N')'$, $\boldsymbol{\theta}^{(-i)} = (\boldsymbol{\theta}_1', \ldots, \boldsymbol{\theta}_{i-1}', \boldsymbol{\theta}_{i+1}', \ldots, \boldsymbol{\theta}_N')'$, and $f(\boldsymbol{y}_i|\boldsymbol{\theta}_i)$ is the sampling distribution of $\boldsymbol{y}_i$. We normalize the values q_j and Mq_0 to obtain the selection probabilities $p_i, i = 0, \ldots, N-1$, in the Polya urn scheme described above. In addition, δ_s is a degenerate distribution with point mass at s, and $g_0(\cdot)$ is the density corresponding to the probability measure $G_0(\cdot)$. Finally, $q_j = f(\boldsymbol{y}_i|\boldsymbol{\theta}_j)$, $j = 1, \ldots, i-1, i+1, \ldots, N$, and $q_0 = \int f(\boldsymbol{y}_i|\boldsymbol{\theta}) g_0(\boldsymbol{\theta})\, d\boldsymbol{\theta}$.

To demonstrate the MDP model, we consider the seminal example of Escobar (1994) and Escobar and West (1995). Suppose that y_i has a univariate normal distribution with unknown mean θ_i and known variance σ_y^2. In this case, we have $n_i = 1$, $i = 1, \ldots, N$. Also assume that each θ_i has a univariate normal distribution. Then (10.4.1) becomes

$$\begin{aligned} &\text{Stage 1:} \quad [y_i|\theta_i, \sigma_y] \sim N(\theta_i, \sigma_y^2), \\ &\text{Stage 2:} \quad [\theta_i|\mu, \sigma_\theta] \sim N(\mu, \sigma_\theta^2). \end{aligned}$$

The MDP model removes the assumption of normality at the second stage, resulting in

$$\begin{aligned} &\text{Stage 1:} \quad [y_i|\theta_i, \sigma_y] \sim N(\theta_i, \sigma_y^2), \\ &\text{Stage 2:} \quad \theta_i|G \sim G, \\ &\text{Stage 3:} \quad [G|M, \boldsymbol{\psi}_0] \sim DP(M \cdot G_0(h_2(\boldsymbol{\psi}_0))). \end{aligned} \tag{10.4.4}$$

10.4.1 Conjugate MDP Models

Suppose $G_0 = N(\mu, \sigma_\theta^2)$ in (10.4.4) so that $\boldsymbol{\psi}_0 = (\mu, \sigma_\theta^2)$. In this case, the unnormalized selection probability q_j is equal to $f(y_i|\theta_j) = \phi(y_i|\theta_j, \sigma_y^2)$, where $\phi(\cdot|\mu, \sigma^2)$ denotes the normal density with mean μ and variance σ^2. With probability proportional to q_j, $\theta_i \sim \delta_{\theta_j}$, which means that $\theta_i = \theta_j$ with probability 1. The unnormalized selection probability q_0 is given by

$$q_0 = \int f(y_i|\theta, \sigma_y^2) g_0(\theta|\boldsymbol{\psi}_0)\, d\theta = \int \phi(y_i|\theta, \sigma_y^2)\phi(\theta|\mu, \sigma_\theta^2)\, d\theta.$$

With probability proportional to Mq_0,

$$[\theta_i|y_i] \sim g_0(\theta) f(y_i|\theta) = N(\theta|\mu, \sigma_\theta^2) N(y_i|\theta, \sigma_y^2),$$

where $N(y_i|\mu, \sigma^2)$ indicates that y_i has a normal distribution with mean μ and variance σ^2. Then

$$[\theta_i|y_i] \sim N\left([(\sigma_\theta^2 + \sigma_y^2)^{-1} \sigma_\theta^2 \sigma_y^2] \left(\frac{\mu}{\sigma_\theta^2} + \frac{y_i}{\sigma_y^2} \right), (\sigma_\theta^2 + \sigma_y^2)^{-1} \sigma_\theta^2 \sigma_y^2 \right).$$

In the example above, selecting G_0 to be normal when the sampling distribution of the data is normal emulates the conjugate relationship between sampling distribution and prior in the usual Bayesian hierarchy. In the MDP case, the sampling distribution is conjugate to the base measure. MacEachern (1994) calls MDP models with base measures and sampling distributions that are conjugate in this fashion "conjugate MDP models." The computational advantages of the conjugate MDP model are clear from the example. First, q_0 has a closed form. Second, the distribution of θ_i corresponding to q_0 is from the same exponential family as the base measure.

As a result, Gibbs sampling in the conjugate model described above can proceed in a relatively straightforward fashion, as described in detail in Kleinman and Ibrahim (1998a).

10.4.2 Nonconjugate MDP Models

When we do not assume conjugacy, the integral needed for q_0 typically has no closed-form solution. Since we must evaluate this integral N times within each Gibbs cycle, the cost in time of numerical integration is compounded, as is the cost in accuracy of approximations. Several attempts to avoid this integration have been made. For example, West, Müller, and Escobar (1994) approximate q_0 with $f(\boldsymbol{y}_i|\boldsymbol{\theta}_i)$, where $\boldsymbol{\theta}_i \sim G_0(\cdot)$. This is certainly simple, but unfortunately, the stationary distribution underlying the Gibbs sampler is no longer the posterior distribution we desire. In fact, the stationary distribution may be quite different from the posterior. Fortunately, MacEachern and Müller (1998) describe a technique whereby one can fit nonconjugate MDP models without numerical integration or approximation. Other techniques have also been suggested by Walker, Damien, Laud, and Smith (1999) and Damien, Wakefield, and Walker (1999). Some additional notation is necessary for the exposition of the MacEachern and Müller method. Recall that when the $\boldsymbol{\theta}_i$'s are known, the observations are grouped into clusters which have equal $\boldsymbol{\theta}_i$'s. There will be some number k, $0 < k \leq N$, of unique values among the $\boldsymbol{\theta}_i$'s. Denote these unique values by $\boldsymbol{\gamma}_l$, $l = 1, \ldots, k$, and recall from the Polya urn scheme that the $\boldsymbol{\gamma}_l$ are independent observations from $G(\cdot)$. Let n_l be the number of observations that share the value $\boldsymbol{\gamma}_l$. Additionally, let l represent the set of subjects with common random effect $\boldsymbol{\gamma}_l$. Note that knowing the $\boldsymbol{\theta}_i$'s is equivalent to knowing k, $\boldsymbol{\gamma}_l$, n_l, and the cluster memberships l, $l = 1, \ldots, k$.

The routine of MacEachern and Müller (1998) is closely intertwined with the Gibbs sampler it generates. The method relies on the augmentation of the k independent $\boldsymbol{\gamma}_l$'s with an additional $N - k$ independent samples from $G_0(\cdot)$ at the start of each loop of the Gibbs sampler. Label these additional draws $\boldsymbol{\gamma}_{k+1}, \ldots, \boldsymbol{\gamma}_N$. Then the routine proceeds in the following fashion. If $n_l > 1$, $i \in l$, meaning that at least one other subject has the same value of $\boldsymbol{\theta}$ as subject i, then $\boldsymbol{\theta}_i$ has the distribution

$$\pi(\boldsymbol{\theta}_i|\boldsymbol{\theta}^{(-i)}, \boldsymbol{y}) \propto \sum_{l=1}^{k} n_l^- q_l \delta_{\boldsymbol{\gamma}_l} + \frac{M}{k^* + 1} q_{k+1} \delta_{\boldsymbol{\gamma}_{k+1}}, \tag{10.4.5}$$

where $k^* = k$ and n_l^- is the number of observations sharing $\boldsymbol{\gamma}_l$ when we exclude observation i. Note that this means $n_l^- = n_l$, except when $i \in l$, in which case $n_l^- = n_l - 1$. Also, $q_l = f(\boldsymbol{y}_i|\boldsymbol{\gamma}_l), l = 1, \ldots, k+1$. In other words, with probability proportional to $n_l^- f(\boldsymbol{y}_i|\boldsymbol{\gamma}_l)$, $\boldsymbol{\theta}_i$ is equal to $\boldsymbol{\gamma}_l$ with probability 1, $l = 1, \ldots, k$. With probability proportional to $[M/(k^*+1)]f(\boldsymbol{y}_i|\boldsymbol{\gamma}_{k+1})$, $\boldsymbol{\theta}_i$ is distributed $\delta_{\boldsymbol{\gamma}_{k+1}}$, meaning that $\boldsymbol{\theta}_i = \boldsymbol{\gamma}_{k+1}$ with probability 1. If $n_l = 1$, $i \in l$, then only subject i has the value $\boldsymbol{\theta}_i$. In this case, we do the following. With probability $k^*/(k^* + 1)$, leave $\boldsymbol{\theta}_i$ unchanged. Otherwise, with probability $1/(k^* + 1)$, $\boldsymbol{\theta}_i$ is distributed according to (10.4.5), with the modification that $k^* = k - 1$.

If it should occur that this routine causes a cluster to disappear, meaning that $n_{l'} = 0$ for some $l' \leq k$, switch the cluster labels of l' and k. Notice that k decreases as a result of this process. Another important point is that the value $\boldsymbol{\gamma}_{l'}$ is not removed, but becomes $\boldsymbol{\gamma}_{k+1}$ in the distribution of $\boldsymbol{\theta}_{i+1}$. Once we have completed an iteration of the Gibbs sampler, we discard the augmentary values $\boldsymbol{\gamma}_{k+1}, \ldots, \boldsymbol{\gamma}_N$.

10.4.3 MDP in Normal Random Effects Models

First, we define the normal linear random effects model, then introduce random effects into generalized linear models. For individual i, with n_i repeated measurements, the normal linear random effects model for outcome vector $\boldsymbol{y}_i$ is given by

$$\boldsymbol{y}_i = X_i\boldsymbol{\beta} + Z_i\boldsymbol{b}_i + \boldsymbol{e}_i, \quad i, \ldots, N,$$

where $\boldsymbol{y}_i$ is $n_i \times 1$, X_i is an $n_i \times p$ matrix of fixed covariates, $\boldsymbol{\beta}$ is a $p \times 1$ parameter vector of regression coefficients, commonly referred to as fixed effects in these models, Z_i is an $n_i \times v$ matrix of covariates for the $v \times 1$ vector of random effects $\boldsymbol{b}_i$, and $\boldsymbol{e}_i$ is an $n_i \times 1$ vector of errors. It is standard in implementations of this model to assume $\boldsymbol{e}_i$ and $\boldsymbol{b}_i$ are independent and that both are distributed normal, with $\boldsymbol{e}_i \sim N_{n_i}(0, \sigma^2 I_{n_i})$ and $\boldsymbol{b}_i \sim N_v(0, V)$, where I_{n_i} is the $n_i \times n_i$ identity matrix. Under these assumptions,

$$[\boldsymbol{y}_i|\ \boldsymbol{\beta}, \boldsymbol{b}_i] \sim N_{n_i}(X_i\boldsymbol{\beta} + Z_i\boldsymbol{b}_i, \sigma^2 I_{n_i}). \tag{10.4.6}$$

For the sake of convenience, we call model (10.4.6) the normal random effects model.

Bush and MacEachern (1996) describe a semiparametric Bayesian version of the normal random effects model, where the normal assumption on the random effects is relaxed. Kleinman and Ibrahim (1998a) consider a more general covariance structure.

To this end, we relax the normal assumption for the $\boldsymbol{b}_i$, and allow $\boldsymbol{b}_i \sim G$, where G is a general distribution. If we assume the sampling distribution for $\boldsymbol{y}_i$ to be normal, then a normal base measure for the random effects completes a conjugate MDP model. Let the distribution of the vector of outcomes $\boldsymbol{y}_i$ for subject i be

$$[\boldsymbol{y}_i|\boldsymbol{\beta}, \boldsymbol{b}_i, \sigma^2] \sim N_{n_i}(X_i\boldsymbol{\beta} + Z_i\boldsymbol{b}_i, \sigma^2 I_{n_i}). \tag{10.4.7}$$

Letting $\tau = \sigma^{-2}$, the prior specifications are

$$\tau \sim \mathcal{G}\left(\frac{\alpha_0}{2}, \frac{\lambda_0}{2}\right),$$

where $\mathcal{G}(\alpha_0/2, \lambda_0/2)$ denotes the gamma distribution,

$$\boldsymbol{\beta} \sim N_p(\boldsymbol{\mu}_0, \Sigma_0),$$

$$\boldsymbol{b}_i \sim G,$$

and

$$G \sim DP(M \cdot N_v(0, V)). \tag{10.4.8}$$

The model (10.4.7) implies that there are p "fixed" effects and v random effects.

When G is a fully parametric prior the joint posterior can easily be found, as in Wilks, Wang, Yvonnet, and Coursaget (1993). Then, following the usual algebraic routes, the full conditionals for $\boldsymbol{\beta}$ and τ are

$$[\boldsymbol{\beta}|\boldsymbol{b}, \tau, \boldsymbol{y}] \sim N_p(\hat{\boldsymbol{\beta}}, T), \tag{10.4.9}$$

where $\boldsymbol{b} = (\boldsymbol{b}_1', \boldsymbol{b}_2', \ldots, \boldsymbol{b}_N')'$, $\boldsymbol{y} = (\boldsymbol{y}_1, \boldsymbol{y}_2, \ldots, \boldsymbol{y}_N)$, $T = (\tau \sum_{i=1}^N X_i'X_i + \Sigma_0^{-1})^{-1}$, and $\hat{\boldsymbol{\beta}} = T\sum_{i=1}^N X_i'(\boldsymbol{y}_i - Z_i\boldsymbol{b}_i) + \Sigma_0^{-1}\boldsymbol{\mu}_0$, and

$$[\tau|\boldsymbol{\beta}, \boldsymbol{b}, \boldsymbol{y}] \sim \mathcal{G}\left(\frac{n + \alpha_0}{2}, \frac{\sum_i \boldsymbol{r}_i'\boldsymbol{r}_i + \lambda_0}{2}\right), \tag{10.4.10}$$

with $\boldsymbol{r}_i = \boldsymbol{y}_i - X_i\boldsymbol{\beta} - Z_i\boldsymbol{b}_i$, and $n = \sum_{i=1}^N n_i$. These full conditionals are unchanged by the MDP model.

Applying the usual MDP results, we find, as in West, Müller, and Escobar (1994),

$$\begin{aligned}\pi(\boldsymbol{b}_i|\boldsymbol{\beta}, \tau, \boldsymbol{y}, \boldsymbol{b}^{(-i)}) \propto &\sum_{j \neq i} \phi_{n_i}(\boldsymbol{y}_i|X_i\boldsymbol{\beta} + Z_i\boldsymbol{b}_j, \tau^{-1}I_{n_i}) \cdot \delta_{\boldsymbol{b}_j} \\ &+ \left\{M \int \phi_{n_i}(\boldsymbol{y}_i|X_i\boldsymbol{\beta} + Z_i\boldsymbol{b}_i^*, \tau^{-1}I_{n_i})\phi_v(\boldsymbol{b}_i^*|0, V)\, d\boldsymbol{b}_i^*\right\} \\ &\times \phi_{n_i}(\boldsymbol{y}_i|X_i\boldsymbol{\beta} + Z_i\boldsymbol{b}_i, \tau^{-1}I_{n_i})\phi_v(\boldsymbol{b}_i|0, V),\end{aligned}$$

where $\boldsymbol{b}^{(-i)}$ denotes the random effects for the subjects excluding subject i, and the multivariate normal density $\phi_{n_i}(\boldsymbol{y}_i|X_i\boldsymbol{\beta}+Z_i\boldsymbol{b}_i,\tau^{-1}I_{n_i})$ and $\phi_v(\boldsymbol{b}_i|0,V)$ are defined by (9.2.4). After some algebra, we get

$$\begin{aligned}\pi(\boldsymbol{b}_i|\boldsymbol{\beta},\tau,\boldsymbol{b}^{(-i)},\boldsymbol{y})&\\ \propto\Bigg(\sum_{j\neq i}\tau^{n_i/2}\exp&\left[\frac{-\tau}{2}(\boldsymbol{y}_i-X_i\boldsymbol{\beta}-Z_i\boldsymbol{b}_j)'(\boldsymbol{y}_i-X_i\boldsymbol{\beta}-Z_i\boldsymbol{b}_j)\right]\cdot\delta_{\boldsymbol{b}_j}\Bigg)\\ +\ M|Q_i|^{1/2}|V|^{-1/2}\tau^{n_i/2}&\exp\left\{\frac{\tau}{2}\left[(\boldsymbol{y}_i-X_i\boldsymbol{\beta})'U_i(\boldsymbol{y}_i-X_i\boldsymbol{\beta})\right]\right\}\\ \times\ \phi_{n_i}(\boldsymbol{y}_i|X_i\boldsymbol{\beta}&+Z_i\boldsymbol{b}_i,\tau^{-1}I_{n_i})\phi_v(\boldsymbol{b}_i|0,V),\end{aligned}\tag{10.4.11}$$

where $Q_i = (V^{-1}+\tau Z_i'Z_i)^{-1}$ and $U_i = (\tau Z_iQ_iZ_i' - I_{n_i})$. So with probability proportional to

$$\tau^{n_i/2}\exp\left\{\frac{-\tau}{2}(\boldsymbol{y}_i-X_i\boldsymbol{\beta}-Z_i\boldsymbol{b}_j)'(\boldsymbol{y}_i-X_i\boldsymbol{\beta}-Z_i\boldsymbol{b}_j)\right\},$$

we select from distribution $\delta_{\boldsymbol{b}_j}$, which means that we set $\boldsymbol{b}_i = \boldsymbol{b}_j$. Also, with probability proportional to

$$M|Q_i|^{1/2}|V|^{-1/2}\tau^{n_i/2}\int\phi_{n_i}(\boldsymbol{y}_i|X_i\boldsymbol{\beta}+Z_i\boldsymbol{b}_i,\tau^{-1}I_{n_i})\phi_v(\boldsymbol{b}_i|0,V)\,d\boldsymbol{b}_i,$$

we select from

$$\pi(\boldsymbol{b}_i|\boldsymbol{\beta},\tau,\boldsymbol{y}_i)\propto\phi_v(\boldsymbol{b}_i|0,V)\phi_{n_i}(\boldsymbol{y}_i|X_i\boldsymbol{\beta}+Z_i\boldsymbol{b}_i,\tau^{-1}I_{n_i}),$$

meaning we sample $\boldsymbol{b}_i$ from its full conditional,

$$[\boldsymbol{b}_i|\boldsymbol{\beta},\tau,\boldsymbol{y}_i]\sim N_v(\tau Q_iZ_i'(\boldsymbol{y}_i-X_i\boldsymbol{\beta}),Q_i).$$

This results in a mixture distribution where one piece is a normal distribution and all of the others are point masses. There is some plausible intuition behind the above mixture scheme. If subject i has a relatively large residual using subject j's random effect $\boldsymbol{b}_j$, then $\boldsymbol{b}_j$ is relatively less likely to be chosen as the random effect for subject i. Conversely, if subject i has a relatively small residual using subject j's random effect, then the random effect $\boldsymbol{b}_j$ is relatively more likely to be chosen as the random effect for subject i. On the other hand, the greater the residuals for subject i, assuming its random effect parameters are all 0, the greater the probability that subject i gets a new value as its random effect.

Typically, the covariance matrix V in the base measure of the Dirichlet Process in model (10.4.8), is unknown, and therefore, a suitable prior distribution must be specified for it. Note that once this has been accomplished, the base measure is no longer marginally normal.

For convenience, suppose

$$V^{-1}\sim W_v(d_0,c_0R_0),$$

where $W_v(d_0, c_0R_0)$ denotes a Wishart distribution defined by (8.2.11), $d_0 \geq v$, $c_0 > 0$, and R_0 is a $v \times v$ positive definite matrix. Then a priori

$$\pi(V^{-1}|d_0, c_0, R_0) \propto |V^{-1}|^{(d_0-v-1)/2} \exp\left\{\frac{-1}{2}\mathrm{tr}((c_0R_0)^{-1}V^{-1})\right\}.$$

After choosing random effects for each subject, the subjects will be grouped into clusters in which the subjects have equal $\boldsymbol{b}_i$'s. That is, after selecting a new $\boldsymbol{b}_i$ for each subject i in the sample, there will be some number k, $0 < k \leq N$, of unique values among the $\boldsymbol{b}_i$'s. Denote these unique values by $\boldsymbol{\gamma}_l$, $l = 1, \ldots, k$. Additionally, let l represent the set of subjects with common random effect $\boldsymbol{\gamma}_l$. Note that knowing the random effects is equivalent to knowing k, all of the $\boldsymbol{\gamma}_l$'s, and the cluster memberships l. Then for the purposes of calculating the full conditionals of V^{-1}, the $\boldsymbol{\gamma}_l$'s are k independent observations from $N_v(0, V)$. Thus, as in West, Müller, and Escobar (1994),

$$\begin{aligned}\pi(V^{-1}|\boldsymbol{b}, \boldsymbol{\beta}, \tau, \boldsymbol{y}) &= \pi(V^{-1}|\boldsymbol{\gamma}, \boldsymbol{\beta}, \tau, \boldsymbol{y}) \\ &\propto |V^{-1}|^{(d_0+k-v-1)/2} \exp\left\{-\tfrac{1}{2}\mathrm{tr}((c_0R_0)^{-1}V^{-1} - \frac{1}{2}\sum_{l=1}^{k} \boldsymbol{\gamma}_l' V^{-1}\boldsymbol{\gamma}_l)\right\},\end{aligned}$$

so that

$$[V^{-1}|\boldsymbol{b}, \boldsymbol{\beta}, \tau, \boldsymbol{y}] \sim W_v\left(d_0 + k, \left(\frac{1}{c_0R_0} + \sum_1^k \boldsymbol{\gamma}_l\boldsymbol{\gamma}_l'\right)^{-1}\right). \tag{10.4.12}$$

One additional piece of the model is recommended by Bush and MacEachern (1996) as an aid to convergence for the Gibbs sampler. To speed mixing over the entire parameter space, they suggest moving around the $\boldsymbol{\gamma}$'s after determining how the $\boldsymbol{b}_i$'s are grouped. The conditional density of $\boldsymbol{\gamma}_l$ is

$$\pi(\boldsymbol{\gamma}_l|\boldsymbol{\beta}, \tau, \boldsymbol{b}, V, \boldsymbol{y}) \propto \phi_v(\boldsymbol{\gamma}_l|0, V) \prod_{i \in l} \phi_{n_i}(\boldsymbol{y}_i|X_i\boldsymbol{\beta} + Z_i\boldsymbol{b}_i, \tau^{-1}I_{n_i}),$$

which implies that

$$[\boldsymbol{\gamma}_l|\boldsymbol{\beta}, \boldsymbol{b}, \tau, \boldsymbol{y}] \sim N_v\left(\tau Q_l \sum_{i \in l} Z_i'(\boldsymbol{y}_i - X_i\boldsymbol{\beta}), Q_l\right), \tag{10.4.13}$$

where $Q_l = (V^{-1} + \tau\sum_{i \in l} Z_i'Z_i)^{-1}$.

10.4.4 MDP for Generalized Linear Mixed Models

Suppose the sampling distribution of y_{it}, $t = 1, \ldots, n_i$, is from the exponential family, so that

$$f(y_{it}|\,\theta_{it}, \tau) = \exp\left\{\tau\left[y_{it}\theta_{it} - q(\theta_{it})\right] + c(y_{it}, \tau)\right\},$$

where

$$\mu_{it} = E(y_{it}|\ \theta_{it}, \tau) = \frac{dq(\theta_{it})}{d\theta_{it}},$$

$$v_{it} = \text{var}(y_{it}|\ \theta_{it}, \tau) = \tau^{-1}\frac{d^2q(\theta_{it})}{d\theta_{it}^2},$$

and τ is a scalar dispersion parameter.

In the generalized linear mixed model, the canonical parameter θ_{it} is related to the covariates by

$$\theta_{it} = h(\eta_{it}),$$

where

$$\eta_{it} = \boldsymbol{x}'_{it}\beta + \boldsymbol{z}'_{it}\boldsymbol{b}_i,$$

$\boldsymbol{x}'_{it}$ and $\boldsymbol{z}'_{it}$ are rows of the X_i and Z_i matrices, $h(\cdot)$ is a monotonic differentiable function, often referred to as the θ-link, and η_{it} is called the linear predictor. Throughout, we write

$$f(y_{it}|\theta_{it}, \tau) \equiv f(y_{it}|\boldsymbol{\beta}, \boldsymbol{b}_i, \tau),$$

where

$$f(y_{it}|\boldsymbol{\beta}, \boldsymbol{b}_i, \tau) = \exp\{\tau[y_{it}h(\eta_{it}) - q(h(\eta_{it}))] + c(y_{it}, \tau)\}. \tag{10.4.14}$$

When $\theta_{it} = h(\eta_{it}) = \eta_{it}$, then the link is said to be the canonical link. Note that the GLMM imitates the normal random effects model in that we assume that, conditional on the random effect $\boldsymbol{b}_i$, the repeated observations on subject i are independent. Thus the likelihood for N subjects in the GLMM is

$$f(\boldsymbol{y}|\boldsymbol{\beta}, \boldsymbol{b}, \tau) \propto \prod_{i=1}^{N}\prod_{t=1}^{n_i} f(y_{it}|\boldsymbol{\beta}, \boldsymbol{b}_i, \tau), \tag{10.4.15}$$

where $\boldsymbol{b} = (\boldsymbol{b}'_1, \ldots, \boldsymbol{b}'_N)'$ and $\boldsymbol{y} = (y_{11}, \ldots, y_{Nn_N})'$. Again, we assume that V^{-1} has a Wishart prior and we relax the normal assumption for the $\boldsymbol{b}_i$, and allow

$$\boldsymbol{b}_i \sim G,$$

where G is a general distribution. Assume that the base measure for the $\boldsymbol{b}_i$'s is normal. Then, any exponential family sampling distribution completes a MDP GLMM. This will be a nonconjugate MDP model except when the data have a normal sampling distribution. Let the distribution of the outcome y_{it} for subject i at time t be $f(y_{it}|\boldsymbol{\beta}, \boldsymbol{b}_i, \tau)$ as given in (10.4.14). Following Kleinman and Ibrahim (1998b), the prior specifications for the parameters of the MDP GLMM are

$$\begin{aligned}\tau &\sim \mathcal{G}(\alpha_0, \lambda_0),\\ \boldsymbol{\beta} &\sim N_p(\boldsymbol{\mu}_0, \Sigma_0),\\ \boldsymbol{b}_i &\sim G,\end{aligned}$$

and

$$G \sim DP(M \cdot N_v(0, V)). \tag{10.4.16}$$

When G is a fully parametric prior, we can write down the joint posterior density up to a constant of proportionality. Suppose G is a v-dimensional normal distribution with mean 0 and covariance matrix V, as in the standard (fully parametric) GLMM. Given V, the joint posterior for the parameters is

$$\begin{aligned}\pi(\boldsymbol{\beta}, \boldsymbol{b}, \tau|\boldsymbol{y}) &\propto \exp\{\ln f(\boldsymbol{y}|\ \boldsymbol{\beta}, \boldsymbol{b}, \tau)\}\pi(\boldsymbol{\beta}, \boldsymbol{b}, \tau)\\ &\propto \exp\left\{\sum_{i=1}^{N}\sum_{t=1}^{n_i} \ln f(y_{it}|\boldsymbol{\beta}, \boldsymbol{b}_i, \tau) - \tfrac{1}{2}(\boldsymbol{\beta} - \boldsymbol{\mu}_0)'\Sigma_0^{-1}(\boldsymbol{\beta} - \boldsymbol{\mu}_0)\right\}\\ &\quad \times \exp\left\{-\tau\lambda_0 - \frac{1}{2}\sum_{i=1}^{N} \boldsymbol{b}_i' V^{-1}\boldsymbol{b}_i\right\}\tau^{\alpha_0 - 1},\end{aligned} \tag{10.4.17}$$

where $\pi(\cdot)$ denotes the joint prior density. However, if G has the form of (10.4.16), it is impossible to write down the joint posterior density of the parameters, because there is not a common dominating measure. The special case where $G = N_v(0, V)$ is included here because the conditional distributions of β and τ can be found through it in the usual way.

From (10.4.17) and the usual MDP results, we can get the full conditional distributions needed for Gibbs sampling.

Following the usual algebraic routes, we get

$$\pi(\boldsymbol{\beta}|\boldsymbol{b}, \tau, \boldsymbol{y}) \propto \exp\left(\sum_{i=1}^{N}\sum_{t=1}^{n_i} \ln f(y_{it}|\boldsymbol{\beta}, \boldsymbol{b}_i, \tau) - \tfrac{1}{2}(\boldsymbol{\beta} - \boldsymbol{\mu}_0)'\Sigma_0^{-1}(\boldsymbol{\beta} - \boldsymbol{\mu}_0)\right).$$

Unless y_{it} has the normal distribution, sampling from this full conditional will not be straightforward. But it can still be accomplished, using for example a Metropolis–Hastings step given in Section 2.2. The full conditional distribution of τ is

$$\begin{aligned}&\pi(\tau|\boldsymbol{\beta}, \boldsymbol{b}, \boldsymbol{y})\\ &\quad \propto \tau^{\alpha_0 - 1}\exp\left\{\sum_{i=1}^{N}\sum_{t=1}^{n-i} c(y_{it}, \tau)\right\}\exp\left\{\sum_{i=1}^{N}\sum_{t=1}^{n_i}[y_{it}\theta_{it} - a(\theta_{it})] - \tau\lambda_0\right\}.\end{aligned}$$

Sampling from the full conditional distribution of τ can also be accomplished through a Metropolis–Hastings step, unless $\ln[c(y_{it}, \tau)]$ takes a form proportional to $\tau^{g(y_{it})}$. In such a case,

$$[\tau|\boldsymbol{\beta}, \boldsymbol{b}, \boldsymbol{y}] \sim \mathcal{G}\left(\alpha_0 + \sum_{i=1}^{N}\sum_{t=1}^{n_i} g(y_{it}), \lambda_0 - \sum_{i=1}^{N}\sum_{t=1}^{n_i} [y_{it}\theta_{it} - a(\theta_{it})]\right).$$

Using the MDP results in Kleinman and Ibrahim (1998b), we have

$$\pi(\boldsymbol{b}_i|\boldsymbol{\beta}, \tau, \boldsymbol{y}, \boldsymbol{b}^{(-i)}) \propto \sum_{j\neq i}^{N} \exp\left\{\sum_{t=1}^{n_i} \ln f(y_{it}|\boldsymbol{\beta}, \boldsymbol{b}_j, \tau)\right\} \cdot \delta_{\boldsymbol{b}_j}$$
$$+ \left[M \int \exp\left\{\sum_{t=1}^{n_i} \ln f(y_{it}|\boldsymbol{\beta}, \boldsymbol{b}_i^*, \tau)\right\} \phi_v(\boldsymbol{b}_i^*|0, V)\, db_i^*\right]$$
$$\times\, \phi_v(\boldsymbol{b}_i|0, V) \prod_{t=1}^{n_i} f(y_{it}|\, \boldsymbol{\beta}, \boldsymbol{b}_i, \tau), \qquad (10.4.18)$$

where $\boldsymbol{b}^{(-i)}$ denotes the random effects for the subjects excluding subject i. The intuition behind (10.4.18) is identical to that in the normal random effects model.

When the sampling distribution is not normal, q_0 generally will not have a closed form. To avoid numerical integration or approximation, we use the algorithm of MacEachern and Müller (1998). Recall that there are $k \leq N$ unique random effects among the N subjects. These random effects, which we label γ_l, $l = 1, \ldots, k$, are independent draws from $G_0(\cdot)$ which in this case is $N_v(0, V)$. The algorithm requires that we sample an additional $N - k$ values from $N_v(0, V)$; we label these values $\gamma_{k+1}, \ldots, \gamma_N$. Then, if $n_l > 1$, $i \in l$, we sample from the following full conditional:

$$\pi(\boldsymbol{b}_i|\boldsymbol{\gamma}, \boldsymbol{\beta}, \tau, \boldsymbol{y}) = \sum_{l=1}^{k} n_l^- \prod_{t=1}^{n_i} f(y_{it}|\boldsymbol{\beta}, \gamma_l, \tau)\delta_{\boldsymbol{\gamma}_l}$$
$$+ \frac{M}{k^*+1} \prod_{t=1}^{n_i} f(y_{it}|\boldsymbol{\beta}, \gamma_{k+1}, \tau)\delta_{\boldsymbol{\gamma}_{k+1}}, \qquad (10.4.19)$$

where $k^* = k$ and n_l^- is the number of subjects sharing the random effect γ_l excluding subject i. The value of $\prod_{t=1}^{n_i} f(y_{it}|\boldsymbol{\beta}, \gamma_l, \tau)$ is the likelihood of subject i's data using the random effect belonging to some group of subjects. Thus the effect of the distribution (10.4.19) has a sensible interpretation. The greater subject i's likelihood with random effect γ_l and the greater number of other subjects who share that random effect, the more likely it is that γ_l will be selected as subject i's random effect. On the other hand, the scalar parameter M regulates the probability that subject i gets a new random effect, meaning that they start a new cluster. If $n_l = 1$, $i \in l$, then with probability $k/(k+1)$ we leave $\boldsymbol{b}_i$ unchanged. Otherwise, we let $\boldsymbol{b}_i$ be distributed according to (10.4.19) except with $k^* = k - 1$.

We may end up with one fewer cluster after drawing $\boldsymbol{b}_i$ from (10.4.19), though this can only happen when $n_l = 1$, $i \in l$. In other words, we may have the case that $n_l = 0$ after drawing from the conditional distribution of $\boldsymbol{b}_i$. If this occurs, we switch the values γ_l for the empty group and γ_k for the last group. The set memberships l and k are also switched. Before drawing from the full conditional in such a case, the number of clusters is k, and afterward there are $k-1$ clusters. Before the draw, there were n_k subjects in set k sharing the random effect γ_k. After the draw and the switching, the set these subjects are in simply has a different label l, $l < k$, and the random effect formerly held by subject i is labeled γ_k. In the full conditional of $\boldsymbol{b}_{i+1}$, there are only $k-1$ clusters, thus the value γ_k from the full conditional of $\boldsymbol{b}_i$ will be used as γ_{k+1} in drawing b_{i+1} from (10.4.19).

As in Subsection 10.4.3, we place a Wishart prior on V^{-1} with the result that

$$[V^{-1}|\boldsymbol{b}, \boldsymbol{\beta}, \tau, \boldsymbol{y}] \sim W_v\left(d_0 + k, \left(\frac{1}{c_0 R_0} + \sum_1^k \gamma_l \gamma_l'\right)^{-1}\right). \quad (10.4.20)$$

Additionally, we again shuffle the γ_l's. The conditional density of γ_l is

$$\pi(\gamma_l|\boldsymbol{\beta}, \tau, \boldsymbol{b}, V, \boldsymbol{y}) \propto \phi_v(\gamma_l|0, V)\left\{\prod_{i\in l}\prod_{t=1}^{n_i} f(y_{it}|\boldsymbol{\beta}, \gamma_l, \tau)\right\}.$$

A Metropolis–Hastings algorithm or some other technique must be applied to draw a sample from this distribution as well. We now consider two examples to illustrate the methods presented in this section.

Example 10.6. AIDS ACTG 116B/117 data. This example contains an analysis of a longitudinal repeated measurements data set. The data come from a study of AIDS patients performed by the AIDS Clinical Trials Group of the National Institute of Allergy and Infectious Disease. The data are public, and come from the study labeled ACTG 116B/117. For a full description of the study, see Kahn, Lagakos, and Richman et al. (1992).

The study was intended to test the effectiveness of switching from zidovudine (AZT) to didanosine (ddI), in light of the fact that the effectiveness of zidovudine is known to diminish with time. The design called for subjects who had been taking zidovudine for at least 4 months prior to enrollment in the study. After enrolling in the study, subjects were randomized to receive a continuation of zidovudine, 500 milligrams per day of didanosine, or 750 milligrams per day of didanosine. As part of the data collection, CD4 cell counts were measured at baseline and at 2, 8, 12, 16, and 24 weeks after enrollment in the study.

For the purposes of simplifying the example, only the zidovudine group and the 750 mg didanosine group are included in this analysis. Additionally, subjects were further required to have been taking zidovudine for 6 months in order to be included in the analysis. Finally, at least two CD4 count measurements were required for inclusion. These restrictions left a total of 151 individuals with 659 measurements between them.

We fit a model to the log CD4 cell counts including an intercept (x_0), time in weeks (x_1), a treatment group indicator (x_2), and a time by treatment interaction (x_3) as fixed covariates; an intercept (z_0) and time in weeks (z_1) are included as covariates for the random effects. The time is centered around its mean in both the fixed and random covariate matrix.

The data from the 500 mg didanosine group, which is not used in the analysis, is used to elicit parameters for the prior distribution of the covariance matrix V in the base measure. This elicitation technique is analogous to using data from a previous experiment to specify prior distributions. For more information about elicitation procedures, see Ibrahim and Laud (1994), Laud and Ibrahim (1995), Ibrahim, Ryan, and Chen (1998), and Chen, Ibrahim, and Yiannoutsos (1999). We emphasize that the data used to generate the priors are not part of the data used in the analysis. In any case, this elicitation is for illustrative purposes. Prior parameters for the Wishart prior on V^{-1} are obtained in the following manner. First, d_0 is chosen to be 10, and $c_0 = 1$. Then $d_0^{-1}R_0$ is taken to have the same diagonal elements as $\hat{V}^{-1}$, where $\hat{V}$ is the maximum likelihood estimate of V for the 500 mg didanosine group. The off-diagonal elements of R_0 are taken to be 0. Thus

$$R_0 = \begin{pmatrix} 0.0926 & 0 \\ 0 & 113.9 \end{pmatrix}.$$

Though it might be desirable in some circumstances to have a flatter prior on the covariance matrix in the base measure, this can lead to nonconvergence in parametric random effects models. (See Cowles, Carlin, and Connett (1996) for an example.)

TABLE 10.2. Posterior 2.5, 50, and 97.5 Percentiles for Various Parameters from the MDP Model.

Parameter	$M = 1.25$	$M = 5$
β_0	$(2.67, 3.52, 4.30)$	$(2.98, 3.63, 4.50)$
β_1	$(-0.0488, -0.0282, -0.0082)$	$(-0.0441, -0.0280, -0.0111)$
β_2	$(-0.295, 0.446, 0.623)$	$(-0.294, 0.375, 0.500)$
β_3	$(-0.0022, 0.0091, 0.0208)$	$(-0.0021, 0.0095, 0.0220)$
σ^2	$(0.165, 0.188, 0.214)$	$(0.158, 0.181, 0.207)$
$b_{0,148}$	$(-1.39, -0.495, 0.534)$	$(-1.53, -0.559, 0.213)$
$b_{0,149}$	$(0.184, 0.838, 0.1.95)$	$(0.0804, 0.803, 1.57)$
$b_{1,149}$	$(-0.0337, 0.0058, 0.0386)$	$(-0.0324, 0.0042, 0.0362)$
$V(0,0)$	$(0.839, 1.53, 3.22)$	$(0.799, 1.37, 2.40)$
$V(0,1)$	$(-0.019, 0.00127, 0.0214)$	$(-0.0146, 0.00064, 0.0163)$
$V(1,1)$	$(0.00038, 0.00073, 0.00166)$	$(0.00038, 0.00068, 0.00173)$
k	12.0	21.2

TABLE 10.3. Posterior 2.5, 50, and 97.5 Percentiles for Various Parameters from the MDP and Fully Parametric Normal Models.

Parameter	$M = 27$	Fully Parametric Model ($M = \infty$)
β_0	$(3.22, 3.74, 4.28)$	$(3.40, 3.67, 3.94)$
β_1	$(-0.0394, -0.0273, -0.0148)$	$(-0.0374, -0.0276, -0.0178)$
β_2	$(-0.383, 0.0803, 0.529)$	$(-0.331, 0.0293, 0.388)$
β_3	$(-0.00365, 0.00992, 0.0229)$	$(-0.00327, 0.0103, 0.0240)$
σ^2	$(0.153, 0.175, 0.201)$	$(0.147, 0.168, 0.192)$
$b_{0,148}$	$(-1.38, -0.709, -0.00444)$	$(-1.15, -0.628, -0.0739)$
$b_{0,149}$	$(0.333, 0.887, 1.42)$	$(0.586, 1.01, 1.42)$
$b_{1,149}$	$(-0.0325, 0.00176, 0.0323)$	$(-0.0281, 0.00456, 0.0367)$
$V(0,0)$	$(0.795, 1.20, 1.86)$	$(0.863, 1.07, 1.34)$
$V(0,1)$	$(-0.00959, 0.00082, 0.0103)$	$(-0.00557, 0.00067, 0.00735)$
$V(1,1)$	$(0.00034, 0.00059, 0.0010)$	$(0.00036, 0.00058, 0.00090)$
$\bar{k}$	48.0	151

Relatively flat priors are chosen for all other parameters. In particular, $\boldsymbol{\mu}_0 = (0,0,0,0)'$, $\Sigma_0 = 10000 I_4$, $\alpha_0 = 2$, and $\lambda_0 = 0.0002$. A range of values for the parameter M are chosen to reflect small, moderate, and large departures from normality for the distribution of the random effects. A value of $M = 27$ reflects a small departure from normality, with the average number of clusters $\bar{k} \approx 50$. A value of $M = 5$ reflects a moderate departure from normality, with $\bar{k} \approx 25$. A value of $M = 1.25$ reflects a large departure from normality, with $\bar{k} \approx 12$. Tables 10.2 and 10.3 show three posterior percentiles for the parameters in MDP and fully parametric models using several values of M. The Gibbs sampler is run for 22000 iterations, with the first 500 being discarded as a burn-in period. In addition, due to high autocorrelation, every tenth iteration is used, and the rest discarded, making a total sample size of 2150. Convergence of the Gibbs sampler is assessed via the Geweke (1992) method, using the CODA (Best, Cowles, and Vines 1995) suite of diagnostics in S-plus. Most of the parameters have Geweke statistics within ± 1.96, indicating convergence is plausible. A more appropriate measure might be the technique of Raftery and Lewis (1992), which is designed for testing the convergence of estimates of percentiles. However, results from this technique depend on the amount of autocorrelation in the iterates. Thus in this case, it indicates that infeasibly large runs of the Gibbs sampler would be necessary for convergence.

In Tables 10.2 and 10.3, β_0 is the intercept, β_1 is the slope over time, β_2 is the treatment effect, β_3 is the slope for the treatment–time interaction, σ^2 is the error variance, $b_{0,i}$ is the intercept for subject i, and $b_{1,i}$ is its slope over time. Also, $V(0,0)$ is the variance of the intercepts in the base measure, $V(1,1)$ is the variance of the slopes, and $V(0,1)$ is their covariance. $\bar{k}$ is the

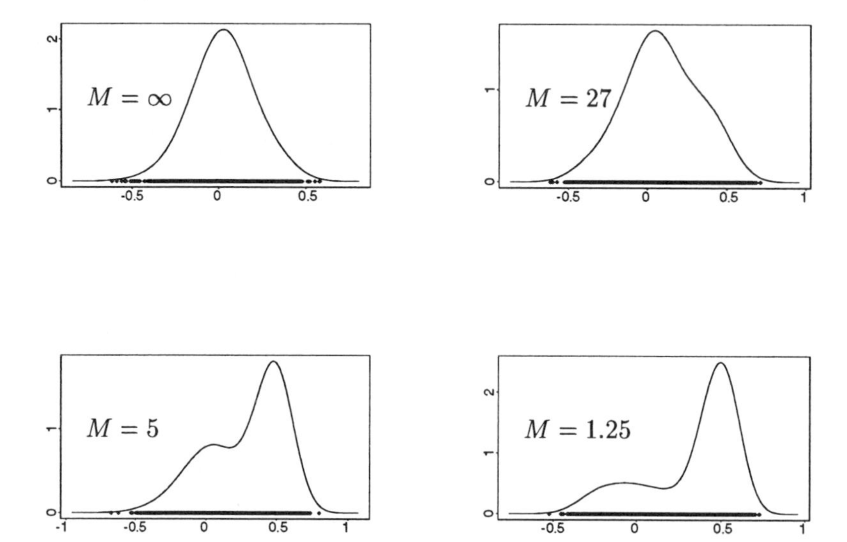

FIGURE 10.4. Vague priors on β.

average number of clusters observed in the course of sampling. The values in Tables 10.2 and 10.3 show an unusual result. Except for β_2, the coefficient for the treatment indicator, the medians of the posterior distributions of the regression coefficients $\boldsymbol{\beta} = (\beta_0, \beta_1, \beta_2, \beta_3)'$ remain approximately the same. The reason for this deviation is shown in the density estimates presented in Figure 10.4. We see that while there is a piece of the density which is near 0 for all values of M, that as M decreases, the distribution of β_2 takes on a bimodal appearance with a great deal of weight centered around 0.5. While the 95% credible intervals include 0 for all the values of M used here, it is reasonable to suppose that for a suitably small M, the analysis would indicate that a treatment difference of 0 was unlikely.

This is a clear example of why it is important to model correctly the distribution of the random effects; very different results may be obtained as a result of using the MDP model rather than the fully parametric model. Thus, the MDP model we have presented is certainly valuable in this case, and may be useful in others as well. The 750 mg didanosine group has been coded as "1" in this example, and the zidovudine group as "0", so these results suggest that in fact switching to 750 mg of didanosine may be better than staying on zidovudine, a fact not in evidence using a fully parametric analysis. Note that the time covariate has been centered, so that this represents the group difference at the middle of the study.

From the posterior distribution of the selected random effects, different facts are revealed. Not only are the Bayesian credible intervals different, but the median values are very different as well. This is to be expected, as the random effects are directly affected by the relaxation of the normal assumption. Some experimentation with smaller data sets shows that the subjects random effects tend to be shrunken from ordinary least squares regression estimates for a subject toward the nearest largest mode in the distribution of the random effects. The shrinkage is more pronounced in subjects where the deviations of the single measurements from a straight line are large. This behavior seems intuitive in light of the mixing distribution shown in (10.4.11). The elements of the matrix V are not easy to interpret in the MDP model, since they have a very complex role in the marginal posterior distribution of the $\boldsymbol{b}_i$.

Example 10.7. Respiratory data. This example presents an analysis of longitudinal repeated binary measurements. Zeger and Karim (1991) analyze a subset of data from a study of respiratory infections in Indonesian children. An analysis of the full data set can be found in Sommer, Katz, and Tarwotjo (1983). The children, all preschoolers, were seen quarterly for up to six quarters. At each examination, the presence or absence of respiratory infection was noted and is the outcome in this analysis. The covariates modeled by Zeger and Karim (1991) are an intercept, age in months, presence/absence of xeropthalmia, cosine and sine terms for the annual cycle, height for age as a percentage of the National Center for Health Statistics standard, and presence/absence of stunting, defined as being below the 85th percentile in height for age. Age in months is centered at 36 and height for age is centered at 90%. Xeropthalmia is a symptom of chronic vitamin A deficiency and height for age is an indicator of long-term nutritional status. In addition, Zeger and Karim (1991) model a random intercept for each child. To facilitate comparison with the results of Zeger and Karim (1991), we use the same model that they use. The original study followed 3000 children. Zeger and Karim (1991) use a subset of 250 of these children. To speed the computations, we take a random subset of 50 from the set of Zeger and Karim.

Since no prior information regarding respiratory infections in this population is available, parameters for the Wishart prior on V^{-1} are chosen in the following fashion. First, d_0 is chosen to be 10. Based on experience with the fully parametric logistic GLMM, we want $d_0^{-1}R_0$, the prior expected value of V^{-1}, to be 0.5. Thus we choose $c_0 = 1$ and $R_0 = 5$. Note that since V is a scalar, this is equivalent to a gamma prior on V^{-1}. Relatively flat

TABLE 10.4. Posterior 2.5, 50, and 97.5 Percentiles for Various Parameters from the MDP Logistic GLMM.

Parameter	$M = 0.75$	$M = 200$
β_0	(−7.03, −3.76, −1.97)	(−5.06, −3.47, −2.26)
β_1	(−0.09, −0.05, −0.01)	(−0.09, −0.05, −0.01)
β_2	(−1.08, 1.15, 3.12)	(−0.84, 1.44, 3.43)
β_3	(−1.58, −0.26, 0.86)	(−1.94, −0.52, 0.77)
β_4	(−2.18, −1.08, −0.11)	(−2.23, −1.14, −0.19)
β_5	(−2.01, −0.97, −0.05)	(−2.16, −0.99, −0.00)
β_6	(−0.36, −0.15, 0.03)	(−0.35, −0.14, 0.04)
β_7	(−2.43, −0.19, 2.10)	(−2.20, 0.05, 2.20)
V	(0.36, 0.79, 2.22)	(0.50, 1.26, 3.41)
b_1	(−1.02, 1.22, 4.58)	(−0.87, 1.09, 3.45)
b_2	(−2.32, 0.46, 4.24)	(−3.16, −0.01, 2.66)
b_3	(−0.78, 1.38, 4.56)	(−0.73, 1.26, 3.53)
$\bar{k}$	4.47	19.0

priors are chosen for the other parameters. We let $\boldsymbol{\mu}_0 = (0,0,0,0,0,0,0,0)'$ and $\Sigma_0 = 10000 I_8$. This is equivalent to saying that the a priori probability of respiratory infection is 0.5 for all subjects across all seasons, but that great uncertainty exists as to the accuracy of this assumption. Without previous experience in this population, this vague prior seems appropriate.

Three values of the parameter M are chosen to reflect large, moderate, and small departures from normality for the distribution of the random effects. A value of $M = 0.75$ reflects a large departure from normality with the average number of clusters $\bar{k} \approx 5$. A value of $M = 200$ reflects a moderate departure from normality with $\bar{k} \approx 20$. A value of $M = 10^8$ suggests that the distribution of the random effects is very nearly normal with $\bar{k} \approx 45$. Finally, the fully parametric case is also modeled by choosing M large enough so that $\bar{k} = 50$.

In Tables 10.4 and 10.5 we present results from the MDP GLMM analysis along with the fully parametric GLMM results. The Gibbs sampler is run for 25000 iterations, with the first 3000 discarded as a burn-in. In addition, due to high autocorrelation, only every tenth iterate is used, with the remainder discarded. This makes for a total sample size of 2200.

The results in Tables 10.4 and 10.5 can be read as follows. In both tables, β_0 is the intercept, β_1 is the effect of age, β_2 is the effect of xeropthalmia, β_3 is the gender effect, β_4 is the effect of the seasonal cosine, β_5 is the effect of the seasonal sine, β_6 is the effect of height for age, β_7 is the effect of stunting, and b_i is the random intercept for subject i. For the MDP models, $V(0,0)$ is the variance of the random effects in the base measure. For the fully parametric model, V is the variance of the random effects. $\bar{k}$ is the average number of clusters observed in the course of sampling.

TABLE 10.5. Posterior 2.5, 50, and 97.5 Percentiles for Various Parameters from the MDP and Fully Parametric Logistic GLMM's.

Parameter	$M = 10^8$	Fully Parametric Model ($M = \infty$)
β_0	$(-4.56, -3.27, -2.25)$	$(-4.56, -3.29, -2.24)$
β_1	$(-0.09, -0.05, -0.01)$	$(-0.09, -0.05, -0.01)$
β_2	$(-0.65, 1.50, 3.48)$	$(-0.54, 1.32, 3.30)$
β_3	$(-1.69, -0.31, 0.93)$	$(-1.65, -0.34, 0.91)$
β_4	$(-2.14, -1.08, -0.14)$	$(-2.17, -1.09, -0.13)$
β_5	$(-2.07, -0.94, 0.01)$	$(-2.08, -0.97, -0.08)$
β_6	$(-0.36, -0.16, 0.01)$	$(-0.36, -0.16, 0.02)$
β_7	$(-2.49, -0.12, 1.92)$	$(-2.24, -0.04, 1.86)$
V	$(0.45, 0.98, 2.34)$	$(0.48, 0.99, 2.32)$
b_1	$(-2.16, 0.31, 3.34)$	$(-2.06, 0.26, 2.46)$
b_2	$(-3.06, 0.02, 2.31)$	$(-2.36, -0.05, 2.28)$
b_3	$(-1.78, 0.52, 2.91)$	$(-1.73, 0.57, 3.05)$
k	43.2	50

In general, many of the medians and 95% Bayesian credible intervals for the population-mean effects are strikingly similar. The exceptions to this rule are the effects for gender, xeropthalmia, stunting, and the intercept. The posterior median of the intercept is similar in all four models, but the 2.5 percentile is progressively more negative as the distribution of the random effects becomes less normal. The same may be said for the effects of xeropthalmia. There is no discernible pattern for the effects of gender or stunting. In no case does the 95% credible interval change from excluding 0 to including it across the models, with the exception of the seasonal cosine, where the 95% credible interval hovers around 0 in all the models. The posterior distributions are most affected by the changing model if the covariates are binary. These parameters are the ones with the highest correlation with the intercept, the continuous covariates being roughly centered at 0. Since it is the distribution of the random intercepts which are directly affected by the changing models, it is unsurprising that the posterior distributions of parameters that are highly correlated with the population-mean intercept should be most affected.

The largest effect of introducing the nonparametric piece of the model is on the intercept, where it indicates that an even more extreme value may be the population mean. In this model, this means that the probability of respiratory infection, when all the other covariates are 0, may plausibly be smaller under the MDP model than under the fully parametric GLMM. This is also demonstrated in the kernel estimates of the posterior distributions presented in Figures 10.5 and 10.6. In comparing the distributions in Figures 10.5 and 10.6, we see that the marginal posterior distribution of β_0

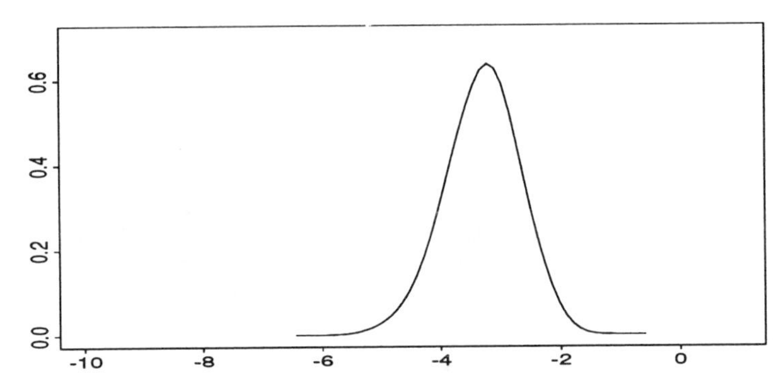

FIGURE 10.5. Posterior distribution of the intercept: Fully parametric logistic GLMM model.

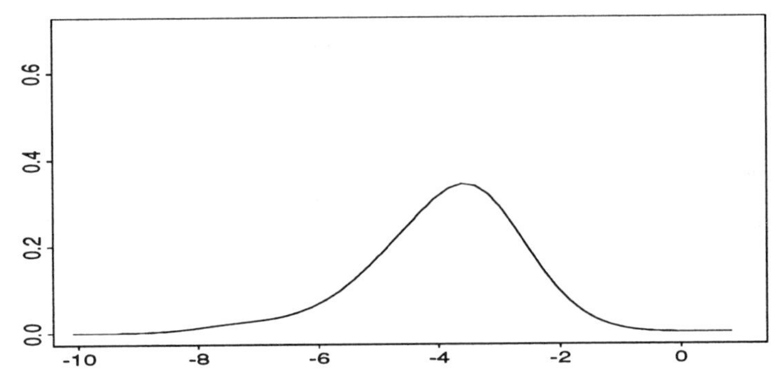

FIGURE 10.6. Posterior distribution of the intercept: MDP logistic GLMM model with $M = 0.75$.

based on the MDP model (Figure 10.6) has much heavier tails than the one based on the fully parametric model (Figure 10.5). Also, we see that the distribution in Figure 10.5 appears to be symmetric, while the distribution in Figure 10.6 is quite asymmetric. However, the medians and modes of the two distributions are similar.

The introduction of the MDP stage in the model introduces larger changes to the posterior distributions of the random effects. For the three particular random effects tabulated, the medians are markedly different under each of the models. If one were interested in the probability that a particular child would have a respiratory infection, the MDP models would give results very unlike those from the fully parametric model. Finally, the posterior distribution of V^{-1} seems different under the MDP models, but the role of this parameter is not the same under the MDP and fully parametric models, and therefore no straightforward comparisons can be made.

Exercises

10.1 In Example 10.1, consider the following checking functions: $g_i(z_i, y_i) = 1\{z_i \le y_i\}$ and $g_i(z_i, y_i) = 1\{f(z_i|\boldsymbol{x}_i, D^{(-i)}) \le f(y_i|\boldsymbol{x}_i, D^{(-i)})\}$.

(a) For each checking function, develop a Monte Carlo procedure for computing $E(g_i(z_i, y_i)|\boldsymbol{x}_i, D^{(-i)})$ by using an MCMC sample from the joint posterior distribution $\pi(\boldsymbol{\beta}, \sigma^2|D)$ or $\prod_{i=1}^n f(z_i|\boldsymbol{\beta}, \sigma^2, \boldsymbol{x}_i) \times \pi(\boldsymbol{\beta}, \sigma^2|D)$. Is one checking function easier to compute than the other?

(b) Propose a criterion for assessing the goodness of fit based on the values of $E(g_i(z_i, y_i)|\boldsymbol{x}_i, D^{(-i)})$.

(c) Using the checking function that is easiest to compute, recheck the adequacy of the constrained multiple linear regression model for the New Zealand data.

10.2 Nonlinear Mixed Effects Models

Draper and Smith (1981, p. 524) present a data set consisting of the trunk circumferences (in millimeters) of five orange trees over time (in days). The response variable is recorded seven times for each tree. The data are given in Table 10.6.

Dey, Chen, and Chang (1997) reanalyze this orange tree data by considering the following nonlinear mixed effects models:

$$\begin{aligned}
\mathcal{M}_1\colon\ & y_{ij} = \frac{\theta_1 + b_i}{1 + \theta_2 e^{\theta_3 t_j}} + \varepsilon_{ij},\\
\mathcal{M}_2\colon\ & y_{ij} = \theta_1 + b_i + \varepsilon_{ij},\\
\mathcal{M}_3\colon\ & y_{ij} = \theta_1 + \theta_2 t_j + b_i + \varepsilon_{ij},\\
\mathcal{M}_4\colon\ & y_{ij} = \frac{\theta_1}{1 + \theta_2 e^{\theta_3 t_j}} + \varepsilon_{ij},
\end{aligned}$$

where t_j is the time, b_i is a random effect such that $b_i \sim N(0, \sigma_b^2)$, ε_{ij} are independent and normal with mean zero, and variance σ^2 for $i = 1, 2, \ldots, 5$ and $j = 1, 2, \ldots 7$.

Let $\boldsymbol{\theta}$ be the vector of θ_j's. Suppose we take independent noninformative priors for $\boldsymbol{\theta}$, σ^2, and σ_b^2 such that $\pi(\boldsymbol{\theta}) \propto 1$, $\pi(\sigma^2) \propto (\sigma^2)^{-(\nu_1+1)} \exp(-1/\tau_1\sigma^2)$, and $\pi(\sigma_b^2) \propto (\sigma^2)^{-(\nu_2+1)} \exp(-1/\tau_2\sigma^2)$, where $\nu_j > 0$ and $\tau_j > 0$ are prespecified hyperparameters. (For the orange tree data, we choose $\nu_1 = \nu_2 = 3$ and $\tau_1 = \tau_2 = 0.01$, which give prior variances of 2500 for σ^2 and σ_b^2.)

(a) Write out the posterior distributions for all four models.

(b) Write out all necessary conditionals required for the Gibbs sampler for each model.

(c) For the orange tree data, compute CPO_{ij} and Bayesian standardized residuals d_{ij} for all four models.

(d) Based on the CPO_{ij} and d_{ij} values, determine which model fits the data best.

TABLE 10.6. Orange Tree Growth Curve, Trunk Circumference in Millimeters.

	Response for Tree No.				
Time (t)	1	2	3	4	5
118	30	33	30	32	30
484	58	69	51	62	49
664	87	111	75	112	81
1004	115	156	108	167	125
1231	120	172	115	179	142
1372	142	203	139	209	174
1582	145	203	140	214	177

Source: Draper and Smith (1981, p. 524).

10.3 Derive (10.1.27), (10.1.28), and (10.1.29) for the probit link. What should these formulas be for the other links?

10.4 Use (10.1.27) and the CMDE method given in Section 4.3 to obtain an estimate of the posterior distribution of the latent residual ϵ_i based on the Gibbs sample $\{(\boldsymbol{\beta}_t, \boldsymbol{z}_t),\ t = 1, 2, \ldots, T\}$ from the posterior distribution given by (10.1.30).

10.5 Let $\{y_i,\ i = 1, 2, \ldots, n\}$ be a random sample from a normal distribution $N(\theta, \sigma^2)$. Assume that we take independent prior distributions for (θ, σ^2) such that $\pi_1(\theta) \propto 1$, and $\pi_2(\sigma^2) \propto (\sigma^2)^{-(\nu+1)} \exp(-\tau/\sigma^2)$, where $\nu > 0$ and $\tau > 0$ are two prespecified hyperparameters. Let $D = (y_1, y_2, \ldots, y_n)$ denote the data, and let $\pi(\theta, \sigma^2|D)$ denote the posterior distribution. Use the Lindley–Smith optimization algorithm to find the joint posterior mode of (θ, σ^2).

10.6 Verify (10.2.6) and (10.2.8).

10.7 Show that the conditional density $\pi(\boldsymbol{\beta}|\boldsymbol{\delta}, D)$ given by (10.3.14) is log-concave in each component of $\boldsymbol{\beta}$.

10.8 Formally show that as $M \to \infty$, then $G \to G_0$ in (10.4.2).

10.9 Consider the MDP model given by (10.4.4). Suppose we add another stage to (10.4.4) by specifying a gamma prior distribution on M, that is, $M \sim \mathcal{G}(\nu_0, \lambda_0)$. Derive $\pi(\boldsymbol{\theta}_i|\boldsymbol{\theta}^{(-i)}, \boldsymbol{y})$.

10.10 Derive (10.4.11).

10.11 Consider the following simulation. Generate

$$\boldsymbol{y}_i = X_i\boldsymbol{\beta} + \boldsymbol{b}_i + \boldsymbol{\epsilon}_i, \quad i = 1, \ldots, 30,$$

where $\boldsymbol{b}_i$ is a 2×1 vector of unobserved random effects, $\boldsymbol{y}_i$ is 2×1, $\boldsymbol{\beta} = (\beta_0, \beta_1)' = (-1, 1)'$, $\boldsymbol{\epsilon}_i \sim N_2(0, 4I_2)$, and X_i is a 4×2 matrix taking the form

$$X_i = \begin{pmatrix} 1 & (-1)^i \\ 1 & i \\ 1 & 0 \\ 1 & 2i \end{pmatrix}.$$

(a) Suppose $\boldsymbol{b}_i \sim N_2(0, V)$, where $V = \begin{pmatrix} 1 & 1 \\ 1 & 4 \end{pmatrix}$. Using the MDP model outlined in Subsection 10.4.3, derive and plot the marginal posterior distribution of β_1 for $M = 1, 3, 5, 10, 100, 10000$. How do these results compare with the fully parametric model, i.e., $M = \infty$?

(b) Suppose $\boldsymbol{b}_i \sim 0.3N_2(0, V) + 0.7N_2(0, V_1)$, where V is given in Part (a) and $V_1 = \begin{pmatrix} 3 & 2 \\ 2 & 2 \end{pmatrix}$. Using the MDP model outlined in Subsection 10.4.3, derive and plot the marginal posterior distribution of β_1 for $M = 1, 3, 5, 10, 100, 10000$. How do these results compare with the fully parametric model which assumes $\boldsymbol{b}_i \sim N_2(0, V)$?

10.12 Consider the following simulation. Generate independent Bernoulli random variables y_{ij}, with success probability

$$p_{ij} = P(y_{ij} = 1) = \frac{\exp\{\beta_0 + \beta_1 x_{ij} + b_{ij}\}}{1 + \exp\{\beta_0 + \beta_1 x_{ij} + b_{ij}\}},$$

$i = 1, \ldots, 30$, $j = 1, 2$, where $\boldsymbol{b}_i = (b_{i1}, b_{i2})'$ is a 2×1 vector of unobserved random effects, $\boldsymbol{y}_i = (y_{i1}, y_{i2})'$ is 2×1, $\boldsymbol{\beta} = (\beta_1, \beta_2)' = (-1, 1)'$, and $X_i = [x_{ij}]$ is a 4×2 matrix taking the form

$$X_i = \begin{pmatrix} 1 & (-1)^i \\ 1 & i \\ 1 & 0 \\ 1 & 2i \end{pmatrix}.$$

(a) Suppose $\boldsymbol{b}_i \sim N_2(0, V)$, where $V = \begin{pmatrix} 1 & 1 \\ 1 & 4 \end{pmatrix}$. Using the MDP model outlined in Subsection 10.4.4, derive and plot the marginal posterior distribution of β_1 for $M = 1, 3, 5, 10, 100, 10000$. How do these results compare with the fully parametric model, i.e., $M = \infty$?

(b) Suppose $\boldsymbol{b}_i \sim 0.3N_2(0, V) + 0.7N_2(0, V_1)$, where V is given in Part (a) and $V_1 = \begin{pmatrix} 3 & 2 \\ 2 & 2 \end{pmatrix}$. Using the MDP model outlined in Subsection 10.4.4, derive and plot the marginal posterior distribution of β_1 for $M = 1, 3, 5, 10, 100, 10000$. How do these results compare with the fully parametric model which assumes $\boldsymbol{b}_i \sim N_2(0, V)$?

References

Agresti, A. (1990). *Categorical Data Analysis.* New York: Wiley.

Akaike, H. (1973). Information theory and an extension of the maximum likelihood principle. In *International Symposium on Information Theory* (Eds. B.N. Petrov and F. Csaki). Budapest: Akademia Kiado, pp. 267–281.

Albert, J.H. (1988). Computational methods using a Bayesian hierarchical generalized linear model. *Journal of the American Statistical Association* **83**, 1037–1044.

Albert, J.H. and Chib, S. (1998). Sequential ordinal modeling with applications to survival data. *Technical Report.* Olin School of Business, Washington University.

Albert, J.H. and Chib, S. (1995). Bayesian residual analysis for binary response regression models. *Biometrika* **82**, 747–759.

Albert, J.H. and Chib, S. (1993). Bayesian analysis of binary and polychotomous response data. *Journal of the American Statistical Association* **88**, 669–679.

Atkinson, C. and Mitchell, A.F.S. (1981). Rao's distance measure. *Sankyā A* **43**, 345–365.

Barker, A.A (1965). Monte Carlo calculations of the radial distribution functions for a protonelectron plasma. *Australian Journal of Physics* **18**, 119–133.

Bayarri, M.J. and Berger, J.O. (1999). Quantifying surprise in the data and model verification. In *Bayesian Statistics* **6** (Eds. J.M Bernardo, J.O.

Berger, A.P. Dawid, and A.F.M. Smith). Oxford: Oxford University Press, pp. 53–82.

Bedrick, E.J., Christensen, R., and Johnson, W. (1996). A new perspective on priors for generalized linear models. *Journal of the American Statistical Association* **91**, 1450–1460.

Bélisle, C.J.P., Romeijn, H.E., and Smith, R.L. (1993). Hit-and-Run algorithms for generating multivariate distributions. *Mathematics of Operations Research* **18**, 255–266.

Bennett, C.H. (1976). Efficient estimation of free energy differences from Monte Carlo data. *Journal of Computational Physics* **22**, 245–268.

Berger, J.O. (1993). The present and future of Bayesian multivariate analysis. In *Multivariate Analysis: Future Directions* (Ed. C.R. Rao). Amsterdam: North-Holland, pp. 25–53.

Berger, J.O. (1985). *Statistical Decision Theory and Bayesian Analysis.* Second Edition. New York: Wiley.

Berger, J.O. and Chen, M.-H. (1993). Predicting retirement patterns: Prediction for a multinomial distribution with constrained parameter space. *The Statistician* **42**, 427–444.

Berger, J.O. and Pericchi, L.R. (1996). The intrinsic Bayes factor for model selection and prediction. *Journal of the American Statistical Association* **91**, 109–122.

Besag, J. and Green, P.J. (1993). Spatial statistics and Bayesian computation. *Journal of the Royal Statistical Society, Series B* **55**, 25–37.

Best, N.G., Cowles, M.K., and Vines, S.K. (1995). *CODA: Convergence Diagnostics and Output Analysis Software for Gibbs Sampling Output.* Version 0.3. Cambridge: MRC Biostatistics Unit.

Blackwell, D. and MacQueen, J.B. (1973). Ferguson distributions via Polya urn schemes. *The Annals of Statistics* **1**, 353–355.

Bondesson, L. (1982). On simulation from infinitely divisible distributions. *Advances in Applied Probability* **14**, 855–869.

Boneh, A. and Golan, A. (1979). Constraints' redundancy and feasible region boundedness by random feasible point generator (RFPG). *Third European Congress on Operations Research*, EURO III, Amsterdam (April 9–11).

Box, G.E.P. (1980). Sampling and Bayes' inference in scientific modelling and robustness (with Discussion). *Journal of the Royal Statistical Society, Series A* **143**, 383–430.

Box, G.E.P. and Tiao, G.C. (1992). *Bayesian Inference in Statistical Analysis.* New York: Wiley.

Bratley, P., Fox, B.L., and Schrage, L.E. (1987). *A Guide to Simulation.* Second Edition. New York: Springer-Verlag.

Broffitt, J.D. (1984). A Bayes estimator for ordered parameters and isotonic Bayesian graduation. *Scandinavian Actuarial Journal* **4**, 231–247.

Brooks, S.P. and Gelamn, A. (1998). General methods for monitoring convergence of iterative simulations. *Journal of Computational and Graphical Statistics* **7**, 434–455.

Brooks, S.P. and Roberts, G.O. (1998). Diagnosing convergence of Markov chain Monte Carlo algorithms. *Statistics and Computing* **8**, 319–335 r.

Bush, C.A. and MacEachern, S.N. (1996). A semiparametric Bayesian model for randomized block designs. *Biometrika* **33**, 275–285.

Carlin, B.P. and Chib, S. (1995). Bayesian model choice via Markov chain Monte Carlo methods. *Journal of the Royal Statistical Society, Series B* **57**, 473–484.

Casella, G. and Berger, R.L. (1990). *Statistical Inference.* Belmont, CA: Duxbury Press.

Casella, G. and George, E.I. (1992). Explaining the Gibbs sampler. *The American Statistician* **46**, 167–174.

Casella, G. and Robert, C.P. (1998). Post-processing accept-reject samples: recycling and rescaling. *Journal of Computational and Graphical Statistics* **7**, 139-157.

Casella, G. and Robert, C.P. (1996). Rao–Blackwellization of sampling schemes. *Biometrika* **83**, 81–94.

Chen. M.-H. (1994). Importance-weighted marginal Bayesian posterior density estimation. *Journal of the American Statistical Association* **89**, 818–824.

Chen, M.-H. (1993). Monte Carlo Markov chain sampling for Bayesian computation, with applications to constrained parameter spaces. *Unpublished Ph.D. Dissertation.* Department of Statistics, Purdue University.

Chen, M.-H. and Deely, J.J. (1996). Bayesian analysis for a constrained linear multiple regression problem for predicting the new crop of apples. *Journal of Agricultural, Biological and Environmental Statistics* **1**, 467–89.

Chen, M.-H. and Dey, D.K. (1998). Bayesian modeling of correlated binary responses via scale mixture of multivariate normal link functions. *Sankhyā, Series A* **60**, 322–343.

Chen, M.-H. and Dey, D.K. (1996). Bayesian analysis and computation for correlated ordinal data models. *Technical Report #96-42.* Department of Statistics, University of Connecticut.

Chen, M.-H., Dey, D.K., and Shao, Q.-M. (1999). A new skewed link model for dicthotomous quantal response data. *Journal of the American Statistical Association* **94**. To appear.

Chen, M.-H., Ibrahim, J.G., and Yiannoutsos, C. (1999). Prior elicitation and Bayesian computation for logistic regression models with applications to variable selection. *Journal of the Royal Statistical Society, Series B* **61**, 223–242.

Chen, M.-H. and Liu, C. (1999). Discussion on "Simulated sintering: Markov chain Monte Carlo with spaces of varying dimensions" by J.S. Liu and C. Sabbatti. In *Bayesian Statistics 6* (Eds. J.M. Bernardo, J.O.

Berger, A.P. Dawid, and A.F.M. Smith). Oxford: Oxford University Press, pp. 402–405.

Chen, M.-H., Manatunga, A.K., and Williams, C.J. (1998). Heritability estimates from human twin data by incorporating historical prior information. *Biometrics* **54**, 1348–1362.

Chen. M.-H., Nandram, B., and Ross, E.W. (1996). Bayesian prediction of the shelf-life of a military ration with sensory data. *Journal of Agricultural, Biological and Environmental Statistics* **1**, 377–392.

Chen, M.-H. and Schmeiser, B.W. (1998). Towards black-box sampling: A random-direction interior-point Markov chain approach. *Journal of Computational and Graphical Statistics* **7**, 1–22.

Chen, M.-H. and Schmeiser, B.W. (1996). General Hit-and-Run Monte Carlo sampling for evaluating multidimensional integrals. *Operations Research Letters* **19**, 161–169.

Chen, M.-H. and Schmeiser, B.W. (1993). Performance of the Gibbs, Hit-and-Run, and Metropolis samplers, *Journal of Computational and Graphical Statistics* **2**, 251–272.

Chen, M.-H. and Shao, Q.-M. (1999a). Existence of Bayes estimators for the polychotomous quantal response models. *Annals of the Institute of Statistical Mathematics.* To appear.

Chen, M.-H. and Shao, Q.-M. (1999b). Monte Carlo estimation of Bayesian credible and HPD intervals. *Journal of Computational and Graphical Statistics* **8**, 69–92.

Chen, M.-H. and Shao, Q.-M. (1999c). Weighted Monte Carlo estimators for computing posterior quantities. *Technical Report MS-06-99-23.* Department of Mathematical Sciences, Worcester Polytechnic Institute.

Chen, M.-H. and Shao, Q.-M. (1998). Monte Carlo methods on Bayesian analysis of constrained parameter problems. *Biometrika* **85**, 73–87.

Chen, M.-H. and Shao, Q.-M. (1997a). On Monte Carlo methods for estimating ratios of normalizing constants. *The Annals of Statistics* **25**, 1563–1594.

Chen, M.-H. and Shao, Q.-M. (1997b). Estimating ratios of normalizing constants for densities with different dimensions. *Statistica Sinica* **7**, 607–630.

Chen, M.-H. and Shao, Q.-M. (1997c). Performance study of marginal posterior density estimation via Kullback–Leibler divergence. *Test, A Journal of the Spanish Society of Statistics and O.R.* **6**, 321–350.

Chib, S. (1995). Marginal likelihood from the Gibbs output. *Journal of the American Statistical Association* **90**, 1313–1321.

Chib, S. and Greenberg, E. (1998). Bayesian analysis of multivariate probit models. *Biometrika* **85**, 347–361.

Chib, S. and Greenberg, E. (1995). Understanding the Metropolis–Hastings algorithm. *The American Statistician* **49**, 327–335.

Chib, S. and Greenberg, E. (1994). Bayes inference in regression models with ARMA $(p,\ q)$ errors. *Journal of Econometrics* **64**, 183–206.

Chipman. H.A., George, E.I., and McCulloch, R.E. (1998). Bayesian CART model search (with Discussion). *Journal of the American Statistical Association* **93**, 935–960.

Chipman. H.A., Kolaczyk, E.D., and McCulloch, R.E. (1997). Adaptive Bayesian wavelet shrinkage. *Journal of the American Statistical Association* **92**, 1413–1421.

Choy, S.T.B. (1995). Robust Bayesian analysis using scale mixture of normals distributions. *Unpublished Ph.D. Dissertation.* Department of Mathematics, Imperial College, London.

Christian, J.C., Carmelli, D., Castelli, W.P., Fabsitz, R., Grim, C.E., Meaney, F.J., Norton Jr, J.A., Reed, T., Williams, C.J., and Wood, P. D. (1990). High density lipoprotein cholesterol: A 16-year longitudinal study in aging male twins. *Arteriosclerosis* **10**, 1020–1025.

Clayton, D.G. (1991). A Monte Carlo method for Bayesian inference in frailty models. *Biometrics* **64**, 141–151.

Clyde, M.A. (1999). Bayesian model averaging and model search strategies. In *Bayesian Statistics 6* (Eds. J.M. Bernardo, J.O. Berger, A.P. Dawid, and A.F.M. Smith). Oxford: Oxford University Press, pp. 157–185.

Clyde, M.A., Desimone, H., and Parmigiani, G. (1996). Prediction via orthogonalized model mixing. *Journal of the American Statistical Association* **91**, 1197–1208.

Cover, T.M. and Thomas, J.A. (1991). *Elements of Information Theory.* New York: Wiley.

Cowles, M.K. (1996). Accelerating Monte Carlo Markov chain convergence for cumulative-link generalized linear models. *Statistics and Computing* **6**, 101–111.

Cowles, M.K. and Carlin, B.P. (1996), Markov chain Monte Carlo convergence diagnostics: A comparative review. *Journal of the American Statistical Association* **91**, 883–904.

Cowles, M.K. and Rosenthal, J.S. (1998). A simulation approach to convergence rates for Markov chain Monte Carlo algorithms. *Statistics and Computing* **8**, 115–124.

Cowles, M.K., Carlin, B.P., and Connett, J.E. (1996). Bayesian tobit modeling of longitudinal ordinal clinical trial compliance data with nonignorable missingness. *Journal of the American Statistical Association* **91**, 86–98.

Cox, D.R. (1975). Partial likelihood. *Biometrika* **62**, 269–276.

Cox, D.R. (1972). Regression models and life tables. *Journal of the Royal Statistical Society, Series B* **34**, 187–220.

Csörgő, M. and Horváth, L. (1993). *Weighted Approximations in Probability and Statistics.* New York: Wiley.

Damien, P., Laud, P.W., and Smith, A.F.M. (1995). Approximate random variate generation from infinitely divisible distributions with applications to Bayesian inference. *Journal of the Royal Statistical Society, Series B* **57**, 547–563.

Damien, P., Wakefield, J., and Walker, S.G. (1999). Gibbs samling for Bayesian nonconjugate and hierarchical models using auxiliary variables. *Journal of the Royal Statistical Society, Series B* **61**, 331–344.

Dellaportas, P., Forster, J.J., and Ntzoufras, I. (1997). On Bayesian model and variable selection using MCMC. *Technical Report.* Department of Statistics, Athens University of Economics and Business, Greece.

Devroye, L. (1986). *Non-Uniform Random Variate Generation.* New York: Springer-Verlag.

Devroye, L. and Wagner, T.J. (1980). The strong uniform consistency of kernel density estimates. In *Multivariate Analysis V* (Ed. P.K. Krishnaiah). Amsterdam: North-Holland, pp. 59–77.

Dey, D.K., Chen, M.-H., and Chang, H. (1997). Bayesian approach for the nonlinear random effects models. *Biometrics* **53**, 1239–1252.

Dey, D.K., Kuo, L., and Sahu, S.K. (1995). A Bayesian predictive approach to determining the number of components in a mixture distribution. *Statistics and Computing* **5**, 297–305.

DiCiccio, T.J., Kass, R.E., Raftery, A., and Wasserman, L. (1997). Computing Bayes factors by combining simulation and asymptotic approximation. *Journal of the American Statistical Association* **92**, 903–915.

Dickey, J. (1971). The weighted likelihood ratio, linear hypotheses on normal location parameters. *The Annals of Statistics* **42**, 204–223.

Draper, N.R. and Smith, H. (1981). *Applied Regression Analysis.* New York: Wiley.

Escobar, M.D. (1994). Estimating normal means with a Dirichlet process prior. *Journal of the American Statistical Association* **89**, 268–277.

Escobar, M.D. and West, M. (1995). Bayesian density estimation and inference using mixtures. *Journal of the American Statistical Association* **90**, 578–588.

Feinleib, M., Garrison, R.J., Fabsitz, R.R., Christian, J.C., Hrubec, Z., Borhani, N.O., Kannel, W.B., Roseman, R., Schwartz, J.T., and Wagner, J.O. (1977). The NHLBI twin study of cardiovascular disease risk factors: Methodology and summary of results. *American Journal of Epidemiology* **106**, 284–295.

Ferguson, T.S. (1973). A Bayesian analysis of some non-parametric problems. *The Annals of Statistics* **1**, 209–230.

Finkelstein, D.M. and Wolf, R.A. (1985). A semiparametric model for regression analysis of interval-censored failure time data. *Biometrics* **41**, 933–945.

Frenkel, D. and Smit, B. (1996). *Understanding Molecular Simulation.* New York: Academic Press.

Gamerman, D. (1997). *Markov Chain Monte Carlo.* London: Chapman & Hall.

Garren, S.T. and Smith, R.L. (1995). Estimating the second largest eigenvalue of a Markov transition matrix. *Research Report #95-18.* Statistical Laboratory, University of Cambridge.

Geisser, S. (1993). *Predictive Inference: An Introduction.* London: Chapman & Hall.

Geisser, S. (1987). Influential observations, diagnostics and discordancy test. *Applied Statistics* **14**, 133–142.

Geisser, S (1980). In discussion of G. E. P. Box. *Journal of the Royal Statistical Society, Series A* **143**, 416–417.

Gelfand, A.E. and Banerjee, S. (1998). Computing marginal posterior modes using stochastic approximation. *Technical Report #98-25.* Department of Statistics, University of Connecticut.

Gelfand, A.E. and Dey, D.K. (1994). Bayesian model choice: Asymptotics and exact calculations. *Journal of the Royal Statistical Society, Series B* **56**, 501–514.

Gelfand, A.E., Dey, D.K., and Chang, H. (1992). Model determinating using predictive distributions with implementation via sampling-based methods (with Discussion). In *Bayesian Statistics* **4** (Eds. J.M. Bernado, J.O. Berger, A.P. Dawid, and A.F.M. Smith). Oxford: Oxford University Press, pp. 147–167.

Gelfand, A.E. and Ghosh, S.K. (1998). Model choice: A minimum posterior predictive loss approach. *Biometrika* **85**, 1–13.

Gelfand, A.E., Sahu, S.K., and Carlin, B.P. (1996). Efficient parametrisations for generalized linear mixed models (with Discussion). In *Bayesian Statistics* **5** (Eds. J.M. Bernardo, J.O. Berger, A.P. Dawid, and A.F.M. Smith). Oxford: Oxford University Press, pp. 165–180.

Gelfand, A.E., Sahu, S.K., and Carlin, B.P. (1995). Efficient parametrisations for normal linear mixed models. *Biometrika* **82**, 479–488.

Gelfand, A.E. and Smith, A.F.M. (2000). *Bayesian Computation.* New York: Wiley. To appear.

Gelfand, A.E. and Smith, A.F.M. (1990). Sampling based approaches to calculating marginal densities. *Journal of the American Statistical Association* **85**, 398–409.

Gelfand, A.E., Smith, A.F.M., and Lee, T.M. (1992). Bayesian analysis of constrained parameter and truncated data problems using Gibbs sampling. *Journal of the American Statistical Association* **87**, 523–532.

Gelman, A. (1992). Iterative and non-iterative simulation algorithms. *Computing Science and Statistics (Interface Proceedings)* **24**, 433–438.

Gelman, A. and Meng, X.-L. (1998). Simulating normalizing constants: From importance sampling to bridge sampling to path sampling. *Statistical Science* **13**, 163–185.

Gelman, A., Meng, X.-L., and Stern, H.S. (1996). Posterior predictive assessment of model fitness via realized discrepancies (with Discussion). *Statistica Sinica* **6**, 733–807.

Gelman, A., Carlin, J.B., Stern, H.S., and Rubin, D.B. (1995). *Bayesian Data Analysis.* London: Chapman & Hall.

Gelman, A. and Rubin, D.B. (1992). Inference from iterative simulation using multiple sequences. *Statistical Science* **7**, 457–511.

Geman, S. and Geman, D. (1984). Stochastic relaxation, Gibbs distributions and the Bayesian restoration of images. *IEEE Transactions on Pattern Analysis and Machine Intelligence* **6**, 721–741.

George, E.I. and McCulloch, R.E. (1997). Approaches for Bayesian variable selection. *Statistica Sinica* **7**, 339–373.

George, E.I. and McCulloch, R.E. (1993). Variable selection via Gibbs sampling. *Journal of the American Statistical Association* **88**, 881–889.

George, E.I., and McCulloch, R.E., and Tsay, R.S. (1996). Two approaches to Bayesian model selections with applications. In *Bayesian Analysis in Econometrics and Statistics – Essays in Honor of Arnold Zellner* (Eds. D.A. Berry, K.A. Chaloner, and J.K. Geweke). New York: Wiley, pp. 339–348.

Geweke, J. (1994). Bayesian comparison of econometric models. *Technical Report 532.* Federal Reserve Bank of Minneapolis and University of Minnesota.

Geweke, J. (1992). Evaluating the accuracy of sampling-based approaches to the calculation of posterior moments. In *Bayesian Statistics* **4** (Eds. J.M. Bernardo, J.O. Berger, A.P. Dawid, and A.F.M. Smith). Oxford: Oxford University Press, pp. 169–193.

Geweke, J. (1991). Efficient simulation from the multivariate normal and Student-t distributions subject to linear constraints. In *Computing Science and Statistics: Proceedings of the Twenty-Third Symposium on the Interface.* Fairfax Station, VA: Interface Foundation of North America Inc., pp. 571–578.

Geweke, J. (1989). Bayesian inference in econometrics models using Monte Carlo integration. *Econometrica* **57**, 1317–1340.

Geyer, C.J. (1995a). Conditioning in Markov chain Monte Carlo. *The Journal of Computational and Graphical Statistics* **4**, 148–154.

Geyer, C.J. (1995b). Estimation and optimization of functions. In *Markov Chain Monte Carlo in Practice* (Eds. W.R. Gilks, S. Richardson, and D.J. Spiegelhalter). London: Chapman & Hall, pp. 241–258.

Geyer, C.J. (1994). Estimating normalizing constants and reweighting mixtures in Markov chain Monte Carlo. *Revision of Technical Report No. 568.* School of Statistics, University of Minnesota.

Geyer, C.J. (1992). Practical Markov chain Monte Carlo. *Statistical Science* **7**, 473–511.

Geyer, C.J. and Thompson, E.A. (1995). Annealing Markov chain Monte Carlo with applications to ancestral inference. *Journal of the American Statistical Association* **90**, 909–920.

Gilks, W.R. and Wild, P. (1992). Adaptive rejection sampling for Gibbs sampling. *Applied Statistics* **41**, 337–348.

Gilks, W.R., Richardson, S., and Spiegelhalter, D.J. (1996). *Markov Chain Monte Carlo in Practice.* London: Chapman & Hall.

Gilks, W.R., Roberts, G.O., and George, E.I. (1994). Adaptive direction sampling. *The Statistician* **43**, 179–189.

Godsill, S.J. (1998). On the relationship between MCMC model uncertainty methods. *Technical Report CUED/F-INFENG/TR.305.* Signal Processing Group, Cambridge University Engineering Department.

Goldsman, D. and Meketon, M.S. (1986). A comparison of several variance estimators. *Technical Report J-85-12.* School of Industrial and Systems Engineering, Georgia Institute of Technology.

Goodman, J. and Sokal, A.D. (1989). Multigrid Monte Carlo method. *Physical Review D* **40**, 2035–2072.

Green, P.J. (1995). Reversible jump Markov chain Monte Carlo computation and Bayesian model determination. *Biometrika* **82**, 711–732.

Green, P.J. (1992). Discussion of the paper by Geyer and Thompson. *Journal of the Royal Statistical Society, Series B* **54**, 683–684.

Green, P.J. and Murdoch, D.J. (1999). Exact sampling for Bayesian inference: Towards general purpose algorithm. In *Bayesian Statistics 6* (Eds. J.M. Bernardo, J.O. Berger, A.P. Dawid, and A.F.M. Smith). Oxford: Oxford University Press, pp. 301–322.

Grenander, U. (1983). Tutorial in pattern theorey. *Technical Report.* Providence, R.I.: Division of Applied Mathematics, Brown University.

Hall, P. (1992). On global properties of variable bandwidth density estimators. *The Annals of Statistics* **20**, 762–778.

Hall, P. (1987). On Kullback–Leibler loss and density estimation. *The Annals of Statistics* **15**, 1491–1519.

Hamada, M. and Wu, C.F.J. (1995). Analysis of censored data from fractionated experiments: A Bayesian approach. *Journal of the American Statistical Association* **90**, 467–477.

Hammersley, J.M. and Handscomb, D.C. (1964). *Monte Carlo Methods.* London: Methuen.

Hannan, E.J. (1970). *Multiple Time Series.* New York: Wiley.

Hastings, W.K. (1970). Monte Carlo sampling methods using Markov chains and their applications. *Biometrika* **57**, 97–109.

He, X. and Shao, Q.-M. (1996). A general Bahadur representation of M-estimators and its application to linear regression with nonstochastic designs. *The Annals of Statistics* **24**, 2608–2630.

Hills, S.E. and Smith, A.F.M. (1992). Parameterization issues in Bayesian inference (with Discussion). In *Bayesian Statistics* **4** (Eds. J.M. Bernardo, J.O. Berger, A.P. Dawid, and A.F.M. Smith). Oxford: Oxford University Press, pp. 641–649.

Hjort, N.L. (1990). Nonparametric Bayes estimators based on beta processes in models for life history data. *The Annals of Statistics* **18**, 1259–1294.

Hyndman, R.J. (1996). Computing and graphing highest density regions. *The American Statistician* **50**, 120–126.

Ibrahim, J.G. and Chen, M.-H. (1998). Prior distributions and Bayesian computation for proportional hazards models. *Sankhyā, Series B* **60**, 48–64.

Ibrahim, J.G., Chen, M.-H., and MacEachern, S.N. (1999). Bayesian variable selection for proportional hazards models. *The Canadian Journal of Statistics* **27**. To appear.

Ibrahim, J.G., Chen, M.-H., and Ryan, L.-M. (1999). Bayesian variable selection for time series count data. *Technical Report MS-01-99-18*. Department of Mathematical Sciences, Worcester Polytechnic Institute.

Ibrahim, J.G., Chen, M.-H., and Sinha, D. (1998). Criterion based methods for Bayesian model assessment. *Technical Report MS-07-98-13*, Department of Mathematical Sciences, Worcester Polytechnic Institute.

Ibrahim, J.G. and Laud, P.W. (1994). A predictive approach to the analysis of designed experiments. *Journal of the American Statistical Association* **89**, 309–319.

Ibrahim, J.G., Ryan, L.-M., and Chen, M.-H. (1998). Use of historical controls to adjust for covariates in trend tests for binary data. *Journal of the American Statistical Association* **93**, 1282–1293.

Ibrahim, J.G., Sinha, D., and Chen, M.-H. (2000). *Bayesian Survival Analysis*. New York: Springer-Verlag. To appear.

Janssen, P., Jureckova, J., and Veraverbeke, N. (1985). Rate of convergence of one- and two-step M-estimators with applications to maximum likelihood and Pitman estimators. *The Annals of Statistics* **13**, 1222–1229.

Jeffreys, H. (1961). *Theory of Probability*. Third Edition. Oxford: Clarendon Press.

Johnson, V.E. (1998). A coupling-regeneration scheme for diagnosing convergence in Markov chain Monte Carlo algorithms. *Journal of the American Statistical Association* **93**, 238–248.

Johnson, V.E. (1992). A technique for estimating marginal posterior densities in hierarchical models using mixtures of conditional densities. *Journal of the American Statistical Association* **87**, 852–860.

Johnson, W. and Geisser, S. (1983). A predictive view of the detection and characterization of influential observations in regression analysis. *Journal of American Statistical Association* **78**, 137–144.

JRSSB (1993). Discussion on the meeting on the Gibbs sampling and other Markov chain Monte Carlo methods. *Journal of the Royal Statistical Society, Series B* **55**, 53–102.

Kahn, J.O., Lagakos, S.W., Richman, D.D. et al. (1992). A controlled trial comparing zidovudine with didanosine in human immunodeficiency virus infection. *New England Journal of Medicine* **327**, 581–587.

Kalbfleisch, J.D. (1978). Non-parametric Bayesian analysis of survival time data. *Journal of the Royal Statistical Society, Series B* **40**, 214–221.

Kalish, L.A. (1992). Phase III multiple myeloma: Evaluation of combination chemotherapy in previously untreated patients. *Technical Report # 726E*. Department of Biostatistics, Dana-Farber Cancer Institute.

Kass, R.E. (Moderator), Carlin, B.P., Gelman, A., and Neal, R.M. (Panelists) (1998). Makov chain Monte Carlo in practice: A roundtable discussion. *The American Statistician* **52**, 93–100.

Kass, R.E. and Raftery, A.E. (1995). Bayes factor. *Journal of the American Statistical Association* **90**, 773–795.

Kaufman, D.E. and Smith, R.L. (1998). Optimal direction choice for Hit-and-Run sampling. *Operations Research* **46**, 84–95.

Kleinman, K.P. and Ibrahim, J.G. (1998a). A semiparametric Bayesian approach to the random effects model. *Biometrics* **54**, 921–938.

Kleinman, K.P. and Ibrahim, J.G. (1998b). A semi-parametric Bayesian approach to generalized linear mixed models. *Statistics in Medicine* **17**, 2579–2596.

Krall, J.M., Uthoff, V.A., and Harley, J.B. (1975). A step-up procedure for selecting variables associated with survival. *Biometrics* **31**, 49–57.

Larose, D. and Dey, D.K. (1996). Weighted distributions viewed in the context of model selection: A Bayesian perspective. *Test, A Journal of the Spanish Society of Statistics and O.R.* **5**, 227–246.

Laud, P.W. and Ibrahim, J.G. (1995). Predictive model selection. *Journal of the Royal Statistical Society, Series B* **57**, 247–262.

Laud, P.W., Damien, P., and Smith, A.F.M. (1998). Bayesian nonparametric and covariate analysis of failure time data. In *Practical Nonparametric and Semiparametric Bayesian Statistics* (Eds. D.K. Dey, P. Müller, D. Sinha). New York: Springer-Verlag, pp. 213–225.

Laud, P.W., Smith, A.F.M., and Damien, P. (1996). Monte Carlo methods for approximating a posterior hazard rate process. *Statistics and Computing* **6**, 77–83.

Law, A.M. and Kelton, W.D. (1991). *Simulation Modeling and Analysis.* Second Edition. New York: McGraw-Hill.

Liang, K.-Y. and Zeger, S.L. (1986). Longitudinal data analysis using generalized linear models. *Biometrika* **73**, 13–22.

Liew, C.K. (1976). Inequality constrained least-squares estimation. *Journal of American Statistical Association* **71**, 746–751.

Lin, Z.Y. and Lu, C.R. (1996). *Limit Theory for Mixing Dependent Random Variables.* New York: Kluwer Academic.

Lindley, D.V. and Smith, A.F.M. (1972). Bayes estimators for the linear model (with Discussion). *Journal of the Royal Statistical Society, Series B* **34**, 1–41.

Liu, C. (1998). Covariance adjustment for Markov chain Monte Carlo—A general frame work and the covariance-adjusted data augmentation algorithm. *Techical Report.* Bell Laboratories, Lucent Technologies, USA.

Liu, C., Liu, J.S., and Rubin, D.B. (1992). A variational control variable for assessing the convergence of the Gibbs sampler. In *Proceedings of the American Statistical Association, Statistical Computing Section*, pp. 74–78.

Liu, J.S. (1994). The collapsed Gibbs sampler in Bayesian computations with applications to a gene regulation problem. *Journal of the American Statistical Association* **89**, 958–966.

Liu, J.S., Liang, F., and Wong, W.H. (1998a). The use of multiple-try method and local optimization in Metropolis sampling. *Technical Report.* Department of Statistics, Stanford University.

Liu, J.S., Liang, F., and Wong, W.H. (1998b). Dynamic weighting in Markov chain Monte Carlo. *Technical Report.* Department of Statistics, Stanford University.

Liu, J.S., Wong, W.H., and Kong, A. (1995). Covariance structure and convergence rate of the Gibbs sampler with various scans. *Journal of the Royal Statistical Society B* **57**, 157–169.

Liu, J.S., Wong, W.H., and Kong, A. (1994). Covariance structure of the Gibbs sampler with applications to the comparisons of estimators and augmentation schemes. *Biometrika* **81**, 27–40.

Liu, J.S. and Sabatti, C. (1999). Simulated sintering: Markov chain Monte Carlo with spaces of varying dimensions (with Discussion). In *Bayesian Statistics 6* (Eds. J.M. Bernardo, J.O. Berger, A.P. Dawid, and A.F.M. Smith). Oxford: Oxford University Press, pp. 389–413.

Liu, J.S. and Sabatti, C. (1998). Generalized multigrid Monte Carlo for Bayesian computation. *Technical Report.* Department of Statistics, Stanford University.

Liu, J.S. and Wu, Y. (1997). Parameter expansion scheme for data augmentation. *Technical Report.* Department of Statistics, Stanford University.

MacEachern, S.N. (1994). Estimating normal means with a conjugate style Dirichlet process prior. *Communications in Statistics* **23**, 727–741.

MacEachern, S.N. and Müller, P. (1998). Estimating mixture of Dirichlet process models. *Journal of Computational and Graphical Statistics* **7**, 223–238.

Madigan, D. and Raftery, A.E. (1994). Model selection and accounting for model uncertainty in graphical models using Occam's window. *Journal of the American Statistical Association* **89**, 1535–1546.

Madigan, D. and York, J. (1995), Bayesian graphical models for discrete data. *International Statistical Review* **63**, 215–232.

Marinari, E. and Parisi, G. (1992). Simulated tempring: A new Monte Carlo scheme. *Europhysics Letters* **19**, 451.

Mason, D. (1982). Some characterizations of almost sure bounds for weighted multidimensional empirical distributions and a Glivenko–Cantelli theorem for sample quantiles. *Zeitschrift für Wahrscheinlichkeitstheorie und Verwandte Gebiete* **59**, 505–513.

Meketon, M.S. and Schmeiser, B.W. (1984). Overlapping batch means: Something for nothing? In *Proceedings of the Winter Simulation Conference*, pp. 227–230.

Meng, X.-L. (1994). Posterior predictive p-values. *The Annals of Statistics* **22**, 1142–1160.

Meng, X.-L. and Schilling, S. (1996a). Bridge sampling after transformation. *Technical Report 376*. Department of Statistics, The University of Chicago.

Meng, X.-L. and Schilling, S. (1996b). Fitting full-information factor models and an empirical investigation of bridge sampling. *Journal of the American Statistical Association* **91**, 1254–1267.

Meng, X.-L. and Wong, W.H. (1996). Simulating ratios of normalizing constants via a simple identity: A theoretical exploration. *Statistica Sinica* **6**, 831–860.

Meng, X.-L. and van Dyk, D. (1999). Seeking efficient data augmentation schemes via conditional and marginal augmentation. *Biometrika* **86**, 301–320.

Mengersen, K.L., Robert, C.P., and Guihenneuc-Jouyaux, Ch. (1999). MCMC convergence diagnostics: A Reviewww (with Discussion). In *Bayesian Statistics 6* (Eds. J.M. Bernardo, J.O. Berger, A.P. Dawid, and A.F.M. Smith). Oxford: Oxford University Press, pp. 415–440.

Merigan, T. C., Amato, D.A., Balsley, J., Power, M., Price, W.A., Benoit, S., Perez-Michael, A., Brownstein, A., Kramer, A.S., Brettler, D., Aledort, L., Ragni, M.V., Andes, A.W., Gill, J.C., Goldsmith, J., Stabler, S., Sanders, N., Gjerset, G., Lusher, J., and the NHF-ACTG036 Study Group (1991). Placebo-controlled trial to evaluate zidovudine in treatment of human immunodeficiency virus infection in asymptomatic patients with hemophilia. *Blood* **78**, 900–906.

Metropolis, N., Rosenbluth, A.W., Rosenbluth, M.N., Teller, A.H., and Teller, E. (1953). Equations of state calculations by fast computing machines. *Journal of Chemical Physics* **21**, 1087–1092.

Meyn, S.P. and Tweedie, R.L. (1993). *Markov Chains and Stochastic Stability.* New York: Springer-Verlag.

Mitchell, T.J. and Beauchamp, J.J. (1988). Bayesian variable selection in linear regression (with Discussion). *Journal of the American Statistical Association* **83**, 1023–1036.

Müller, P. (1991). A generic approach to posterior integration and Gibbs sampling. *Technical Report #91-09.* Department of Statistics, Purdue University.

Müller, P. and Roeder, K. (1998). A Bayesian semiparametric model for case-control studies with errors in variables. *Biometrika* **84**, 523–537.

Mykland, P., Tierney, L., and Yu, B. (1995). Regeneration in Markov chain samplers. *Journal of the American Statistical Association* **90**, 233–241.

Nachbin, L. (1965). *The Haar Integral.* Princeton, N.J.: Van Nostrand.

Nandram, B. and Chen, M.-H. (1996). Reparameterizing the generalized linear model to accelerate Gibbs sampler convergence. *Journal of Statistical Computation and Simulation* **54**, 129–144.

Nelson, B.L.(1990). Control variate remedies. *Operations Research* **38**, 974–992.

Nemhauser, G.L., Rinnooy Kan, A.H.G., and Todd, M.J. (1989). *Optimization.* Amsterdan: North-Holland.

Newton, M.A. and Raftery, A.E. (1994). Approximate Bayesian inference by the weighted likelihood bootstrap (with Discussion). *Journal of the Royal Statistical Society, Series B* **56**, 1–48.

Oh, M.-S. (1999). Estimation of posterior density functions from a posterior sample. *Computational Statistics and Data Analysis* **29**, 411–427.

O'Neill, R. (1971). Algorithm AS47-function minimization using a simplex procedure. *Applied Statistics* **20**, 338–345.

Peligrad, M. and Shao, Q.-M. (1994). Self-normalizing central limit theorem for sums of weakly dependent random variables. *Journal of Theoretical Probability* **7**, 309–338.

Peligrad, M. and Shao, Q.-M. (1995). Estimation of the variance of partial sums for ρ-mixing random variables. *Journal of Multivariate Analysis* **52**, 140–157.

Peng, L. (1998). Normalizing constant estimation for discrete distribution simulation. *Unpublished Ph.D. Dissertation.* Department of Management Science and Information System, University of Texas at Austin.

Peskun, P.H. (1973). Optimum Monte–Carlo sampling using Markov chains. *Biometrika* **60**, 607–612.

Polson, N.G. (1996). Convergence of Markov chain Monte Carlo algorithms (with Discussion). In *Bayesian Statistics* **5** (Eds. J.M. Bernado, J.O. Berger, A.P. Dawid, and A.F.M. Smith). Oxford: Oxford University Press, pp. 297–322.

Prentice, R.L. (1988). Correlated binary regression with covariate specific to each binary observation. *Biometrics* **44**, 1033–1048.

Priestley, M.B. (1981). *Spectral Analysis and Time Series.* London: Academic Press.

Raftery, A.E. (1996). Approximate Bayes factors and accounting for model uncertainty in generalised linear models. *Biometrika* **83**, 251–266.

Raftery, A.E. and Lewis, S. (1992). How many iterations in the Gibbs sampler? In *Bayesian Statistics* **4** (Eds. J.M. Bernardo, J.O. Berger, A.P. Dawid, and A.F.M. Smith). Oxford: Oxford University Press, pp. 763–773.

Raftery, A.E., Madigan, D., and Hoeting, J.A. (1997). Bayesian model averaging for linear regression models. *Journal of the American Statistical Association* **92**, 179–191.

Raftery, A.E., Madigan, D., and Volinsky, C.T. (1995). Accounting for model uncertainty in survival analysis improves predictive performance.

In *Bayesian Statistics 5* (Eds. J.M. Bernardo, J.O. Berger, A.P. Dawid, and A.F.M. Smith). Oxford: Oxford University Press, pp. 323–350.

Rao, M.M. (1987). *Measure Theory and Integration.* New York: Wiley.

Rashid, M.M., Chen, M.-H., and Ganter, S.L. (1999). A nonparametric analysis of a multi-group incompletely ranked item response data. *Journal of Nonparametric Statistics.* To appear.

Ripley, B.D. (1987). *Stochastic Simulation.* New York: Wiley.

Ritter, C. and Tanner, T.A. (1992). The Gibbs stopper and the griddy-Gibbs sampler. *Journal of the American Statistical Association* **87**, 861–868.

Robbins, H. and Monro, S. (1951). A stochastic approximation method. *Annals of Mathematical Statistics* **22**, 373–405.

Robert, C.P. (Ed.) (1998). *Discretization and MCMC Convergence Assessment.* New York: Wiley.

Robert, C.P. and Casella, G. (1999). *Monte Carlo Statistical Methods.* New York: Springer-Verlag.

Robert, C.P. and Hwang, J.T.G. (1996). Maximum likelihood estimation under order restrictions by the prior feedback method. *Journal of the American Statistical Association* **91**, 167–172.

Roberts, G.O. (1994). Methods for estimating L^2 convergence of Markov chain Monte Carlo. In *Bayesian Statistics and econometrics: Essays in Honor of Arnold Zellner* (Eds. D. Berry, K. Chaloner, and J. Geweke). Amsterdam: North-Holland, pp. 373–384.

Roberts, G.O., Gelman, A., and Gilks, W.R. (1997). Weak convergence and optimal scaling of random walk Metropolis algorithms. *Annals of Applied Probability* **7**, 110–120.

Roberts, G.O. and Gilks, W.R. (1994). Convergence of adaptive direction sampling. *Journal of Multivariate Analysis* **49**, 287–298.

Roberts, G.O. and Polson, N.G. (1994). On the geometric convergence of the Gibbs sampler. *Journal of the Royal Statistical Society, Series B* **56**, 377–384.

Roberts, G.O. and Sahu, S.K. (1997). Updating schemes, correlation structure, blocking and parameterization for the Gibbs sampler. *Journal of the Royal Statistical Society, Series B* **59**, 291–317.

Roberts, G.O. and Tweedie, R.L. (1996). Geometric convergence and central limit theorems for multidimensional Hastings and Metropolis algorithms. *Biometrika* **83**, 95–110.

Robertson, T., Wright, F.T., and Dykstra, R.L. (1988). *Order Restricted Statistical Inference.* New York: Wiley

Rosenthal, J.S. (1995a). Rates of convergence for Gibbs sampling for variance component models. *The Annals of Statistics* **23**, 740–761.

Rosenthal, J.S. (1995b). Minorization conditions and convergence rates for Markov chain Monte Carlo. *Journal of the American Statistical Association* **90**, 558–566.

Ross, E.W., Klicka, M.V., Kalick, J., and Branagan, M.T. (1987). A time-temperature model for sensory acceptance of a military ration. *Journal of Food Science* **52**, 1712–1717.

Rubinstein, R.Y. (1981). *Simulation and the Monte Carlo Method.* New York: Wiley.

Schervish, M.J. and Carlin, B.P. (1992). On the convergence of successive substitution sampling. *Journal of Computational and Graphical Statistics* **1**, 111–127.

Schmeiser, B.W. (1982). Batch size effects in the analysis of simulation output. *Operations Research* **30**, 556–568.

Schmeiser, B.W. and Chen, M.-H. (1991). On Hit-and-Run Monte Carlo sampling for evaluating multidimensional integrals. *Technical Report 91-39.* Department of Statistics, Purdue University.

Schmeiser, B. W. and Song, W.-M.T. (1987). Correlation among estimators of the variance of the sample mean. In *Proceedings of the Winter Simulation Conference*, pp. 309-317.

Schmeiser, B.W., Avramidis, A.N., and Hashem, S. (1990). Overlapping batch statistics. In *Proceedings of the 1990 Winter Simulation Conference*, pp. 395–398.

Schwarz, G. (1978). Estimating the dimension of a model. *The Annals of Statistics* **6**, 461–464.

Scott, D.W. (1992). *Multivariate Density Estimation.* New York: Wiley.

Sen, P.K. and Singer, J.M. (1993). *Large Sample Methods in Statistics.* New York: Chapman & Hall.

Serfling, R.J. (1980). *Approximation Theorems of Mathematical Statistics.* New York: Wiley.

Silverman, B.W. (1986). *Density Estimation for Statistics and Data Analysis.* London: Chapman & Hall.

Sinha, D, Chen, M.-H., and Ghosh, S.K. (1999). Bayesian analysis and model selection for interval-censored survival data. *Biometrics* **55**, 585–590.

Sinha, D. and Dey, D.K. (1997). Semiparametric Bayesian analysis of survival data. *Journal of the American Statistical Association* **92**, 1195–1212.

Smith, R.L. (1984). Efficient Monte Carlo procedures for generating points uniformly distributed over bounded regions. *Operations Research* **32**, 1297–1308.

Smith, R.L. (1980). A Monte Carlo procedure for the random generation of feasible solutions to mathematical programming problems. *Bulletin of the TIMS/ORSA Joint National Meeting*, Washington, DC, p. 101.

Sommer, A., Katz, J., and Tarwotjo, I. (1983). Increased mortality in children with vitamin A deficiency. *American Journal of Clinical Nutrition* **40**, 1090–1095.

Song, W.-M.T. (1988). Estimators of the variance of the sample mean: Quadratic forms, optimal batch sizes, and linear combinations. *Un-*

published Ph.D. Dissertation. School of Industrial Engineering, Purdue University.

Song, W.-M.T. and Schmeiser, B.W. (1995). Optimal mean-squared-error batch sizes. *Management Science* **41**, 110–123.

Song, W.-M. T. and Schmeiser, B.W. (1993). Variance of the sample mean: Properties and graphs of quadratic-form estimators. *Operations Research* **41**, 501–517.

Song, W.-M. T. and Schmeiser, B.W. (1988a). On the dispersion matrix of estimators of the variance of the sample mean in the analysis of simulation output. *Operations Research Letters* **7**, 259–266.

Song, W.-M. T. and Schmeiser, B.W. (1988b). Minimal-mse linear combinations of variance estimators of the sample mean. In *Proceedings of the Winter Simulation Conference*, pp. 414–421.

Stark, P.C., Ryan, L.-M., McDonald, J.L., and Burge, H.A. (1997). Using meteorologic data to model and predict daily ragweed pollen levels. *Aerobiologia* **13**, 177–184.

Tanner, M.A. (1996). *Tools for Statistical Inference.* Third Edition. New York: Springer-Verlag.

Tanner, T.A. and Wong, W.H. (1987). The calculation of posterior distributions by data augmentation. *Journal of the American Statistical Association* **82**, 528–549.

Thisted, R.A. (1988). *Elements of Statistical Computing – Numerical Computation.* London: Chapman & Hall.

Tierney, L. (1994). Markov chains for exploring posterior distributions (with Discussions). *The Annals of Statistics* **22**, 1701–1762.

Tierney, L. and Kadane, J. (1986). Accurate approximations for posterior moments and marginal densities. *Journal of the American Statistical Association* **81**, 82–86.

Torrie, G.M. and Valleau, J.P. (1977). Nonphysical sampling distributions in Monte Carlo free-energy estimation: Umbrella sampling. *Journal of Chemical Physics* **23**, 187–199.

Trotter, H.F. and Tukey, J.W. (1956). Conditional Monte Carlo for normal samples. In *Symposium on Monte Carlo Methods* (Ed. H.A. Meyer). New York: Wiley, pp. 64–79.

Tsiatis, A.A. (1981). A large sample study of Cox's regression model. *The Annals of Statistics* **9**, 93–108.

Verdinelli, I. and Wasserman, L. (1996). Bayes factors, nuisance parameters and imprecise tests. In *Bayesian Statistics* **5** (Eds. J.M. Bernado, J.O. Berger, A.P. Dawid, and A.F.M. Smith). Oxford: Oxford University Press, pp. 765–772.

Verdinelli, I. and Wasserman, L. (1995). Computing Bayes factors using a generalization of the Savage–Dickey density ratio. *Journal of the American Statistical Association* **90**, 614–618.

Volberding, P.A., Lagakos, S.W., Koch, M.A., Pettinelli, C., Myers, M.W., Booth, D.K., Balfour, H.H., Reichman, R.C., Bartlett, J.A., Hirsch,

M.S., Murphy, R.L., Hardy, D., Soeiro, R., Fischl, M.A., Bartlett, J.G., Merigan, T.C., Hylsop, N.E., Richman, D.D., Valentine, F.T., Corey, L., and the AIDS Clinical Trials Group of the National Institute of Allergy and Infectious Diseases (1990). Zidovudine in asymptomatic human immunodeficiency virus infection. *New England Journal of Medicine* **322**, 941–949.

Volinsky, C.T. Madigan, D., Raftery, A.E., and Kronmal, R.A. (1997). Bayesian model averaging in proportional hazards models: Assessing the risk of a stroke. *Applied Statistics* **46**, 433–448.

Voter, A.F. (1985). A Monte Carlo method for determining free-energy differences and transition state theory rate constants. *Journal of Chemical Physics* **82**, 1890–1899.

Walker, S.G., Damien, P., Laud, P.W., and Smith, A.F.M. (1999). Bayesian nonparametric inference for random distributions and related functions (with Discussion). *Journal of the Royal Statistical Society, Series B* **61**, 485–528.

Wei, G.C.G. and Tanner, M.A. (1990). Calculating the content and boundary of the highest posterior density region via data augmentation. *Biome- trika* **77**, 649–652.

West, M. (1985). Generalized linear models: Scale parameters, outlier accommodations and prior distributions. In *Bayesian Statistics* **2** (Eds. J. Bernardo, M.H. DeGroot, D.V. Lindley, and A.F.M. Smith). Amsterdam: North-Holland.

West, M., Harrison, P.J., and Migon, H.S. (1985). Dynamic generalized linear models and Bayesian forecasting (with Discussion). *Journal of the American Statistical Association* **80**, 73–97.

West, M., Müller, P., and Escobar, M.D. (1994). Hierarchical priors and mixture models, with applications in regression and density estimation. In *Aspects of Uncertainty: A Tribute to D.V. Lindley* (Eds. A.F.M. Smith and P.R. Freeman). New York: Wiley.

Whitt, W. (1991). The efficiency of one long run versus independent replications in steady-state simulation. *Management Science* **37**, 645–666.

Wilks, W.R., Wang, C.C., Yvonnet, B., and Coursaget, P. (1993). Random effects models for longitudinal data using Gibbs sampling. *Biometrics* **49**, 441–453.

Wolpert, R.L. (1991). Monte Carlo importance sampling in Bayesian statistics. In *Statistical Multiple Integration* (Eds. N. Flournoy and R. Tsutakawa). *Contemporary Mathematics* **116**, 101–115.

Wong, W.H. and Liang, F. (1997). Dynamic weighting in Monte Carlo and optimization. *Proceedings of the National Academy of Science* **94**, 14220–14224.

Yang, R. and Berger, J.O. (1994). Estimation of a covariance matrix using the reference prior. *The Annals of Statistics* **22**, 1195–1211.

Yang, Y. and Chen, M.-H. (1995). Bayesian analysis for random coefficient regression models using noninformative priors. *Journal of Multivariate Analysis* **55**, 283–311.

Yu, B. and Mykland, P. (1998). Looking at Markov samplers through cusum path plots: A simple diagnostic idea. *Statistics and Computing* **8**, 275–286.

Zeger, S.L., (1988). A regression model for time series of counts. *Biometrika* **75**, 621–629.

Zeger, S.L. and Karim, M.R. (1991). Generalized linear models with random effects: A Gibbs sampling approach. *Journal of the American Statistical Association* **86**, 79–86.

Zeger, S.L. and Liang, K.-Y. (1986). Longitudinal data analysis for discrete and continuous outcomes. *Biometrics* **42**, 121–130.

Zellner, A. and Rossi, P.E. (1984). Bayesian analysis of dichotomous quantal response models. *Journal of Econometrics* **25**, 365–393.

Author Index

Subject Index

Springer Series in Statistics

(continued from p. ii)

Ramsay/Silverman: Functional Data Analysis.
Rao/Toutenburg: Linear Models: Least Squares and Alternatives.
Read/Cressie: Goodness-of-Fit Statistics for Discrete Multivariate Data.
Reinsel: Elements of Multivariate Time Series Analysis, 2nd edition.
Reiss: A Course on Point Processes.
Reiss: Approximate Distributions of Order Statistics: With Applications to Non-parametric Statistics.
Rieder: Robust Asymptotic Statistics.
Rosenbaum: Observational Studies.
Rosenblatt: Gaussian and Non-Gaussian Linear Time Series and Random Fields
Särndal/Swensson/Wretman: Model Assisted Survey Sampling.
Schervish: Theory of Statistics.
Shao/Tu: The Jackknife and Bootstrap.
Siegmund: Sequential Analysis: Tests and Confidence Intervals.
Simonoff: Smoothing Methods in Statistics.
Singpurwalla and Wilson: Statistical Methods in Software Engineering: Reliability and Risk.
Small: The Statistical Theory of Shape.
Stein: Interpolation of Spatial Data: Some Theory for Kriging.
Tanner: Tools for Statistical Inference: Methods for the Exploration of Posterior Distributions and Likelihood Functions, 3rd edition.
Tong: The Multivariate Normal Distribution.
van der Vaart/Wellner: Weak Convergence and Empirical Processes: With Applications to Statistics.
Weerahandi: Exact Statistical Methods for Data Analysis.
West/Harrison: Bayesian Forecasting and Dynamic Models, 2nd edition.